Cerebral Palsy

A Johns Hopkins Press Health Book

Cerebral Palsy

A Complete Guide for Caregiving

SECOND EDITION

Freeman Miller, M.D.
Steven J. Bachrach, M.D.

with Marilyn L. Boos, R.N.C., M.S.

Kirk Dabney, M.D.

Linda Duffy, B.S., P.A.-C.

Robin C. Meyers, M.P.H., R.D.

Douglas T. Pearson, Ph.D.

Kathleen Trzcinski, R.N., M.S.N., C.R.N.P.

Rhonda S. Walter, M.D.

Joan Lenett Whinston

THE JOHNS HOPKINS UNIVERSITY PRESS

BALTIMORE

NOTE TO THE READER

This book embodies our approach to cerebral palsy *in general*. It was not written about *your* child. While we believe and practice its philosophy, we adjust our approach to suit each child's particular need and each family's situation. We would not treat your child without first learning a great deal about him or her, and so your child's treatment should not be based solely on what is written here. It must be developed in a dialogue between you and your child's physician. Our book is written to help you with that dialogue.

9 8 7 6 5 4 3 2 1

The Johns Hopkins University Press
2715 North Charles Street
Baltimore, Maryland 21218-4363

Library of Congress Cataloging-in-Publication Data

Miller, Freeman.
   Cerebral palsy : a complete guide for caregiving / Freeman Miller, Steven J.
Bachrach ; with Marilyn L. Boos . . . [et al.].—2nd ed.
      p. ; cm.
   "A Johns Hopkins Press health book"
   Includes bibliographical references and index.
   ISBN 0-8018-8354-7 (alk. paper)—ISBN 0-8018-8355-5 (pbk. : alk. paper)
   1. Cerebral palsied children. 2. Cerebral palsy—Popular works. I. Bachrach,
Steven J. II. Title. III. Series.
   [DNLM: 1. Cerebral Palsy. 2. Caregivers. WS 342 M647c 2006]
RJ496.C4M53 2006
618.92'836—dc22   2005052683

A catalog record for this book is available from the British Library.

The preparation of illustrations for this book was supported in part by funding from the Nemours Research Programs of the Nemours Foundation. Illustrations on pages vi, viii, 2, 16, 40, 96, 122, 144, 166, 206, 228, 246, 256, and 268 are by Kathleen King; all other illustrations are by Jacqueline Schaffer.

Contents

PART 3 CEREBRAL PALSY ENCYCLOPEDIA

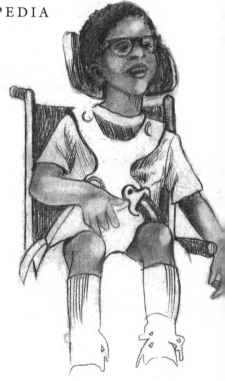

Foreword

♦ PROBABLY EVERY PARENT of every child who has a health problem remembers the first time someone gave that problem a name. It may have been in the hospital, soon after the baby was born, or it may have been months, or even years, later. Hearing those words about your child, and wanting so much for them not to be true, is something that stays forever in your mind.

For my husband and me, that moment occurred more than twenty-five years ago. It was when our son Joshua was six months old. We suspected something was wrong with Josh, and our pediatrician had recommended that we consult with a specialist. But we were not prepared to have the doctor tell us that Josh had cerebral palsy, and that his development was going to be delayed.

Cerebral palsy. We had heard the words, of course, but they had never before had any relation to us. What did these words mean for the future of our precious son? As time went on, we found out that it's difficult to know, in the early years of childhood, just what cerebral palsy does mean for an individual child. With cerebral palsy, as with many things in life, only time will tell. But waiting, and not knowing, is a very difficult thing when it involves your child.

While we were searching for answers, my husband and I met Dr. Freeman Miller and Dr. Steven Bachrach. We were so impressed with the concern and sensitivity they showed toward Josh, and toward us, that we knew we'd found the doctors who not only would help our family through the difficult times but would cheer along with us when times were good. Their medical advice proved to be among the most valuable we'd ever received, and their open, caring, and honest approach let us know that they would be there for us when we needed them. Drs. Bachrach and Miller have been there all through the years, even after Josh was no longer eligible for treatment at the Alfred I. duPont Hospital for Children because of age restrictions. Both my husband and I shall be ever appreciative and grateful.

Sound professional advice and a caring commitment to do what's best for your child. That's what anyone who is the parent of a child with cerebral palsy wants. And that's what Drs. Miller and Bachrach and their colleagues offer in this book. They will help you understand cerebral palsy and how it affects your child. They will answer your questions. They will help you cope. They will show you on every page that they understand, at least a little bit, what it's like to be the parent of a child with cerebral palsy. Perhaps most importantly, they will do all this because they care so much about the children.

Whether you've just learned that your own precious child has cerebral palsy, or whether you and your family have been living with this condition for several years, you will find that this book is a wonderful resource, as valuable to someone with an infant as to someone with a young adult. I still open the pages and glance through it from time to time. I still learn from its masters, and it's still a timely fit. I urge you not to put it on your bookshelf, but to keep it handy, and turn to it often. The information it provides will give strength and hope and courage, to both you and your child.

I wish you luck and success in your journey.

Joan Lenett Whinston

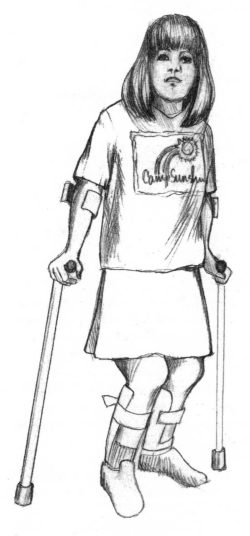

Preface

♦ THE INFORMATION in these pages represents the current thinking of professionals who specialize in the medical, psychological, educational, and legal aspects of caring for children who have cerebral palsy. The book was written for everyone who provides the daily care of a child with cerebral palsy, whether parent, grandparent, great-grandparent, brother, sister, aunt, or uncle. We hope that teachers, physicians, and anyone else who cares about the well-being of such a child will also benefit from it. Our goal in writing this book is to help those who care for a child with cerebral palsy understand the child's needs and how these needs can best be met. In helping the caregivers, of course, our ultimate goal is to help the child.

By learning about CP and the many options for treatment, parents and others will be better prepared to ask direct questions of the professional, who will probably respond by providing additional information or clarification. Thus, one of our purposes in writing this book is to improve communication between the professional and the caregiver—again, resulting in better treatment for and care of the child.

Cerebral Palsy: A Complete Guide for Caregiving is arranged in three parts. The first part is composed of chapters that address a range of issues, usually progressing in sections by the chronological age of the child. You may want to read this part of the book from beginning to end, or you may prefer to turn to the specific section of this part of the book that addresses the issues that are relevant for your child right now. For example, if your child is 5 years old and has a hemiplegic pattern of involvement, you may want to begin by reading the introduction to Chapter 5, plus the section of that chapter that focuses on children with hemiplegia from age 4 to age 6.

The twelve chapters in Part I are arranged as follows: Chapter 1 provides an overview of cerebral palsy, and Chapter 2 presents normal developmental milestones from a pediatric perspective, including a discussion of normal and abnormal behavior. Chapters 3 and 4 describe medical problems and intellectual and psychosocial issues associated with CP. Specific patterns of involvement are discussed in Chapters 5, 6, and 7. Although problems encountered in childhood provide the primary focus of this book, one chapter—Chapter 8—looks at issues confronted by the adult with CP. Chapter 9 describes the medical system and introduces the various kinds of professional caregivers you and your child may meet. In Chapter 10, health insurance and other financial aspects of care are addressed. Finally, Chapters 11 and 12 explain how the educational and legal systems can benefit your child—and how you can make sure that they do.

Part 2 provides practical information for the caregiver. Subjects covered range from wheelchair maintenance to daily hygiene tips such as toothbrushing, and entries are intended to help caregivers provide exceptional care for children with cerebral palsy. We must add a word of caution here, and that is that caregivers need to learn the techniques described in this section *from an experienced professional.* The instructions in Part 2 are *memory refreshers* for those who have already been taught these caregiving techniques by professionals.

Part 3 of the book is an encyclopedia, arranged in alphabetical order. Listed, defined, and described in this section are the medical terms and diagnoses and the medical and surgical procedures that are encountered by families and others who provide care to children with cerebral palsy. Parents can use this reference as a guide, and can consult it when new problems arise or new treatments are being considered. Those caring for a child whose doctor recommends that a *pelvic osteotomy* be performed, for example, can find out what this procedure involves, why and when it is recommended, and what the preoperative and postoperative course will be like for the child.

The Resources section at the back of the book lists the names, addresses, phone numbers, and web pages of organizations that provide professional support for children with CP and their caregivers. Finally, additional information about many of the topics in this book may be found in the books and Web sites listed in the Recommended Reading section.

A final thought before we begin: Each child is an individual, and no book can provide information that applies specifically to an individual child at any given time. We have written this book to provide information that applies generally to all children with CP, but specific information about *your child* can only be obtained directly from a medical professional who knows the child.

Acknowledgments

♦ AS WE NOTED in the first edition, a work of this scope depends on the efforts and contributions of many people. We thank the following colleagues and health care professionals for their contributions to this new edition:

Michael Alexander, M.D.
Benjamin Alouf, M.D.
Ellen Arch, M.D.
Joan Blair, M.S.N., R.N., A.P.R.N.-B.C.
Millie Boettcher, M.S.N., C.P.N.P., C.N.S.N.
Mary Bolton, P.T.
Winslow Borkowski, M.D.
Aaron Chidekel, M.D.
Steven Cook, M.D.
Maureen Edelson, M.D.
Stephen Falchek, M.D.
T. Ernesto Figueroa, M.D.

Rochelle Glidden, Psy.D.
H. Theodore Harcke, M.D.
Douglas Huisenga, P.T., A.T.C.
Heidi Kecskemethy, R.D., C.S.P.
Maura McManus, M.D.
Ralph Milner, M.D.
Robert O'Reilly, M.D.
Denise Peischl, B.S.B.M.E.
Joseph Queenan, M.D.
Mena Scavina, D.O.
Ellen Scharff, M.S.W.
David Sheslow, Ph.D.
Susan Stine, M.D.
Philip Wolfson, M.D.

Special thanks go to Josh Whinston, Bart Stevens, Ch.L.A.P., Diane Gallagher, Ed.D., and Brian J. Hartman, Esq., for significant contributions to chapters 8, 10, 11, and 12 respectively. Special thanks also to Rochelle Sassler for her major contribution of time and effort with typing, editing, and coordinating this project.

We acknowledge the major contributions of our fellow authors, who helped write and edit major portions of this book. We also acknowledge the support of our editors at the Johns Hopkins University Press, especially Jacqueline Wehmueller, who has been with this project since the first edition was proposed.

We especially acknowledge our families for their patience and support as we worked on this project.

We also acknowledge the many patients and their families who have helped us understand what they want to know about caring for their child with cerebral palsy and have encouraged us to write this book.

Finally, we acknowledge the help and support of the Nemours Foundation, the Nemours Children's Clinic–Wilmington, and the Alfred I duPont Hospital for Children, whose support was crucial to this second edition. We especially acknowledge Roy Proujansky, M.D., Chief Executive of the Practice and J. Carlton Gartner, M.D., Chairman of the Pediatrics Department, for giving Dr. Bachrach the time to work on this second edition. We must also thank Dr. Bachrach's colleagues in the Division of General Pediatrics who helped care for his patients and covered his administrative duties while he was away. These include Benjamin Alouf, M.D., Gary Frank, M.D., J. Carlton Gartner, M.D., Sandra Hassink, M.D., J. Jeffrey Malatack, M.D., Keith Mann, M.D., Maureen McMahon, M.D., Amy Renwick, M.D., Joanne Woodbridge, M.D., Kathleen Trzcinski, M.S.N., C.R.N.P., and Marilyn Boos, R.N.C., M.S.

Steven J. Bachrach, M.D.
Freeman Miller, M.D.

Contributors

Steven J. Bachrach, M.D., is Chief of the Division of General Pediatrics and Co-Director of the Cerebral Palsy Program at the Alfred I. duPont Hospital for Children, Wilmington, Delaware, and Clinical Professor of Pediatrics at Jefferson Medical College, Philadelphia, Pennsylvania.

Marilyn L. Boos, R.N.C., M.S., is a pediatric clinical nurse specialist for the Cerebral Palsy Program at the Alfred I. duPont Hospital for Children, Wilmington, Delaware.

Kirk Dabney, M.D., is Co-Director of the Cerebral Palsy Program, Department of Orthopaedics, at the Alfred I. duPont Hospital for Children, Wilmington, Delaware; Assistant Professor of Orthopaedic Surgery at Jefferson Medical College, Philadelphia, Pennsylvania; and Assistant Professor of Orthopaedic Surgery at Georgetown University Medical School, Washington, DC.

Linda Duffy, B.S., P.A.-C., is staff physician's assistant in the Cerebral Palsy Program, Department of Orthopaedics, at the Alfred I. duPont Hospital for Children, Wilmington, Delaware.

Robin C. Meyers, M.P.H., R.D., is a pediatric dietician at the Alfred I. duPont Hospital for Children, Wilmington, Delaware.

Freeman Miller, M.D., is Co-Director of the Cerebral Palsy Program at the Alfred I. duPont Hospital for Children, Wilmington, Delaware; Assistant Professor of Orthopaedic Surgery at Jefferson Medical College, Philadelphia, Pennsylvania; and Adjunct Assistant Professor of Mechanical Engineering at the University of Delaware.

Douglas T. Pearson, Ph.D., is a retired child psychologist. He is currently involved in teaching and volunteering his expertise in inner-city day care centers.

Kathleen Trzcinski, R.N., M.S.N., C.R.N.P., is a nurse practitioner in the Cerebral Palsy Program at the Alfred I. duPont Hospital for Children, Wilmington, Delaware.

Rhonda S. Walter, M.D., is the Chief of the Division of Developmental Medicine at the Alfred I. duPont Hospital for Children, Wilmington, Delaware.

Joan Lenett Whinston currently serves as the New Jersey State Representative of the Amputee Coalition of America. She also serves on the Camden County Disabilities Board of Directors of New Jersey. She is the author of *Grandma Has One Leg* and *I'm Joshua and "Yes I Can,"* which she wrote for her son who has cerebral palsy.

Part One

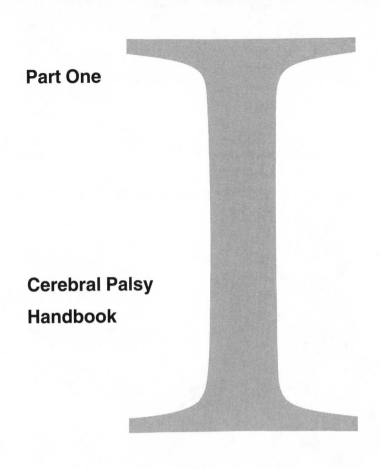

**Cerebral Palsy
Handbook**

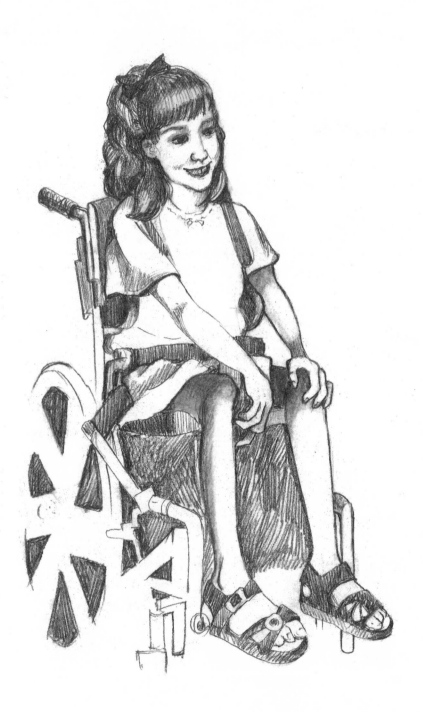

What Is
Cerebral
Palsy?

I

♦ CEREBRAL PALSY is a collection of motor disorders result-ing from damage to the brain that occurs before, during, or after birth. The damage to the child's brain affects the motor system, and as a result the child has poor coordination, poor balance, or abnormal movement patterns—or a combination of these characteristics.

Cerebral palsy (CP) is a *static* disorder of the brain, not a progressive dis-order. This means that the disorder or disease process will not get worse as time goes on. Nor are the motor disorders associated with cerebral palsy temporary. Therefore, a child who has temporary motor problems, or who has motor problems that get worse over time, does not have cerebral palsy. Children with cerebral palsy may have many other kinds of problems, in-cluding medical problems. Most of these problems are related to brain in-jury. They include epilepsy, mental retardation, learning disabilities, and/or attention deficit–hyperactivity disorder.

Congenital cerebral palsy (or cerebral palsy that exists from birth) is re-sponsible for the largest proportion of cases of cerebral palsy. For a small per-centage of children, injuries sustained during the birthing process or in early childhood may be considered the cause of cerebral palsy. When motor dis-orders appear after age 5, they are slightly different from the motor disorders of cerebral palsy and are usually diagnosed as they would be in an adult, as stroke or traumatic brain injury.

Cerebral palsy is one of the more common congenital problems: of every 2,000 infants born, 5 are born with cerebral palsy. This incidence had re-mained constant for over 30 years, despite advances in obstetrical and pedi-atric care, but began to rise slightly in the last years of the twentieth century in the United States and other industrialized countries. Although improve-ments in medical care have decreased the incidence of CP among some chil-dren who otherwise would have developed the disorder, medical advances have also resulted in the survival of children who previously would have died at a young age, and many of these children survive with an impairment or a disability such as cerebral palsy.

What has also changed is the *type* of cerebral palsy that is most prevalent in the developed Western world. In the 1960s in the United States 20 percent of all children with cerebral palsy had *athetoid* cerebral palsy, a type of CP caused by *hyperbilirubinemia* and characterized by slow, writhing involuntary movements. Today only 5 or 10 percent of children have this type of CP, and 80 to 90 percent have spastic CP. The decrease is mainly due to advances in the treatment of hyperbilirubinemia. At the same time, *spastic* cerebral palsy, characterized by rigidity in muscles, which causes stiffness and restricted movement, has become more prevalent because intensive care for newborns has resulted in higher survival rates for very small premature babies. These babies are at high risk of developing spastic cerebral palsy: between 5 and 8 percent of premature infants under 1,500 grams (3 lb. 5 oz.) who survive have cerebral palsy.

What causes cerebral palsy?

When cerebral palsy was first described in the 1880s, it was believed to be caused by lack of oxygen for the infant at birth. We now know that this is the cause in only a small minority, approximately 10 percent, of children with CP. The great majority of CP is caused by damage to the brain during fetal development, well before the birth process begins. Although the cause of this damage is usually not known (the medical term for "unknown cause" is *idiopathic*), we know from modern imaging techniques (computerized tomography and magnetic resonance imaging) that some cases of CP are caused by strokes or hemorrhaging in the brain in the late stages of fetal development. Others are caused by abnormal development of the brain in the early stages of fetal development (what is called a *malformation* or *birth defect of the brain*). The brain damage that leads to CP can be caused by:

Idiopathic (no known cause of damage to brain during pregnancy)—still the most common cause

A viral infection during pregnancy, such as cytomegalovirus (CMV) or rubella

Hydrocephalus, either before or after birth

A blood clot in the fetus's brain causing a stroke while in utero

Bleeding into the brain: While in utero, this could be due to a bleeding disorder; after birth, this can be seen as a complication of extreme prematurity.

Prolonged period of asphyxia (lack of oxygen) from, for example, abruptio placenta, when the placenta tears away from the uterine wall during labor, cutting off the baby's blood supply.

Bacterial meningitis after birth

Head trauma from shaken baby syndrome (child abuse) during the first year of life

Lead poisoning during the first two years of life

There is no way to predict which children's brains will be damaged by one of these factors, or what the extent of the damage will be. However, none of these factors always results in brain damage, and even when brain damage occurs, the damage does not always result in CP. Some children may have an isolated hearing loss from their meningitis, others will have severe mental retardation, and some will have CP (either alone, or with these other problems, too).

The most recent theory on the cause of idiopathic CP is that something (possibly an infection in the amniotic fluid that surrounds the fetus in the womb) sets off an inflammatory reaction in the brain of the fetus, and this inflammation causes the brain damage resulting in CP. While not fully proven, some experimental evidence supports this theory. This inflammation may also be the cause of premature labor in many cases, which may explain why CP and prematurity often occur in the same child.

What are the different types of cerebral palsy?

Cerebral palsy is classified by the type of movement problem (spastic, athetoid, hypotonic, or mixed) and by the body parts involved (legs only, one arm and one leg, or all four limbs). Motor ability and coordination vary greatly from one child to another, and there are very few statements that hold true for *all* children with cerebral palsy. Thus, generalizations about children with cerebral palsy can only have meaning within the context of the subgroups described below. That's why subgroups are used in this book whenever treatment and outcome expectations are discussed. Most professionals who care for children with cerebral palsy are familiar with these diagnoses and use them to communicate about a child's condition.

Spasticity refers to the inability of a muscle to relax, while *athetosis* refers to an inability to control the movement of a muscle. Infants who at first are *hypotonic,* or very floppy, may later develop spasticity. *Hemiplegia* is cerebral palsy that involves one arm and one leg on the same side of the body, whereas *diplegia* primarily involves both legs. *Quadriplegia* refers to a pattern involving all four extremities as well as trunk and neck muscles. Generally a child with quadriplegia does not walk independently. Another frequently used classification is *ataxia,* which refers to balance and coordination problems.

Although almost all children with cerebral palsy can be classified as having hemiplegia, diplegia, or quadriplegia, there are significant overlaps that have led to the use of additional terms, some of which are confusing. Occasionally you'll encounter terms like *paraplegia, double hemiplegia, triplegia,* and *pentaplegia;* these classifications are also based on the parts of the body involved. For simplicity, however, most of the discussion of CP is limited to the three broader categories.

The word for the dominant type of movement or muscle coordination problem is often combined with the word for the component that seems to be most problematic for the child. The result is a more specific descriptive term. For example, the child with *spastic diplegia* has mostly spastic muscle problems, and his legs are mainly affected, although he may also have athetosis and balance problems. The child with *athetoid quadriplegia*, on the other hand, has involvement of both arms and legs, primarily with athetoid muscle problems, but he or she often also has some ataxia and spasticity.

To summarize, we can classify different kinds of cerebral palsy according to the type of movement the child makes or to the part of the body that is most involved, or both:

By type of movement

Spastic	too much muscle tone
Athetoid	no muscle control
Hypotonic	decreased muscle tone (not enough tone)
Ataxic	balance and coordination problems
Mixed	mixture of two or more of the above

By involved body parts

Hemiplegia	one arm and one leg on the same side of the body
Diplegia	predominantly both legs (arms also involved)
Quadriplegia	all four extremities

Other terms used to define specific problems of movement or muscle function include *dystonia, tremor, ballismus,* and *rigidity.* The words *severe, moderate,* and *mild* are also often used in combination with both anatomical pattern and motor function classification terms (severe spastic diplegia, for example), but these qualifying words do not have any specific meaning. They are subjective words, and their meaning varies depending upon the person who is using them.

What are the right words to use when referring to children with cerebral palsy?

Cerebral palsy is the term used to describe the motor impairment resulting from brain damage in the young child, regardless of the cause of the damage or its effect on the child. *Impairment* is the correct term to use to define a deviation from normal, such as not being able to make a muscle move or not being able to control an unwanted movement. *Disability* is the term used to define a restriction in the ability to perform a normal daily activity that someone of the same age is able to perform. (For example, a 3-year-old child who is not able to walk has a disability because normal 3-year-olds can walk independently.) *Handicap* is the term used to describe the condition of a child or adult who, because of the disability, is unable to achieve a normal role in society appropriate to his or her age and environment.

A 16-year-old who is unable to prepare his own lunch or brush his teeth is handicapped. But a 16-year-old who walks with the assistance of crutches, attends a regular school, and is fully independent in daily activities is disabled, not handicapped. Thus, a person can be impaired and not necessarily be disabled, and a person can be disabled without being handicapped.

Impaired means a deviation from normal;
Disabled denotes restricted ability to perform normal activities of daily living; and
Handicapped means being unable to achieve an age-appropriate role in society.

In the past there was a lack of awareness and sensitivity among the general public with respect to the words used to describe people with disabilities. Over the past years, however, an increasing amount of attention has been paid to such language, and recently a great deal of attention has been given to issues of education, employment, and public access for individuals with disabilities. Because of this evolving awareness and respect, it is no longer acceptable to refer to individuals by their disability (in other words, as "the epileptic," "the spastic," or "the retarded child"). While it may take years for a country's language to catch up with society's changing views, the current acceptable terminology stresses the *individual person* and then mentions the disability that the person has: a girl with spastic diplegia, or a boy with mental retardation. Clearly, this language acknowledges that there is much more to a person than his or her disability. Other terms that have recently come into use represent an even more enlightened view; for example, some people may refer to a child as mentally challenged rather than mentally retarded.

In this book, we have chosen to use respectful language that presents information in a way that can be understood by the general reader. Although there may be newer, even better terms to use, we haven't used them because they often create confusion.

What medical problems will my child encounter?

The following list presents the medical problems most often associated with cerebral palsy. These problems (and other, less common problems) are discussed in detail in Chapter 3.

Neurological problems
Mental retardation
Learning disabilities
Attention deficit–hyperactivity
　disorder
Seizure disorder (epilepsy)
Visual impairment
Swallowing difficulties
Speech impairment (dysarthria)
Hearing loss

Orthopedic problems
Scoliosis
Hip dislocation
Contractures of joints
Discrepancy in leg length

Secondary effects
Communication disorder
Drooling
Poor nutrition
Depression
Fragile bones and frequent fractures
Cavities
Constipation

What are some disorders that look like cerebral palsy but are in fact a different problem?

Children with different kinds of disabilities have many problems in common, especially in interacting with family members and society. Although the physical and medical difficulties of children with disabilities vary widely, some of the characteristics of various disorders *resemble* those of cerebral palsy. It isn't until after closer examination that the medical issues turn out to be quite distinct.

Children with spinal cord dysfunction, for example, face medical problems such as a lack of feeling in their skin and lack of bowel and bladder control, which differ markedly from the medical problems faced by children with cerebral palsy. Spinal cord dysfunction may be a result of spinal cord injury, spina bifida (a defect in the formation of the spinal *column*), or a congenital spinal cord malformation (a defect in the formation of the spinal *cord*). Other children who may look similar to children with cerebral palsy are children with temporary motor problems resulting from closed head injuries, seizures, drug overdoses, or some brain tumors. The medical issues for this group of children are also different from the medical issues for children with cerebral palsy, because these injuries can occur at any age, and the severity of the problems caused by these injuries changes over time.

Disorders that are primarily of muscle, nerve, and bone are not cerebral palsy. Such conditions include muscular dystrophy, peripheral neuropathies such as Charcot-Marie-Tooth disease, and osteogenesis imperfecta. All of these conditions are associated with specific medical problems.

Children with progressive neurological disorders (including Rett syndrome, leukodystrophy, and Tay-Sachs disease) also have medical needs that differ from those of children with cerebral palsy. Some children with chromosomal anomalies (for example, trisomy 13 and 18) or congenital disorders (hereditary spastic paraplegia, for example) may appear similar to children with cerebral palsy; others, such as children with Down syndrome, appear very different but may have some issues in common with children who have cerebral palsy. They also have problems that are unique to children with that specific disorder.

Can cerebral palsy be prevented?

When a physician diagnoses a baby with CP, the mother and father often feel guilty and wonder what they did to contribute to their child's disorder. While it is certainly true that good prenatal care is an essential part of preventing congenital problems, these "birth defects" often occur even when the mother has strictly followed her physician's advice in caring for herself and the developing infant. Since the cause of most cases of CP is still not understood (see page 4), prevention in most cases is not yet possible. However, when there are specific known causes, the possibility of prevention exists.

Infections such as rubella (German measles), toxoplasmosis (a disease caused by the invasion of parasitic microorganisms), and the virus known as cytomegalovirus can cause brain damage in the fetus. Rubella can be prevented by immunization (a woman should be immunized *before* becoming pregnant), and the chances of becoming infected with toxoplasmosis can be minimized by not handling the feces of cats and by avoiding raw or undercooked meat. There is no immunization for CMV. Bacterial meningitis can cause severe brain damage in young infants after birth and is caused by a number of different bacteria. There is an immunization for some of these bacteria, including *haemophilus influenzae* type B and some strains of pneumococcus, which should prevent infection and thus protect the child from meningitis due to these organisms.

Premature infants are at a much higher risk for developing cerebral palsy than full-term babies, and the risk increases as the birthweight decreases. Between 5 and 8 percent of infants weighing less than 1,500 grams (3 lb. 5 oz.) at birth develop cerebral palsy, and infants weighing less than 1,500 grams are 25 times more likely to develop cerebral palsy than infants who are born at full term weighing more than 2,500 grams (5 lb. 8 oz.). Many premature infants suffer bleeding within the brain, called *intraventricular hemorrhages,* or *intracranial hemorrhages.* Again, the highest frequency of hemorrhages is found in babies with the lowest weight: the problem is rare in babies who weigh more than 2,000 grams (4 lb. 6 oz.). This bleeding may damage the part of the brain that controls motor function and thereby lead to cerebral palsy. If the hemorrhages result in destruction of normal brain tissue (a condition called *periventricular leukomalacia*) and the development of small cysts around the ventricles and in the motor region of the brain, then the infant is more likely to have CP than an infant with hemorrhages alone. While we do not yet know the cause of premature labor, available treatments sometimes succeed in stopping such labor, or at least delaying delivery of the infant for a while. Prevention of early delivery, along with medicines to help mature the lungs, may prevent some of the severe medical and neurological problems associated with premature birth.

What circumstances in the birthing process might cause a newborn to have cerebral palsy?

In the nineteenth century, William John Little, M.D., described cerebral palsy and stated that in most cases the condition was due to birth injury. Sigmund Freud, M.D., who was a prominent neurologist before he entered the field of psychiatry, also investigated the causes of cerebral palsy. Dr. Freud thought that the condition was due to something that occurred before the child's birth. He argued that the problems seen at birth were often due to an abnormality present in the baby before birth and were not caused by the birthing process. Freud's view was greatly ignored for nearly one hundred years but recent research has lent support to the idea that cerebral palsy is more often a result of a congenital abnormality than an injury sustained at birth.

The birthing process can be traumatic for an infant, however, and injuries occurring during birth do sometimes cause cerebral palsy. Modern prenatal care and improved obstetrical care have significantly reduced the incidence of birth injury, but it is unlikely that it will ever be completely eliminated.

There are no specific events that, if they occur during pregnancy, delivery, or infancy, always cause cerebral palsy. One large study, for example, indicates that more than 60 percent of all pregnancies have at least one complication, and that most of these complications cause no problems. For instance, 25 percent of all the newborns in the study had the umbilical cord wrapped around their neck, and 16 percent passed meconium (had the first bowel movement) at the time of birth. Fortunately, these common "birth events" and the development of CP have only a small correlation.

On the other hand, newborns in this study who had very low Apgar scores for a prolonged period (less than 3 at 20 minutes) had a risk of developing cerebral palsy that was 250 times greater than infants with normal Apgar scores. (An Apgar score is a system for assessing the condition of a newborn baby by scoring respiration effort, heart rate, color, muscle tone, and motor reactions, usually at 1 and 5 minutes after birth.) An Apgar score of less than 3 at 20 minutes after birth suggests that the infant suffered severe asphyxia during birth (asphyxia is a lack of sufficient oxygen to the brain). Half of the infants who suffered severe asphyxia during birth did *not* develop cerebral palsy, however.

When CP is diagnosed in childhood, it is often found that the child suffered asphyxia at birth. The asphyxia, however, is often considered the *symptom* of an otherwise sick baby with a neurological problem, not the primary *cause* of CP. In a number of studies, only about 9 percent of children with CP were thought to have CP directly and exclusively related to asphyxia at delivery. Ninety-one percent of the babies had other inherent causes that led to their brain damage, unrelated to their birth experience. This is apparently why the incidence of CP in undeveloped and poverty-stricken countries, where infant mortality is very high, is the same as in northern Europe, where infant mortality is the lowest in the world. It may also explain why modern obstetrical care, including monitoring and a high rate of cesarean section, has lowered infant mortality rates but not the incidence of cerebral palsy.

What might cause a child between birth and the age of 2–3 years to develop CP?

During infancy and early childhood, a child is completely dependent on others for his or her safety and protection, and shielding a child from injury is one of the most important responsibilities of a child's caregivers. An injury like asphyxia damages the brain in a variety of ways, and it is the number one cause of CP in this age group. Asphyxia is most commonly caused by poisoning, near-drowning, and choking on foreign objects such as toys and pieces of food (including peanuts, popcorn, and hot dogs).

The brain may also be damaged when it is physically traumatized as a result of a blow to the head. A child who falls, is involved in a motor vehicle accident, or is the victim of physical abuse may suffer irreparable injury to the brain. One form of child abuse is the shaken baby syndrome, in which the caretaker is trying to quiet the baby by shaking him but shakes him too vigorously, causing the infant's brain to strike repeatedly against the skull under high pressure. This kind of abuse can damage the brain.

Severe infections, especially *meningitis* or *encephalitis,* can also lead to brain damage in this age group. Meningitis is inflammation of the meninges (the covering of the brain and the spinal cord), usually caused by a bacterial infection. Encephalitis is brain inflammation that may be caused by bacterial or viral infections. Either of these infections can cause disabilities ranging from hearing loss to CP and severe retardation.

How does a physician diagnose cerebral palsy?

Many of a child's normal developmental milestones, such as reaching for toys (3 to 4 months), sitting (6 to 7 months), and walking (10 to 14 months), are based on motor function. A physician may suspect cerebral palsy if a child is slow to develop these skills. In making a diagnosis of cerebral palsy, the physician takes into account the delay in developmental milestones as well as physical warning signs such as abnormal muscle tone, abnormal movements, and persistent infantile reflexes.

Making a definite diagnosis of cerebral palsy is not always easy, however, especially before the child's first birthday. In fact, diagnosing cerebral palsy usually involves a period of waiting for the definite and permanent appearance of specific motor problems. Most children with cerebral palsy can be diagnosed by the age of 18 months, but this is a long time for parents to wait for a diagnosis, and it is understandably a difficult and trying period.

Making a diagnosis of cerebral palsy is also difficult when, for example, a 2-year-old has suffered a head injury. The child may appear to be severely injured in the period immediately after the trauma, and three months after the injury he may have symptoms that are typical of a child with cerebral palsy. But one year after the injury the child may be completely recovered, and it's clear that he doesn't have cerebral palsy. Although he has a scar on his brain, the scar is not permanently impairing his motor activities. During the year between the injury and the diagnosis of no permanent injury, the parents will have a difficult time waiting. No matter how frustrating this period of waiting and observing is, however, it must pass before the diagnosis can be made.

Do x-rays or other tests help in the diagnosis?

In making a diagnosis of cerebral palsy, the most meaningful aspect of the examination is the physical evidence of abnormal motor function. A diagnosis of cerebral palsy cannot be made solely on the basis of an x-ray or a blood test, though the physician may order such tests to exclude other neurological diseases that could cause similar symptoms.

Blood tests and chromosome analysis are helpful in diagnosing hereditary conditions that may be the cause of the abnormal motor function. It is important to diagnose these conditions for the child's sake, to understand the cause of her problems and the possible prognosis. It is also important for the family, because it may influence the parents' decision to have more children. When the tests indicate that a child's condition is something other than cerebral palsy and that the condition is inherited, family members often benefit from genetic counseling. Cerebral palsy is not a hereditary condition, however, and a normal genetic test or normal chromosomes neither establish nor rule out a diagnosis of CP.

Magnetic resonance imaging (MRI) or computerized tomography (CT) scans are often ordered when the physician suspects that the child has cerebral palsy. These tests may provide evidence of a malformation of the brain (such as lissencephaly), of an intrauterine stroke, periventricular leukomalacia (PVL), hydrocephalus, or a bleed into the brain.

Seeing these abnormalities on the MRI of a child who has abnormal tone lends support to the possible diagnosis of CP, and sometimes may explain the nature and timing of the brain injury. Sometimes, these scans show evidence of a progressive neurological disease, which rules out a diagnosis of CP. Sometimes the scan appears normal. A normal scan tells us that the structure of the brain appears normal. However, the function of the brain at the level of connections between nerves may still be abnormal, so a normal scan does not mean that the child has no problems. The physical examination and the child's delay in development is the best indicator of neurologic problems. These scans, even when abnormal, also cannot predict how a specific child will function as he or she grows. Thus, children with normal scans may have severe cerebral palsy, and children with clearly abnormal scans occasionally appear totally normal or have only mild physical evidence of cerebral palsy. A child with an abnormal scan might appear normal until she begins school, for example, when significant learning problems may surface.

As a group, children with cerebral palsy do have brain scars, cysts, and other changes that show up on scans more frequently than in children without cerebral palsy. Therefore, when an abnormality is seen on a CT scan of the brain of a child whose physical examination suggests he may have cerebral palsy, it is one more indication that the child is likely to have motor problems in the future.

My infant has just been diagnosed with cerebral palsy. What can I expect for her future?

The first questions usually asked by parents after they are told their child has cerebral palsy are, "What will my child be like?" and "Will she walk?" Predicting what a young child with cerebral palsy will be like or what he or she will or will not do (this prediction is called the *prognosis*) is very difficult. Any predictions for an infant under 6 months of age are little better than guesses, and even for children younger than 1 year it is often difficult to predict the severity of CP. By the time the child is 2 years old, however, a qualified physician can determine whether the child has hemiplegia, diplegia, or quadriplegia. Based on this involvement pattern, some predictions can be made.

Remember, children with cerebral palsy do not stop activities once they have begun them. Such a loss of skills, called *regression,* is not characteristic of this disorder. If regression does occur, a different explanation for the child's problems should be sought.

For a child to be able to walk, some major events in motor control have to occur. A child must be able to hold up his head before he can sit up on his own, and he must be able to sit independently before he can walk on his own. It is generally assumed that if a child is not sitting up by himself by age 4 or walking by age 8, he will never be an independent walker. But a child who starts to walk at age 3 will certainly continue to walk and will be walking for the rest of his life.

It is even more difficult to make early predictions of speaking ability or mental ability than it is to predict motor function. Here, too, evaluation is much more reliable after age 2, although a motor disability can make the evaluation of intellectual function quite difficult. Sometimes "motor-free" tests, which can assess intellectual ability without the child using his hands, are administered by psychologists who are experts in this type of testing. Overall, a child's intellectual ability, far more than his physical disability, will determine the prognosis. In other words, mental retardation is far more likely to impair a child's ability to function in the world than is cerebral palsy.

What can *my doctor tell me about my newborn's neurological problems?*

As a parent, you're naturally concerned when your newborn has problems. Although your child's physician needs to evaluate your child's condition and prognosis and discuss this with you, the outcome cannot be predicted. Remember, although an increased risk of CP can sometimes be identified at birth, an actual diagnosis of cerebral palsy cannot be made at birth, and certainly the extent and severity of involvement that an individual child might eventually have is impossible to assess at birth.

Some neonatologists (doctors who specialize in the care of newborn infants) may avoid discussing the infant's problems in detail with the parents. They do this because they are aware of the normal interaction and bonding that occurs between the newborn and parents, and they don't want to do anything to interfere with that healthy interaction. The presumption of a bleak future for a child sometimes causes parents to withdraw from the child, and this can have a significant negative effect on the child.

Physicians usually communicate their concerns in terms of the child's symptoms, such as muscle problems, and prepare parents for the possibility of neurological damage. Clearly, it is part of the physician's role to inform parents, but the variability of outcome makes it virtually impossible for the physician to predict the future, and so the physician must weigh the need to inform (and the imprecision of the information that is available) against the need for the parents to have hope for, and become close to, their child.

Given all these uncertainties, what kind of medical treatment should a sick newborn receive?

Many times when a child is 2 or 3 years old and has a severe disability, parents begin to wonder whether treatment should have been less aggressive during those first few years. Given the tremendous uncertainties in outcome, physicians and parents often choose to treat newborns and preserve life with the hope that the outcome will be a good one. There are clearly exceptions, such as when the baby has a known chromosomal defect (such as trisomy 18), where a poor prognosis is known and very aggressive treatment may be futile. However, in the majority of cases, neither the doctor nor the parents know what the outcome will be, and they must do the best they can with the limited information they have.

Often the prognosis is based on information from studies of a large number of babies with similar birthweights. The chance of an individual baby having cerebral palsy or mental retardation (expressed as a percentage) is derived from these studies. Nevertheless, it is impossible to know whether an individual infant will fit into the 70 to 90 percent group that has a good outcome or the 10 to 30 percent group with a poor outcome.

The role of the physician is to gather as much information about the child's condition as possible and to convey this information to families, along with the best information available about chances of outcome. The role of the family is to help in the decision-making process, especially when decisions must be made about further aggressive treatment. Ultimately, treatment decisions are medical ones, but they should be made with input from the family. The relationship between physician, patient, and family should be one of mutual respect, where each member of the "team" is working toward the patient's common good. Only with an open exchange of information and communication is this possible.

The problem is trying to figure out what is best for the child. At the time the decisions must be made it is often very difficult to know what will ultimately be best. A decision to treat aggressively usually involves the use of sophisticated equipment, although the availability of such technology does not mean that it must always be used, and there are clearly times when it is more humane to withhold or withdraw aggressive treatment. These are never easy decisions to make. Clergy, social workers, ethicists, and other health care workers who have come to know the patient and family often help in making decisions.

As parents reflect back over previous treatments, they should remember all these uncertainties and focus on the fact that decisions were made based on the best information available at the time. Focusing on decisions that in hindsight are thought to have been wrong is not beneficial to anyone. Similarly, the treatment plan should be a flexible one, and parents and medical specialists should not be afraid to alter the course as new information becomes available.

As parents, how can we work with doctors to set realistic goals for our child?

When it comes to expectations and questions of what the future holds for the child with CP, a combination of optimism and realism is probably your best bet. Consider that the parents of a 3-year-old without a disability who hope and expect that the child will go to college and law school, enter politics, and eventually become president of the United States have a vision for their child that combines realism and fantasy. Rather than map out a child's career path in this way, it would be far better for parents to care for the child as a 3-year-old—not as a college student or as a budding politician. It is equally important for the parent of a child with a disability to understand the child's present and future abilities, and to develop a set of realistic goals to live by.

Occasionally difficulties in communication arise when parents, educators, and medical care providers discuss the child's present abilities. It's often a challenge to improve communication so that everyone involved in the decision-making process is heard. People who are involved in making difficult decisions in an emotionally charged atmosphere must know that they will have a chance to express their opinions regarding the child's treatment, and that these opinions will be taken seriously. Parents know their child best, but their judgment may be clouded by fantasy; physicians need to help parents develop realistic goals without quashing their hope. Sometimes parents don't have high *enough* expectations for their child, and in this case doctors need to provide encouragement to the parents to help them help their child achieve everything that he or she is able to.

An attempt to define future expectations is usually most important in the teenage years and beyond, when function is better defined and the future looks clearer to everyone involved. However, if everyone keeps their sights set on the primary goal—helping the child function at his or her maximum ability—then a team spirit is often a natural result.

The next chapter describes the general patterns of "normal" pediatric development. These patterns provide a basis of comparison for parents whose child has problems associated with cerebral palsy. By comparing their own child's development with that of the child whose development is proceeding as expected, parents whose child has CP can sometimes be comforted by seeing that their child is developing along certain avenues just as he or she is expected to do. If, on the other hand, the child is experiencing developmental delays, parents can bring the problems to the attention of their child's physician, who can then work with the parents to determine the best course of action.

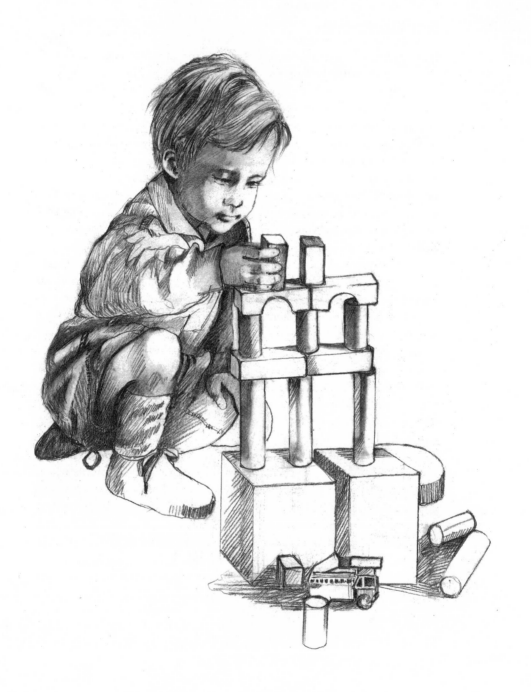

An Overview of Early Child Development

2

♦ WHEN WE TALK about the changes that an individual goes through while maturing from infancy into being a toddler, a child, an adolescent, and, finally, an adult, we sometimes use the words *growth* and *development*. When we use the word *growth,* we are referring to an increase in physical size, but when we talk about *development,* we mean an increase in control over body movements. In this chapter, we will be focusing on this second aspect of the maturation process.

A newborn infant responds primarily in an involuntary, or reflexive, way to his or her environment, but over the next few years a combination of physical growth and learning experiences will enable the child to participate actively in the world. The child will learn to run, talk, and think creatively, and this development will occur step by step, in a sequential fashion.

Many parents have their own ideas about "normal development"—that is, what a "normal" child should do at any given age. This perception is based on common family experiences, on what the parents have read in parenting books, and on the advice they have received from pediatricians and other professionals. While most books caution parents about comparing their child's development with the "norms," it is only natural for parents to consider their child as either advanced or delayed in comparison to their perception of "normal."

It's important to keep in mind that each baby develops in his or her own way. Although there is a sequential unfolding of developmental milestones, most parents, educators, and professionals who spend time around children know that different children develop at different rates. These developmental differences may be due to an inborn "inner nature" that is influenced by the environment in which the child grows. Clearly, however, there are some children whose development is delayed to the point where the parents begin to worry, and some children's development differs from the range of norms in a way that interferes with an orderly acquisition of skills.

The growth and development of infants born with disabilities or chronic or life-threatening illnesses may be erratic, showing normal patterns of development in some areas but not in others. It is at these points of perceived delay that parents need to become concerned, seek professional advice, investigate the problem, and, if necessary, obtain remedial help for the child. While their infant is maturing, it's worthwhile for parents to keep in mind some general principles of development. In this way, they are more likely to recognize when their child may need some help.

First, parents need to view development as a continuous process, from conception to maturity, rather than as a series of milestones. Before such markers are reached, a child proceeds through many stages of development, and as a parent you need to observe not only *what* a child does, but *how* he does it. It is important to know that development depends on the maturation of the nervous system. Until that has occurred, no amount of practice or coaching can make a child learn a skill that his brain is not yet capable of directing.

While the *sequence* of development is the same for all children, the *rate* of development varies from child to child. For example, a child learns to sit before he walks, but the age at which different children learn to sit and walk varies considerably. Certain so-called primitive reflexes need to be lost before voluntary movement can develop. (In children with severe motor disabilities, these primitive reflexes are likely to persist beyond the usual age and may, in fact, impede normal development.)

Finally, the direction of development is *cephalocaudal*—that is, from head to toe. The child must be able to control his head before he can control the spinal muscles; ultimately he will gain control of the extremities as he progresses through the developmental stages and begins walking.

Remember that developmental "norms" are not absolutes. Your child may gain individual skills earlier or later than other children. In children with cerebral palsy, neurological problems accompany the primary motor disability. In fact, many of the problems associated with CP (such as mental retardation, communication or learning disorders, disturbances of hearing or vision, emotional problems, seizures, and orthopedic complications) have a greater effect on development than the primary motor dysfunction does. This does not mean to imply that each and every child who is given the diagnosis of cerebral palsy is going to experience difficulties in all areas of development. Nor does it mean that your child, or any child with CP, will experience any or all of the associated dysfunctions. But as a parent, you need to educate yourself about delays in development and potential difficulties in various parts of the body, and be ready to investigate if you become concerned. This chapter will help you do that.

What specific skills do children generally master during development?

Early child development involves gaining mastery of four major types of skills: gross motor, fine motor, communication, and social. Development in these areas occurs simultaneously to prepare the child to meet physical, social, linguistic, and emotional demands. Gross motor skills such as postur-

Table 1   Overview of Developmental Milestones

Age	Gross Motor	Visual/Fine Motor	Language	Social
1 month	Prone, lifts head	Hands usually fisted; stares at objects	Soothes to voice	Regards face
3 months	Supports chest in prone position	Grasps placed rattle; follows slow-moving objects with eyes	Coos/laughs	Smiles easily, spontaneously
6 months	Rolls and sits well, without support	Reaches and grasps, transfers hand to hand	Babbles; plays peek-a-boo	Fear of strangers; smiles at self in mirror
12 months	Walks alone	Pincer grasp of raisin	Says "mama," "dada," + 2 other words	Shy, but plays game, gives affection
18 months	Walks up steps	Stacks 3 blocks; manages spoon	Points to named body parts; follows simple command	Helps with simple tasks; imitates play
24 months	Alternates feet on stairs; kicks ball	Stacks 6 cubes; turns book pages	At least 50-word vocabulary; understands 2-step commands	Washes/dries hands; helps get dressed
30 months	Jumps with both feet	Holds pencil in hand, not fist	Uses pronouns "I," "you," "me" correctly; states full name	Plays tag; asserts personality
36 months	Balances on 1 foot, 5 sec.; rides tricycle	Imitates block bridge; buttons	Recognizes 3 colors	Plays with children, takes turns

Note: It is not uncommon for a child to lag behind in one area and be advanced in another. However, there are generally accepted limits for what is considered "normal development."

Source: Adapted from *The Harriet Lane Handbook,* 17th ed. (Philadelphia, Elsevier Mosby, 2005).

ing, locomotion, and coordination require the use of large muscles to sit, crawl, stand, walk, and run, as well as other activities (table 1).

Fine motor or adaptive skills include manipulative skills, such as those used for feeding and dressing, skills that are necessary to interact effectively with the environment. Fine motor activities involve the use of small muscles in the fingers and hands, in tasks such as picking up small objects.

Communication skills are the capacities needed to understand others and express oneself. Communication skills are both verbal and nonverbal and are used in understanding both simple and complex instructions. This area encompasses the development of receptive language—the ability to receive and process information, and understand its meaning. Communication also

Table 2   Developmental Red Flags

Milestone	"Normal"	Concern if Not Acquired By
GROSS MOTOR		
Head up/chest off in prone position	2 months	3 months
Rolls front to back, back to front	4–5 months	6–8 months
Sits well unsupported	6 months	8–10 months
Creeps, crawls, cruises	9 months	12 months
Walks alone	12 months	15–18 months
Runs; throws toy, from standing without fall	18 months	21–24 months
Walks up and down steps	24 months	2–3 years
Alternates feet on stairs; pedals tricycle	3 years	3½–4 years
Hops, skips; alternates feet going down stairs	4 years	5 years
FINE MOTOR		
Unfists hands, touches object in front of them	3 months	4 months
Moves arms in unison to grasp	4–5 months	6 months
Reaches either hand, transfers	6 months	6–8 months
Pokes forefinger; pincer grasp; finger feeds; holds bottle	9 months	1 year
Throws objects, voluntary release; mature pincer grasp	12 months	15 months
Scribbles in imitation; holds utensil	15 months	18 months
Feeds self with spoon; stacks 3 cubes	18 months	21–24 months
Turns pages in books; is steady cup drinker; removes shoes and socks	24 months	30 months
Unbuttons; has adult pencil grasp	30 months	3 years
Draws a circle	36 months	4 years
Buttons clothes; catches a ball	4 years	5 years

Continued on next page

includes expressive language—the ability to transmit information. Social skills are the skills required to interact with other individuals.

What are some signs of developmental problems?

Significant delays in early child development are "red flags" that should prompt parents to discuss their concerns with the child's doctors (table 2). Significant delays in gross motor development include the inability to hold the head up securely by about age 3 months, to sit independently when placed in a sitting position by 10 months, or to walk independently by 18 months. Warning signs of fine motor problems include the inability to bring hands to midline (to center the hands in front of the body) or objects to the mouth by 6 months. A child who persistently keeps her hands fisted should also be checked. Babies generally pass out of the hand-clenching stage by 3 to 4 months of age. Persistence of this posture will interfere with both fine and gross motor development, and any child who is consistently keeping her hands clenched should be investigated for underlying abnormal neurological tonal imbalance.

Table 2 — Continued

Milestone	"Normal"	Concern if Not Acquired By
LANGUAGE		
Smiles socially after being talked to	6 weeks	3 months
Coos	3 months	5–6 months
Orients to voice	4 months	6 months
Babbles	6 months	8 months
Waves bye-bye; says "dada," "mama" indiscriminately	8–9 months	12 months
1–2 words other than dada/mama; follows 1-step command with gesture	12 months	15 months
7–20 words; knows 1 body part; uses mature jargoning	18 months	21–24 months
2-word combinations; 20 words; points to 3 body parts	21 months	24 months
50 words; 2-word sentences; pronouns (inappropriate); understands 2-step commands	24 months	30 months
3-word sentences; plurals; minimum 250 words	36 months	3½–4 years
Knows colors; asks questions; multiple-word sentences (tells story)	4 years	5 years
SOCIAL		
Regards face	1 month	1–2 months
Recognizes parents	2 months	2–3 months
Enjoys viewing surroundings	4 months	5–6 months
Recognizes strangers	6 months	7–8 months
Reciprocal games: so big, pat-a-cake	9 months	12 months

Delays that are a cause of concern in language development include lack of babbling, making raspberries, or cooing by 8 months, no intelligible words by 15 months, and no two-word distinct combinations by 2 years. Any child with these types of language delays should be investigated for problems with hearing. In addition, a young infant who is not easily startled at loud sounds, a 6-month-old who does not turn toward a voice, or a 1-year-old who does not appear to respond to her name when called requires a hearing evaluation. Questions or concerns about an infant's vision should be raised if by approximately 3 months of age the infant does not focus on a person's face or follow moving objects or people with his or her eyes. If a child has random eye movements (nystagmus), the parents should call the child's pediatrician.

"Red flag" concerns about social and emotional development are often more difficult to identify than physical ones because there are wide variations in cultural, ethnic, and familial expectations about a child's emotional makeup and temperament. However, we can say that if an infant by several months of age does not smile when talked to by family or friends, that infant ought to be examined. The same thing applies to an infant who in the first six months of life appears to stiffen when held, or is extraordinarily "unhuggable." Such a child is distinctly different from a motor-impaired child with tonal abnormalities; the latter is physically unable to hug, whereas the former is capable of reciprocating a hug or an endearing gesture but appears totally uninterested in doing so. Children generally enjoy making eye contact with parents and others they are comfortable with. A child at any stage of development after the first several months of infancy who cannot make or who actually appears to avoid making eye contact with familiar people should be examined for a potential social or emotional problem.

Concerns about developmental delays should be discussed with your child's physician. Depending on your child's age and other factors, several options are available, from a full neurodevelopmental evaluation to a watch-and-wait-and-see approach. Often your doctor can reassure you that your child's progress is within the range of normal development.

Birth to One Year

The first year of life is filled with advances in all aspects of development. Parents expect their baby to progress on to walking (or close to it), talking (one or more words), and semi-independence in feeding skills (introduction of cup, holding of spoon). For many parents of children ultimately diagnosed as having cerebral palsy, the first year of life may be the beginning of their realization that their own child's development "is not quite right." They notice that their child's progress is not exactly what their parents, friends, experiences with other children, or consultation with baby books predict.

What follows is a discussion of the first-year milestones, based on norms of child development. We do not mean to imply that your child's development should adhere to these norms. Remember, each child develops at his or her own rate, all the while following a sequential pattern. There is a wide range of "normal," from the very precocious child who rolls over, sits up, crawls, and walks and talks at a much younger age than the average, to the child who does all of these things later than most other children do.

The following discussion should be used as a guide, then, for becoming aware of patterns of development. These discussions may alert you to a problem in your child's overall development or to a problem in one of the areas of development, at which point you may want to discuss the problem with your child's physician. What follows may also enhance your knowledge of what your child may be capable of at a given stage, thereby helping to guide your interaction and play time with your child.

During the first 4 weeks of life (the neonatal period), the infant's large and fine motor movements are primarily reflexive. That is, they are controlled by persistence of automatic responses to situations and stimuli. The newborn baby lies primarily in a flex position (the so-called fetal position), keeps his hands in tight fists, and has little head control when held in a sitting position. Lying on his stomach, a newborn may be able to turn his head from side to side, and during the first four weeks will begin to be able to lift his head briefly.

Newborn infants can briefly fix their eyes on an object in their line of vision (that is, an object held in the direction their eyes are facing). They focus best on objects that are about 8 to 14 inches away. It is not unusual for a newborn to sleep for about 75 percent of a 24-hour day. Newborns go through several states of arousal, including lying quietly, being intensely active, and crying—seemingly inconsolably—for what seems to be long periods of time. Infants can require as many as eight feedings a day, or an average of one feeding every three hours (but rarely is a newborn's feeding schedule so predictable, as any mother will tell you). Babies often don't seem to react much to noises when they are "sleeping right through things," but in fact most babies will react to loud noises by acting startled, or by changing their "arousal state." While it is difficult to describe a newborn infant's social or emotional development, it does seem that infants respond to human voices more than to other noises. And most newborns soon begin to show visual preference for a human face.

By the second month, or between 4 and 8 weeks of age, infants become more socially interactive. By approximately 6 weeks the so-called social smile emerges. Generally by the eighth week of life an infant will return a person's gaze and give the appearance of smiling or even of giggling. There are also significant developments in gross and fine motor skills. Specifically, when placed on her stomach, an infant of between 4 and 8 weeks of age can begin to lift her chin off a flat surface so that her face is at a 45-degree angle from the flat surface. When the infant is pulled to a sitting position from lying down, the infant's head does not lag quite as much as it did in early infancy. The hands generally are still persistently fisted, but infants may begin to study their own hand movements (often looking quite "serious" while doing this). Eyes that previously wandered and occasionally crossed may appear to focus and in fact begin to follow an object briefly in a limited range.

Children between 4 and 8 weeks may be able to express distress or delight, and be soothed by a familiar person's touch. Some children by 8 weeks will in fact appear to listen to voices and actually to coo in response (most specialists call this "pre-cooing," to distinguish it from the various pitched squeals that older infants make).

At 3 months, or around 12 weeks, the infant may produce a series of gurgling and cooing sounds. The baby's fingers usually begin to relax, and fisting is no longer commonplace. A 3-month-old generally can make sustained social contact in the sense of smiling easily and spontaneously, and barring any visual problem, an infant of this age can follow slow-moving objects. Some infants may in fact begin to recognize and differentiate family members from strangers. There is much greater head control as the infant is pulled up from a lying to a sitting position.

Placed on her stomach, a 3-month-old can lift her head and chest with her arms extended. Infants at this stage may begin to swing at or reach toward (and miss) objects. There is a general diminishment of the so-called primitive reflexes, and the infant may actually make defensive movements or selective withdrawal reactions. By the end of the third month, the infant's suck-and-swallow feeding from either bottle or breast is coordinated to the point of seeming effortless. Those who choke, gag, cough, and sputter, or who do not appear to have mastered their breathing and eating patterns or who persist in making seemingly odd, high-pitched, or guttural sounds while eating, should be seen by a physician.

Somewhere near 4 months of age, infants begin to roll (front to back, back to front). A 4-month-old will react to sound and may turn to a familiar voice: the infant in the crib hears her mother's voice, for example, and turns in her direction before she comes into sight. The infant's ability to follow movement visually in all directions should be more accurate and active.

By 6 months the infant's language has developed from pre-coo to cooing, and then to continuous vowel sounds. True babbling emerges (vowel-consonant combinations expressed repetitively, such as "ma-ma-ma-ma-ma"). The 6-month-old may truly begin to show fear of strangers and appear shy. In addition, a personality emerges, as the baby begins to show likes and dislikes for certain positions, sounds, and foods (by now most children will have added cereals and various purees to bottle or breast).

By 7 months, most infants can bear some weight on their legs when held upright, should be able to sit without support, and may even be able to pull to standing from sitting as well as get into a sitting position from the stomach. At this age, a child may try to grab a toy that is placed out of reach, hold a block or rattle in one hand, and rake up small objects such as raisins with his fist. An infant between 7 and 8 months is able to grasp objects with his thumb and forefinger, and is able to "isolate his forefinger," meaning that he can poke at objects with his index finger.

The infant may begin to crawl at this age, as she pulls herself forward with her hands and slithers on her belly, pulls up on her knees to crawl, or moves forward in some modified style, often called "commando crawling" (since it imitates the movement of a soldier crawling on his arms in a crouched position). By 9 months the infant begins to play games such as patty-cake or waving bye-bye.

An infant between 7 and 8 months of age should definitely be able to turn in the direction of a loved one's voice and may begin to respond to the sound of her own name. Language continues to be a progression of repetitive consonant-vowel sounds, and distinct "mamas" and "dadas" begin to be heard, although not necessarily referring to the child's mother or father. By the end of 8 months, most children look for a dropped object by playing "over-the-edge," and many infants of this age begin throwing things off the highchair. An infant between 7 and 8 months of age may truly begin to develop "stranger anxiety," although this aversion to strangers may in fact have been surfacing for several months.

By 10 months an infant's gross motor development should include crawling backward and forward using reciprocal movements; assuming the sitting position and sitting with the back straight; and pulling to stand. There are certainly 10-month-olds who can stand with or without support, and there are children who by the end of the tenth month stand with little support. Infants at this age also tend to explore in a poking fashion, beginning to master what developmental specialists call the "pincer grasp": the thumb and index finger meet in a way that allows significant control of an object.

At 10 months, infants are interested in fitting things together, and some may enjoy splashing in water and messing up their food. Searching for hidden objects, enjoying peek-a-boo and patty-cake games, and inviting a parent or other friendly person to play are all characteristic of a 10-month-old. The baby's language continues to progress, perhaps to the point where the baby can say "dada" or "mama" discriminately and understand the word "no" (although she may choose not to obey it).

By the end of the first year of life most infants can stand alone, and most take a step or two without holding on to anything for support. Many 1-year-olds walk in some combination of standing, "cruising" along furniture, and taking independent steps. Reaching becomes much more accurate as a child searches for objects that are farther away. Objects held in the two hands can be brought together purposely (banging cymbals, for example), and the infant can purposefully release an object from his grasp.

At age 1 the infant begins to distinguish himself as separate from others (matching objects that are his), seek approval and avoid disapproval, and most likely understand the meaning of "no" more fully. Some 12-month-olds also cooperate in dressing and understand a one-step command when it is accompanied by a gesture such as "Give me that toy." Spoken language at a year is highly variable, and may include "mama" and "dada" as well as one or two other single words. One-year-olds freely show affection and also show attachment to favorite objects such as stuffed animals or blankets.

How may the development of a child with cerebral palsy differ from this?

Developmental delays are anticipated for the child with CP, and these are perhaps most easily recognized when the child does not reach milestones when expected. The child with cerebral palsy most often does not accomplish gross motor tasks at the same rate as the child without CP, for example. Differences in the pattern of movement may be seen as well. Due to increased tone, or spasticity, some children with CP may not be able to fully separate the movement of their heads from the movement of the rest of their bodies, making their limbs feel and look stiff when they are rolling, attempting to sit, or trying to walk. The child who is "floppy" or who has low tone may not be able to generate the forces necessary to hold his head up or roll in a smooth pattern. This child may slump when seated or placed to sit and may buckle or collapse at the knees when attempting to stand.

In terms of fine motor skills, small muscles in the hand that are used to manipulate objects are often affected by tone imbalances in children with cerebral palsy. In children with spasticity, or increased tone, impairment may begin at the shoulder, with the inability to extend the arm to reach for an object. The hand itself may be less controlled in fine regulation of movement, making it difficult for the child to reach and grasp. In children with an athetoid component, the "fine tuning" required to coordinate reaching, grasping, and releasing may be missing.

The child with a known or emerging hemiplegic pattern may prefer to use one hand over the other. Parents may think that their child is a "lefty" when in fact the function of the child's right hand is affected by the cerebral palsy. Hand preference usually doesn't emerge until about 18 months, so if your child does not use both hands equally when he or she is younger than 18 months, you should mention this to your child's doctor.

Language development and problem-solving abilities are not necessarily affected in the young child with cerebral palsy, although language delay and mental retardation do sometimes accompany cerebral palsy. You need to be aware of normal milestones and bring to the doctor's attention any behavior that is significantly behind what you perceive to be normal for a child of this age.

Many children with cerebral palsy are active and very social in the first years of life. A child with physical limitations, just like other children, seeks and needs verbal and physical affection in order for his personality and identity to develop. Visually impaired children, for example, often need more touching and verbal feedback than other children, since they can't rely on their sight to pick up a parent's soothing expressions.

You may find, however, that your child is less "huggable" and cannot return your embraces, but you shouldn't necessarily view this as your child's choice. A very small percentage of children with cerebral palsy exhibit autistic-like tendencies in the first year of life. These children appear to be in a "world of their own," neither seeking nor returning affection, eye contact, or social contact. This behavior should be brought to the attention of the child's physician, and counseling may be initiated to help stimulate the parent-child interaction.

Ages One to Three

The child entering his or her second year truly becomes a toddler, with significant strides made in the area of locomotion—getting around, walking, and "getting into everything." Over the next several years, the child begins to develop a sense of self-mastery and tries to understand her "fit" in the world around her, composed of parents, siblings, and perhaps an emerging peer group.

Many parents describe the period between 12 and 15 months as one of the most pleasurable in the raising of their children. Language is beginning to emerge, a sense of curiosity is exploding, and the physical ability to get around has developed to the point where the child is truly exploring his environment. By 15 months, most children are walking without support (although they may hold their arms up, in a high position) and are beginning to creep upstairs (and therefore need to be watched carefully). Fine motor skill increases as an infant is able to solve simple games, successfully nest, or stack, objects inside each other, and grasp a crayon with enough coordination to make a mark on a piece of paper.

While the child may make known the vast majority of her needs by pointing and gesturing, many children 15 to 16 months old have a spoken vocabulary of four to six words. Often, parents describe gibberish that actually has the rhythm and flow of speech, but with very few intelligible words. A 15-month-old can follow simple commands and should have a clear understanding of the concept "no." Socially the infant is much more available: he often hugs his parents spontaneously and reciprocates affection, either by blowing kisses or by responding to commands such as "give mommy a hug." Hiding objects and throwing them continue to be a favorite pastime as the child develops a sense of difference between an inanimate object and himself. The child also understands the concept of retrieving an object—although often it is the parent, not the child, who retrieves it.

The parent-child interactions that emerge at 15 months continue to develop as the child reaches 18 months of age, including hugging and reciprocal affection involving parents, siblings, and inanimate objects (the child begins to lug around her favorite doll or other toy). Children are also now more capable of feeding themselves (mastering a spoon and generally a "sipee" or spouted cup) and may seek help or consolation when in trouble and look to others for entertainment or amusement. Walking should be more steady by this time. Many 18-month-olds have mastered the ability to seat themselves in child-sized chairs, throw a ball in response to "Let's play catch," and make towers of cubes.

At this age, many children love to scribble (although in an imitative fashion), and prefer to use either the left or the right hand to do most things. Although hand preference may begin to appear at age 18 months, it is usually not fully emerged until about age 2. The average 18-month-old's spoken vocabulary is composed of 7 to 20 words, a mixture of understandable words mixed in with gibberish. Most 18-month-olds can identify one or two familiar objects by pointing to pictures, and they can identify several parts of the body. While it is somewhat early for the "terrible twos," 18-month-olds may begin to show their temper by either playfully or willfully refusing to comply with what a parent asks of them.

By age 2, most toddlers are very assertive and independent. While the terrible twos don't strike with the same intensity in all children, it is perfectly normal for 2- and 3-year-olds to refuse to comply with demands and to test the boundaries that their parents have set. While this may be incredibly frustrating at times, parents need to remember that the child is becoming a person, with a mind of her own—and is more than capable of letting her druthers be known in a specific situation.

The 2-year-old has begun to run well (only infrequently falling), kick a large ball, walk up and down stairs one at a time while holding on to a railing, and open and close doors. His fine motor abilities have expanded to include circular scribbling with a crayon, helping to dress and undress himself, feeding himself with less spilling, and successfully drinking from a sip cup. Children of this age begin to be able to name body parts, associate use with objects, and listen to stories. They can identify more pictures. In terms of spoken language, the average 2-year-old has at least 200 to 250 words in her vocabulary and can form two-word sentences, although the voice pattern will be somewhat broken in rhythm when compared to adult speech. Most 2-year-olds begin to make known their toileting needs. Issues of toileting sometimes become a large struggle in the quest for independence.

As a child progresses to age 2½, he starts to master coordination, including jumping up and down and walking backwards. Pencil or crayon grasp is also much more steady. Most 2-and-a-half-year-olds refer to themselves as "I" or "me" and know their first and last names. Spoken vocabulary starts to expand and may include repetition of simple nursery rhymes. Between ages 2 and 3, children become much more "helpful" (for example, they will help put toys away), and they demonstrate some imagination (they "pretend") when playing with objects or other people.

By 3 years of age children can go up and down stairs alternating feet, ride a tricycle, stand on one foot, and attempt to throw a ball overhand. Feeding is much neater, most buttons can be negotiated to the point of unbuttoning, and shoes and socks can be pulled on. They may engage in some simple tasks of body grooming such as washing and drying their hands and imitating combing their hair. Three-year-olds begin to play simple games with other children. They should begin to know their age and differentiate between the sexes, count to three, and be able to use sentences of three or more words. Most 3-year-olds can name several colors and understand three prepositions (most likely *under, over,* and similar prepositions), and are extremely curious, asking endless questions.

Parents can expect 3-year-olds to have some awareness of a dangerous situation (they may say "That's hot," for example). By age 3 most children start to use the toilet, with some help, although the age when bodily functions are mastered varies greatly from child to child. In general, as compared to the 2-year-old, the 3-year-old is slightly more cooperative and eager to please. Sharing and turn taking become more acceptable.

Three-year-olds may be much more fearful than 2-year-olds, however, and may express displeasure at new situations. Many have difficulty separating from their parents at bedtime. Fortunately, most 3-year-olds can also better understand explanations for the cause of their fears. Their average vocabulary is somewhere between 800 and 900 words, with four-word sentences and the ability to tell simple stories and understand actions and picture telling. By the end of the third year, as the child progresses to preschool, many parents say they have lost their "baby" and now have a "little person" capable of thinking and talking his way through situations.

My toddler has CP. How might his development differ from this?

Generally, children with increased tone (spasticity) experience delays in walking. A general rule is that children who sit unsupported by age 2 will most likely be walking (with or without braces or assistive devices) by age 4. Most "tight" children may appear to roll on time or close to it (due to excess tone, they may actually "flip") but then make no further developmental progress for many months, not crawling or pulling to stand until well after their first birthday. Hypotonic or "floppy" children may actually stand with support (they may cruise around the coffee table) close to the appropriate age, but they have long lags before developing enough stability in the trunk to walk independently.

Children with cerebral palsy often have small or fine motor developmental delays. In the toddler years, this is typically seen in their feeding and dressing skills. The child may not have full command of the ability to grasp objects between thumb and index finger and therefore may have to rely on clumsier, raking movements to grasp objects. Holding a bottle may be difficult, and steadiness with cup drinking may be delayed or impossible. Both snapping snaps and tying knots rely on smooth, fine motor control and good hand-eye coordination, so a child with cerebral palsy whose control is affected may have difficulty dressing herself. The ability to grasp a pencil, generally in place by age 2 or 3, may elude children with CP.

Children with severe cerebral palsy also experience delays in language and problem-solving abilities. In the toddler years, this may be most noticeable because the child uses only a limited number of words, or it might be most apparent because the child is unable to combine words into phrases or sentences. Children with cerebral palsy may understand what they are being asked to do but be physically limited in their ability to carry out these tasks. Thus, the child may appear dull because he doesn't respond, when what's really going on is that he is physically unable to carry out the task.

On standard IQ testing for the 1- to 3-year-old, much of the testing material involves tasks requiring the child to use motor skills and to perform in response to commands; the results of such a test for the child with CP may be misleading. For one thing, the child's language skills may be underestimated if his disability prevents him from forming words. We recommend that parents have their child tested by professionals who are skilled in interpreting results of "standard IQ" tests in children with cerebral palsy, with an emphasis on nonverbal performance standards. This kind of specialized testing may not be available in the school diagnostic setting. In this case, outside (independent) evaluation should be sought to obtain an accurate picture of the child's abilities.

The world of a 1-, 2-, or 3-year-old involves play and the beginning of social interaction. At first a child just plays alongside other children (this is called *parallel play*) or by imitating what another child is doing (*imitative play*), but later on she will begin to play *with* other children, in *interactive play*. A youngster with a significant motor disability is physically unable to keep up with the other active toddlers and must be encouraged to persist in activities to help foster social skills such as taking turns and sharing. Circle games, storytelling, acting out characters, sing-alongs—all are examples of less physically demanding activities that can help the child with cerebral palsy, with or without cognitive limitations, learn social skills.

Are there any guidelines for toilet training?

By the time a child is 2 years old, most parents are anxiously anticipating the start of toilet training and the end of diapering. But a child must be temperamentally, physically, and cognitively ready to accept toilet training in order to have any success at the task. Daytime bladder control can usually be achieved by 32 months (the range is from 18 to 40 months) and bowel control by 29 months (with a range from 16 to 48 months). Most experts (and parents looking back on the experience) agree that the best approach to toilet training is a fairly casual, nonconfrontational introduction to the process. Indications of readiness include a child's ability to understand that he is "wet" or "soiled" and an ability to communicate this information, through gesture or word, to the caregiver.

A child probably cannot voluntarily control the functioning of bowel or bladder until age 18 months. Before that age, or for a child who is mentally disabled, toilet training is more a reflexive act than a cognitive act. The child who is put on the potty seat will sometimes by coincidence relax her sphincter tone and produce a bowel movement, but this is very different from voluntarily directing her muscles to relax so she can evacuate her bowels.

How does a child's cerebral palsy affect toilet training?

Training the child with cerebral palsy may involve several difficulties. A child may physically be unable to sit on a toilet seat, for example, and therefore will have a difficult time getting urine or a bowel movement into the bowl. This problem is best remedied by using one of the many adaptive potty seat systems available. A physical or occupational therapist can provide guidance in the selection and purchase of these systems.

Many children have a fear of losing a part of their body as they see their bowel movements flushed away. Although most children come to terms with this in a matter of a few weeks, some children continue to imagine that part of them may be "flushed away." This fear may be accentuated in the child with CP, whose unsteadiness on the potty may lead to falls. Unsteadiness during elimination can be very scary to a young child. To overcome this, usually all that is needed is reassurance by the parents that all is well and that they will not let the child be harmed or flushed away. A child with a persistent fear of toileting may be helped by a physician or a behavioral therapist.

The child with cerebral palsy and mental retardation poses an additional challenge regarding toileting, in that the child may not understand the need to eliminate in a bathroom setting. These children often respond best to a program that incorporates "clock timing," whereby the child is placed on the toilet half an hour or an hour after each meal every day. Parents can ask the physician or other health care provider to give them a detailed description of this method of toilet training, sometimes called *habit training*.

How do I handle my child's temper tantrums?

All children go through periods of having temper tantrums, most commonly in the second year of life. Most tantrums arise from frustration or the inability to communicate wants or needs through words and gestures. Some tantrums seem to arise out of the blue, apparently unprovoked, and may purely be a child's way of testing his parent's or caretaker's limits. Parental response to tantrums should allow children to regain their sense of self-control.

Physical punishment rarely has an effect on tantrum throwing. Physically punishing the child may bring that particular tantrum to an end, but the long-term pattern of throwing tantrums will not be broken by spanking. Rather, the parent should attempt to distract the child and get him or her involved in a more appropriate or more easily handled activity. If this fails, then isolating the child in a "time out" situation will usually be effective in sending the message that the given behavior is unacceptable.

Setting limits is accomplished by displaying a mixture of consistent disappointment with unacceptable behavior and praise for demonstrating acceptable behavior. Rewards are also useful, as are behavior systems such as "point cards," which award prizes once goals are reached. Rewards can serve as meaningful reminders to children that they *can* behave and they *can* stop tantrums, if they want to.

How does cerebral palsy affect temper tantrums?

As a parent of a child with physical limitations, you must realize that your child is just as prone to temper outbursts and tantrums as any other child. Certainly tantrums may arise from a child's frustration surrounding his inability to be understood, especially when receptive abilities (understanding language) exceed expressive capabilities (speaking or communicating). Extra time may be needed to figure out your child's communicative intent—to "crack the code" of what he is frustrated about. However, escalation of behaviors to get your attention may cross the line into harm to self or others. You need not feel guilty for imposing appropriate limits on your child or for discussing intolerable behavior with him. Applying consistent, loving rules is the best approach when children act up. Should the child's behavior become harmful to him or to others, you may want to seek professional counseling for the child.

What about sleep disturbances?

One of the most sought-after developmental milestones in any home is the child's ability to sleep through the night. Almost three-quarters of all infants will sleep at night without interruption for six or seven hours by 6 months of age. When a young infant wakes up during the night, it is usually because he or she is uncomfortable—hungry, wet, or badly positioned—and needs someone to respond or soothe him or her back to sleep. In the second year of life, some children develop problems getting to sleep, often because of anxiety over separation. Setting routines and rituals (reading a story, having a regular bath time, drinking a cup of juice or milk) often goes a long way toward soothing a child with separation issues at sleep time.

How can CP affect sleep?

For children with a physical disability, fear of separation may be compounded by a sense that they are helpless to get up and reach their parents. Should your child's anxieties become intense, you may need to reassure your child that you check on him frequently while he sleeps. Because some nighttime awakening can be due to the need for position changes in children with CP (due to muscle tone imbalance), repositioning your child and comforting him may be helpful. Using an intercom or a baby monitor may be helpful, because it allows your child to realize that you will hear him and be able to respond should he need you in the middle of the night.

Should I be concerned about my child's masturbation?

Exploration of the body, including the genital or "private" areas, is a natural, healthy occurrence in children of all ages. While many theories and cultural or religious biases exist to explain or condemn masturbation, most developmental experts agree that discovery of the genitals and manipulation of them for pleasure is a natural process, occurring in all children regardless of physical or mental limitations. Perhaps the best approach for parents of a young child (age 3 to 4) is to ignore the behavior. As children get older, they can be told that certain parts of the body are private and should be touched by them in a private place such as the bathroom or bedroom, not in front of playmates. Most children in the preschool years do not make the mental connection between masturbation and sexual pleasure. That is, they may touch themselves out of habit, perhaps as a way of self-soothing, but they are not consciously teaching themselves to achieve sexual satisfaction.

How parents react to masturbation in an older child is often colored by the parent's own feelings, cultural practices, or family experiences. There are no data to suggest that masturbation leads to or comes from perverted thoughts or is associated with sexual aggressiveness. Parents should discuss with their children the concept of taking care of bodily functions in private.

In addition, parents should instruct children that there are inappropriate social settings for masturbation. If necessary, guidance can be sought from a pediatrician or a developmental counselor.

Ages Four to Six

Somewhere around the fourth year of life, children develop the ability to play with several children in a cooperative setting, and they are able to share with others more readily. The vast majority of 4-year-olds are toilet trained and can feed themselves and generally amuse themselves in a situation that is structured and supervised by adults. Their language has progressed, and use of plurals, different tenses (distinguishing present and future, for example), and opposites has emerged, as has the ability to tell stories. Children at this age are capable of dressing and undressing with supervision and can copy simple shapes, draw stick figure people, and imitate simple block designs. The child can now throw a ball overhand or underhand, and can climb in a coordinated way.

A 4-year-old may be much more verbal about his fears, but he will probably separate more easily from his mother than will a younger child, because he can understand that his mother will return. Four-year-olds are generally less eager to conform and please than children at 3 years of age, because the desire to assert their own will reemerges, although not usually as strongly as during the "terrible twos." Four-year-olds tend to understand special friendships and seek out play eagerly. Language develops rapidly to the point where four- and five-word sentences are used, simple words can be defined, and stories are listened to enthusiastically. Many 4-year-olds can follow multiple-stage, rapid-fire commands, know at least four colors and the difference between night and day, and recognize some capital letters as well as shapes.

The 5-year-old can skip, kick a ball several feet, and run and jump. This is the age when children begin to ride a bike with training wheels. Five-year-olds can hold a pencil using the thumb and index and middle fingers (as an adult does), can eat with a knife and fork, and know how to spread butter. Tying shoes is still difficult for a child at this age, and the child may still reverse letters and numbers. The child's knowledge expands to include names of siblings (and often their ages) as well as the child's own address and phone number and basic colors and shapes. A 5-year-old's language expands to where it may include five- and six-word sentences.

Social interaction is better developed. Most 5-year-olds want to be "good," and they actually seek out adult approval. Small group play is generally favored, but 5-year-olds also enjoy "team" games and sports. Fears resurface: the child may worry about separation from his mother, lightning and thunder, or becoming lost. Generally, however, 5-year-olds "go with the flow" and can be led back from their fears with gentle reassurance, since they have the ability to understand past, present, and future, and to understand that separations will not be permanent.

The seventh year of life, between age 6 and age 7, is often one of significant transition, falling between the preschool and school years. Many children at age 6 are easily excitable and tend to show off and act silly, with occasional spells of more mature behavior. The inconsistency in behavior is probably the result of trying to fit themselves into the tasks of schooling and new regimentation. Six-year-olds are ready to attend a full day of school but still need a good deal of physical activity to burn off excess energy. They are notorious for procrastinating but form friendships easily and readily join in enjoyable activities.

Most 6-year-olds can describe how several objects are different or alike, begin to have an understanding of the concept of time, and know the alphabet. While a 5-year-old can count aloud to 20, a 6-year-old understands the concepts of numbers up to 10, knows all the primary colors, and understands simple money concepts. Gross motor skills are much smoother, as balance emerges along with true physical independence in purposeful activities. In the fine motor sphere, around 6 years of age, the child begins to develop skill at grasping a pencil like an adult, although he or she will press fairly hard while writing.

Six-year-olds are totally independent in self-care and are able to handle simple household tasks. The average vocabulary consists of approximately 1,500 to 2,000 words, but the *receptive* fund of knowledge (words whose meaning the child understands, as demonstrated by pointing to pictures) may be much greater: 10,000 to 13,000 words. Language is now used in a much more social way, to include others and to express ideas, especially by children who have early school experiences and who have come to understand that words are listened to while gestures are often ignored.

How might the development of a child with CP be different from this?

The child with physical limitations may have a hard time keeping up with the explosion of physical activity that occurs during the preschool years. Verbally talented youngsters with cerebral palsy may begin to express their frustration over this and may even begin to ask, "Why me?" Parents need to provide alternative activities for the child, such as swimming, adaptive horseback riding, and participation in Special Olympics. Despite these outlets, the preschool child with CP may realize that his disability may restrict him from fully participating in activities. Bicycle riding may be difficult, coordinated self-feeding next to impossible, and handwriting unintelligible. Occupational therapists can help by recommending adaptive equipment such as computers and special eating utensils.

Daily living activities such as bathing and toileting may become more cumbersome during these years, as the child grows physically larger and may be having difficulty positioning himself for these tasks. Bath chairs, potty seats, home lifts, and van modifications are often helpful. Most gross and fine motor skill patterns are set by this time, so the aims of therapy are to maximize the child's potential in his or her environment through adaptive equipment modifications.

The child who had expressive speech and language delays prior to the preschool years may now obviously appear to be a slow talker compared to his peers, who tell stories and engage in more adultlike conversation. Children whose speech is hampered by tone or a difficulty in articulating words can learn to communicate more effectively during the preschool years using a combination of signing and communication boards and computer-assisted devices. A common misconception is that a child who is taught sign or picture language will then "forget" how to talk or become too lazy to use spoken words. Actually, alternative means of communication often provide these youngsters with an avenue for expression, and this helps relieve their frustrations over not being understood. When the child is able to speak, the child's speech will progress along with the other means of communication.

At this age the sense of self or identity emerges, adding to children's security in themselves, their family, their school world, and their peer world. Children with severe motor disabilities may experience a sense of loss at their inability to mix with others and may withdraw or, conversely, act out. Parents can help their child feel as if she belongs by fostering a "can do" attitude regarding their child's desire to be with others. Children need group experiences in outings, scouting organizations, church groups, and elsewhere as they pass from preschool into the elementary school years, so that the foundation for personal growth and exploration is set. Put more simply, a child with physical limitations should not be protected from or excluded from age or cognitively matched social experiences just because his parents feel he is different and might be sensitive to mixing with other, perhaps more able-bodied, children. Parent support groups and other resources often offer suggestions for activities suitable for children with motor disabilities, and these should be explored. If summer camp opportunities exist, they should be pursued (even at this age), since they are usually nonthreatening for the child.

Ages Six to Twelve

As the child grows older, he not only matures physically but is expected to perform in a school setting. From age 6 to age 12 children attend elementary school and are exposed to the "rules of learning" and the whole idea of a social world outside the family and immediate neighborhood friends. Seven- and 8-year-olds are generally fairly anxious to please—they may even be somewhat perfectionist in this sense—and are fairly self-confident. The younger 7-year-old will be somewhat sensitive to praise and blame, concerned about right and wrong. A sense of humor in most children emerges by about the eighth year of life. Eight-year-olds are thought to have the capacity for self-evaluation. Participation in group activities, including team sports, becomes important, and participation in organized activities is often extremely important to this age group.

Eye-hand coordination improves at this age, and by 7 years of age most children have learned the days of the week, can tell time, and are beginning to think in concrete terms. Handwriting skills are perfected, and the child can now correct something that doesn't "look right" on the written page. Seven-year-olds generally read and write between the first and second grade level. Written letters may occasionally be reversed, although this mistake generally disappears by 8 years.

Adult concerns about the child's learning abilities begin to surface as school tasks progress from word decoding and basic addition and subtraction to actual reading comprehension and applying of math principles. Any developmental lag as it relates to a child's ability to understand directions may show up as academic or behavioral difficulties in the classroom; such a lag may be simply a learning inefficiency, or it may be a true learning disability. In either case, it needs to be closely monitored.

The 9-year-old's language ability differs slightly from that of younger children. True sequencing, such as day, month, and year, as well as ordering of information, can be understood by the 9-year-old. Simple multiplication and division concepts also appear to make sense to most children at this age. Balance and coordination have progressed to the point where the child can stand on one leg, can play follow the leader, and can play backyard games such as kickball.

Significant sex differences begin to appear in the tenth year of life, as girls generally begin to appear more mature than boys, with some girls beginning to show physical signs of sexual maturation. Most 10-year-olds understand rules and will follow them. Lasting friendships are formed that replace the earlier, temporary, "play friends." Ten-year-olds begin to understand simple fractions, including parts of an hour, and are able to understand the concept of higher numbers and possibly begin to think in abstract terms.

The ability to think abstractly fully surfaces in the preadolescent youth (11 to 12 years of age). Preadolescents begin to reason through problems and situations, understand social and political issues, and perhaps even form an opinion on family matters. Preadolescents are joiners of groups and clubs. At this point in development girls begin to fall behind in physical strength, although they are generally taller than boys for the next several years.

How might the development of a child with CP differ from this?

The increasing hand-eye coordination that occurs in the school-age years may be significantly limited in the child with physical disabilities, and the ability to write legibly may be hampered by fluctuations in tone (increased or decreased) in children with cerebral palsy. Many children find the computer tremendously helpful in compensating for difficulties with writing, and the computer may be especially helpful for the child with athetoid movements, for whom an adapted keyboard may make a significant difference in communication skills.

Differences in physical ability, particularly at team sports, become clear among school-age children. A child's self-esteem is often derived from his perception of how others view him. For this reason, children with cerebral palsy who have normal cognitive abilities need to receive continued reassurance that they can master some physical activities. Even significantly disabled children can engage in supervised adaptive aquatics and bowling and modified dance routines.

The child with hemiplegia has some unique fine and gross motor limitations that may become strikingly evident in the school years. *Hemiatrophy* (poor development of musculature and bone structure) on the side of the involved limb may appear more obvious as the child's growth spurt begins. The child may be unable to keep up in activities such as physical education, climbing, and throwing or batting a ball. Adaptations made for doing things (such as using Velcro or loops instead of buttons) may function well but may make the child self-conscious; she may wonder why she can't button her clothes. Sometimes it's helpful to buy the child clothes like those her classmates are wearing, explaining that hers are specially tailored for her.

Many children with hemiplegia can use their uninvolved side for writing and for performing most fine motor tasks, so the child can do most activities of daily living, such as dressing, eating, and teeth brushing, without assistance from parents. Subtle learning difficulties and true learning disabilities will surface during the school years. Even children with cerebral palsy who have so-called normal intelligence must be monitored closely if they perform poorly in school. Parents need to determine whether the child is performing less well than expected because of anxiety (the child may be wondering why he is different, causing his attention to wander from schoolwork), or whether the child might truly be unable to master higher academic concepts due to a learning block or disability. (A learning block may be global, meaning that all areas are affected, or it may be specific to one academic area.) The child may be performing poorly in school because she is mentally limited compared to her classmates. Psychological testing can help sort these issues out, and more accurate class placement and utilization of special education resources help such children reach academic goals.

From age 6 to age 12, the child with cerebral palsy may perceive himself to be different and begin to isolate himself from social situations so he doesn't feel hurt when others make comments or exclude him from team play. These are the years when parents can have the most profound impact on the child's emerging identity. Frank discussion—being honest about the child's limitations—is probably best, although overpraising for a job well done can occasionally bolster a child's self-esteem. Even very cognitively limited children respond to praise and reward, and detect even the slightest amount of parental criticism or disapproval. The school-age years for the child with cerebral palsy may be a time when the family chooses to seek counseling or to reactivate themselves in family support groups to obtain new strategies to bolster their child's positive sense of self.

Ages Thirteen to Eighteen

The adolescent years are years of physical and sexual maturity and intellectual and social expansion. Increases in height and weight occur earlier in girls than in boys. The so-called growth spurt in girls may begin from age 10 to age 11, and generally is nearly completed by age 13 to age 14. In contrast, boys begin rapid growth between 13 and 15 years of age. Sexual maturation is a gradual process in both sexes. In girls, sexual maturity is accompanied by the growth of pubic hair, widening of the hips and pelvis, and development of mature breasts with projecting nipples. Boys grow pubic as well as body and facial hair, and the penis and testes grow and mature.

Along with the physical changes of sexual maturation comes the ability to produce children—the stage of maturation defined as puberty. Puberty in girls is defined as beginning at *menarche,* the first menstrual period. No such clear beginning for puberty is noted in boys, but most pediatricians would agree that growth of the testes in the scrotal sac and growth of the penis are signs that puberty has begun.

Gains in height, weight, and physical sexual maturity are only part of the changes that occur in adolescence. As every person who has ever been through adolescence, and every parent who has raised teenagers, will tell you, these years are among the most confusing for a young person searching for his or her identity. Psychologists have long considered adolescence a period of potential turmoil. From being completely dependent on the family, the individual begins to turn increasingly to friends, and the evolution of his own identity continues. All individuals, whether able-bodied or physically limited, can experience anxiety and mood changes as they try to make sense of their adolescent world.

How might cerebral palsy affect the adolescent?

Discussions of adolescence in children with cerebral palsy are few and far between, probably at least in part because the focus for many years has been on physical maturation rather than on psychosocial development (see Chapter 4). Some children with cerebral palsy experience precocious puberty, a hormone-induced early onset of sexual maturation. The child's body undergoes all of the aforementioned physical changes prematurely. In girls, breast development and pubic hair can appear at a young age (even in the infancy or toddler stages). In boys, enlargement of the penis and testes can occur at very young ages as well.

Signs of precocious puberty should be brought to the physician's attention, so that underlying causes can be investigated. The changes of puberty normally occur under the control of the pituitary, or hypothalamic, and gonadal glands. The more unusual causes of precocious puberty include endocrine (hormonal) imbalance, lesions or disturbances of the central nervous system, and genetic syndromes. Generally, however, precocious puberty in the child with cerebral palsy is not due to a rare disease. In "normal" children, 50 to 75 percent of precocious puberty exists without other pathological findings. Perhaps the brain lesion or injury associated with CP also contributes to the disordered hormonal signal that triggers early sexual maturation.

While some children with cerebral palsy undergo precocious puberty, others may experience delayed sexual maturation well into their teens or early twenties. Some girls with CP never menstruate. The reason for delays or absences is unclear. The vast majority of adolescents with delayed puberty will, however, eventually achieve sexual maturation. In girls who are severely physically disabled, the delayed or absent menstruation can be an advantage for reasons of hygiene. Generally, a major medical exam is undertaken only if a girl reaches age 13 or 14 without breast buds (breast buds generally develop one and a half to two years before the onset of periods). It may be helpful to consult with your child's physician as the teenage years approach. If necessary, a specialist in puberty such as an endocrinologist may be asked to help evaluate the delay.

Support groups, social activities with peers, and a supportive school and home environment can be crucial to the adolescent's emotional well-being. Counseling should be sought if suicidal, hopeless, or self-abusive or self-injurious behavior (including substance abuse) surfaces during this time. Parents may also experience much joy as they watch their youngsters turn into men or women. Praise and admiration for jobs accomplished, academic achievement, and exploration of new ideas is always helpful to a teen's self-esteem when it comes honestly from a parent.

Career counseling for potential academic pathways should begin early in adolescence. The teen who has cerebral palsy and good cognitive ability might be guided to a college preparatory academic curriculum or to job training such as apprenticeships. The teen needs to know that his or her physical limitations don't have to block the pathway to achievement of personal growth in academic or employment pursuits. For teens with cerebral palsy and some cognitive limitations or retardation, emphasis should be placed on mastering daily living skills. Employment opportunities, including "sheltered workshops," can be offered to help the adolescent make the transition from a school to a work environment.

In this chapter we have seen the variability within normal child development as well as the variety of effects which cerebral palsy can have on development. Most importantly, we see the marvelous uniqueness that is part of each child.

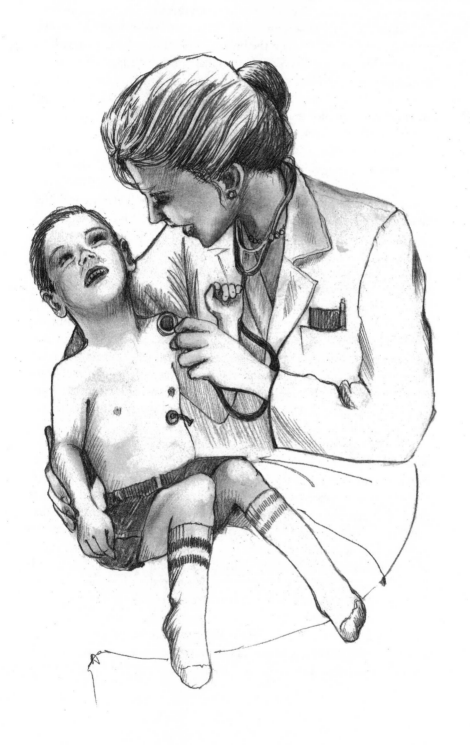

Medical Problems Associated with Cerebral Palsy

3

♦ B E C A U S E cerebral palsy is a condition caused by damage to the central nervous system, many of the complications of cerebral palsy are neurological. Children with CP may also have orthopedic problems—problems that affect the spine, bones, joints, muscles, or other parts of the skeletal system. And they may have problems that are considered to be "secondary" to the neurological and orthopedic problems. One example of a secondary effect of CP is poor nutrition caused by the child's difficulty in swallowing.

For some children, one of these other kinds of problems may dominate, and the cerebral palsy will be a relatively minor issue. For example, for a child with CP who is able to walk and who has few physical limitations but is severely retarded mentally, the focus of care will be on the mental disability rather than on the cerebral palsy.

In this chapter we consider the neurological and secondary problems associated with cerebral palsy. (The orthopedic aspects of CP are covered in Chapters 5 through 7.) Neurological problems associated with cerebral palsy include:

Seizures and epilepsy
Mental retardation
Learning disabilities
Attention deficit–hyperactivity
    disorder
Hydrocephalus

Behavior problems
Visual impairment
Hearing loss
Speech impairment
Swallowing difficulties

The secondary effects of cerebral palsy include:

Poor growth
Poor nutrition
Aspiration pneumonia
Gastroesophageal reflux
Frequent fractures
Constipation
Drooling

Sleep disorders
Upper airway obstruction
Communication disorder
Tooth decay and gum disease
Hernia
Bladder control problems

Primary Care Issues

What's the role of the doctor in caring for the child with cerebral palsy?

The primary care physician (the pediatrician or family practitioner) is the doctor who provides first contact care, preventive care, and continuity of care over time, no matter how complex. The primary care physician should play a central role in caring for a child with a developmental disability such as cerebral palsy, and should remain in contact with the family as the child matures through the years. Thus, the pediatrician or family practitioner should play the same role he or she plays for any pediatric patient. The child with cerebral palsy should receive the same care from his or her primary care physician that every other child does.

Even when the child is being seen by various specialists, the pediatrician or family practitioner should remain at the center of medical activity, acting as the medical coordinator. The specialist sends information on to the primary care physician so that he or she can explain the various care options to the family and help the family decide between various treatment options.

The primary care physician remains the advocate for the child within the medical care system. The parents are advocates for the child, as well; they need to help the child navigate the educational system and the working world, too, if that's appropriate. The pediatrician helps the family find an appropriate physician when the child becomes too old to stay with the pediatrician. Parents also must begin to anticipate, as the adolescent approaches adulthood, when it is time to help the young adult leave home and begin to function in the adult world. A sheltered setting or an institutional setting is appropriate for some individuals, though other people with cerebral palsy can achieve full independence. And for them to achieve full adulthood, independence is a necessity.

Why does my child need regular checkups if she's already seeing a specialist?

While many of the concerns related to CP (such as seizures and orthopedic problems) are addressed during a visit to the specialist, primary care issues need to be reviewed when your child visits his or her pediatrician. The pediatrician monitors physical growth (by measuring and recording the child's height, weight, and head circumference), general developmental progress (especially in areas other than the motor area, which is expected to be delayed in cerebral palsy), and immunizations, while providing counseling on such issues as accident prevention (tables 3, 4). The pediatrician provides vision and hearing screening, both of which are extremely important, particularly for children with an increased risk of sensory deficits, such as children who were born prematurely.

The primary care physician's role in providing guidance to both caregiver and child evolves over the years. For toddlers, providing parents with guidance about accident prevention is most important. Behavioral issues gain importance for the preschool and school-age child, and issues involving sexuality must be addressed for the adolescent and young adult.

Should my child with cerebral palsy receive the same immunizations as other children?

Yes. In the United States today, infants are routinely immunized against diphtheria, pertussis, tetanus, polio, Hemophilus influenza, measles, mumps, rubella, hepatitis B, varicella (chickenpox), and pneumococcus. Thus, by the time the child has reached the age of 18 months—whether or not the child has CP—he or she should be protected against all these diseases.

The child with CP should receive all these immunizations, as should premature infants, and at the same age as other children. In addition, consideration should be given to administering the influenza vaccine each winter to children with CP, especially to children who cannot walk. (Someone who spends most of the time in bed or in a wheelchair is likely to get sicker from influenza than someone who is up walking, because such a person doesn't breathe as deeply as an active person does.)

Are there any vaccines that should be avoided because my child has CP?

The only vaccines that might be considered controversial are the vaccines against pertussis (whooping cough) and measles. Pertussis vaccine has routinely been given in combination with vaccines for diptheria and tetanus in the immunization known as DPT. For many years the pertussis component of this vaccine was blamed for the onset of neurological problems, including severe brain damage, in some children. A number of studies published in the 1990s cast doubt on this picture, however, and suggested that the pertussis vaccine rarely if ever causes neurological problems. Nevertheless, concern about this vaccine led to the manufacture of a new form of the pertussis vaccine (known as acellular pertussis vaccine) which is not made from the bacteria itself as the original vaccine had been. This new vaccine has been found to have fewer side effects than the original DPT vaccine, including less frequent fever and febrile seizures. The measles vaccine has been blamed by some for autism or pervasive developmental disorders in children. A number of good scientific studies have failed to find a link between autism and vaccines. The incidence of autism does seem to have risen in the past ten years, for reasons that are not known, but measles or measles-mumps-rubella (MMR) vaccine would not appear to be one of them.

The Committee on Infectious Diseases of the American Academy of Pediatrics, which advises on immunization practices, recommends that the pertussis component of the DPT vaccine not be given to children who have a progressive neurological disease, that is, a disease that is ongoing and causing loss of function. By definition, CP is a *nonprogressive* condition. Therefore, this recommendation does not apply to children with a diagnosis of CP. With the new acellular DPT vaccine and the new data that disprove that the pertussis vaccine was ever a problem, there is no reason to avoid immunizing a child with CP against all childhood illnesses, including pertussis and measles. In a child who is somewhat debilitated or is bed-bound, the risk from pertussis or measles (or any of the illnesses that these immunizations prevent) is far greater than the risk from the immunization. Any of these illnesses can result in hospitalization and, in severe cases, death.

Table 3 *Recommended Evaluations/Health Maintenance Schedule for Children with Cerebral Palsy*

Procedure	0–3 mo	6 mo	9 mo	12 mo	18 mo	24 mo	36 mo	3–5 yr	5–10 yr	10–15 yr	15–20 yr
Medical evaluation											
Initial/interval history and physical examination						All visits					
Developmental/behavioral assessment						All visits					
Orthopedic evaluation (see table 4)						All visits					
Measurements											
Height and weight						All visits					
Weight for height or BMI						All visits					
Head circumference	X	X	X	X	X	X	X				
Blood pressure								X	X	X	X
Laboratory											
Hereditary/metabolic screening	X			(Should be done according to state law)							
Hemoglobin or hematocrit			X	Then as clinically warranted							
Urinalysis								X	Then as clinically warranted		
Lead, cholesterol, TB screening	Testing should be done for high-risk patients, as determined by the child's physician.										
Immunizations				Per AAP Guidelines (www.cdc.gov)							
Referral to education program — early intervention with primary therapies (P.T., O.T., speech/language) and/or Part H Eligibility programs	X	X	X	As early as clinically suspected so eligibility can be established							
Referral to cerebral palsy team	X	X	X	As early as clinically suspected so diagnostic workup, evaluation, and treatment recommendations can be formulated and clinical course followed							
Nutrition evaluation											
Intake assessment				All visits							
Anthropometrics				As clinically warranted							

Hearing assessment/screening				All visits				
OAE testing	X							
Pneumatic otoscopy	X	As clinically indicated						
Audiometry ⎱		X	X	X	X	X	X	X
Tympanometry ⎰								
BAER		As clinically warranted, especially if screening failed						
Vision assessment/screening					All visits			
Ophthalmic evaluation					All visits			
		Earlier referral to a specialist and more frequent screening if any ophthalmologic abnormality suspected or if history of premature birth and/or low birthweight						
Dental evaluation (every six months)			X	X	X	X	X	X
Anticipatory guidance				All visits				
Family support services e.g., parent groups, formal counseling, Part H eligibility access to SSI/MA, sibling support				All visits				
Oral motor/swallowing		As clinically warranted, or if failure to thrive, dysphagia (choking/gasping on food), or frequent congestion present						
Review education program						X	X	X
Psychometrics (psychoeducational testing) at school entry or at any time learning problems are identified or suspected.						X		
Review puberty, sexuality (gynecological issues for girls)						X	X	X

Note: BMI, body mass index; TB, tuberculosis; AAP, American Academy of Pediatrics; P.T., physical therapy; O.T., occupational therapy; OAE, otoacoustic emissions; BAER, brainstem auditory evoked response; SSI/MA, Supplemental Security Income/Medical Assistance.

Source: Adapted from AAP Policy on Preventive Pediatric Health Care, (RE9939), March 2000.

Table 4   Recommended Evaluations of Musculoskeletal Function in Children with Cerebral Palsy

	Age (Months)										
	1	2	4	6	9	12	15	18	24	36	48
Musculoskeletal Motor Development	A	A	A	A	B	C	C	C	D	E	E

A. Newborn hip examination: Check for hypotonia, hypertonicity. Use ultrasound for any questionable abnormalities; orthopedic referral if any abnormality on ultrasound.
B. Hip abduction: Check with hip and knee extended. If less than 45° each, hips need x-ray.
C. Same as B: If not sitting independently, needs to be fitted with adaptive seating for feeding and play. Refer for seating to P.T., O.T., or seating clinic.
D. Same as above: All children should now be standing; refer for stander evaluation if nonambulatory. Referral for orthotic assessment should be made by orthopedist or physiatrist. If nonambulatory, hip x-ray is required.
E. If nonambulatory: Hip exam and x-ray are required every 6 months; if greater than 45° abduction, orthotic check every 6 months. Gait problems requiring assistive devices or orthotics should also be evaluated every 6 months by orthopedist or physiatrist.

	Age (Years)												
5	6	7	8	9	10	11	12	13	14	15	16	17	18
F	F	F	F	G	G	G	G	H	H	H	H	H	H

F. Orthopedic surgery, baclofen pump, or dorsal rhizotomy may be considered to improve gait. Power wheelchair prescription usually first considered. All other information as above.
G. Continue hip exam: But x-ray only yearly. Examine for scoliosis; x-ray if definitely present.
H. If nonambulatory: Progressive scoliosis needs fusion. If ambulatory: Needs final gait correction. Either should be seen yearly by orthopedist or physiatrist.

In conclusion, we will say that if your child has new-onset neurological problems such as seizures and you have not been given a definite diagnosis of CP, or if the diagnosis is in doubt, then your child should receive a vaccine *without* the pertussis component. In any case, parents should discuss the advantages and disadvantages of this vaccine with their child's pediatrician. No other vaccines need to be avoided in a child who has CP.

What are the provisions of the National Childhood Vaccine Injury Act?

In 1986 Congress passed a law that funds a program to compensate parents of children who suffered neurological damage from vaccines that are required by state law. The purpose of the law is to keep parents whose children suffer neurological damage from such a vaccine from having to go through the court system to sue an individual physician or manufacturer of the vaccine. Instead, the government pays the family for expenses related to the neurological damage and loss of future earning ability. There are specific symptoms that qualify a family for compensation under this law if the symptoms occur very close to the time of immunization. If you believe that your child has suffered neurological damage because of an immunization, your doctor can call in a report to the Department of Health and Human Services. Or you can call this number yourself: 1-800-338-2382.

Epilepsy/Seizure Disorder

What are seizures?

The brain normally has electrical activity going on within it in a controlled manner. A *seizure* is a sudden out-of-control event that can cause involuntary movements and/or behavior changes, and a change in awareness. It occurs when there are bursts of abnormal electrical activity in the brain which interfere with normal brain functioning. *Epilepsy* is a group of disorders characterized by recurrent seizures. Epilepsy is not a disease.

What causes a seizure?

In many cases of epilepsy, no cause for the seizure is ever found. Cases in which the cause is known include the following:

- *Gestational.* When a woman is pregnant, the fetus may be harmed by an insult to the brain such as a viral infection of the mother or bleeding in the brain of the fetus. Abnormal brain development can also occur during this time. The same list of possible causes of CP listed in chapter 1 could also cause epilepsy.
- *Genetic.* There may be causes that are handed down from parents to children through genes. Frequently, neither parent has a recognized history of epilepsy.
- *Metabolic disorders.* These are problems that can occur when certain enzymes in the body are abnormal, resulting in an accumulation of abnormal proteins. These are genetic disorders.
- *Infection.* The aftereffects of *meningitis,* an infection in the brain or spinal cord, or *encephalitis,* an infection in the brain.
- *Traumatic.* The result of severe head trauma from a fall, child abuse, sports injury, or bike or car accident. The injury can cause scarring in the brain.
- *Neoplastic.* Brain tumors, leukemia, or other cancers.
- *Vascular.* A problem with the veins or arteries in the brain.
- *Intraventricular hemorrhage.* A bleed in the brain often related to prematurity.
- *Asphyxia.* A lack of oxygen to the brain that can occur before, during, or after the child is born.
- *Poisoning.* Ingestion of lead, alcohol, or other substances that are toxic to the brain.

Cerebral palsy (CP) is also associated with scarring or some form of brain abnormality. Therefore, CP is often associated with seizures.

How common are seizures?

In the general population, the incidence of epilepsy is 0.5 to 3 percent. Among children with cerebral palsy, however, the incidence is increased to approximately 30 to 50 percent. Epilepsy is more common in the child with the spastic quadriplegic or hemiplegic forms of cerebral palsy. Complex partial seizures are the most common type of seizures in the person with cerebral palsy.

How are seizures and epilepsy diagnosed?

Seizures are diagnosed based on the history of the event, medical history, and physical and neurological examination and tests. Information obtained about the seizure event include the timing of the event, warning signs before the event, parts of the body involved, awareness during the event, loss of bowel or bladder control, length of the event, presence of weakness on one side of the body after the event, appearance of the child once the event is over, memory of the event, and presence of fever or illness at the time of the event. The neurological examination tells the health care provider how certain parts of the brain function.

What kinds of tests are performed when someone is being evaluated for seizures?

Diagnostic testing can help make the diagnosis of seizures or epilepsy. The testing may help the health care provider find out what problem is in your child's brain, or what the reason is for your child's seizures. Numerous tests are available.

An *electroencephalogram* (EEG) is done to look for abnormal brain activity by recording the brain's electrical activity. It is usually done with the child who has been sleep deprived the night before the test, both awake and asleep. In certain cases the child is given medicine when he arrives to help him sleep. Sometimes a longer tracing of the brain activity (lasting 24 to 72 hours) is necessary, so an *ambulatory EEG* is performed during the child's normal waking activities and sleep. The child is set up with the EEG and then goes home. Sometimes a video-recording machine is used with this test; this is called *intensive video EEG monitoring*. The child is admitted to the hospital for this test. It is important to know that a child can have a normal EEG (no seizure activity on the EEG) and still have epilepsy.

Brain-imaging techniques, such as *computerized tomography (CT scan)*, *magnetic resonance imaging (MRI)*, *positron emission tomography (PET scan)*, and *single photon emission computed tomography (SPECT scan)* of the brain (to name a few) may also be used. These tests give information about the structure and activity of the brain. The CT and MRI show physical structures of the brain, whereas the PET and SPECT show metabolic activity in the brain. In children who have both cerebral palsy and seizures, chances of finding an abnormality on the test are increased. The most common abnormality is cortical atrophy (or shrinkage) of the brain's gray matter. No specific treatment is available for most of the abnormalities that are found in a child with cerebral palsy.

The child's health care provider may order various blood tests to determine the reason for your child's problem. The type of blood tests ordered depends on the child's medical history.

What are the different kinds of seizures?

Seizures can be either partial seizures or generalized seizures. *Partial seizures* occur when the bursts of abnormal electrical activity are confined to one part of the brain. The right side of the brain usually controls the left side of the body, and the left side of the brain usually controls the right side of the body. If the abnormal activity occurs in the right side of the brain, you may see movement on the left side of the body. Partial seizures can cause *motor* symptoms such as jerking, twitching, or shaking; *somatosensory* symptoms such as a change in the way things look, sound, smell, or taste; *autonomic* symptoms such as becoming pale or flushed; or *psychic* symptoms such as fear, anger, hallucinations, or déjà vu (reliving an experience one had in the past). Sometimes after a partial seizure is over the child has a weakness of one side of the body that can last up to 24 to 48 hours. This is called a *Todd's paralysis.*

A *simple partial seizure* occurs when the abnormal activity in the brain occurs in one part of the brain but consciousness is not affected. Therefore, the person is aware during the event and can carry on a conversation, but they cannot control the symptoms that occur.

Complex partial seizures, once known as psychomotor or temporal lobe seizures, occur when the electrical activity in the brain occurs in one part of the brain, but consciousness is also affected. No complete loss of consciousness occurs, however. Complex partial seizures can have all the same symptoms of simple partial seizures, but the child is also confused, disoriented, or unresponsive. The child may hear you talk but cannot answer you. He or she may be unable to follow directions. The child may move or wander around and mumble. After the seizure is over, the child may be aware that the seizure occurred or she may have no memory of the seizure.

An *aura* is a "warning" some people have before a seizure. It can be a smell, feeling, visual change, and so on. This aura is usually a type of simple partial seizure.

A *generalized seizure* occurs when the abnormal electrical activity in the brain occurs over the whole brain all at one time. The entire body is affected equally (both sides) and there is a complete loss of consciousness. During this type of seizure the child cannot talk or respond, is unaware of his/her surroundings, and has no memory of the seizure afterward. There may be a loss of bowel or bladder control during this type of seizure. There are many types of generalized seizures.

Absence seizures, once known as "petit mal" seizures, occur for brief periods in which the child will suddenly stare and be unaware of her environment. The child is unable to talk or respond. There can be *automatisms,* such as eye fluttering or mouth movements. These seizures can last up to twenty seconds. They interrupt a child's concentration and can happen very often (up to hundreds of times a day). The child always returns to her previous activity after the seizure is over, without awareness of the seizure.

During a *tonic seizure* the child's body gets rigid. He may have slight tremors or fine shaking. A *postictal state* can occur after this type of seizure. This is a period of time where the child may sleep after the seizure is over.

Tonic-clonic seizures were once known as "grand mal" seizures. The child's body stiffens and then jerks in a rhythmic pattern. Breathing can become shallow during this type of seizure. The child can go into a *postictal state* after this type of seizure also.

Myoclonic seizures are brief, very quick, forceful muscle jerks that the child cannot control. They often involve the arm or face but may also involve the whole body. A myoclonic seizure looks like a quick startle. These seizures are not triggered by any type of event, such as a loud noise, light, or a sudden movement.

Akinetic seizures are also known as drop attacks because the child suddenly and forcefully drops to the ground. He then immediately gets back up. Children who have these types of seizures may sustain head or face injuries from the sudden fall, so it is recommended that they wear a helmet to lessen the chance of injury.

Atonic seizures result in a sudden loss of muscle tone. The child suddenly drops or "melts" to the ground and is limp for a period of time. Children who have these types of seizures also may sustain head or face injuries from the fall, so it is recommended that they wear a helmet to lessen the chance of injury.

Infantile spasms are seen in children who are less than one year of age. These spasms occur in clusters and are very quick. There are three different types of infantile spasms:

- *Flexor spasms* are abrupt flexing or bending spasms of the neck, trunk, arms, and legs. They are often called *jack-knife seizures* or *salaam seizures*. The child looks as if she is suddenly bending in half.
- *Extensor spasms* are the least common. They are abrupt extension or straightening spasms involving movement of the neck, trunk, arms, and legs. They are often called *cheerleader spasms*.
- *Mixed spasms* are the most common. They usually include flexion of the neck, trunk, and arms and extension of the legs.

Seizures can spread from a simple partial seizure to a complex partial seizure and then to a generalized seizure.

What can trigger a seizure?

Many things can trigger a seizure in a child who already has a seizure disorder. *Illness,* especially when accompanied by fever, can cause an increase in the number and severity of seizures. It is important to treat illness aggressively as directed by your child's health care provider. *Lack of sleep* can be a triggering event for some people with seizures. If a child needs eight hours of sleep a night, and then for one or two nights gets only five or six hours, the child may have increased seizures. It is important for your child to get adequate nightly sleep. *Stress,* which can result in a lack of sleep, can cause increased seizures a day or so after the event. Stress can be good stress (Christmas, birthdays, trip to the amusement park) or bad stress (death in the family, divorce). It is not the actual stressful event that causes the seizures, but rather the lack of sleep the child may get during this time. *Certain sounds or flickering lights* can be triggers for a small number of children with a certain kind of epilepsy. Television, video games, and strobe lights are common sources of flickering lights.

These triggers are not the cause of seizures, but they can cause an increase in the number and severity of seizures in a child who has epilepsy.

What is it like for the parents or caregivers when their child is having a seizure?

It is very frightening for the parent or caregiver the first time they see their child have a seizure. They may think the child is going to die. The more educated parents are about seizures, the better they will respond. They should be instructed that most seizures are over in less than five minutes. The health care provider will teach the family seizure precautions and first aid for seizures (discussed later). Most parents and caregivers eventually overcome their anxiety about seizures. It is important for the parent and caregiver to try to remain calm during the child's seizure.

What is it like for the child when she is having a seizure?

The child may or may not be aware of the seizure, but she will not be able to control the symptoms. During a simple partial seizure, the child will be aware of the seizure and have memory of the seizure after it is over. During a complex partial seizure, the child may or may not be aware during the seizure and may or may not have memory of the seizure when it is over. During a generalized seizure the child will have a total loss of consciousness and will be unaware during the seizure, having no memory of the event once it is over.

The seizure itself is not painful, but depending on what type of seizure the child is having, the child may be injured. The child's reaction after the seizure is over will depend on how the people around him react during the seizure. To help with the child's anxiety about the seizure, it is best to teach the child about his seizures and what they look like.

How are seizures treated?

There are various options for treatment of seizures. Pharmacological treatment consists of antiepileptic drugs (AEDs) and nonpharmacological treatments consist of the ketogenic diet, the Vagal Nerve Stimulator (VNS), and brain surgery. Some families have also elected to treat seizures with alternative therapies such as herbal preparations and supplements. The decision to treat should be made after discussion with your child's health care provider.

AEDs raise the seizure threshold by decreasing the electrical impulses of the cells in the brain to try to stop the seizure from occurring or from spreading. The primary goal of therapy is to have complete seizure control with no medication side effects. If this goal is not attainable, then the secondary goal of therapy is to reduce the number of seizures, decrease the frequency of the seizures, decrease the duration of the seizures, and decrease the side effects of the AEDs. There are numerous AEDs that your health care provider can choose from when treating your child's seizures. Each AED will have two names. The drug company's brand name for the drug is the *trade name,* and the chemical name of the drug is the *generic name.* Your health care provider will try to treat your child's seizures with *monotherapy,* meaning the use of a single AED. However, sometimes *polytherapy,* the use of several AEDs, is necessary. For successful therapy, the AED should be taken properly by following the correct schedule and taking the correct dose. Your child should continue on medication even when he becomes seizure free. Your child should never stop taking AEDs abruptly, because this can possibly result in sudden increased seizures, or even *status epilepticus,* a seizure that does not stop. Your health care provider will provide you with further information about the medication that your child will be taking.

Depending on the AED your child is taking, your child may need to get *blood levels* checked. This is the measurement of the amount of the drug that is in the body. It can take one to two weeks for the medication level to rise in the blood and then level off; this is called the *steady state.* AEDs have *peaks* (the highest level in the blood) and *troughs* (the lowest level in the blood). Drug levels are usually drawn as trough levels, first thing in the morning before the morning dose of medication. Peak levels are drawn when side effects are a problem for the child. The *therapeutic range* is the range of the level of the AED in the blood, determined during drug trials, that gave the majority of people good seizure control with minimal side effects. Your child's medication dose may be changed depending on the result of the blood levels.

The *Ketogenic Diet* is a special diet that is used to try to gain improved seizure control. The diet is high in fat and low in carbohydrates and protein combined. The diet keeps the body in a fastlike state that makes the body burn fat for energy, instead of sugar. The diet also keeps the body in a partially dehydrated state by limiting fluid intake. *A neurologist and dietitian who are well educated in the diet must manage the ketogenic diet.* You should never attempt to try this diet on your own without the help of these professionals.

The *Vagal Nerve Stimulator* (VNS) can also be used to try to control seizures. This is a small device that is surgically placed under the skin in the left chest area with wires that thread under the skin to the vagus nerve in the left neck area. The vagus nerve is a link to the brain. When this nerve is stimulated by the device, it stimulates the base of the brain and sometimes can help to control seizures. The device stimulates the vagus nerve at preset intervals throughout the day. The family is also given a special, very strong magnet that they can pass over the device in the chest to give an extra "dose" of stimulation to prevent or stop a seizure.

Brain surgery is performed in some people when all other methods fail. The individual must have a *focus* or a specific spot from which the seizures originate. Brain surgery involves removing the part of the brain identified as the area that is producing the seizures.

More people are using *alternative therapies,* such as *herbal preparations* and *supplements,* to treat medical problems. A number of herbs have been labeled as being effective in controlling seizures; however, none are recommended for use in children. An important fact to keep in mind is that herbal preparations and supplements are also medications, and as such they have potential side effects. These preparations can interact with the body and with other medications the individual may already be taking.

What are the first aid procedures for seizures?

The main things to remember in any seizure are to prevent injury to the child and to monitor the seizure. It is important to remain with the child during the seizure. It is also important to make the environment safe during a seizure by moving sharp objects and furniture out of the way if possible. Once the seizure is over, do not rush your child to stand up, walk, drink, or eat something until he is fully awake.

For generalized seizures:
- Stay with the child during the seizure.
- Gently lower the child to the floor, if she is not already there.
- Position the child on her side.
- Support the child's head so it is in straight alignment with her body. You can use a jacket, towel, small pillow, or your hand to do this.
- Do not put anything into the child's mouth (including a finger or hard object).
- Loosen any tight clothing around the neck, chest, and abdomen.
- Do not restrain the child.
- Move furniture and sharp objects away from the child, if possible.

For complex partial seizures:
- Stay with the child during the seizure.
- Do not restrain the child.
- Speak softly.
- If the child is walking, place your hands on the child's shoulders from behind and gently guide the child away from a dangerous situation.
- If the seizure spreads to a generalized seizure, follow the first aid guidelines for a generalized seizure.

Once the seizure is over, the child may sleep for a period of time. Once he is awake, the child can resume his previous activity.

For absence seizures:
- Stay with the child.
- Do not restrain the child.
- Reorient the child to his surroundings after the seizure is over.

Sometimes when a seizure starts, there is no way to stop it without special medications. Many physicians recommend giving *Diastat* rectally if a child has a seizure that lasts five minutes or longer. This is valium that is premeasured in a rectal syringe. This medication usually stops a seizure within five to ten minutes of giving the medication. *If the seizure does not stop with Diastat, if a seizure lasts longer than five minutes and you don't have Diastat to give, if seizures occur one right after another, or if your child has breathing difficulties once on his side, call 911, or emergency services in your area.*

What are some important seizure precautions?

To keep your child safe, some precautions are necessary for the child with seizures. You must be very careful with your child around *water.* Your child should take showers instead of baths, if she is able and old enough. Be sure your bathtub drain works well. If your child is taking a bath, you must be present and watching at all times to prevent drowning if a seizure occurs.

Your child should not lock the bathroom door or take a shower or bath when she is home alone. Your child must be watched at all times with one-to-one supervision by an adult when swimming. If a seizure occurs while the child is in the water swimming, the adult can get the child out of the water immediately. Contact your health care provider if a seizure occurs while your child is in the water.

If your child's seizures are not controlled, he should not be climbing in *high places.* If going on amusement park rides, your child must be securely strapped into the ride and should not go alone. If your child is playing on park equipment, be sure there is soft ground beneath and appropriate adult supervision.

When cooking at home be sure the pot and pan handles are turned inward, to the center of the stove. If your child is near the stove, be sure someone is present. If your child is at a campfire or bonfire, be sure she is far enough away from the fire so if she had a seizure, she would not fall into the fire.

If your child's seizures are not controlled he should not be near or use electrical or mechanical equipment. If using this equipment, an adult should be present at all times.

If your child rides a horse, he must wear a helmet at all times. Check with your health care provider before you allow your child on a horse. When bike riding or skating, your child should wear a helmet at all times and not bike or skate on busy streets.

If there is an activity your child would like to do other than what is discussed here, and you are not sure if he should be allowed to do it, check with your health care provider.

Where can I get further information about seizures?

You can get further information about your child's seizures from your child's health care provider or neurologist. You can also obtain further information about epilepsy and your child's seizures by contacting the *Epilepsy Foundation of America (EFA)* at 1-800-332-1000. They will be able to tell you how to contact the local chapter of the EFA in your area. You can also look in the phone book for the local EFA chapter.

Mental Retardation, Learning Disabilities, and ADHD

I've heard the term "developmental delay" used. What does it mean?

Developmental delay is a descriptive term that refers to a lag in developmental milestones in an infant or young child. This delay could be in just one area of development, such as motor skills, as in a child with cerebral palsy, or language skills, as in a child who has a hearing deficit. Alternatively, there could be a delay in all areas of development, including gross and fine motor skills, language, and social-adaptive development. If such a global developmental delay persists beyond age 4 and is confirmed by formal psychological testing, it is called mental retardation.

What is mental retardation?

Mental retardation is below average intellectual functioning as measured on a standard test of intelligence. It reflects deficits in both cognitive functioning, otherwise known as thinking skills, and adaptive behavior, or one's ability to adapt to the environment. Average intellectual functioning is measured by an IQ of 100; mental retardation is defined as having an IQ below 70.

What are the different categories of mental retardation?

There are four categories of mental retardation. They are: (1) mild mental retardation, defined as an IQ between 55 and 69; (2) moderate mental retardation, defined as an IQ between 40 and 54; (3) severe mental retardation, defined as an IQ between 25 and 39; and (4) profound mental retardation, defined as an IQ below 25. Someone with mild mental retardation is considered to be an educable mentally retarded person, and someone who has moderate mental retardation is considered to be a trainable mentally retarded person.

What are the implications of these categories?

People with severe or profound mental retardation (about 5 percent of the mentally retarded population) cannot function outside of the home. That is, they cannot hold a job or live independently, and they need lifelong supervision by their families or an institution. Those with moderate mental retardation (about 10 percent of the retarded population) can be trained to do a job while under supervision (usually a repetitive, unskilled task). They can care for themselves with supervision and are often able to live in a group home with supervision. Those with mild mental retardation (85 percent of the retarded population) can live independently. Eighty percent of them hold jobs that don't require high intellectual functioning, and can live independently. More than 80 percent of these individuals are married.

What are the causes of mental retardation?

There are many possible causes, including all the factors that can cause brain damage of any sort. They include (1) factors that are present prior to or at the time of conception, such as genetic disorders, brain malformation, or metabolic disorders; (2) factors that affect the developing brain during pregnancy, such as alcohol, infections such as rubella (German measles), and malnutrition of the fetus caused by medical illness of the mother; (3) factors at the time of delivery, such as poor oxygenation of the brain, trauma, or infection; and (4) factors affecting the young child, such as lead intoxication, severe nutritional deficiencies, infections such as meningitis, and trauma from an automobile accident or child abuse. For more than 60 percent of people who have mental retardation, no cause can be identified.

Is there a difference between mental retardation and cerebral palsy?

Yes, there is a difference. Mental retardation implies an impairment of cognitive and adaptive functioning, or a limitation of intellectual capabilities. Cerebral palsy implies an impairment of motor function, meaning that use of the muscles in the arms or legs is impaired. Someone can have CP and have normal intelligence, and someone can have mental retardation but have no physical impairment. Mental retardation and CP do not necessarily go together, but mental retardation and cerebral palsy often occur together.

Approximately two-thirds of people with cerebral palsy have mental retardation. One-third of children with CP have mild mental retardation, one-third have moderate to severe mental retardation, and one-third have a normal IQ. Children with spastic quadriplegia are more likely to have mental retardation than those with hemiplegia or diplegia. Even children with CP who have normal intelligence, however, are at risk for learning disabilities or attention deficit disorders.

What is a learning disability?

By definition, children with learning disabilities have normal intelligence but have an impairment or disorder in one or more of the psychological processes involved in understanding or using written or spoken language. As a result, their ability to listen, think, speak, read, write, spell, or do mathematical calculations is impaired. This means that, despite normal cognitive potential, there is an interference in learning abilities in subjects such as reading, writing, or mathematics or in the skills necessary for academic performance such as thinking, listening, and speaking. This interference is due to a dysfunction of the central nervous system. Learning problems are often caused by perceptual difficulties or a difficulty in processing information.

What is attention deficit–hyperactivity disorder?

Attention deficit–hyperactivity disorder (ADHD) is a disorder of the executive function of the brain that allows a person to focus and organize. It is a developmental disability that occurs in approximately 3 to 5 percent of children overall, but it is more common in children who have CP (or any other disorder of the brain) and in children who were born prematurely. It is characterized by inattention, distractibility, and impulsivity, and it interferes with learning in the classroom and results in low academic achievement. There are three major types of ADHD: predominantly inattentive type, predominantly hyperactive-impulsive type, and the combined type. Sometimes, however, these symptoms are a side effect of a medication the child is taking (such as phenobarbital), a learning disability, anxiety, depression, or neglect.

Children with ADHD may fidget with their hands or feet when sitting, have difficulty remaining seated, be easily distracted, have difficulty waiting for their turn in a game, or have difficulty playing quietly. In the classroom they may talk excessively, blurt out answers to questions before the question has been completed, have a hard time following through on instructions, or fail to finish chores. They may shift from one uncompleted task to another, frequently lose things necessary for tests or activities at school or home, and engage in physically dangerous activities because they have not considered the possible consequences.

Many children with ADHD have poor social skills, resulting in difficulties making friends, playing with others, and sticking to the rules while playing games. In the classroom they may act out and become the class clown because they aren't able to pay attention to the teacher and to the work at hand. They may be singled out as disruptive or lazy, and this may lead to feelings of low self-esteem. Similar problems can occur in the family setting, as the child's poor social skills interfere with interactions in the home.

How are learning disabilities treated?

The major focus of the treatment is to ensure that the child gets into the proper educational environment. Appropriate management of learning disabilities includes a comprehensive, coordinated approach to educational, parental, and child issues. Parents and teachers must not incorrectly perceive the child as lazy, stubborn, or incorrigible. Developing a thorough understanding of the child's learning abilities and disabilities, as well as an educational program devised to match the child's specific learning style, is of paramount importance.

How is attention deficit–hyperactivity disorder treated?

Modification of the learning environment is the primary treatment. The optimal setting is a highly structured environment with minimal distractions and a considerable amount of small group or one-on-one instruction. To help the child manage organizational difficulties, she or he can be taught management techniques such as regular daily routines at home and in the classroom; short, concentrated work periods; and the use of calendars and communication books.

Many children with ADHD may also be treated with medications. Approximately 80 percent of children with ADHD will respond dramatically to stimulant medications. These include methylphenidate (Ritalin) and its long-acting forms, such as Concerta, and dextroamphetamine (Dexedrine) and Adderall (which is a mixture of amphetamines and includes a long-acting form). Other drugs, such as atomoxetine (Strattera) and other classes of medications in addition to stimulants also may prove beneficial. However, medication alone is not sufficient. While the medications help improve the attention level and decrease the impulsivity of many children, the child with ADHD continues to face many social and learning problems. Teaching him specific learning strategies to address learning difficulties and counseling the parents and teachers to help shape more appropriate behavior are important parts of management. An individualized educational program is vital for the child with ADHD or learning disabilities.

What are the significant side effects of stimulant medications?

Many children show signs of insomnia (difficulty in getting to sleep) and decreased appetite, with resultant mild growth delay. In addition, some children develop a tic—a rapid, repetitive, stereotyped movement. While it is not believed that the medication causes tics, the medication may hasten the appearance of a tic that was going to appear later. The appearance of tics may be a reason to discontinue the stimulant medication. There is concern that the stimulant medication might lower the seizure threshold in children with seizure disorders and result in worse seizure control.

Hydrocephalus

What is hydrocephalus?

Hydrocephalus is an enlargement of the fluid-filled spaces in and around the brain known as ventricles, combined with signs and symptoms of increased intracranial pressure. It is caused by an imbalance in the production and absorption of cerebrospinal fluid (CSF), usually brought about by blockage in the normal circulation of this fluid. If the normal flow of CSF is blocked, the fluid backs up into the ventricles of the brain. The brain continues to produce CSF, however, causing the ventricles to enlarge and put pressure on the brain. Unless this pressure is treated, brain damage can result.

What conditions cause hydrocephalus?

Sometimes the channel through which CSF normally passes from the third ventricle to the fourth is not properly formed. This is called *aqueductal stenosis.* Sometimes tumors or congenital malformations block the outflow of CSF. There is also a form of hydrocephalus that results when the CSF is blocked from being reabsorbed. This can result from meningitis, trauma, or bleeding within the ventricles of the brain (this bleeding, called *intraventricular hemorrhage,* is a common cause of hydrocephalus in premature infants).

How is hydrocephalus treated?

To correct the damaging effects of the fluid buildup, a surgical procedure is performed involving placement of a *shunt.* A shunt is a tube; one end of the shunt is inserted into the ventricles in the head, and the other end is inserted into another cavity in the body. The purpose of the shunt is to bypass the obstruction and drain the cerebral spinal fluid into a place where the body can dispose of it.

The most commonly used body cavity is the *peritoneal cavity,* the space inside the abdomen. This space can accept the daily fluid production and absorb it. This shunt is called a *ventriculo-peritoneal shunt,* or V-P shunt. A less commonly used option is to insert the shunt into the *jugular vein* or right atrium to allow fluid to drain into the bloodstream. These are known as *ventriculojugular shunts* or *ventriculoatrial shunts*. Another option is the placement of the shunt tube into the pleural spaces around the lungs. This is called a *ventriculopleural shunt.*

Another option for the treatment of hydrocephalus is to perform an endoscopic third ventriculostomy. This procedure creates an internal bypass, allowing the fluid to escape the third ventricle. It is utilized in obstructive forms of hydrocephalus.

How is the shunt inserted?

A shunt is implanted during a surgical procedure performed under general anesthesia. This procedure is well tolerated and can be performed even on newborn babies. Once the anesthesia takes effect, a small incision is made in the scalp and a small hole is made through the skull. The shunt tubing is inserted into the ventricles; for a VP shunt, tubing is then tunneled under the skin until it comes out through the incision in the abdomen, where it is inserted into the peritoneal cavity.

A valve is usually connected internally, within the tubing, with a small, bubble-like dome in the valve which allows the functioning of the shunt to be assessed periodically. This dome can be accessed to provide information about the function of the shunt. It can also allow us to measure the intracranial pressure and to remove spinal fluid. There is little reason to "pump" a shunt, because pumping has not been shown to provide any useful information and has been associated with shunt malfunction.

What are the possible complications from a shunt?

Sometimes shunts become clogged. When this occurs, the shunt has to be surgically repaired or replaced. Symptoms of shunt obstruction include persistent headaches and vomiting as well as changes in mental status or increased irritability. A shunt can also become infected. Infection may remain confined to the shunt tubing itself, but infection can spread into the nervous system, causing meningitis (infection and inflammation of the *meninges,* or membranes that surround the brain), which is a serious condition that needs to be recognized and treated promptly.

Even with the most advanced technology, shunts are prone to problems, and it is likely that one or more surgical revisions will be performed following the initial placement of a shunt. About 50 percent of shunts will fail within two years, and more than 90 percent will fail within five years of insertion.

Behavioral Issues

What are self-injurious behaviors?

Self-injurious behaviors, also called SIB, are repetitious and chronic behaviors that a person inflicts upon himself or herself in order to cause physical harm. Some common forms of SIB include biting oneself; pinching, scratching, or pulling on a body part; striking oneself (head banging or face slapping); repeated vomiting or rumination (self-induced vomiting); and severe pica (eating nonedible substances such as paint chips or dirt).

Many of these behaviors can be seen in the course of normal development in up to 20 percent of infants and preschool children. Such behaviors as body rocking, head rolling, and head banging often appear at around 8 to 9 months of age and disappear under normal circumstances by age 4. These behaviors almost always disappear as the child develops more sophisticated means of communication and stimulation.

Do these behaviors ever persist?
In people with developmental disabilities, such behaviors may persist for long periods and can result in serious tissue damage. Self-injurious behaviors that cause tissue damage have been described in 3 to 4 percent of children under 10 who have developmental disabilities, in 8 percent of 10- to 15-year-olds with developmental disabilities, and in 12 percent of people over 15 with developmental disabilities. This behavior is most common in people with severe or profound mental retardation.

There are specific but rare disorders that are associated with such behaviors, especially the *Lesch-Nyhan syndrome,* which is caused by a gene mutation resulting in a specific enzyme deficiency. In the typical patient with cerebral palsy and severe mental retardation, these behaviors may start as self-stimulatory activities and may then be reinforced because they attract the attention of parents and caregivers.

I've heard of behavior management as a treatment for SIB. How does it work?
Behavior management strategies are the primary treatment strategies for children with SIB. They may be used in conjunction with education and treatment with drugs. The key to any behavioral program is positive reinforcement for desired behaviors. Reinforcement increases the likelihood that the desired behaviors will occur and decreases the likelihood that the undesired behaviors will occur.

All too often, parents and other adults respond only when the child does something "wrong." This reaction, even if a scolding, may represent the attention that the child wants, and as a result the child will repeat the behavior to get more attention. In contrast, when a child is playing quietly by himself, a parent often chooses that moment to do a chore or make a phone call, and as a consequence the child receives no attention or reward for this "good" behavior.

In a behavior modification program, good behavior is rewarded, either with verbal feedback ("Johnny, I'm so glad to see you playing nicely with your sister") or with a concrete reward, like an ice cream cone or permission to watch a special show on television. Alternatively, this positive reinforcement might come in the form of a token that can later be traded for a desired reward. Negative reinforcement, on the other hand, is lack of reward for poor behavior. A child who is having a temper tantrum should be ignored (not rewarded with attention) as long as he is not hurting himself. If a child is banging his head, the parent may need to move him to a carpeted floor, but the parent should do as little, and react as little, as possible.

Aside from behavior modification, what else can be done to manage SIB?

Behavior modification is sometimes not effective in treating SIB, especially when the behavior is maintained by internal cues rather than by social reinforcement. A variety of medications have been used to treat SIB with varying success. Some drugs commonly used to treat other conditions have been used with some success in this disorder including oral medications and application of a local anesthetic cream. It is sometimes necessary for a person to wear protective equipment to protect him or herself from further injury. Such protective equipment should be used as part of a program designed to increase adaptive behavior. For instance, helmets can be used to protect the head when head banging or head hitting is likely to occur. Elbow splints can be used to keep the person's arms extended and prevent head hitting, eye gouging, and hand biting. Gloves, padded clothing, and goggles can also be used.

Another treatment of SIB is more controversial than protective equipment. This is the application of aversive stimuli such as bitter substances, water mist, or mild electric shock to the skin. These stimuli are sometimes used when the person's behavior has not responded to other, conventional treatments and the person is at high risk for injury from the behavior. This approach should be reserved for only the most serious situations and used only after the techniques have received approval from an outside agency or advisory panel not directly involved in the care of the child.

Besides SIB, what other behavioral concerns may arise in children with CP?

Children with CP (or any neurological impairment) may be more prone to having problems controlling their impulses, as well as having difficulties with focus and attention that may have an impact on language, learning, and developmental progress. A thorough evaluation by a mental health professional (psychologist or clinical social worker) may be helpful in assessing the child's behavior in the context of overall intellectual functioning, individual temperament, and parent-child interaction.

How can such behavior be managed?

The first strategy is to structure the environment based on the child's developmental abilities. This means setting consistent limits at home and at school and using rewards that have meaning for that particular child. There are children who require medication to help regulate their behaviors, because they are at risk of doing harm to themselves or others, or they are missing opportunities for developmental growth because of their attention difficulties. As previously discussed, stimulant medications are utilized to maximize focus (and often decrease hyperactivity) by stimulating that area of the brain that helps in attention regulation. Other classes of medications act as mood stabilizers, helping to modulate a child's reaction to his environment, while others can be used to prevent outbursts or impulsive behavior that could result in harm, as well as stimulate social awareness of consequences to actions. The use of medications for behavior management needs to be individualized, and needs to be discussed with a physician familiar with their use in children with developmental disabilities. Not all medication used for behavior management in adults can or should be used in young children, because of different side effect profiles. The goal should always be judicious use of medication to maximize developmental progress without blunting the child's personality and spontaneity.

Visual Impairment

What is the definition of visual impairment and blindness?

The term *blindness* refers to complete impairment of vision, when the person sees no light whatsoever. *Visual impairment* refers to diminished vision (or "low vision") but not total blindness. A child with visual impairment, who can be described as *partially sighted,* has visual acuity that is better than 20/200 without eyeglasses but worse than 20/70 even with correction (eyeglasses).

Legal blindness is defined as a visual acuity of 20/200 or less in the better eye after the best possible correction, or a visual field of 20 degrees or less. This definition is used by the federal government and other agencies to determine eligibility for federal programs such as SSI.

In terms of the educational system, a child with a visual impairment is one whose visual limitations interfere with his ability to learn. There is no specific level of visual impairment a child must have in order to qualify for services. Usually, visual services for children can be obtained when visual acuity is 20/60 or less.

What kind of visual problems do children with cerebral palsy have?

Nearly half of all children with spastic cerebral palsy have an eye muscle imbalance problem known as *strabismus,* commonly called "cross-eye." Strabismus causes one of the eyes to turn outward or inward. Children who were born prematurely and were exposed to oxygen are at risk for developing *retinopathy of prematurity,* a condition that in its severest form can cause blindness in one or both eyes. Children with severe asphyxia (lack of oxygen) may also suffer from blindness along with their other deficits.

As many as 75 to 90 percent of children with CP may suffer from *amblyopia* ("lazy eye"), *optic atrophy* (a shrinking of the optic nerve due to damage), *nystagmus* (jerking movements of the eye in a vertical or horizontal direction), visual field defects (loss of one side of the visual field) or *refractive errors* (near- and farsightedness and astigmatism, or distorted or blurred vision).

What can be done for children with severe visual impairment or blindness?

Special educational techniques are vitally important to a child with severe visual impairment. The child may need to attend a special class in a regular school or may require special education throughout his or her educational career, depending on whether visual impairment is the only disability or is just one of several handicaps. If visual problems are accompanied by other disabilities such as mental retardation, the visual impairment adds to the burden on the child and makes education that much more difficult. It is estimated that between 30 percent and 70 percent of children with severe visual impairment have other disabilities in addition to visual ones. Regardless of visual acuity, any child with normal cognitive and social skills can legally attend public school and expect to have the benefit of appropriate visual and educational aids. As discussed in Chapter 11, Public Law 94-142 requires that states provide a free and appropriate education to all children, regardless of their disability.

How is visual function assessed in the newborn?

There are a number of ways to assess visual functioning in the newborn. *Optico-kinetic nystagmus* is a reflex that is normally present in newborns, and can help the pediatrician assess the pathways leading to the visual part of the brain. A drum with alternating black and white lines is rotated in front of the baby, with both of the baby's eyes opened or one eye patched. A positive reflex is seen when there are horizontal jerks in the eye as the eye tries to follow and then pulls back, with the fast component being in the direction opposite to the rotation. This reflex can be seen in premature babies as early as 30 weeks' gestation (born after 30 weeks in the womb).

Other aspects of visual function can be measured by a baby's blink response to light, which develops at approximately 25 weeks' gestation. The pupils constrict in response to light at 29 to 31 weeks' gestation. Some discriminatory visual function appears by 31 to 32 weeks' gestational age. Tests using *preferential looking* (where the baby chooses to focus on a more interesting or more appealing picture) can estimate the actual visual acuity of a newborn.

Visual-evoked potential (VEP) or visual evoked response (VER) have also been used to assess the integrity of the entire system up to the cortex, but their usefulness is limited because the exact site in the brain where the abnormal response occurs cannot be determined. A visual-evoked potential is an electroencephalogram used in combination with a computer to assess the brain's response to visual stimuli such as a flashing light, or a checkerboard pattern. To test vision, the baby's responses are compared with those of children known to have normal vision.

How is visual function assessed in young children?

There are two basic kinds of vision tests, those that require minimal cooperation and those that require active participation by the child. In young children, Allen cards and the illiterate E game are the vision tests most commonly used. Allen cards are cards printed with objects familiar to children (such as a teddy bear, a telephone, or a birthday cake), and designed for use at 20 feet or less. The child is asked to identify the pictures on the cards. In the E game, the letter E is presented in different directions and the child is instructed to mimic the direction by pointing his or her hand or arm. In children who are a bit older and know the alphabet, the Snellen letters remain the standard test, using a chart with nine lines of letters measuring acuity from 20/10 to 20/200.

When should my child's eyes first be tested, and how often should they be examined after that?

A child with cerebral palsy, just like any other child, should have his or her eyes examined when there is any deviation from normal. Deviations include crossed eyes, roving eyes, or an abnormal appearance of the eyes. The examination is initially done by the primary care physician; if an abnormality is confirmed, the child is usually referred to an eye specialist—the ophthalmologist.

For children with significant physical risks, such as infants with a very low birthweight who were exposed to oxygen, the initial eye exam is usually done in the nursery by an ophthalmologist. Except for these children, who continue to see an ophthalmologist, children with cerebral palsy can be evaluated routinely by their primary care physicians at each visit and can be referred to an ophthalmologist if an abnormality is noted.

The exam should include an evaluation of the way the eyes move (specifically looking for crossing of the eyes) and a sense of visual acuity, that is, how well the child is seeing and following with his or her eyes. If the child is referred to an ophthalmologist, the ophthalmologist will dilate the pupil with eye drops in order to examine for refractive errors (farsightedness, nearsightedness, or astigmatism) and to evaluate the retina and internal structures of the eye. The dilated pupil evaluation will also help in evaluation of amblyopia ("lazy eye").

How is strabismus treated?

There are three goals for any child with cross-eye. These goals are the same regardless of whether the child has cerebral palsy or not. They are: (1) good and equal visual acuity in each eye, (2) ocular alignment (meaning getting the eyes straight, both for cosmetic reasons and for functional reasons), and (3) being able to use both eyes together. Strabismus is normally treated by correcting the visual acuity in each eye, either with glasses or by patching. If a significant strabismus remains even after these therapies, then surgery is indicated.

What is the surgery for strabismus?

Operations for strabismus are done under general anesthesia in an operating room. The eye muscles are either tightened or loosened. The main risk to a child from this operation is the anesthetic one. The complications of the operation itself are exceedingly rare and primarily involve infection. The most common complication is either incomplete or overcorrection of the crossed eyes. Approximately 70 to 75 percent of children respond to the initial surgical intervention with good alignment of their eyes, but one out of every four or five children requires more than one surgical procedure. For this reason, if there is any possibility that nonsurgical treatment such as glasses or patching will work, then these are tried first.

What are the different forms of blindness, and which ones do children with CP have?

For a person to be able to see, several things must occur. First, the person must have a clear optical structure, meaning that there are no cataracts or opacities (conditions that block light) that obstruct vision of the eye itself. Second, the person must be able to focus on an object, which sometimes requires wearing corrective glasses. Third, the person's eye must be able to pick up the light and transfer it into energy to send the image to the brain. The retina picks up the light and transfers this light stimulus to the optic nerve, which then conducts the nerve impulse to the back of the brain. Finally, the back of the brain, specifically the occipital lobe, must translate these electrical impulses into visual stimuli, which are then interpreted by the brain.

In optic nerve atrophy, the third process described above is impaired. That is, the optic nerve itself is injured and the light image cannot get from the eye to the brain. In cortical blindness, the ocular apparatus (the eye, retina, and nerve) is normal but the part of the brain which should pick up the visual stimuli is not working properly and cannot convert the electrical energy into a visual image. In children with cerebral palsy, blindness can be a result of damage to the retina, the optic nerve, or the occipital lobe of the brain. Premature infants who were exposed to oxygen may suffer a severe form of retinopathy resulting in retinal detachment, which interferes with the reception of light by the retina due to damage to the photoreceptor cells, and obstructs transmission of light to the optic nerve. Other children with cerebral palsy may have suffered lack of oxygen or blood supply at birth or in the months thereafter, resulting in damage either to the optic nerve or to the occipital area of the brain—or both.

Can head banging or rubbing the eyes cause blindness?

Repeated trauma from severe head banging can lead to a tear in the thin retinal surface, which will allow the membrane to detach. Once the retina is detached, it starves from lack of nutrients from its blood supply and rapidly degenerates. This process leads to blindness if not corrected quickly. For this reason, retinal detachment needs to be diagnosed and repaired promptly.

It is rare for permanent damage to occur from eye rubbing, however. While conjunctivitis and recurrent eye infections can be caused by constant rubbing, especially when dirt is introduced into the eye from the child's hands, eye rubbing will not cause blindness. It is common for children who have poor vision or who are blind to rub their eyes as a stimulating tactic (known as "blindism"). If the cornea of the eye gets scratched and an infection results, then the cornea can form an ulcer and deep scarring can occur.

Hearing Impairment and Otitis Media

Should my child be screened for hearing problems?

Severe to profound hearing loss affects 1 or 2 out of every 1,000 children. Inherited factors are thought to account for approximately 30 percent to 50 percent of children with hearing loss. Approximately 25 percent of childhood hearing loss is thought to result from environmental causes; in another 25 percent the cause is unclear. Approximately 15 percent of children with cerebral palsy have a hearing impairment.

The key to early detection of hearing problems is identifying children at high risk, including those with any of the following risk factors: (1) a family history of childhood hearing impairment, (2) congenital infections, (3) malformations that involve the head and neck, (4) a birthweight under 1,500 grams (3 lb. 5 oz.), (5) bacterial meningitis, (6) jaundice, or (7) severe asphyxia. Even when none of these risk factors is present, parents should bring any concerns regarding their child's hearing to the attention of their primary care physician. If the child does not act startled or turn his or her head toward loud noises, the physician may want to screen the child or recommend a more formal hearing test by an audiologist. Any failure of a newborn to "pass" a screening test for hearing should be pursued with the child's physician.

How is hearing tested?

The most commonly used test, the *behavioral audiogram,* is usually administered by a well-trained pediatric audiologist who during the test will ask the child to respond directly to word or sound cues. For an infant younger than 6 months, hearing is gauged by observing the infant's responses to sounds of various intensities and frequencies—responses such as widening her eyes, blinking, becoming quiet as she pays attention, or turning her head.

From 6 to 24 months, a visual re-enforcer, known as *visual re-enforced audiometry,* can be used to test hearing. In this approach, a flashing light or animated toy is used to re-enforce a response to sounds of controlled intensities and frequencies. When the child looks in the direction of a sound, a toy or bright light is presented in the same place to encourage the child to look again when he or she hears the sound. Between the ages of 2 and 5, children are usually tested by a technique called *conditioned play audiometry,* where they engage in a play activity such as putting a block in a box each time a sound is heard.

A child who is developmentally delayed will be tested based on his developmental abilities rather than his chronological age. For children who cannot cooperate or who give inconsistent responses, a *brainstem auditory evoked response* (BAER) is often used. This is a type of EEG that establishes a threshold of loudness below which the child cannot hear. Its limitations are that it primarily tests high-frequency sounds, sedation is often required to administer it, and it is more expensive than other methods of testing hearing. An additional method of objective hearing testing is to measure *otoacoustic emissions* (OAE). These are sounds produced by the outer hair cells of the cochlea, which can be measured in the ear canal. The ability to detect these sounds indicates cochlear health and, in general, a normal hearing threshold. It is being used as a routine screening test for newborns in many nurseries.

What are the different types of hearing impairment?

Hearing impairment is usually classified as one of two types, conductive or sensorineural. *Conductive* hearing loss occurs when there is a problem in the outer or middle ear preventing sound from being conducted normally into the inner ear and auditory nerve. *Sensorineural* hearing loss occurs when there is damage to the inner ear or auditory nerve itself. If both conductive and sensorineural hearing loss are present, the hearing loss is said to be mixed.

How are the different degrees of hearing impairment classified?

Hearing impairment ranges from slight to profound, based on the threshold (the minimum loudness) of sounds that the child hears. Table 5 identifies the kinds of assistance that will prove beneficial to people with various degrees of hearing impairment.

How are type and degree of hearing loss determined in children?

Once it is established that a child has a hearing loss, the next step is to determine the type and degree of hearing impairment. The degree is determined by testing and, as noted above, is described as a threshold at which sound is heard. The type (conductive, sensorineural, or mixed) is assessed by measuring middle ear pressure and eardrum mobility through a test called *tympanometry*. Hearing can also be tested using *air* conduction (the child wears earphones, and sound is conducted down the ear canal to the middle ear) or *bone* conduction (the sound is conducted to the middle ear by vibrations against the skull).

Table 5   Ranges of Hearing Impairment

Level of Hearing Loss (Hz)	Description	Sounds Heard	Possible Needs
15–25 dB	Slight hearing loss	Hears vowels clearly	Preferential seating
25–40 dB	Mild hearing loss	Hears only some louder-voiced speech sounds	Hearing aid, lip reading, auditory training, speech therapy, FM system
40–65 dB	Moderate hearing loss	Misses most speech sounds at normal conversational level	All of the above, plus consideration of special classroom situation
65–95 dB	Severe hearing loss	Hears no speech sounds of normal conversation	All of the above, plus probable assignment to special classes, possible cochlear implantation
More than 95 dB	Profound hearing loss	Hears no speech or other sounds	All of the above, plus probable assignment to special classes

*How can children
with hearing
impairment
be helped?*

At the time of initial diagnosis a medical evaluation should look for under-lying diseases, some of which may be treatable, as well as for genetic fac-tors, which may affect other children in the family or future children. For most children with conductive hearing loss, medical or surgical intervention should restore most, if not all, of the hearing to normal. On the other hand, a sensorineural hearing loss is rarely treatable, and the hearing loss is almost always permanent. The child's hearing impairment in this case is treated through amplification with a hearing aid. With a mixed hearing loss the con-ductive impairment needs to be treated aggressively, so as to minimize the hearing loss based on the sensorineural component.

Children of any age, even infants, can successfully use a hearing aid, which is essentially a miniature public address system with a microphone (to pick up the sound and amplify it to make the sound louder) and a loudspeaker (to deliver the amplified sound to the ear). The two most commonly used hear-ing aids in children are body-style hearing aids and behind-the-ear hearing aids. Even with these devices, however, hearing is still far from perfect. Hear-ing aids tend to amplify *all* sounds, including undesirable noises, and they don't clarify the sound; they simply amplify it.

For a child with a severe hearing impairment of the sensorineural type, there is almost always some degree of language delay because so many of the auditory cues and experience that are necessary to language development have been missed. Even after diagnosis is made, learning continues to be a struggle for many children, especially those with a more severe and pro-found hearing loss. Most children with sensorineural hearing loss need the benefits of early intervention programs designed for children with hearing impairments. In addition, special supportive services or special education may be necessary throughout the school years, particularly for children who have hearing impairment as part of a multihandicapping condition such as cerebral palsy or mental retardation, or if they also have visual impairment.

In select children with severe to profound hearing loss, consideration can be given to cochlear implantation. This is a surgical procedure in which a de-vice is implanted into the deaf ear, allowing the hearing nerve to be directly stimulated electrically. It can be done as early as 7 months of age but typically is performed between 1 and 2 years of age. With intensive rehabilitation, these children will often develop normal hearing thresholds and speech and language on par with their peers. However, not all children with severe to profound hearing loss are candidates for cochlear implantation, and for them, alternative modes of communication must be developed, including cued speech or American Sign Language. Unfortunately, sign language may not be a practical option for a child whose CP affects his hand functions.

*What causes hear-
ing loss?*

By far the most common cause of conductive hearing impairment in chil-dren is middle ear disease or otitis media (middle ear infection). Other causes include congenital malformations of the middle ear or obstruction of the ear canal by cerumen (earwax). Sensorineural hearing impairment may be present at birth; it may be inherited; or it may be caused by a maternal viral infection or a drug, particularly one ingested during the first trimester which interferes with the normal development of the inner ear. Acquired causes include a lack of oxygen at some time, either during the birth process or shortly afterward; head trauma; and other perinatal difficulties. Certain medications, including some that may have been used in the newborn nursery, or high bilirubin levels (causing jaundice) may also cause hearing loss, as can meningitis or mumps acquired later in life. Since many of these factors can also contribute to cerebral palsy, hearing impairment and cerebral palsy are often found together.

What is otitis media?

Otitis media is the medical term for a middle ear infection. It is a very common problem in children, second only to the common cold in frequency as the reason for illness-related visits to the pediatrician. Risk factors for developing otitis media include going to sleep with a bottle, bottle as opposed to breast-feeding, male gender, environmental smoke, pacifier use, and day care attendance. Estimates are that more than 90 percent of all children have had at least one such infection by age 5.

How is otitis media diagnosed?

Children with acute otitis media often complain of an earache. They may rub or tug at their ears, may have drainage from their ears, and may have a fever. Sometimes none of these symptoms is present, however. Upon examination with an otoscope (an instrument with a probe, a light, and a magnifying lens) a physician sees a red, bulging, immobile eardrum. Such an infection is commonly treated with antibiotics, even though some ear infections are caused by viruses, in which case antibiotics are ineffective. The accepted approach is to treat acute otitis media with an antibiotic, since such infections usually respond well to these medications. Fluid in the middle ear may persist for weeks or even months following the acute infection. This persistent fluid collection, known as serous otitis media or otitis media with effusion, may make the child more susceptible to recurrent infections as well as to hearing problems.

What is serous otitis media?

Serous otitis media is a chronic condition of the middle ear whose most obvious characteristic is fluid in the middle ear. The condition usually results from poor functioning of the eustachian tube. (The eustachian tube normally equalizes pressure between the middle ear and the atmosphere and permits secretions to drain from the middle ear.) When this tube does not work well or when it is blocked (most commonly when nasal tissues swell due to a cold or an allergy), fluid can accumulate in the middle ear.

If fluid remains in the middle ear for a time, disease-producing bacteria and viruses can cause an active infection leading to acute otitis media. Acute otitis media itself is always accompanied by middle ear fluid, and the fluid in the middle ear can persist long after the infection has been effectively treated with antibiotics. So serous otitis media can make a person more likely to develop an acute ear infection, and an acute infection, even when treated, can leave a person with serous otitis media.

How does serous otitis media affect hearing?

While the degree of hearing loss from serous otitis media can vary from mild to severe, the mild to moderate range of impairment is most common. It can cause obvious difficulty in hearing for a child who was hearing well before, or even greater loss of function for a child who already had some hearing impairment. Because serous otitis media is most common in children under 2 years of age, and because language takes shape during these first years of life, serous otitis media can interfere with the development of language, which is dependent upon hearing. There have been concerns raised that serous otitis media and hearing loss at this age can lead to long-term learning disabilities in children of school age, but this position has not been proven.

What other complications of otitis media are there?

One complication, known as *mastoiditis,* occurs when infection spreads from the middle ear into the mastoid bone and the cells behind the ear. This condition is sometimes treated successfully with antibiotics; sometimes successful treatment requires an operation, however.

An acute infection of the middle ear can also lead to perforation of the eardrum, which usually (but not always) will heal on its own. While perforation usually is not serious, it can lead to loss of function and to susceptibility to the formation of cholesteatoma in the middle ear. *Cholesteatoma* is a condition in which surface cells in the external auditory canal grow into the middle ear space and form a tumor that can erode the small bones of the middle ear. Rarely, acute otitis media can lead to meningitis, facial paralysis, brain abscess, or labyrinthitis (inflammation of the structures of the inner ear).

What is the treatment for acute otitis media?

The standard treatment for acute otitis media is antibiotics, which are available in many forms. In most cases the doctor prescribes one of the antibiotics that is effective in combating the three or four bacteria known most commonly to infect the middle ear. In some cases, however, the doctor wants to find out exactly which bacterium is primarily responsible for the infection, and in those cases he or she will insert a needle through the eardrum and extract a small amount of fluid from the middle ear to grow a culture. The choice of antibiotic prescribed in part depends upon the resistance of the bacteria to a specific antibiotic in that part of the country, the cost of the antibiotic, and the history of previous infections in that child.

What is the treatment for serous otitis media?

Many medical treatments for serous otitis media have been tried, including steroids, antihistamines, and decongestants. None of these treatments has been shown to be very effective, and even for children whose problem seemed to get better, the condition recurred fairly quickly. Surgical treatment is an option when serous otitis media is accompanied by hearing loss.

What about recurrent otitis media?

Recurrent otitis media is more difficult to manage. It can be treated either with antibiotics or through a surgical procedure. Low doses of preventive antibiotics (called prophylactic antibiotics) may be prescribed, especially during the winter season when the incidence is highest. However, concern about bacteria developing resistance to antibiotics that are used for a prolonged time has made this practice less common. Surgery involves the placement of tympanostomy tubes in the eardrum, to allow continuous drainage and provide for ventilation of the middle ear space.

What factors contribute to the development of recurrent otitis media with effusion?

The child under age 2 years is the one who most often develops recurrent (or persistent) otitis media with effusion (also called serous otitis media). The risk factors for developing otitis media with effusion include developing a first episode of otitis before six months of age, as well as those mentioned for otitis media (see page 69). Winter is the most common season for children to become infected.

When are tympanostomy tubes used?

Tubes are recommended when antibiotic treatment of recurrent otitis media has failed. For persistent effusion, tubes are considered appropriate if the effusion is accompanied by hearing loss of at least 20 decibels and has lasted for at least three to four months. However, because there are many different opinions about when tympanostomy tubes are called for, it's best to consult your child's physician.

How are tympanostomy tubes placed in the ear?

The procedure is formally known as a *myringotomy,* which is done under general anesthesia and is usually very brief, lasting approximately 10 minutes. This procedure can almost always be done on an outpatient basis, with the child returning home once he or she has awakened and has recovered from general anesthesia. Myringotomy tubes remain in place in the eardrum for 6 to 12 months, and usually fall out by themselves. They usually prevent middle ear infection and accumulation of fluid in the middle ear. When the tubes are present, water must be prevented from entering the ear, since this can cause an infection. Thus, care must be taken when the child is showering or swimming, and ear plugs are often recommended. Tubes are sometimes replaced after they fall out, if ear infections recur frequently after the tubes are no longer there. Some children get ear infections even with the tubes in place.

Issues of Feeding and Nutrition

Does cerebral palsy affect height and weight?

For some children with cerebral palsy, growth is affected. They are much smaller than their same-age friends who do not have CP. In some children, cerebral palsy affects only weight; in other children, both weight and height.

This is especially true for children with spastic quadriplegia, and much less true for those with hemiplegia or diplegia.

What causes this poor growth?

Several factors affect the growth of the child with CP, and not all of them are clearly understood. Primarily, poor growth is caused by an inadequate intake of nutrition. In addition, there apparently are some neurological factors that affect growth, primarily on the basis of hormones that come from the brain and that may be affected by the brain damage that caused the CP.

What causes poor nutrition?

There are multiple factors that interfere with good nutrition in children most severely affected by CP. Many children, especially those with spastic quadriplegia, have *pseudobulbar palsy,* which means that the muscles of their tongue and mouth are affected by their CP. This interferes with the normal coordination of chewing and swallowing, and it causes problems with drooling and poor pronunciation, as well. Many children with this constellation of problems also have a tongue thrust and a tonic bite, meaning that when something is introduced into their mouth, their jaws clench shut and their tongue pushes the food out instead of bringing it in and pushing it back toward their throat.

All these factors make it difficult for the child to receive adequate nourishment and calories. Meals may take over an hour, with much of the food still not ending up in the child's stomach. These same abnormalities make it difficult to brush a child's teeth, and so tooth decay and gum disease may develop. These conditions may compound the problem by making chewing food painful. In addition, many children with CP have tooth defects that make chewing more difficult.

What are the neurological factors that delay growth?

Even when their nutritional deficiency is corrected, some children fail to grow. This is especially true if the nutritional deficiencies are corrected later in childhood rather than in the first two or three years. While the neurological factors are not clearly understood, it has long been thought that damage to the brain affects those areas that produce various hormones, including growth hormone.

What can be done to stimulate the growth of a child with CP?

Since the underlying neurological cause will not improve, there is not much that can be done for that aspect of the growth problem. However, there are various methods available to improve the nutritional intake of a child with cerebral palsy. Sometimes a change in feeding technique is enough to improve the situation. This might mean better seating (a more upright posture will help some children) or special techniques, such as holding the jaw forward. Other children might benefit from a change in texture of the food—for instance, many children with CP cannot swallow liquids or chew solid food, but would do well with puréed foods. And for children who simply cannot take large quantities of food, high-calorie supplements can help them gain weight. This might mean very high calorie foods like butter, cream, or milkshakes, or commercially available nutritional supplements. If the child cannot be adequately fed by mouth, then a feeding tube may be recommended.

How is growth evaluated for the child with CP?

The primary care physician should be measuring the height and weight of the child with CP just as he or she would with any other child. For the child who is able to stand, a standing height is the most accurate. The doctor will try to get the child to stand up as straight as possible. Weights should be measured on the appropriate scale for the age of the child: an infant scale for young children and a standard scale for older children. For the child who cannot stand, a recumbent (lying down) length is measured from the top of the head to the bottom of the foot with the ankle at 90 degrees. This measurement can be done on a special length board or on an examining table or bed. If a wheelchair scale is not available, the child's weight may have to be obtained with the parent holding the child. Growth charts show the normal growth for children in the United States from birth through age 20. These charts are divided into percentiles, which reflect the expected normal growth over time. These percentiles range from the 3rd to the 97th percentile. Anyone over the 97th percentile is overweight or unusually tall. A child who is under the 3rd percentile is underweight or unusually short—although, by definition, 3 percent of the normal population fall into this category.

How can a child who has contractures of the hip, foot, or ankle be measured?

Contractures make it impossible to stretch the legs out and make it nearly impossible to obtain an accurate length. There are several alternate ways to obtain a child's length. The forearm can be measured from the elbow to the tip of the longest finger. Femur length can be measured from the hip to the knee. Tibia length can be measured from the top of the tibia to below the anklebone and knee height can be measured from the top of the knee to the bottom of the foot. All of these are height alternatives. Some, such as tibia length and knee height, can be put into an equation to estimate height. These values can then be plotted on a standard growth chart. For comparison over time the same method of measuring should be used each time, if possible.

Are there other ways to assess the nutritional status of a child with CP?

Triceps skinfold is a measurement of a child's fat stores. Triceps skinfold is helpful for monitoring a child's nutritional status, especially if the child has a weight and length below the 3rd percentile. If the child has a skinfold measurement within the normal range, this indicates good fat stores. The measurement is taken at the back of the upper arm at mid-point with a special caliper. The value is compared to other children of the same age and gender. This measurement can also be used to monitor nutritional status over time.

What if the child's weight is below the third or fifth percentile?

The growth of every child should be plotted on the growth chart during the early years of life. A weight or height that is consistently slightly below the 3rd or 5th percentile in a line parallel to the growth curve might simply mean that the child is growing normally and fits into the smallest 3 or 5 percent of the children his or her age. However, if the child is "falling away from the curve," meaning that he or she is dropping down in percentile, then the physician usually calls for further evaluation. Triceps skinfold and weight for height ratios can also help determine whether further evaluation is needed. If more intervention is needed, your doctor may have you do a diet history, a blood test, x-rays, or some combination of these. Usually the initial evaluation is primarily a nutritional one, since the assumption is that a fall-off in weight is primarily due to inadequate nutrition.

If the problem is nutritional, what other evaluations are done?

If the physician feels that a child's fall-off in weight or poor weight gain is due to poor nutrition, then a detailed nutritional history is obtained. This may be done by the physician or by a nutritionist, who will determine the number of calories and amount of minerals, vitamins, and micronutrients the child is getting compared to how many the child needs in order to grow and be healthy. If the physician feels that the child is not getting sufficient calories because of *oral motor dysfunction* (which includes poor chewing and swallowing, tongue thrust, tonic bite), then an evaluation by an occupational or speech therapist may be recommended. This evaluation includes a clinical visit, when the therapist watches the feeding of the child and tries to detect special problems. It may also include a modified barium swallow, an x-ray procedure that evaluates the ability of the child to eat and swallow food safely. Recommendations by the therapist to help deal with these problems might include better positioning or use of special techniques such as holding the jaw to help the child swallow better.

What does aspiration mean?

Aspiration is the process whereby food or secretions that are swallowed get into the lungs. Aspiration can result in chronic damage to the lungs. The child with CP may aspirate food into the lungs due to a lack of coordination in swallowing and lack of a protective gag reflex. Some children even aspirate their own saliva. Many children who aspirate have no cough or gag reflex and show no obvious response to the aspiration.

How will I know if my child is aspirating?

The symptoms of aspiration of food may include coughing, gagging, or choking while eating, or having difficulty breathing while eating. Some children aspirate without showing any of these symptoms, however, because they have no gag reflex and the food is getting into the lungs without producing any symptoms. Aspiration is suspected in such cases when the child suffers from repeated episodes of pneumonia. This is called an *aspiration pneumonia,* and it should alert the physician to the possibility that the child is aspirating. Aspiration could be due to problems with swallowing or due to gastroesophageal reflux (when food comes back up the esophagus after having gone down; see page 77).

Are there any tests that indicate whether my child is aspirating?

A regular chest x-ray might show "dirty lungs," a sign of chronic aspiration, but the cause is not clear from a chest x-ray alone. The test that provides information about the child's swallow and evidence of aspiration is the modified barium swallow. This test is done by a radiologist, usually with a speech or occupational therapist present to feed the child different textures to see how he swallows. Having a parent present is also helpful to try to feed the child in the usual manner. In this test, the child is fed the way he is normally fed at home or at school, but a liquid metallic element known as barium is mixed into food of different consistencies, usually liquids, pureed food, and solid food. The child is then fed in the x-ray department, where the x-ray evaluation of the feeding in progress can be recorded on videotape and reviewed. Since the barium shows up on x-ray, it reveals where the food is going when the child swallows, whether into the esophagus (as it should) or into the lungs. Another possible source of aspiration, the child's own saliva, is investigated with a nuclear medicine test called a *salivagram* (see page 83).

What can be done if my child is aspirating food?

If the modified barium swallow shows aspiration primarily of one type of food, then recommendations can be made to avoid this type of food. For instance, if liquids are being aspirated but pureed foods are swallowed correctly, then the recommendation can be made to thicken all liquids and not to give any liquids by themselves. (Liquids are usually more easily aspirated than pureed or solid foods.) The child can then continue to eat by mouth and simply avoid the foods that are hard for him or her to handle. Sometimes the modified barium swallow will show that a change in position or in feeding technique will stop the aspiration, and recommendations can be based on these findings.

If there is evidence that the child is aspirating everything he or she is eating, and if there has been a history of recurrent pneumonias or chronic congestion, then an alternative feeding method may well be recommended. Making a decision to use one of the alternative feeding methods is dependent on the child's and family's lifestyle, and each situation must be evaluated on an individual basis. If the decision is made to recommend an alternative feeding method, then this usually means placement of a gastrostomy tube.

What is a gastrostomy tube?

A *gastrostomy tube* is a tube that goes directly into the stomach through the skin, allowing the person to be fed without having to swallow. The food goes directly into the stomach and then is digested normally through the intestinal system. Liquids and pureed foods can be put through the tube, as can liquid medicines or crushed pills.

How is a gastrostomy tube placed?

There are four ways of placing a gastrostomy tube. A *Stamm gastrostomy* involves placing a tube into the stomach either via an open operation (where the surgeon makes an incision in the abdominal wall) or via a laparoscopic procedure (where the surgeon operates using several thin tubes that are placed through small holes or cuts in the abdominal wall). Both of these methods are done in the operating room. The third method is called a percutaneous endoscopic gastrostomy (PEG), and does not involve opening the abdomen. An endoscope (a long tube) is placed through the mouth and into the stomach. A needle is passed into the stomach from the outside and a tube pulled up from the stomach onto the abdominal wall. These three procedures are done in the operating room with anesthesia. The fourth is done by a radiologist, in a special x-ray room with intravenous sedation and local anesthesia. A needle is passed into the stomach and then the tube is pushed through the opening. Once the child has recovered from the anesthesia, feeding is begun through the tube. Usually, within one to three days the child is getting all the nutrition he or she needs through the gastrostomy tube.

Which method for placing a gastrostomy tube is best?

If the child has significant gastroesophageal (GE) reflux requiring an operation called a *fundoplication* (see below), then usually a Stamm gastrostomy is placed at the same time. The operation involves tightening the lower esophageal sphincter by wrapping the upper part of the stomach around the lower esophagus. It can be wrapped all the way around or partially around. This may be done either by an open procedure or laparoscopically, depending on the preference and skills of the surgeon. If there is no significant reflux and the child only needs a gastrostomy tube for better nutrition, then a PEG may be placed. This procedure should be done by someone who has been trained, either a gastroenterologist or a GI advanced practice nurse (nurse practitioner), who are specialists in caring for children with gastrointestinal diseases.

Can a child with a gastrostomy tube still eat by mouth?

Having a gastrostomy tube does not prevent a person from eating by mouth. If the tube is being placed because the child was unable to eat enough—if it is being used as a *supplement* to feedings by mouth—then certainly the child can continue to eat by mouth as well. If the tube is being placed because the child was aspirating everything he or she was eating, then the recommendation would be not to eat by mouth, though it may be possible for the child to take occasional tastes of food.

What are the side effects of having a gastrostomy tube?

The most common side effect is irritation of the skin around the tube, causing *granulation tissue* (a fleshy projection on the surface of a wound). Infection of the skin can develop at the site where the gastrostomy tube goes into the abdomen, but this is usually a local skin infection and is easily treated with an antibiotic ointment.

There are other, less-common complications: The placement of the gastrostomy tube may worsen or cause GE reflux in the patient who did not have severe reflux prior to having the tube placed. Also, the placement of the tube by Stamm gastrostomy can result in *adhesions,* which are bands of fibrous tissue in the abdomen. This can sometimes lead to bowel obstruction whereby food cannot pass through the intestines. Such a condition would make it necessary for the child to have another operation to relieve the obstruction.

Does the gastrostomy tube have to be changed?

The usual routine for changing a gastrostomy tube is every three months. This schedule will help to prevent the tube from becoming infected. The tube may also need to be changed if it becomes clogged, if the tube gets pulled out accidentally, or if the tube has a balloon that breaks and the tube falls out. G-tubes may be replaced by physicians, nurses, or parents, who can be taught the procedure and made to feel comfortable doing this at home. If a parent does not have a spare tube at home or is unable to replace it, he or she should call the physician or go to the nearest emergency room. Replacing the tube needs to be done quickly to prevent the hole from closing, which can occur in a matter of hours.

Can the child with a gastrostomy tube go swimming?

Yes! The child can shower or bathe, and even can go swimming.

What is a button tube?

A button tube or low-profile tube is the name for a gastrostomy tube that lies flat on the abdomen rather than "hanging" out from the abdomen. Many parents prefer this type of tube because it is less obvious to others that the child has a tube. A low-profile tube is also less likely to be pulled out by the child or by others, or to get caught on clothing or equipment.

Gastroesophageal Reflux

What is gastroesophageal reflux?

Ordinarily, when food is swallowed it goes down a tube in the body called the *esophagus* and then into the stomach. There is a muscle or sphincter at the end of the esophagus that acts as a one-way valve, preventing food from coming back up the esophagus. In many newborn babies this muscle (known as the *lower esophageal sphincter*) is underdeveloped, resulting in what is commonly known as "spitting up." As the child grows and develops, this sphincter gets stronger and eventually stops food from coming up into the esophagus. Thus, usually by age 1 to 1½ years this "spitting up" has stopped. However, in many children with CP this problem continues, though the child may not actually vomit or have food come back up.

This condition, known as gastroesophageal reflux, or GE reflux, can cause inflammation of the esophagus called *esophagitis.* This inflammation occurs because, as the food comes up, so does acid that is normally in our stomachs. Esophagitis causes pain, sometimes to the point where the child refuses to eat. When severe, this condition can cause anemia from blood loss, as well as *strictures,* which is a narrowing of the esophagus caused by chemical burns from stomach acid. Other complications of GE reflux include aspiration pneumonia and an inability to gain or maintain weight.

How is GE reflux diagnosed?

One test used to evaluate causes of GE reflux is a contrast study of the GI tract, or "Upper GI." In this test, the child drinks a milklike substance (barium) and, via x-ray, the radiologist watches it go down into the stomach. This x-ray looks at the anatomy of the GI (gastrointestinal) tract to make sure that there are no twists or narrowed areas (called strictures) that might be causing the reflux. This study only takes about 15 minutes and reflux may not be seen. If this test is normal and your physician still strongly suspects reflux, then other tests may be recommended. These could include a pH probe study and a gastric emptying scan.

What is a pH probe?

A pH probe is a thin wire coated in plastic that is passed like a nasogastric tube, through the nose and into the esophagus, by a radiologist or via a procedure called an upper endoscopy (EGD) by a gastroenterologist. It does not go all the way down to the stomach but remains a few centimeters above the lower esophageal sphincter. This probe remains in place for 16 to 18 hours. The child is fed as usual or with some apple juice, and the probe measures each time the child has a reflux episode and acid comes back up into the esophagus. If your child is already on an acid-reducing medication, the medication needs to be stopped at least five days before the pH probe study.

What is a gastric emptying study?

A gastric emptying (GE) scan (sometimes called a milk scan) is a study done in the nuclear medicine section of the radiology department. This test measures how well the stomach empties. The child is given a certain amount of milk or formula that contains an isotope. The scan lasts for one hour, and the radiologist calculates how fast the stomach empties and also notes any episodes of reflux. Children should empty at least half of what they drink in one hour. Less than half indicates delayed emptying of the stomach, which can make reflux worse.

How can reflux be treated?

There are several ways to help decrease reflux episodes. One conservative method is to hold the child upright for 20 to 30 minutes after feedings. Another is to avoid placing the child in an infant seat to feed, as the child is often bent forward, putting increased pressure on the stomach and making reflux worse. Thickening feedings with cereal or a thickening agent (like Thick-It) can help to keep food in the stomach but can also delay gastric emptying.

Are there medications that treat reflux?

There are medications that can help decrease reflux but do not stop it altogether. Two general types of medications are used. One group comprises prokinetics, which are medications that help make the stomach empty faster;

the second group comprises medications that reduce acid or stop acid production. Examples of prokinetic medications are metoclopramide (Reglan) and bethanechol (Urecholine). These medications work by increasing contractions in the stomach and by acting on the vomiting center in the brain. They have potential side effects, however, including decreased seizure threshold, drowsiness, involuntary movements, decreased urine production, abdominal cramps, and headache.

Two types of medications help reduce acid production: H2 blockers or proton pump inhibitors. Examples of H2 blockers are Ranitidine (Zantac), famotidine (Pepcid), and cimetidine (Tagamet). These medications decrease a child's production of acid and thus decrease acid going into the esophagus with each reflux episode. Since it is the acid that causes all the complications associated with reflux, some children only need to be treated with this type of medication and do not have any further problems. They may continue to reflux or regurgitate but do not have complications.

The second type of medication that reduces acid production is called proton pump inhibitors (PPI), which inhibit the production of acid. This group of medications only comes in capsule or granule form. However, these capsules can be opened up and placed in food or Maalox. Omeprazole (Prilosec) and Prevacid are the only two that have been studied in children and have been approved by the FDA for use in children. The potential side effects include diarrhea, headache, and abdominal pain.

What kind of surgery is done for reflux?

The surgery most commonly done to prevent reflux is a *Nissen fundoplication,* in which a portion of the stomach is wrapped around the lower part of the esophagus. This operation prevents food from coming back out of the stomach. It is still possible to eat after the surgery has been done, since the procedure does not totally close off the esophagus. Instead, it allows food into the stomach but prevents it from coming back up. This procedure can be done as an open procedure (with an incision) or as a laparoscopic procedure. A gastrostomy tube is usually inserted at the time of surgery. An alternative to a fundoplication is placement of a jejunostomy (or J-) tube.

What is a J-tube?

A jejunostomy tube (J-tube) is placed into the part of the small intestine called the *jejunum.* This procedure can be done as a temporary measure or as a more permanent one. In the first procedure, a radiologist passes a tube through the G-tube site, threading it down past the stomach and ending in the small intestine. This procedure must be done in the radiology department and involves radiation exposure for the child. This type of J-tube needs to be replaced every three months in the radiology department and it can easily be dislodged. However, using this type of J-tube can help determine whether the child will tolerate feedings in the small intestine before placing a more permanent tube or can help determine that the child needs a fundoplication. Placement of a permanent J-tube is done by a surgeon by taking a loop of small intestine and stitching it to the skin surface. A low-profile tube may eventually be placed at this site just as at a G-tube site.

What are the possible complications of a fundoplication?

The most common complication is wound infection, which may require local drainage or antibiotic treatment. Rarely, the wrap around the esophagus is too tight, making it difficult for food to get into the stomach. More often, the child may not be able to burp and release air trapped in the stomach. This can easily be treated if a gastrostomy tube is in place by letting the trapped air out through the tube. Intestinal blockage (obstruction) from adhesion formation within the abdomen can occur. These adhesive bands may require surgery to relieve the blockage. The risk of this occurring is 5 to 10 percent. Another possible complication is the dumping syndrome, where food exits the stomach too rapidly; the causes of this phenomenon after a fundoplication are not clear. Finally, over time, the wrap may become undone (especially in a child with a seizure disorder), resulting in a recurrence of the reflux. A reoperation may be necessary.

What is dumping syndrome, and how is it treated?

"Dumping syndrome" can look like recurrence of reflux. This occurs because the shape of the stomach is changed and can no longer act as a reservoir to hold food in the stomach. Therefore, food dumps out immediately from the stomach into the small intestine. This can result in malabsorption of feedings, sweating, increased heart rate, and a sudden increase in blood sugar followed by a sudden drop in blood sugar rather than a gradual drop. This syndrome can be treated with formula changes, by adding complex carbohydrates and increasing fiber or caloric content. If these do not work, then medications can be used to slow gastric emptying.

Is constipation a common problem in patients with CP?

Constipation is not an uncommon problem in any child, but it is even more common among patients with CP, especially those who either are confined to bed or are not taking sufficient liquids—or both. If the child is not taking in enough liquids, for all the reasons discussed earlier, then constipation certainly may be another problem the child has.

How is constipation treated?

Constipation is easier to prevent than to treat, and the first step in doing either one is usually dietary changes. In particular, an increase in fluids and fiber in the diet should help prevent or treat mild constipation. It is important to determine how constipated the child is by obtaining a careful history, taking an abdominal x-ray, and performing a rectal exam. If there is a moderate amount of retained stool, dietary changes will likely not be sufficient. If the child has not had a bowel movement in a week, had fecal soiling, or has been constipated for a long time, most likely he or she will need a "clean out" to rid the entire colon of stool before being successful with a maintenance regimen. A clean out can be done "from below" with enemas, or "from above" via a tube inserted through the nose into the stomach with an infusion of a medication called Go-Lytely. Children with CP may have decreased tone, and because the colon is a muscle it too may have decreased tone. Therefore, the colon may be unable to effectively contract to push the stool out of the rectum. Such children may require a stimulant such as senna or bisacodyl to help these contractions.

Osteopenia/Osteoporosis

Which children are likely to fracture their bones easily?

Not all children with CP are susceptible to fracturing their bones. Some children with CP do seem to be unusually susceptible, however, and will break their bones from a minor fall or minimal trauma or sometimes even with no obvious trauma at all. A number of factors put a person at risk for fracturing bones easily. The more risk factors present, the more susceptible that child is to such fractures. Once a child has had a nontraumatic fracture, his or her risk for additional such fractures is increased considerably. The factor that seems to predict who is at risk is low bone mineral density (called *osteopenia*).

What are the risk factors for low bone mineral density (BMD)?

Multiple factors may affect bone density in children with severe CP. Mechanical factors include the absence of weight-bearing ambulation and periods of immobilization (sometimes in a cast) following orthopedic surgical procedures. Diminished growth, poor nutrition, and low calcium intake are common in this population and contribute to low BMD. Many children with CP take or have taken anticonvulsants, which may adversely affect bone mineralization. Physically impaired individuals are less likely to participate in out-of-doors activities, a factor that could affect bone metabolism, because seasonal sunlight exposure contributes to vitamin D levels. Cerebral palsy is often associated with prematurity, and many low birth-weight premature infants have lower than normal bone mineral content when evaluated as older children (whether or not they have CP). Delayed puberty may also contribute to low bone density in children. Undoubtedly, the underlying pathophysiology of osteopenia in children with CP is complex, but it is clear that the biggest risk factor is nonambulation: that is, children who are primarily in wheelchairs or bed-ridden are the most likely to have osteopenia.

How is bone mineral density (BMD) measured?

The most commonly used method today is a technique called DXA, which stands for Dual Energy X-Ray Absorptiometry. It is a type of x-ray and involves a small amount of radiation exposure. It has been widely used in the elderly adult population and has been found to relate directly to the risk of an osteoporosis-related fracture in that population. This relationship has not yet been proven true in children, though it is assumed that the lower the BMD, the more likely it is that a fracture could occur. Results of the DXA study are given in actual measured density of the bone (grams per square centimeter) but are also reported as z-scores, which is the number of standard deviations above or below normal for age and gender. A z-score of less than –2.0 (that is, more than 2 standard deviations below normal) is the definition of osteopenia. There are other ways of measuring BMD, including quantitative CT scans and ultrasound, but these are not as widely used as DXA.

What can be done to prevent these fractures?

Some of the risk factors mentioned above are not easily avoided. For instance, if a child needs to take seizure medications, the medications should not be stopped because the child has had broken bones. It may be possible for the child's anticonvulsant to be changed to one with less potential interference with vitamin D metabolism. If the problem is nutritional, then some adjustments in the diet (such as adding milk or dairy products or special formulas with extra vitamin D, phosphorus, and calcium) may be helpful. It is also possible to take calcium, phosphorus, and vitamin D supplements, either in liquid or tablet form, on a daily basis. Increased exposure to sun should help the child's body make more vitamin D. It has also been suggested that physical therapy may help improve BMD in children with CP, especially when it improves their potential for standing and ambulation.

Currently the most promising intervention to treat osteopenia in pediatric populations is with the bisphosphonate medications, which are widely used to treat osteoporosis in elderly people. In children with quadriplegic CP, the bisphosphonate that has been used most often is pamidronate, which is given intravenously every three months and has been shown in small trials to significantly improve BMD. Still unknown, however, is the optimal dose and timing for this medication, and whether it actually reduces the risk of fracture.

Drooling and Airway Issues

Why do people with CP drool so much?

Lack of coordination of the muscles in the face, head, and neck can result in a significant amount of drooling. Just as some people can't coordinate their swallowing in order to get adequate food, some people have such poor coordination that they can't even swallow their own saliva. Certain anticonvulsant medications (especially Klonopin) may contribute to drooling by increasing the amount of saliva. Of all people with CP, approximately 35 percent or more drool significantly.

How can this be treated?

To some extent, drooling can be improved by modifying the person's position so that the head does not fall forward. Other measures that may help include better toothbrushing to help eliminate dental disease, correction of orthodontic problems that may interfere with the ability to close the mouth, and elimination of enlarged tonsils or adenoids that may be obstructing the mouth or nose.

Three primary methods have been tried to reduce drooling: (1) oral motor therapy, usually by a speech therapist, to improve tongue and jaw position and mouth closure; (2) medications to decrease the amount of saliva; and (3) surgery, either to decrease the amount of saliva or to divert the saliva toward the back of the throat, where it can more easily be swallowed. A fourth approach is behavior modification with the use of cuing and positive reinforcement. No one of these approaches has been proven to be more effective than another, and both medications and surgery can have significant side effects. Recently, however, the use of glycopyrrolate, an anticholinergic medication, has been shown to be effective, as has injection of botulinum toxin (Botox) directly into the salivary glands.

How does glycopyrrolate work, and what are its side effects?

Glycopyrrolate (Robinul) and other anticholinergic medications have been used to decrease excessive tracheal and bronchial secretions, as well as saliva. Studies of children with CP treated with Robinul have found that most showed a significant decrease in drooling (or tracheal secretions in those who have tracheostomies). Side effects included constipation, behavioral changes, dry mouth (or thick tracheal secretions), flushing, and urinary retention. A small number of those experiencing side effects were switched to an alternative anticholinergic medication. Such alternatives include benztropine (Cogentin), hyoscyamine (Levsin), and the scopolamine patch (Transderm Scop).

How can I tell when my child is aspirating saliva?

When a child has recurrent aspiration pneumonia, the physician usually looks first for aspiration of food, either from swallowing difficulties or from gastroesophageal reflux. If these conditions have been corrected (for instance, with gastrostomy tube feedings and fundoplication) so that there is no possibility that food is going into the lungs, and the pneumonias continue, then the physician usually begins to suspect that the child is aspirating his or her own saliva.

At this point, a test called a *salivagram* is done. This involves placing a small amount of a radioactive material called *technetium 99* on the tongue. The technetium is followed by a special scanning device that sees if the material goes into the stomach, as it should, or into the lungs, as is suspected.

What can be done about aspiration of saliva?

Operations such as a tracheostomy or laryngotracheal separation may need to be considered. A *tracheostomy* involves placing a breathing tube into the trachea (windpipe) at the front of the neck. This procedure is recommended when a child has a breathing obstruction in the upper part of the airway, such as in the mouth, throat, or larynx. A regular tracheostomy does not prevent aspiration and in most cases is used to treat upper airway obstruction rather than aspiration.

A laryngotracheal separation is a more absolute procedure, in that it completely separates the windpipe and lungs from the mouth. It is highly successful in preventing aspiration. The major drawback is that it is permanent and that, after a laryngotracheal separation, the person will never be able to speak. This procedure is therefore reserved for children with severe aspiration and with significant mental impairment who are not expected ever to develop a significant amount of verbal speech.

What care is involved for a child with a tracheostomy?

Caring for the tracheostomy tube can be intimidating at first. Nurses at the hospital, where the procedure is initially done, teach parents and other caregivers how to manage the "trach" tube at home. Routine care involves suctioning the tube and periodically replacing the tube with a new one. The frequency of suctioning can be from as seldom as a few times a day, or just when the child is congested, to as often as once every 1 to 2 hours. The tracheostomy allows secretions from the lungs and airway to be suctioned easily. The presence of a tracheostomy tube may affect the child's acceptance into certain schools that cannot handle the amount of nursing care necessary.

What equipment is needed to care for a tracheostomy?

A child with a tracheostomy usually needs a fair amount of equipment at home, including a humidifier, which provides a mist to help increase the moisture in the air in the child's room. Many children require this only when they sleep. A child may or may not need oxygen with a tracheostomy. Many need a suction machine and suction catheters in order to help suck out the secretions in the tracheostomy tube itself and to keep it from getting plugged up. As part of tracheostomy care, parents may be taught to do chest physiotherapy, which involves pounding on the chest and draining the phlegm in the airway. The tracheostomy tube is changed at a regular interval, usually every week. Some children also may require medications to be delivered through their tracheostomy, often with the use of a *nebulizer* (which is similar to a vaporizer in that it produces a medicated mist). These medications, such as albuterol (known as Ventolin or Proventil) and budesonide (Pulmicort) are given to children who have recurrent wheezing, either on a regular basis or just when they have symptoms.

What is a normal sleep pattern?

Sleeping habits vary widely, but most healthy people get an average of 7½ to 8 hours of sleep per night, with anywhere between 4 and 10 hours considered normal. An individual's needs depend on genetic factors and ingrained rhythms. REM sleep is the stage of dreaming that is associated with deep sleep and is the pattern that usually dominates during the last half of the night. Young children average seven such cycles each night and awaken one to three times per night, whereas adults have fewer REM cycles and typically awaken two to four times per night.

What causes sleep problems, and how are they treated?

A regular sleep pattern is established in the first few years of life. Often, an infant or a 2- to 3-year-old child fights this pattern and wants to stay awake. If this happens, parents should set a specific bedtime, using the time just before it to help the child settle down through quiet activities.

If parents do not set a regular bedtime, or if there is a great deal of nighttime activity, the child may not develop the habit of going to bed and to sleep at the same time every night. Sometimes, too, an established sleep pattern may be disrupted by a major event such as illness or surgery. The changed routine may disrupt the child's sleep pattern even after he returns home.

Some children with CP never develop a sleep pattern—perhaps because of brain immaturity. In this situation, doctors sometimes prescribe a sedative.

When is snoring a problem?

Snoring is very common in adults and not unusual in children, and it generally is no cause for concern. Sometimes snoring is an indication that there is a serious obstruction of the upper airways, however, especially when it is accompanied by episodes of apnea (cessation of breathing). Snoring usually results from a partial obstruction of the airway during sleep, but when the obstruction becomes total, *obstructive sleep apnea* occurs. If left untreated, obstructive sleep apnea can lead to serious heart or lung disorders or even death.

Obstructive sleep apnea is characterized by loud snoring with episodes of silence during which the snorer struggles unsuccessfully to breathe. After several seconds of such effort a loud snort forces open the airway, and breathing resumes. This is often accompanied by the child's awakening partially, sometimes kicking, flailing the arms, or experiencing a total body spasm. The child may then resume sleeping only to experience the same sequence of events again. These problems are considered pathological when apnea lasts longer than 20 seconds and occurs more than 7 to 10 times an hour or 30 times per night.

What causes this obstruction?

One or more factors may contribute to this obstruction of the upper part of the airway, which includes the mouth, throat, and larynx (where the vocal cords are located), resulting in decreased or no movement of air into the lungs. A child's throat muscles may have inadequate tone and poor muscle control, allowing the tongue to fall back into the throat, so that the airway becomes blocked. This is often the cause of the obstruction in children with cerebral palsy. Enlarged tonsils or adenoids can obstruct the airway; in children, this is the most common cause of obstruction. Adenoids, which sit above the roof of the mouth in the back of the nose, may block nasal passages, causing a child to breathe through his or her mouth, especially while sleeping. They also can block normal drainage of fluid from the middle ear and contribute to middle ear fluid and infection. By blocking the oral and nasal airway, enlarged tonsils and adenoids can worsen the mouth breathing that is typical in children with CP, as well as worsen drooling and cause sleep apnea and sleep disturbance. Obstruction of the nasal passages, often secondary to allergies, creates a negative pressure when the patient breathes in and can cause this problem, as can an unusually large soft palate or *uvula,* which obstructs the airway when the patient is lying flat.

Besides snoring, are there other symptoms of obstructive apnea?

A child who hasn't slept well at night might be hyperactive or antisocial, tired, and cranky during the day. Some children with obstructive apnea have a below normal body weight and may be very slow eaters or dislike foods that require chewing—though, as we've seen, there are many other reasons why someone with cerebral palsy might have trouble eating. Another sign is that nighttime bed wetting may reappear in a child who has been dry. A child may chronically breathe from the mouth because of the obstruction, and this can lead to orthodontic malformations and changes in the development of the face known as *adenoid facies,* or long face syndrome.

What is the treatment for obstructive apnea?

The treatment is aimed at relieving the obstruction: if obstruction is due to enlarged tonsils and adenoids, for example, then these are removed. Some children undergo surgical reconstruction of the airway, including a *uvulopalatopharyngeoplasty* (UPPP). If the child is markedly obese, weight loss is the first attempted treatment. Night-time BiPAP, which involves delivering airway pressure through a face mask at night while the child is sleeping, is also a treatment for obstructive sleep apnea. For children whose obstruction is severe and caused by poor muscle control, or for those who don't respond to the less invasive treatments, a tracheostomy may be recommended.

What complications are possible from a tonsillectomy and adenoidectomy?

Commonly, there is a sore throat following this surgery, which may interfere with the child's ability to eat and drink. Bleeding from the throat, although unusual, can occur even two weeks after surgery. In children with CP there are other risks, such as the inability to handle secretions, especially with the sore throat postoperatively, which may increase the possibility of aspiration pneumonia in the days just after surgery. The presence of poor respiratory muscle control and an ineffective cough may also increase the likelihood of pneumonia. These operations pose a special risk for children who are mentally retarded and for very young children. For these children, poor intake of fluids after surgery may put them at significant risk for dehydration, prolonging their hospitalization following surgery. Thus, children having this procedure usually stay in the hospital overnight.

Communication Issues

What are the factors that make it difficult for a child with CP to communicate?

To communicate successfully, a person must be able to receive and interpret language as well as to express it. Cerebral palsy may interfere with both receptive and expressive language skills. Poor attention span, for example, with or without mental retardation, can decrease the ability to process speech from other people. A hearing impairment can also interfere to the point of affecting speech and language development. On the expressive side, neuromuscular disability can interfere with breath control, vocal cord movement, and lip, tongue, and palate motion—all of which can result in articulation problems and difficulty in speaking.

What can be done to help my child communicate?

Early diagnosis and identification of any factors that might be correctable (such as fluid in the ears) is the first step to ensuring good communication. If there are no factors that can be corrected—that is, if the impairment is due to the cerebral palsy itself and not to a correctable hearing problem, for instance—then the child may be referred to a speech therapist, who may help improve communication for the CP patient. For children who have normal or near normal intelligence and the ability to comprehend and express thoughts but who cannot speak because of the cerebral palsy, there are assistive devices, known as *augmentative communication devices,* that can help. These devices, ranging from a simple board with pictures to point to or focus on with the eyes, to very sophisticated electronic devices with synthesized speech, can help a child with cerebral palsy express himself even when he cannot form words with the vocal cords. As a part of the evaluation, speech therapists determine which of these different devices are most appropriate for an individual child.

Dental Issues

At what age should a child with CP have a first dental evaluation?

A child with cerebral palsy should be seen at the age of 18 to 24 months for a first exam, just like any other child. This first visit is even more significant when a child has CP, however, because it enables the dentist and staff to evaluate their ability to treat the child and their interest in accepting the child for treatment. The first visit usually includes a detailed medical and dental history and a thorough examination and dental x-rays. X-rays may need to be taken under sedation if the child cannot sit still.

Do children with CP have more cavities than other children?

Dental cavities depend on the presence of plaque, which is a group of bacteria firmly attached to the tooth structure. There are many factors that can promote the accumulation of plaque and, ultimately, the formation of cavities. For one thing, a defect in the enamel (the outer covering of the tooth) can make the tooth more susceptible to cavities. Such defects are more common in children with cerebral palsy. Also, the arrangement of teeth in the mouth, especially when they are crowded and irregular, can make the teeth more susceptible to cavities because it also makes cleaning these teeth more difficult. Finally, it is very difficult to get a toothbrush into the mouth of a child with CP who has a tonic bite reflex or a strong tongue thrust. Because it is hard to clean the child's teeth, he or she is more likely to get cavities. Cavities can be painful. When a child who cannot communicate is crying, cavities must be considered in the list of possible reasons for the tears.

How can cavities be prevented?

Fluoride is recommended for all children and can be administered through fluoridated water or, if the water system is not fluoridated, through fluoride drops or pills taken daily. In addition, dentists often apply a fluoride coating to the teeth at the time of a child's visit. In the dentist's office, with proper equipment the dentist or hygienist also may be able to clean the teeth more effectively than the parents are able to.

What is gum hypertrophy?

Gum hypertrophy (also called *gingival hypertrophy*) is enlargement of the gums. The enlargement takes the form of a painless mass of tissue which is firm and pink and which may grow over the teeth. It appears more frequently in the front part of the mouth. Areas that are without teeth are rarely involved. If this tissue becomes inflamed as a result of local irritants, the gums may become dark pink or red and bleed easily. They may even become painful.

Gum hypertrophy sometimes develops as a side effect of medications, especially Dilantin. In fact, approximately 40 percent of people taking this medication develop the problem. Symptoms are more prevalent in younger children and occur approximately 2 to 3 months after they start to take the medication. Symptoms reach their worst level after 9 to 12 months.

What's the treatment for swollen gums?

Swollen gums can be treated by eliminating the local irritants with good toothbrushing and tooth cleaning. The most effective method for treating swollen gums is to remove the extra tissue surgically. Even after surgery the tissue can regrow, but it may be less extensive if good toothbrushing is maintained.

Are there other dental abnormalities that are common in children with CP?

Another abnormality is *malocclusion,* meaning poor alignment of the teeth. In malocclusion the upper teeth do not line up evenly opposite their counterparts on the lower jaw. Muscle spasticity has a direct relationship to dental and skeletal formation. The spasticity results in pathological contraction of muscles. Head and neck muscles are all involved, and when the motor nerves that supply the muscles of chewing are in spasm, they can remodel the bones of the face. When this affects the jaw, it can result in malocclusion. Thrusting of the tongue, and mouth breathing, also can affect the shape of the jaw and contribute to malocclusion.

Hernias and Undescended Testicles

Are children with CP more likely to get hernias?

A hernia (or rupture) is a projection of a body part beyond its natural location. The most common type of hernia is an *inguinal hernia,* in which the rupture occurs in the groin region. It appears that the incidence of inguinal hernias in boys with cerebral palsy is higher than that in boys who do not have cerebral palsy. We know that inguinal hernias are more common in premature infants, especially those weighing less than 1,500 grams (3 lb. 5 oz.). But even among these children, the incidence is higher for those who have CP, possibly twice as great as that among premature children without CP. It's not clear why this should be so. In a child with CP, especially a boy who was premature at birth, parents and the physician should be on the alert for signs of an inguinal hernia, especially for swelling, either in the scrotum it-self or, more usually, in the thigh area above the scrotum.

Are undescended testicles a common problem?

Normally, the testicles begin forming in the abdomen of the male fetus prior to birth and descend into the scrotum by the time of birth, if the baby is full term. Thus, premature infants are more likely to have undescended testicles. However, the testicles will often descend on their own into the scrotum by the end of the first year of life. If they do not, surgical correction is recommended, because the undescended testicle can twist on itself, cutting off the blood supply and permanently injuring the testicle. An emergency operation is required if this occurs. An undescended testicle also may develop a tumor later in life. It is easier to detect a testicular tumor if the testicle is in its normal position within the scrotum.

Even if the testicles are normally descended at birth, there can be problems later on. Studies have shown that there is an increased incidence of undescended testicles in teenage boys and young adults with cerebral palsy, with estimates as high as 50 percent of males with CP having this condition. It would appear that spasticity of a muscle known as the *cremasteric muscle* causes a higher position of the testis as the boy with cerebral palsy grows older, thus pulling it out of the scrotal sac.

Retractile testicles are those that are not in the scrotum but can be felt in the groin and brought down into the scrotum by gently pulling with the hand. Retractile testicles do not usually become undescended and do not need surgery.

Do children with cerebral palsy have more trouble with bladder control?

Problems with bladder control are not common in children with cerebral palsy, but they do occur more often among these children than among the general population. These problems can include incontinence (day or nighttime wetting), difficulty starting a urinary stream, or symptoms of urgency, meaning the feeling that one has to urinate immediately, without prior warning. Some children may have subclinical voiding disorders, meaning their bladders do not work entirely normally, but they do not show any symptoms under ordinary circumstances. These children may then develop symptoms, especially an inability to empty the bladder, after surgical procedures.

Issues Regarding Puberty

What physical changes should I expect when my son begins puberty?

In boys, the onset of puberty is marked by the testicles getting larger, followed by pubic hair and the penis getting larger. The age range for the start of puberty in boys is generally between nine and 14 years. It is generally believed that a boy who develops puberty before age nine, or does not develop signs of puberty by age 14, should be evaluated by a doctor for a possible medical problem. It has been found that boys with CP start puberty earlier than boys without CP, but progress through the stages is slower, and puberty ends later.

What physical changes should I expect to see when my daughter begins puberty?

Girls generally begin with breast growth, followed by pubic hair growth, followed by the start of menstrual periods. For girls without CP the starting age of puberty, which begins with breast growth, could be as early as age six years but is generally around age eight years. The end of puberty, considered the time when a young woman gets her first period, is at approximately 12 years of age. From start to finish, puberty takes about two to five years. Nutrition, body fat, racial background, medications, and underlying medical conditions affect a young woman's puberty. No breast growth by age 14 or no periods by age 16 is concerning and should be evaluated by a doctor.

Will CP affect my daughter's puberty?

Although girls with CP start puberty earlier than girls without CP, they end puberty later, with periods generally beginning at age 14. In addition, in girls with CP, pubic hair tends to appear before breasts begin to grow. This is different from girls without CP, in whom breast growth is the first sign of puberty. The average age of the start of breast development in girls with CP is about 10 years, and the average age of the start of pubic hair is about eight years.

How will puberty affect seizures?

In young women with CP and seizures, the onset of menstrual periods can be a cause of worsening seizures. The hormones that control the menstrual cycle also have an effect on the brain. Because of the monthly changes of these hormones, seizures may increase a few days before and a few days into the menstrual bleeding.

What can be done if a girl experiences increasing seizure activity during puberty?

There are several options for managing these seizures. One strategy is to give an extra dose of the prescribed antiseizure medication a few days before the expected start of the period and about two days into the bleeding. Another option is to provide hormonal therapy in the form of a pill or an injection. A change in the dosing of the antiseizure medications may be needed as the way the body handles those medications changes during puberty. This should be discussed with the physician who treats your child's seizures.

What can be done about a change in behavior that occurs around the time of a girl's period?

Premenstrual syndrome (PMS) usually occurs one to two weeks before the onset of bleeding and goes away a few days after bleeding begins. Young women with PMS report a multitude of symptoms, including hot flashes, chills, difficulty concentrating, and mood changes, including irritability and depression. In women and girls with mental retardation, PMS can cause an increase in behavior problems, seizures, aggression, tantrums, crying spells, self-abusive behavior and self-mutilation, restlessness, and agitation. Hormonal contraception, medications such as ibuprofen or naproxen, as well as medications used for depression, can be used for these symptoms.

Talk with your doctor about the options that would be appropriate for your daughter.

What can be done about a girl becoming agitated and seeming to be in pain around the time of her period?

Pain during the time of a period is called *dysmenorrhea*. Usually pain onset is within one to four hours of the start of the period, and lasts for one to two days. In some girls, the pain starts earlier and ends later. Nausea, vomiting, diarrhea, back pain, thigh pain, and headache may also be experienced. Girls who cannot communicate may become very agitated and distressed during their period because of these symptoms. They may thrash around or tense up. Posturing, teeth grinding, and increased irritability may occur as well. Although medications such as ibuprofen and naproxen are very effective for the treatment of dysmenorrhea, if symptoms continue birth control pills may be effective.

What can be done if menstrual bleeding is difficult to manage?

Menstrual hygiene may be an issue for some teenage girls with CP. Although it is felt that with encouragement and teaching most girls with mental retardation can learn to use sanitary napkins, some girls with CP simply cannot change a pad or a tampon. During the first two years of starting to have periods, some girls may bleed unpredictably and heavily at times. This bleeding should be evaluated by a physician. Although most girls will outgrow it, it is a nuisance for families and the child. In such a situation, hormonal contraception as well as surgery, both of which are discussed below, can be used to stop or decrease monthly bleeding.

Do females with cerebral palsy need birth control?

Teenage girls and adults with cerebral palsy are capable of and interested in sexual activity in much the same way other women are. Women who have severe physical limitations may not be able to seek out such activities on their own, but they may be victimized by males in their environment. Studies have shown that girls who are mildly mentally retarded engage in sexual activity, including sexual intercourse, in proportions comparable to the general adolescent population. Those who are moderately or severely retarded do so in much smaller percentages. One-third of mildly retarded and one-fourth of moderately retarded adolescent girls have been reported to be victims of rape or incest.

Teenage girls who are out of the home and are not under the direct supervision of their families may engage in sexual activity, and they need to be protected with birth control. Contraceptive devices include condoms, intrauterine devices (IUD), or hormonal contraception. Hormonal contraception comes either as a pill that needs to be taken daily, an injection that is given every three months, or a patch that is placed on the skin and is changed weekly. The injectable hormone, medroxyprogesterone acetate (Depo-Provera), is given by injection and will protect against pregnancy for three to six months. It also often decreases the amount of menstrual flow considerably, making it easier to manage the period. The intrauterine device

(IUD) providing protection against pregnancy is inserted by a gynecologist and can remain in place for many years. Both of these approaches to birth control are more reliable than birth control pills or condoms in a population that may not remember to take a pill every day.

What are the potential side effects of these birth control methods?

If an IUD gets infected or is causing pain, it needs to be removed. Unfortunately, some girls with CP may not be able to communicate that they are having problems with their IUD. This can lead to medical complications. Neither the IUD nor hormonal treatment will prevent sexually transmitted infections.

The disadvantage of the pill and the patch is that they may cause blood clots. These blood clots can cause severe illness and, in some cases, death. There is also a concern that if there are heart problems, blood clots can develop in the heart which can then travel to the brain and cause a stroke. The lack of mobility seen in many girls with CP, it is thought, may predispose them to get blood clots if they use a contraceptive patch or pill. Although this association has not been definitely proven to be true, it is a reason why many physicians do not prescribe the patch or the pill to young women who have CP.

With the injectable hormone, the likelihood of blood clots is not regarded as a major issue. However, a young girl receiving the injection may gain up to 10 pounds and risks having worsening of osteopenia, which is already a problem for many patients with CP.

Would a young woman need an "internal" exam before starting hormone treatment?

A parent seeking hormonal contraception for the child, hormonal control of the child's period, or control of the symptoms that come with having a period, should consult a physician who is experienced in the use of such methods. There are medical conditions that would exclude some girls from receiving some of these hormonal treatments, but, in general, a therapy can be found that is safe and effective for most women. One concern that arises is the need for a pelvic or "internal" exam to start hormonal therapy. It is generally accepted that if a girl's blood pressure is normal, and a careful medical and family history does not reveal any reasons for refraining from hormonal therapy, a breast and pelvic exam is not required.

If medications are not an option, is surgery a possibility?

Surgical options are available but are a difficult issue. The two procedures performed are hysterectomy, which is removal of the uterus, and endometrial ablation. Endometrial ablation involves the destruction of the inside lining of the uterus so that bleeding is decreased or stopped altogether. Not all women stop bleeding right away or even have a decrease in their bleeding, so it is not guaranteed to work. Sometimes it needs to be repeated to obtain the desired result.

Endometrial ablation is also controversial because a woman can still become pregnant after she has the procedure. A woman who becomes pregnant after such a procedure is at risk for problems with her pregnancy. It has been recommended that a woman be sterilized if she has endometrial ablation.

Can a young woman with cerebral palsy be sterilized at the request of her parents if she is severely retarded?

Some parents would like to have their daughters sterilized surgically, by having a hysterectomy performed or having their daughter's fallopian tubes tied so that becoming pregnant would never be an option. This is especially true of parents of severely retarded women who would not be capable of caring for a child. Whereas years ago many retarded women and men were sterilized against their will, doing this is much more difficult today. A parent must go through the courts to obtain permission to have the procedure done, primarily because society feels that being able to bear a child is an inalienable right. In the case of a retarded individual, the burden is on the parents or others to prove that bearing a child is not in the best interests of the woman who is to undergo sterilization; in general, having cerebral palsy in and of itself would probably not be enough of a reason. Profound mental retardation and the possibility of being sexually abused would need to be entered as reasons in addition to CP for this procedure to be approved.

When people with CP have children, what is the risk that their babies will have CP?

Since CP is not a genetic disorder, there is no genetic reason that the disorder would be passed on to the next generation. There has been concern that a problem with the woman's placenta might affect the baby, but recent studies indicate that this is not so. Also, the frequency of miscarriages and toxemia are no greater for women with CP than for other women. The majority of disabled adults have normal children, though parents with CP have more children with abnormalities of all kinds than the norm.

Life Span

What is the expected life span of someone with cerebral palsy?

In recent years, children with cerebral palsy have been surviving to adulthood in much greater numbers than ever before. In the general population of children, more than 99 percent survive to age 20, whereas approximately 90 percent of children with cerebral palsy survive to age 20. Those with no severe functional disabilities have a 99 percent survival to age 20, compared with those with severe functional limitations in all three major areas (ambulation, manual dexterity, and mental ability), whose survival is only 50 percent at age 20. Death is usually due to respiratory illness, often aspiration pneumonia or upper airway obstruction. As physicians become more vigorous in treating aspiration and gastroesophageal reflux with gastrostomy tubes and fundoplications, and in treating obstruction with tracheostomies, there is a greater chance that many more children with CP will survive into adulthood.

Sometimes a family is faced with having to decide whether to let their chronically ill child die or whether to introduce new and more intensive treatments, such as using a ventilator. Some families will choose to provide comfort to the child without any intensive intervention, while others will elect to do everything possible. Parents need to think about this issue *before* a crisis arises. It's helpful to talk it over with those who can provide emotional support, such as other family members, the family's or child's physician, or clergy. If possible, discuss it with the child herself. While there is no one right answer for all patients and their families, many families have to face making this decision at some point, and it is helpful to have thought about it in advance. You may also want to put your wishes into a document called an "Advanced Directive," which specifies what kind of treatments a patient would and would not want when being admitted to the hospital. A parent (or any adult) who is the guardian of a disabled child can complete this form on their child's behalf.

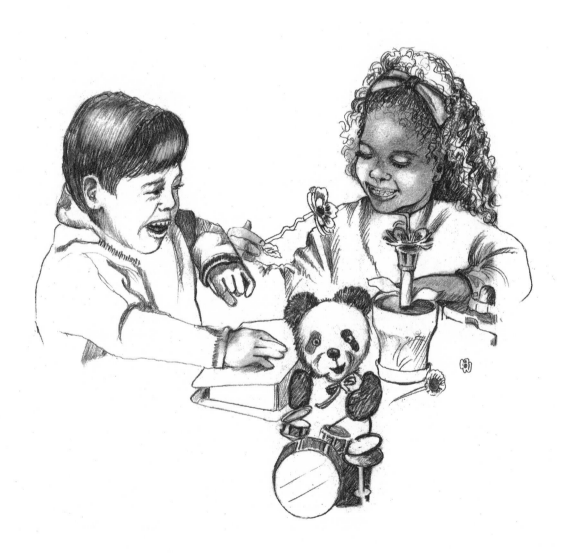

Intellectual, Psychological, and Social Development

♦ THIS CHAPTER explores how cerebral palsy affects the intellectual and psychological development of the individual from infancy, toddlerhood, and childhood through adolescence and young adulthood. We focus on the emotional and social development of children with cerebral palsy, and we also look at how children develop intellectually. We explore how cerebral palsy affects psychological development differently in different children, depending upon what part of the child's body is affected and how profound the involvement is. Family functioning is important to the well-being of a child with cerebral palsy, so in this chapter we pay attention to both the family and the child. In fact, since problems in the newborn are so devastating for families, we begin the chapter with a look at how families function.

Birth to One Year

The hallmark of emotional development during this period is the growing attachment between parents and their new baby. This attachment is dependent upon the interplay between the infant's characteristics (for example, his or her temperament) and the parents', and the interplay itself influences the child's emotional development. The child's intellectual development, on the other hand, is driven by the infant's motivation to reach out and discover the world by using sensorimotor actions on people and things around him or her. Cerebral palsy can affect the infant's emotional and intellectual development both directly, through the child's limitations, and indirectly, by the way the world responds to the child.

How might parents react when they hear that their child has cerebral palsy?

The discovery that their baby has a disability usually has a significant impact on parents and on how the family functions. Often the disability begins to have an impact before a diagnosis is made. In this case, parents "just know" that their child is not developing or behaving as they expected. They begin to be concerned that something is wrong with the baby, even though the doctor may not yet know whether or not something is wrong. Thus, parents sometimes experience anxiety and fear even before the doctor is finally able to deliver the diagnosis. The tension and fear experienced during this period of uncertainty often lead to stress and may begin to undermine the family unit even before the diagnosis has been made.

When they hear that their baby has cerebral palsy, parents often react by going into a state of shock or disbelief. Such a reaction to threatening and devastating news is natural and, indeed, expected. But individuals who are in this state are likely to experience stress even more keenly than they would if they were able to react normally. Shock and heightened stress often make it difficult for parents to take in all the information that the doctor gives them. Because of this, it's a good idea for parents to return to their doctor to go over information about their child's medical condition.

How does the initial reaction change over time?

As parents become better acquainted with their child and understand more about what cerebral palsy means, they develop different responses to their child's disability. Some parents cope by getting as involved with their infant's care as they can. This means that they investigate the nature of their baby's disability and take an active role in the baby's care and therapy.

For other parents, the grief, pain, and uncertainty that they feel about having a child with a disability is more than they can endure. To cope with these feelings, these parents sometimes either deny that their baby has a disability or they minimize its effect. Such denial is likely to become more apparent as the child gets older and the extent of the involvement becomes clearer. Other parents, laboring under these same stresses and feelings, continue to feel angry about what has happened to them.

Becoming actively involved in the infant's care and therapy is a healthy way of coping with the feelings a parent has when he or she discovers that an infant has cerebral palsy. Denial and anger, on the other hand, can have a negative effect on the child and the parents—indeed, such feelings take their toll on people and relationships throughout the family. Spouses who are persistently under stress, for example, might find that they argue more often. Sometimes the care and the long-term outlook for the disabled child are the source of the conflict. The end result of these reactions is that the parents emotionally distance themselves from the child. This, in turn, means that the much-needed emotional closeness between the parents and the child is diminished.

Families in this situation are vulnerable to continuing discord, which can lead to separation and divorce. Other children in the family can be affected by this persistent discord, too. They are often neglected or shunted aside for periods of time because their parents are preoccupied with the disabled baby. Brothers and sisters of a child with a disability are at higher risk for developing emotional, learning, and behavioral problems.

How does the family's emotional reaction affect the child?

If the parents deny that their child has a problem, they can't really absorb the information provided to them by doctors and other professionals involved in the care and treatment of their child. Without this information, parents may not be in a good position to make decisions about or take part in their child's treatment, or they may be unable to make proper use of the resources available to help.

A parent's negative emotional reaction can also inhibit development of a healthy relationship with the baby. For a few parents the pain and hurt may be so crippling that they become depressed and don't interact with their baby. These parents are psychologically and emotionally unavailable to the child. The result of this is a weakened attachment that may result in the abuse or neglect of the child. In response, the baby typically becomes withdrawn and depressed.

Some parents overprotect the child in situations they view as potentially harmful or dangerous. Overprotection may also stifle the child's development and inhibit the child's efforts to be more independent, which is usually seen in the second year of life.

Finally, some parents may react by overcompensating. They may ask the baby to do too much, or they may have higher expectations for the child's progress at any point in treatment than the child can realistically be expected to meet.

How can the family be helped?

Families need professional help and good support to come to terms with the fact that their baby has a disability. Ideally, help in the form of counseling, therapy, support groups, and sibling groups will be offered to the family within a reasonable time after the diagnosis is made. This help could go a long way toward preventing the development of unhealthy parental coping styles. It also prevents many of the other undesirable consequences mentioned.

How does the emotional tie between parent and child develop?

One important development in the first year of life is the establishment of a lasting tie between the baby and his or her parents in a process known as *attachment*. The strength of this tie is influenced by the way in which the baby and the parents respond to each other. The baby's appearance, vigor, and basic way of responding to the environment (that is, his or her temperament) are important factors, just as are the parents' skillfulness at tuning into the feelings of the baby and "reading" his or her needs. In addition, the parents' ability to adapt to the temperamental style of the infant (especially if he or she is fussy and irritable) plays a large role in the development of this tie. If secure attachments begin to develop with the infant early in life, they are demonstrated in many infants by a fear of strangers (which develops at around 7 to 8 months), by a sense of trust in the parents, and by a mutual love between infant and parent. The sense of trust and security, which for the young child go hand in hand, are of course undermined by parents who are not emotionally available to the baby or who abuse or neglect the baby. Failure to develop this sense of trust is demonstrated when a baby fails to thrive and grow or becomes either very negative or passive and withdrawn.

How are emotions expressed?

A second major development in the infant during this first year is emotional expression—the infant's ability to signal his or her feelings through facial expression, body tone, and activity in a way that is accurately communicated to caretakers. Basic emotional expressions of joy, sadness, and anger are common by the end of this phase of life. The development of the ability to express basic emotions is important because it helps the communication between parent and baby and cements the evolving relationship between them.

What is the relationship between the child's emotions and his or her actions?

A third development that begins to appear in this period is the growth of *motivation*. Motivation is a set of feelings that makes the baby act. The important motivational factors that develop during this period are the need to relate to others, the need to learn to use the body to get around, and the need to use toys and other materials and understand how they work. The development of motivational factors during this period of life is one of the building blocks for later emotional, social, and intellectual growth.

How does cerebral palsy affect these areas of emotional growth?

The influence of cerebral palsy on emotional growth during the first year of life depends on two factors: how parents cope with having an infant with a disability, and personal characteristics of the individual infant. The role of parental coping strategies has already been discussed; the baby's role is influenced by his or her temperament and the extent of the cerebral palsy.

An infant who has an engaging style of responding to his family, regardless of how much disability he might have, may conquer his parents' pain and fears and weave them into a tapestry of mutual love which will promote attachment and security. On the other hand, an infant who has a mild degree of disability but who nevertheless has a difficult temperament may intensify his parents' pain and fears and thereby frustrate his own emotional growth.

Much of the emotional development that takes place during the first year of life depends upon the infant's ability to signal needs and express emotions to his parents. This ability may be impeded in an infant who has either extremely low or high tone. For example, a baby who is very floppy and flaccid may not have the muscle strength to express emotions or needs in a way that will produce interaction with a parent. For an infant with very high tone (such as a child with spastic quadriplegia), the inability to control movement could inhibit or distort emotional expression. In either case, the lack of or distortion of the expression of emotions and needs may make it seem that the infant is not really responding when a parent is trying to "read" the baby and interpret his needs. This can be frustrating to parents and can lead them, over time, to spend less time interacting with the baby. This in turn can jeopardize attachment and security, and it can ultimately jeopardize the infant's emotional development.

What can parents do to cope with their child's expressive disability?

A parent whose child has either lack of or distortion of expression can be helped. The parent of a very low-toned infant can be taught to read the diminished or muted cues of the baby so that satisfying interaction takes place.

The parent of an infant who is severely involved (who has very high tone) can be taught to work with the infant by anticipating the baby's schedule and providing what the infant probably needs. Likewise, parents can learn to use a variety of soothing techniques to quiet a stiff, irritable child and to arouse their infant in a way that will promote love and communication. In addition, a consultation with a qualified mental health or health professional may be useful in helping parents work with these kinds of problems.

How can parents motivate the infant with cerebral palsy?

Cerebral palsy also has an impact on the baby's motivation to interact with her surroundings. Its effect is apparent in the infant's desire to master her body in order to move about and reach and grasp, and to make things work or happen: to play with toys, for example. The impulse to move about and explore is thwarted if the child has very low muscle tone. Alternatively, a child may have so much spasticity (tightness) that she can't move about or reach out, grasp, and manipulate toys and other objects. In either case, parents need to bring the world to the child. This means moving the baby to different rooms in the house or having the baby "ride along" when common household routines like cooking or cleaning are taking place. It also means presenting the baby with appropriate toys (like a rattle), showing the infant how the toy works (shaking the rattle to make a noise), and assisting the infant in her attempts to play with the toy.

Some babies with low tone may be less inclined to move about and manipulate toys. In this case parents can put desirable toys just out of reach, to motivate the baby to move and reach and grasp. It's especially important to teach the baby to be persistent in overcoming obstacles in order to attain a goal. The baby may have the desire to move about or to manipulate toys but may find it difficult to do this because of spasticity. In this case parents need to assist the baby in his efforts in a way that helps the baby reach his goal. This does not mean doing it for the baby; it means providing the minimal amount of support and assistance needed. For example, when the child learns that he can propel himself forward on his own to get a toy, or can grasp and move a rattle with his hand to produce a sound, he will feel a sense of accomplishment and will be encouraged to try other things. The baby's motivation to persist and to try to master tasks should be supported in a way that allows the baby to deal with a tolerable level of frustration and yet be successful. Parents may find it helpful to consult with an appropriate professional, such as a physical or occupational therapist, for ideas and help in these areas.

How does intelligence develop?

The development of intelligence during this period of life depends to a great extent on the infant's ability to anticipate regularly occurring events (so-called contingent relationships) and to use her sensorimotor system to explore objects, to discover the permanence of objects, and to come to recognize the uses of some objects commonly found in her environment (like toys).

The capacity of the baby to anticipate regularly occurring events comes about when the baby learns, for example, that crying and thrashing about will bring her contentment in the form of food, a diaper change, the chance to sleep, or the experience of being comforted in her mother's or father's arms. Under these conditions the infant learns that she can have an impact on her environment. Just as importantly, this sets the stage for development of trust and security, the beginning of a sense of mastery, and the beginning of the ability to understand cause-and-effect relationships. Of course, this early line of development depends on the parents' ability to understand the baby's cues and respond to them in a sensitive and suitable manner. Consistent failure by parents to respond in this manner may interfere with this line of growth. Difficulties of this sort may be overcome by consulting a qualified mental health professional.

How does discovering the world help a child develop intelligence?

The other major intellectual development during infancy is the baby's ability to discover the world of toys and other objects, including people. This begins before the baby can use his hands. It starts with the baby's looking at things and people and tracking them with his eyes as they move around. Indeed, by the time he is 3 or 4 months old, a baby can remember familiar faces and toys. More importantly, the ability to engage in such tracking helps the baby start to develop the concept of spatial relationships and the notion that objects are "real." The idea that objects are real is constructed during this period when the baby becomes aware that objects disappear and reappear as they travel around the environment. When the baby begins to use his or her hands to reach and grasp things, there is a surge in the pace of development.

At this point, when the baby has a toy in his hands, he can look at it, feel it, put it in his mouth, and listen to any noise it might make. In a like manner, the baby discovers that the toy makes a noise or does something else when he moves his hand. In this way the baby uses several sources of information to get an idea of what the toy is like. Thus, the baby begins to form ideas of objects that are similar (such as rattles) because they generally look and feel the same when held, and they make a similar noise when the hand is waved. By the same token, the infant also begins to discover that objects are substantial or real because he can use his hands to recover them when they fall or are dropped. Finally, the infant is further developing his sense of cause and effect, because he discovers that he can make toys do things that are interesting and fun.

How can cerebral palsy affect these experiences of discovery?

Cerebral palsy can have an impact on the infant's ability to develop an awareness of shared relationships. Infants who are very tight and spastic, for example, may have disruptive feeding patterns—they may have difficulty sucking, for example. This could interfere with the baby's ability to recognize that there is a relationship between (1) his or her hunger pangs, (2) crying, and (3) being soothed by food. A child who has very high tone and is tight may also be prone to being fussy and irritable, and therefore may not be able to appreciate his parents' efforts to soothe him at times of distress or upset. He may not be able to recognize the relationship between feelings of distress and their eventual decline.

The motor coordination involved in tracking people and objects as they move about can also be affected by cerebral palsy. The infant with either very low or very high muscle tone may not be able to engage in the kind of coordinated eye and head movement needed to do such tracking. Therefore, the beginning stages of the development of visual memory, spatial relationships, and so-called object permanence (the idea that objects are real and substantial) may be delayed or distorted in some manner.

Cerebral palsy can also disrupt the early growth of object recognition and the understanding of cause-and-effect relationships. The reason is that this early line of development normally hinges on the development of reaching and grasping. The coordination between the feel and sight of the object being grasped and whatever sound or action it produces when the hand is moved or waved is essential. Developmental delays might be expected in particular for infants whose disability affects their ability to use their hands to reach for, grasp, and manipulate toys and other objects. This would be the case when at least a moderate degree of spasticity is present in the upper trunk and upper limbs. Delays may also be seen in babies with extremely low tone, however. In any case, infants can be helped to compensate for this problem. Parents can show an interested infant how a toy like a rattle works, and help the baby play with the toy. Likewise, toys adapted to the infant's needs (such as toys with special switches) can be used to foster this development. Consulting a physical therapist, occupational therapist, or an early education specialist may be useful in helping parents stimulate their baby.

Ages One to Three

At this stage, the child becomes increasingly independent. At the same time, he or she begins to master control of body functions and impulses. Thus, the child learns to use the toilet successfully, and can also postpone gratification to some degree. This, too, is the time when the child begins to play with other children and learns the foundations of give and take.

Intellectually, this period is marked by the child's recognition that people and objects are substantial and real, by a growing sophistication in the understanding of cause-and-effect relationships, and by the ability to imitate. There is also tremendous development in the child's imagination, and she or he begins to use language.

What are the main issues in emotional and social development?

Children at this age display real evidence of emotional and social development: they strive to be independent; they test boundaries and limits; they begin to learn to control their impulses and feelings. This is primarily why children 18 to 36 months of age are described as going through "the terrible two's." This is the period when intense feelings, especially anger, are played out by the child, and children throw temper tantrums as a way of expressing unhappiness and frustration.

Another hallmark of social development during this period is increased socialization with peers. At this age, children move from being the lone actor on the stage (except for interaction with parents) to having at least one playmate. Over the course of these two years the child comes to enjoy being with children, learns how to share toys and other possessions, and learns how to deal with his own feelings and those of other children in the context of budding social relationships.

In some ways this period is marked by the struggle for independence as well as the struggle to find out where the limits are—all influenced by the child's temperament (and his or her parents' temperament) and the child's sense of emotional security. A high-strung and highly active child, for example, is generally more tempestuous and headstrong than a laid-back toddler. A more easygoing toddler may not put up as much resistance to having things done for him or having limits set on his behavior. A lack of security and trust can either intensify or stifle the striving for independence, depending upon whether the child is highly anxious and defensive or not. The rearing styles and personal attributes of parents (their patience and resilience, for example) influence the ease with which both toddler and parent get through this period of development.

How might cerebral palsy affect the child's independence?

The child with cerebral palsy can have a difficult time gaining a sense of independence and learning self-control. Ordinarily children at this age develop a sense of independence by trying to do things for themselves (like using a spoon to feed themselves) and by moving about and exploring the environment. The child who does not have use of her hands or who cannot move around (such as a child with diplegia or quadriplegia) may not be in a position to assert her willfulness or growing sense of independence in a way that would foster both a sense of autonomy and a sense of self-control. Sometimes, too, issues of control between parent and child are played out in an exaggerated fashion in any area where the child does have some power (such as eating).

Other factors, such as mental retardation, can also impede this area of development. Likewise, parents who have a hard time letting go of their child, who cannot see the child as a person in his or her own right, and who foster a great deal of dependence in the child may interfere with or distort the child's progress in this area. Finally, a child who by temperament is very passive or who perhaps has very low tone may find it hard to muster the energy to test limits or to get into things that would bring him into confrontation with a parent and thus eventually promote autonomy and independence.

How might cere-bral palsy affect the child's self-control?

The toddler develops the ability to master feelings (especially anger and frus-tration) and to control impulses by interacting socially with parents, other adults, and other children. To some extent, because a child with cerebral palsy may have restricted use of his hands and limited mobility, he may not develop these skills as readily. However, these restrictions aren't as likely to interfere with the child's development of self-control as much as they are with his development of independence.

Cerebral palsy *is* likely to have an impact on how the parents confront the child when he is angry or out of control, or when he cannot immediately get a desired object at the very moment he wants it. Parents who see the child as an individual, who let the child know they understand these feelings, and who nevertheless, when necessary, exercise appropriate disciplinary tech-niques are going to foster growth and promote the child's ability to master his feelings. On the other hand, parents who believe that they need to cod-dle and cater to their toddler, perhaps because of his disability, are less likely to help the child come to terms with strong feelings and impulses; this ap-proach can delay or distort the child's development of self-control.

What is cerebral palsy's effect on socialization?

The growth of peer socialization which takes place during this time is de-pendent on the child's having access to other children. For a child with cere-bral palsy, this access may be limited by the parents' protectiveness, the atti-tudes of other parents toward having their child play with a child who has a disability, and the child's own ability to keep up with other children in play activities.

At about two years of age is an ideal time for a child to play with or be a part of a peer group that includes children without disabilities, because most children this age are very accepting of children who are different from them. They will usually adapt and adjust to the other child's limitations if helped to do so by a caring adult. This is easier to do with a child who has a mild to moderate degree of motor impairment, but it is even possible to integrate a toddler with a severe disability in the extremities if this is done with careful planning. For the child without a disability, playing with a child who has one teaches tolerance, patience, and generosity. The child with a disability has an opportunity to learn that he can be accepted and to learn social skills.

It is important not to ask the disabled child to play with children who are much older or who are much more advanced in social and intellectual skills. (This is true for children whether they have a disability or not.)

What is normal intellectual devel-opment like at this age?

At this age, most babies go through tremendous changes in their intellectual development. Indeed, the 3-year-old child barely resembles the child she was at 1 year in terms of thinking and problem-solving skills. The major mile-stones of intellectual development that usually occur during this period are the development of a sophisticated understanding of cause-and-effect re-lationships, the ability to imitate what has been seen and heard some time after the incident has occurred, the ability to represent reality in internal thought or images and through the spoken word, and the ability to use speech as a way of communicating ideas and needs to other people.

The child continues to learn the concept of object permanence, which is necessary before she can master verbal, spatial, and mathematical concepts. It is not until the child comes to understand that toys and other objects still exist when they are out of sight (a concept a 1-year-old cannot understand) that she can begin to lump objects together by one or more common features, can start to map out where things belong in the environment, and can begin to count objects or order them along some physical dimension (such as smallest to largest).

How does the understanding of cause and effect develop?

The appreciation of cause-and-effect relationships begins during the first year of life when, for example, the baby aimlessly waves his hand to produce a sound from a rattle, and then realizes that it's the hand shaking that causes the effect (the sound). Children ages 2 and 3 play with much more advanced toys (progressing from a busy box to a wind-up toy) and use more advanced methods of problem solving (for example, to get things that are out of reach). Indeed, this is when children first use tools to solve problems (getting a chair to stand on in order to get something that is out of reach, for example). By the beginning of the third year, the child can solve a problem by thinking about it and then getting what is needed to solve the problem. At this age, solutions to problems are concrete; they are mainly carried out using motor skills and materials available in the surrounding environment. Later the child is able to solve mental problems.

What is the role of imitation and representation?

During this period of development, imitation and representation are tied to each other. Indeed, the ability to represent internally some aspect of reality grows out of imitation. In this case, imitation means that the child can copy an act that he has seen someone else do or repeat something that he has heard someone else say. As the child matures during this period, imitation becomes increasingly more sophisticated in terms of the succession of acts and phrases that can be copied and the amount of time that passes between the time the child notes the activity and repeats it. Thus, imitative activity changes: rather than precisely mimicking an action or spoken phrase immediately after seeing it or hearing it, the child now puts together internal thoughts or images and creates his or her own sentences or actions.

The capacity to form images stems from repeatedly imitating the same acts until, in a sense, they are committed to memory in the form of an internal picture. With maturation the child relies less on repetitive imitation to form such images. These images are pictures or representations of aspects of the growing child's reality. It is the ability to represent reality in the mind that allows a child to engage in different forms of imaginary play, such as playing roles (for example, pretending to be a doctor) or playing make-believe (for example, having a tea party with friends). Of course, the ability to represent reality increases with age and enriches the child's play and thinking.

How does speech develop?

Speech development undergoes a significant evolution during this time frame. For one thing, there is a dramatic increase in the number of words the child can string together. The child progresses from an infant who has a few words at her disposal to the 2-year-old who can combine two or three words. As a 3-year-old she can very nearly hold a conversation: stringing several words together in order to express feelings, thoughts, or needs. The complexity of the communicative intent on the part of the child evolves from one word expressing a need or describing an action to the use of phrases or sentences that aid the child in expressing thoughts and ideas, in communicating present and future needs, and in developing her relationships with adults and peers. Likewise, the child, over this span of time, learns to put spoken words in the correct order so that others can understand her better. The child also develops the ability to engage in the give-and-take of social conversations in a culturally acceptable manner.

How might cerebral palsy affect intellectual development with respect to these skills?

Much of the intellectual development that occurs between 1 and 3 years seems to rely on the coordination of input from the senses with movement (such as crawling or walking) and hand use. This is particularly true for the development of object permanence, cause-and-effect relationships, and representational thought. But it is also true for speech, because much of what a child knows and can talk about at this age comes from what the child learns by doing.

As discussed before, the child with cerebral palsy may meet with difficulties in this area of growth because of limitations in mobility or hand use. Development could be even further jeopardized if there is any reduction or distortion in the input from the senses of vision, hearing, or touch. The child who is disabled in a way that severely restricts her ability to move about could show some delays in the development of object permanence and spatial relationships. However, even in this case, the child who is capable of using her hands can overcome this kind of impediment. Thus, for example, the baby who is able to search for and pick up a toy that falls from behind her is getting the kind of information that will probably allow development in these areas to proceed.

Impaired hand use is often a major obstacle to development in this area. A child who has a great deal of spasticity in the upper extremities or throughout the body may be more hindered in intellectual development than if only his legs were affected. This is because ordinarily the ability to manipulate toys and objects and play with them in both familiar and novel ways is essential to intellectual development. For example, losing and finding objects stimulates the development of object permanence; making the jack-in-the-box pop up stimulates recognition of cause and effect; and giving the dolly a drink is a way to learn imitation and representation. By the same token, delays here can also affect speech development in the sense that the child, because of these drawbacks, may not form the ideas and concepts that most children talk about at this age (not to mention that speech is a highly coordinated motor activity that may be impaired due to the cerebral palsy).

How can a child who is severely affected by cerebral palsy be helped in these areas?

Delays in intellectual development are not always inevitable when a young child with cerebral palsy is severely disabled in hand usage. Some young children who have severe disabilities do overcome such major obstacles and become intellectually competent. How this happens is not entirely understood, although experts believe that the child's inborn intellectual ability may have significant influence. However, it may be the way that parents bring the outside world to such a child or allow the child to interact with toys and people that plays a significant role here.

Parents who help the child play with toys or work with switches may help the child overcome the barriers posed by the disability. By the same token, parents who in a sensitive way help the child cope with the frustration of trying to reach or manipulate toys and other objects are probably encouraging the child's intellectual development. Parents who support efforts on the part of a child who has these kinds of limitations are most likely building the child's sense of mastery over the environment as well as helping the child learn to be persistent and diligent in the face of physical hurdles.

Finally, the process of talking to the child and, most importantly, actively trying to understand the child's attempts to communicate can facilitate the development of ideas that might not otherwise come about in a child with a severe motor impairment. Likewise, listening to such a child in a way that allows the child to communicate, be it with language, gesture, gaze, pointing, or signing, promotes in the young child the idea that communication is an interactive and social activity.

Ages Four to Seven

These years are marked by an increase in the child's investment in peer relationships and forming friendships. It is also a time when the young child begins to develop a sense of identity and a sense of right and wrong. At the same time, the youngster is learning to reason concretely and to solve problems, and is beginning to master academic subjects such as reading and mathematics.

What are the typical social and emotional developments?

The child's desire for autonomy and independence begins to manifest itself in a different way, as the child begins to separate physically from his parents. Socialization includes making friends with peers, typically of the same sex.

Indeed, this is an age when friendships and contacts with peers begin to play an increasingly dominant role in the child's life, starting a trend that will continue to gather strength and direction until at least the time of young adulthood. The move to peer friendships makes it more important than ever that the child learn to share, to take turns in games and other pursuits, and, most importantly, to see things through other persons' eyes.

How does a sense of identity develop?

A major development during this period is the child's increased sense of identity. The identity that begins to take shape at this age will be influential in forming the child's attitudes and aspirations for the future. Identity is often an important factor in shaping the child's idea of what it means to be male or female. Identity formation happens at this age, as the child begins to identify closely with a parent or other significant adult, typically of the same sex. For example, a son may take on the personal characteristics of his father or pretend to do some of the same things that the father does at home and at work. This process continues throughout childhood but becomes suppressed to some extent by the onset of adolescence.

What about the child's sense of morality?

This is the time when the child develops a conscience and a sense of guilt. The development of a moral sense depends upon the child's intellectual capacity, but its shape is a function of the values practiced and taught by parents and other significant adults and, to a lesser extent, by peers.

How might cerebral palsy affect these areas of development?

At this point the impact of having cerebral palsy changes. The child's sensorimotor abilities are less influential on development at this age than they were in earlier developmental stages. Instead, what becomes increasingly important is the child's access to a range of social relationships.

Specifically, children need to be around parental figures or other adults who are nurturing and caring and who will serve as role models to reinforce the child's own identity. Parents and other significant adults should work at instilling pride in the child with respect to his abilities, whatever they might be, and in his physical makeup, even though the child may be different from the majority of people around him. It's important to help such a child recognize his disability and take pride in his accomplishments—it's essential to *maximize self-esteem*. One boy reflected back on his memories of his first awareness that he was different from other children, and the process of coming to terms with that realization:

The first time I realized that something might be wrong with me was when I would go for therapy. At first, I thought it was a normal routine; I thought that everybody did it. Then, as I got older, I realized it wasn't something that other kids were doing. I wondered what was wrong with me. I probably should have asked, but I don't remember asking. I should have, but I think it would have been painful. I was sad. It was hard knowing that something was wrong with me. I remember thinking, "Why me? Why me?"

Another thing that I remember was when I realized that I had to have more operations than other people. That was hard. Why did I have to do this? Why did I have so much pain?

When I was very young, I also noticed that I still crawled while other kids were able to walk. I decided that it just wasn't my time yet to learn how to walk. Later I realized that I wasn't going to be able to walk. That made me sad. Getting a powered wheelchair helped. Things are much better now. I've come to accept my disability, and I will keep trying to fight on to be the best I can be.

Ultimately helping the child understand and own his disability will help the child to cope with any ridicule or rebuff he may encounter as a result of his disability. To do other than help the child maximize self-esteem—and especially to try to make the child pass for being normal—is to lower the child's ability to cope with whatever emotional, social, and physical adversity he encounters while growing up with a disability.

Children with cerebral palsy also need to have the opportunity to be in social settings with children their same age, such as preschools or elementary schools, in order to learn to relate to peers who aren't disabled. The social engineering that must be done to integrate a child into such a setting is far easier at this age than later on. To some extent, moderate to severe sensory or intellectual impairments make this harder to do, but even a child with these impairments will profit from having some kind of access to peers without disabilities.

These arrangements also allow children without disabilities to learn to accept the kinds of differences presented by people with disabilities. Acceptance can be encouraged by providing the child who has a moderate to severe motor impairment with adaptive devices, such as computer-aided communication devices, that make it easier for the child to participate in classroom activities and to communicate with peers and teachers. Children at this age who do not have disabilities can learn to be comfortable with modifications made in classroom activities to accommodate the child with cerebral palsy.

How does a child's ability to think change over time?

At this age, children generally begin to think, reason, and solve problems using their toys and educational materials to help them. For example, preschoolers learn to count and to sort and group objects by use (such as things that bounce), by name (such as cars), and by physical attributes like size and color. Children at this age are able to think about what they are doing with their toys and other objects and sometimes invent new ways of using them. They are also able to think about their friends, recognize that their friends and playmates have feelings of their own, and take these feelings into account in their peer relationships.

In general, this is a period when thinking becomes more abstract, but the child still must rely on objects to support her thinking. The development of such thinking skills is essential to the child's early academics (counting and letter recognition, for example) and to her later ability to think more abstractly.

What is the role of speech?

Language spoken by the 4- to 7-year-old resembles adult forms of speech in terms of grammar, since the child's grammar at this age is nearly as sophisticated as an adult's. By this time most children have acquired an extensive vocabulary corresponding to the world around them, although the child does not yet have the vocabulary of an adult. Finally, it is at this point that the child becomes aware of the speaker-listener relationship and begins to learn the rules of conversation so that he can effectively communicate with others. Development of language skills—grammar, vocabulary, and rules of conversation—is of course important for the child's ability to communicate, but it also plays a significant role in his ability to learn how to read and write.

What kind of impact can cerebral palsy have on these developmental issues?

During this period, intellectual development usually progresses through play and schooling. Cerebral palsy may interfere with development in this area because it may interfere with integration of the child's motor and sensory skills. A child who has severe to moderate impairment (such as spasticity) involving the upper extremities may have difficulty engaging in the kind of play that ordinarily results in the ability to think about how different things relate to one another. Other factors such as native intelligence can work in such a child's favor, that is, the brighter the child, the more likely he is to learn these thinking skills, even with minimum input from his own efforts.

The child's efforts to learn from play should be promoted by parents and others who can support the effort to manipulate educational materials. Professional therapists who work with the child can provide some of this encouragement. Toys and equipment can be adapted, too, to fit the needs of a particular child. She can also be encouraged to experience play vicariously, by watching other children. The overall goal is to help children with an impairment experience this level of play in some way, so that the impediments to intellectual growth posed by their disability are diminished.

Unlike intellectual development, the development of communication skills is very closely tied to social interaction. To develop communication skills, a child with cerebral palsy—especially one with a moderate to severe degree of motor involvement—must have the chance to relate to people in a way that encourages communication and teaches the child the rules of conversation. But speaking is only one way of communicating. The child with cerebral palsy may have to rely on gesture, signing, or a communication device to "talk" to others. All efforts to communicate, whatever form they take, should be encouraged at this age. If language skills and relationships with friends who are not disabled aren't fostered until later on, the child with limited ability to communicate may find that his peers have less patience with his limitations.

Ages Eight to Twelve

During these years the young child is working on peer relationships and refining her sense of right and wrong. It is also a time when the child becomes more independent of her parents in terms of activities and relationships. Finally, it is a time when a great deal of energy is devoted to schooling and to learning the basic academic skills involved in reading, writing, and mathematics.

What are the social and emotional milestones of this age span?

Personality, peer relationships, and the development of a sense of morality take on more importance. In the early years of this period, the family still has a major influence on the child's personality and moral development. Values embraced and expressed by peers also contribute to the child's emotional and social development. Indeed, by age 12, a good deal of a child's personality and moral sense has usually been formed. The child's own inherent or constitutional makeup also influences this development.

Especially toward the end of this period, the child develops relationships and friendships, particularly with children of the same sex, that last for a long time, sometimes for a lifetime. The child's social world begins to be dominated by friends rather than by his parents. The child's friends begin to serve as important models in terms of gender roles and in terms of determining, in some part, the child's interests, social mores, and value systems. Since choice in friends is to some extent influenced by values already established by the family, this wider social network and its influence is typically consistent with the child's family background.

What about increasing freedom at this age?

This is also a period during which the child gains greater freedom from the home and becomes less reliant on parents for entertainment. The child begins to learn how to get around the neighborhood and the community by himself. He may travel to school independently of his parents and, in a few years, he may go shopping or participate in social or sports functions without always having one or both parents present.

How does cerebral palsy affect these developments?

Cerebral palsy can influence social and emotional development since it sometimes has an impact on peer relationships. A child with a motor impairment, especially if it is moderate to severe, may be impeded in her ability to get around with her nondisabled peer group. Also, the kind of activities that bind children together at this age involve the ability to converse freely with one another and often involve the use of both the legs and the hands (in sports activities, for example). Thus, a child who lacks the motor ability to talk, or whose movement is impaired even to a mild extent, may have less access to peers and peer socialization.

Another reason cerebral palsy may affect this line of development is that the child begins to stand out as being different from most children his age, and marked physical and mental differences sometimes result in the child's being rejected by children who don't have disabilities. Even the child with a very mild degree of cerebral palsy may be socially isolated.

What qualities enable the child to cope best with these stresses?

There's no question that the child with cerebral palsy must have a lot of courage and determination to deal with the possible rebuffs, cruelty, and rejection she will encounter. The child must reach out for people in spite of rejection, and must continue to want to achieve in school and other settings. In order to do this the child must already have a very strong, positive self-image. In fact, this is probably the determining factor for keeping the child moving ahead during this and the next phase of life (adolescence).

What can parents do?

To achieve this kind of positive self-image, the child needs to have—and to continue to have—parents or other significant adults who nurture and care about him and who see him as a person in his own right. Parents should promote interactions between their child and adults and other children by introducing him into settings where peer interaction is more likely to be successful. The child may need to use adaptive devices to achieve better communication, mobility, and hand usage. Parents must begin early in their child's life to encourage and reward him for mastering a variety of social and play situations and for all the special talents the child may possess.

During this period, the child with cerebral palsy needs his parents to be available, to listen when he is wounded by peer rebuff or cruelty. Given proper support and encouragement, the child can effectively communicate and vent his feelings. The parent can help the child understand why other children behave this way and, more importantly, can interpret such incidents in a way that does not undermine the child's self-esteem and self-image.

Finally, parents, during this time, must continue to be effective advocates for the child. In the area of social and emotional growth, this means allowing the child access to peers who are likely to be accepting. It may mean, in some instances, fighting hard to prevent the child's segregation into a special school or a restrictive classroom setting: the child who is in a regular classroom benefits from having relationships and friendships with children without disabilities who are at his social and intellectual level. It may also mean that parents and other significant adults have to challenge the child at times to behave in ways that will foster such relationships. Parents may need to seek the help of a skilled counselor to guide them and their child through what can sometimes be a turbulent period of life.

What are the major intellectual tasks at this age?

The major intellectual tasks for children during this age occur at school, where they learn to read, to express themselves in written language, and to perform fundamental mathematical calculations. Additionally, this is the time when the child learns to accept the structure and rules of the classroom and to obey the teacher.

How can this stage of development be affected by cerebral palsy?

Cerebral palsy can affect schooling and classroom learning in a number of ways. The level of the child's intelligence and, as a corollary, the child's ability to learn is scrutinized at this time, especially for children with a severe disability. It is difficult to evaluate the intellectual ability of the child with restricted hand use and limited speech, and it is not uncommon for such children to be judged as intellectually less proficient than they are. Inaccurate assessment frequently results in inappropriate classroom placement.

Many of these children have disabilities that make it difficult to assess what they know and what they have learned. Indeed, it is important to make a distinction here between learning and performance. It is likely that many children with cerebral palsy with moderate to severe impairment can learn, sometimes on a par with their peers. The problem is that the child cannot communicate this to others by writing or speaking.

Children with cerebral palsy may have other subtle impairments that interfere with learning and performance in the classroom. Some children have a learning disability such as dyslexia (normal vision but an inability to interpret written language), which is tied to their central nervous system disorder. Some children may also, for the same reason, have short attention spans or the inability to store or retain knowledge. Finally, the child with cerebral palsy may have a limited ability to accept adult authority and classroom rules and structure, depending upon how much past opportunity the child has had for this kind of interaction.

A child who has had the earlier experiences of learning to share with peers and to accept rules when playing with other children will have an easier time. By the same token, the child who has learned to accept the authority of his parents and to take responsibility for his own acts will find it much easier to be an active and appreciated participant in the classroom.

How can teachers and parents help?

Educators first must identify children who cannot demonstrate their level of learning. Then they must provide the child with the means to get over this barrier. This can be accomplished by providing her with suitable alternatives for expressing or demonstrating what she is learning. The child might do very well working at a computer, for example, or using computer-assisted communication devices. Sometimes a tutorial or one-on-one session between a teacher and the child is the best way to unblock communication. Also, parents need to be aware of possible problems with reading, and teachers should be on the lookout for telltale signs of such problems and be available for extra help. When teachers and parents are insensitive to a child's individual learning capabilities, they may condemn the child unnecessarily to academic failure, and this may lower self-esteem and decrease the motivation to learn.

Ages Thirteen to Eighteen

These years are more often than not marked by emotional turbulence. During this period the adolescent struggles with self-identity, with increased physical and emotional independence from parents and family, with sexual impulses, and with the growing influence of his or her peer group. Likewise, the adolescent's thinking, problem-solving, and reasoning skills often move from the concrete to a more abstract and mature level. Finally, during this time, youngsters are beginning to make career or vocational choices that may carry into adulthood.

What are the primary areas of social and emotional development?

Sooner or later, almost every adolescent goes through a stormy period. The major issues of the turbulent teens include striving for independence and autonomy, the increasing importance of peer relationships, and, most of all, managing the surge of sexual feelings and impulses.

It is during this period that many young people gain a conclusive sense of their own identity and autonomy. It is also the time when young people gain mobility, as they are increasingly able to come and go from their homes and other places in the community without continual adult supervision. Social activities at this age often do not include parents or other family members.

Most young people at this age form long-term friendships with peers that in some cases last a lifetime. Indeed, the young person typically develops a social circle of peers who help define her interests and recreational activities and to some extent dictate who and what is socially acceptable and unacceptable. Being part of a peer group often leads young persons to rebel against family and cultural traditions and expectations.

During this period, sexual feelings and impulses develop, and adolescents begin to recognize and express them. Sexual expression often develops against the backdrop of family, religious, cultural, and peer group values—value systems that are frequently at odds with each other. The young adolescent also begins to recognize his sexual identity and orientation and starts to come to terms with it in some fashion. Adolescents begin to develop relationships that have sexual overtones, typically involving members of the opposite sex. This ushers in a period of dating, of expressing sexuality with someone else (including often deciding if and when one should become sexually active), and moving into short- and long-term relationships with a partner.

In what ways can cerebral palsy have an effect on these areas?

As previously mentioned, motor impairment that interferes with mobility and communication can restrict autonomy as well as access to peers and members of the opposite sex and the expression of sexual feelings and impulses. Likewise, severe or profound intellectual deficiencies often diminish interest in sex and the expression of sexual impulses. But in many cases the impediments to full development in these areas are more emotional and social than physical. The young adult with cerebral palsy may already have encountered so much rebuff and ridicule from peers that he or she is afraid of rejection or failure and therefore is unwilling to take a chance on dating or intimacy. Thus the experiences that normally lead to a mature expression of sexual feelings are often avoided or put off until sometime later.

Growth may also be hindered by lack of social access. For some adolescents, social isolation (due, for example, to the adolescent's need to attend a separate school) may be the reason there is not much opportunity for interaction with peers, and especially with potential sexual partners. But lack of opportunity for interaction may also be due to the fact that young people with cerebral palsy, regardless of type or severity of disability, are often viewed as "different" by able-bodied peers and thus are rejected. Sometimes such a young person is accepted only in a very limited sense—he or she may be seen as a great pal, for example, but not as a prospective dating partner (this is particularly true in early adolescence).

Most young adults with cerebral palsy have the same sexual feelings and impulses as their able-bodied peers. Denying this—which happens frequently—robs young people with cerebral palsy of their dignity and their right to experience the fullness of life. It is therefore essential that parents and other significant individuals give these young adults the opportunity, over time, to explore and express their sexual nature, within the context of the family's value system. Professional advice and counsel can be invaluable here.

What are the major characteristics of intellectual development at this age?

One of the hallmarks of this period is that the young person develops the ability to think abstractly. This means that ideas, words, and other abstract symbols dominate when the individual is trying to solve a problem. The ability to think abstractly is seen in the young person's schoolwork (when doing algebra problems, for example) as well as in social relationships, where more abstract moral and ethical considerations color how young people relate to one another.

Whether or not an individual can reach this stage of thinking is partly dependent on her or his mental abilities. However, every individual needs a great degree of social and intellectual experience, as well as schooling, before being able to reach this stage of thinking. Individuals who are delayed in their intellectual development, and particularly those who are mentally retarded, either will be delayed in reaching this stage of thinking or will never actually reach it.

Another significant milestone that occurs during this period is that young people begin to make and sometimes finalize their vocational and career choices. Adolescents, especially by the time they get to high school, typically start making choices that will lead them into a trade or profession. Choices here are often dictated by the young person's interests and talents, but these factors may be circumscribed by family background and tradition, perceived gender roles, and ethnic and socioeconomic considerations. Encouragement and nurturing from parents, other significant adults, other family members, and friends may also influence a young person's career aspirations.

How might cerebral palsy affect this development?

Cerebral palsy may or may not affect the young person's capacity to engage in abstract thinking and problem solving. For example, the young person who has a disability that has produced moderate to severe intellectual deficits most likely will not attain this level of thinking. Associated visual, hearing, or learning handicaps may also delay or inhibit such development. However, many people with cerebral palsy, even those with significant physical impairment, have normal intellectual abilities and can achieve a great deal, as this letter from one child with CP testifies:

My name is. . . . These are my thoughts on obtaining membership in the Order of the Arrow and the rank of Eagle Scout.

When I was sworn into Scout Troop 652 on . . . , I didn't really know what to expect. I wanted to explore things for a bit. At that time I remember one of my friends was going to get his Eagle rank. I was, of course, happy for him, but I didn't know what it entailed. I went to his ceremony. When I saw all they gave him and did to honor him, for the first time in my life I wanted that—badly. I knew that I would have to try my best to get it. I knew that you couldn't get Eagle after you turned 18, and I was 14. I only had a few years to work on this. After one camping trip, I remember coming home and saying to my father, "Dad, I want to be an Eagle." And so we went to work. Dad agreed to help me. I attacked this like I never worked on anything before. I realized this was something I could do. I can't play football or any other sports, but I knew I could do this.

Now, it is 3½ years later and I am waiting for my ceremony. My badges are complete—25 of them. I worked on three projects for the three highest ranks. For Star projects, I raised $6,500 to have a hydraulic lift installed on the Scout bus. Before that my Scoutmasters would have to lift us, our wheelchairs, and all the gear for the camping trip into the bus. For Life project I painted, with lots of helpers, an auditorium in the church where our troop meets. For Eagle project I realized the need to have badge books put on cassette tapes. This is how I did all my merit badges, because of my vision problems. My father recorded the ones we did at home, and I used those plus several more that Scout friends recorded for me.

On September 18 I passed the Eagle Board of Review, which is the final test before the National Council scrutinizes the folder with the application, the summary of projects, and letters of recommendation. I feel that I have achieved a lifelong dream. It makes me feel fulfilled and proud. This is the one thing that I tried and came out successful. I can say to any other disabled kids who are thinking about doing something and are not sure they can, "Try your best. Don't give up. If you do it, great! If you don't make it, at least you know you tried your darndest."

Many factors influence the young adult's ability to attain the capacity for abstract thought. Previous stimulation and social experience can either aid or stunt such development. Access to appropriate schooling can also promote or arrest the child's progress toward attaining this kind of thinking ability.

The impact of cerebral palsy on vocational and career decisions has many facets. Again, significant impairment in intellectual, learning, visual, or hearing capacity may ultimately restrict the kind of education and training the child receives and, as a result, limit the vocational choices the young person can make. But even the less involved child or the child who is bright but quite physically disabled may face unnecessary limits on choices. In this case, it is vital to recognize, early on, the child's potential and to assist him (with therapy and educational assistance) to overcome these barriers to more fully develop his abilities.

What can be done to help children overcome these problems?

Children with cerebral palsy must be able to obtain an education that will put them into a position to exercise their choices as widely as possible. This again means that parents and other significant adults must, on the one hand, advocate for the child's appropriate educational needs and, on the other hand, provide the child with the assistive devices, aids, and tutors that may be necessary for him to learn and express what he knows. The child needs to be stimulated and challenged educationally while at the same time people who matter to the child must consistently motivate him or her to persist in the face of whatever odds are stacked against short- and long-term success.

It's important not to undersell or oversell the child. Thus, good counseling and assessment are important in the decision-making process. Likewise, every attempt must be made to insure that, as he grows toward adolescence, the child is exposed to the social world in a way that enables him to interact appropriately with people in a variety of situations. Good social skills are a significant determinant of the young person's access to employment. Finally, it's important to know and understand the laws with regard to the disabled person's right to an appropriate education and to employment without discrimination. The parents and child who understand their rights in this regard are going to be in a better position to advocate for the young person with cerebral palsy to attain his or her ultimate career or vocation.

Adulthood

The major issues of adulthood revolve around the formation of long-term relationships such as marriage, the direct expression of love and sexuality, the raising of children, and finding a job or career that will firmly establish independence.

Most adults who are able to express sexual feelings and impulses are interested in settling into a suitable relationship. This involves finding a partner, making a commitment, and, often, working toward making it a long-term relationship. Such relationships are dependent on communication; only through communication can needs of the involved individuals be met. And relationships are composed of practical issues as well as emotional ones. Decisions about child bearing, child rearing, household responsibilities, and finances must be made and carried through.

How might cerebral palsy affect adult developmental issues?

For adults with cerebral palsy who have adequate intellectual skills, quality of life and adjustment are influenced more than anything else by the attitudes they hold about themselves and by the attitudes of able-bodied people toward them. It is true that moderate to severe motor impairment of any kind, particularly if it extends to all areas of functioning, can be a stumbling block in working out a long-term relationship, having sex, and rearing children. However, the willingness of each partner to explore these limitations and to seek out the appropriate professionals (such as physicians, therapists, and psychologists) who can help the couple confront the physical barriers to a meaningful relationship can go a long way to overcome such problems.

What is crucial, then, is a sense of self-esteem and self-worth in the individual adult. For many, if not most, adults with cerebral palsy, it takes a good deal of strength, persistence, and courage to socialize with adults without disabilities, and to reach out to try to form relationships that are deep and lasting. For it is likely that most individuals with cerebral palsy will have encountered, at some time in their lives, some degree of rejection and even cruelty when trying to form friendships.

The physical disability of the adult with cerebral palsy may create some obstacles to employment. The more the impairment limits mobility, hand use, or communication, the greater these obstacles will be. Nevertheless, assistive devices like computers can be used to integrate the adult with cerebral palsy into the workplace. Again, it is important that individuals become familiar with federal and state laws governing employment of the disabled so that they can act to make certain that their opportunities are not being unfairly—and unlawfully—limited.

What tools are most important to the adult with cerebral palsy?

The adult needs the kind of self-esteem and strength that allows her to weather rebuff and rejection while continuing to risk finding friends and partners. The sources of self-esteem and persistence have been discussed throughout this chapter: these attitudes come from being loved and held in high esteem by family members and friends, and from being seen as a person with talent, value, and skills that can be put to use in the everyday world. An infant, child, adolescent, and young adult who has support from parents, friends, and perhaps an encouraging counselor is better prepared to handle problems.

The attitudes of able-bodied people toward the adult with cerebral palsy also play a role. It is likely that some adults with cerebral palsy only find a limited number of people who are available for friendships, and perhaps even fewer who are open to sexual or long-term relationships. Again, high self-esteem, courage, and persistence are important assets for the adult with cerebral palsy. Likewise, such adults benefit from having had experiences with peers in late childhood and in adolescence that taught them appropriate social skills.

Finally, it is important for parents, relatives, and other significant adults in the individual's life to recognize that this person is going to experience the same need for a sexual outlet and a loving relationship as anyone else. Disability should not automatically exclude young adults from experiencing the fullest measure of life possible; therefore parents, relatives, and friends must encourage and pave the way for such experiences, rather than prevent them.

In addition to job-related training, the adult needs good work skills and the ability to get along with others in the workplace, both of which are known to be highly related to success and stability on the job. Again, the experiences the child has all through the growing-up years influence his or her ability to succeed as an adult.

In this chapter we have described how cerebral palsy affects intellectual and psychological development. We have seen clearly that the life pattern for the person with cerebral palsy is set early. In the end, parents and the person with cerebral palsy walk a fine line throughout life in terms of expectations. It is easy to set them either too high or too low. There is no easy way to manage this tightrope act. Seeking appropriate counsel from physicians, therapists, and other professionals along the way is often helpful, but in the final analysis, both parents and child need to know when to forge ahead and when to pull back if the stresses and barriers are unmanageable. The real goal is to help children with cerebral palsy grow into adults who feel good about themselves and their abilities, adults who are fulfilled because they are able to experience the joys and disappointments that life has to offer.

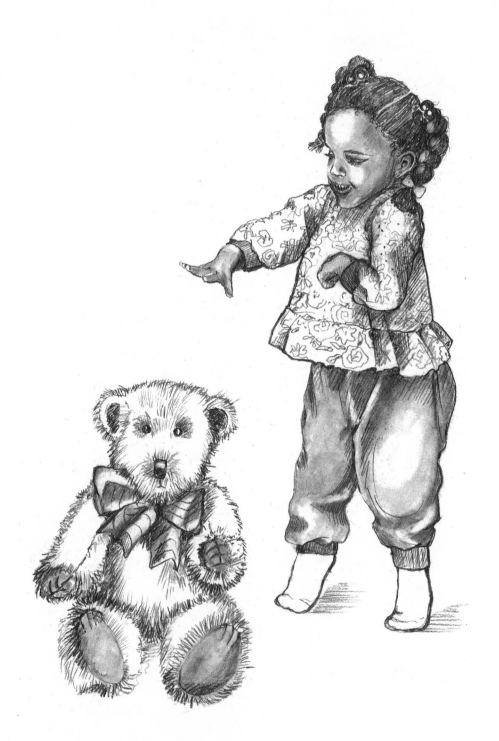

Hemiplegia

5

♦ HEMIPLEGIA is a form of cerebral palsy in which one arm and one leg on the same side of the body are affected. The majority of children with hemiplegia have normal intelligence, go to regular, age-appropriate schools, can expect to have relatively normal function as adults, and have few problems beyond the physical difficulties of the arm and leg that are involved.

The term *hemiplegia* is sometimes more broadly used to describe children with mild involvement of one limb (also called *monoplegia*). A child whose primary motor dysfunction involves both legs and one arm may also be diagnosed with hemiplegia, although this pattern is more properly called *triplegia. Double hemiplegia* is a sometimes confusing term that is used to describe cerebral palsy when it affects all four limbs but with asymmetry between the right and left side. Children with this diagnosis have very different physical problems from the problems of children whose CP involves only one side of the body, and more closely resemble those with diplegia or quadriplegia.

If your child's CP involves one arm more than it involves the legs, then this chapter will appropriately address most of your issues of concern. However, Chapter 6, on diplegia, better addresses issues concerning a child whose more severe involvement is in the legs, and a child with double hemiplegia who can walk. Chapter 7, on quadriplegia, is most relevant if your child cannot walk.

What does hemi-plegia usually look like?

For most children with hemiplegia, the arm is usually more affected than the leg, and the problems are usually worse at the end of the limb. The child with hemiplegia has a harder time with hand and wrist movements than with shoulder function, and problems with the elbow fall somewhere in between. Similarly, the child's foot and ankle present more difficulties than his knee. Hips are seldom significantly involved. The child's most significant problems are usually related to spastic muscles and decreased growth of these spastic muscles. This growth abnormality causes the muscles to be short and the joints to be stiff, so that as the child grows, he has progressively less range of movement in the affected limbs.

Birth to One Year

What physical abilities can the newborn's parents expect to see? At first the infant's hands and legs function only immaturely, and the infant has poor trunk control. As the first year of life progresses, however, the infant rapidly develops many new abilities—though of course different infants develop these abilities at different ages and in different ways. This is an exciting time for parents. Because of the natural variation in development and the rapid changes that are taking place, mild abnormalities often go unnoticed by parents and physicians alike.

Can hemiplegia be diagnosed at this age?

The diagnosis of hemiplegic cerebral palsy is very seldom made in the first year of life, primarily because it is virtually impossible to determine conclusively that a child has hemiplegia at this young age. A child's first year is a difficult time for parents if they suspect that their child has a problem. Because it is often easier to deal with bad news than it is to handle an unknown diagnosis and the waiting that's required before the outcome can be determined, many parents push for an early diagnosis. But the only reliable way to determine the outcome of a child who has a brain injury is to wait and see. That, unfortunately, is what parents of such a child must do.

Predicting the future outcome for the child who has been diagnosed with a birth abnormality that is not specifically related to a syndrome or a more specific diagnosis is only slightly more reliable than an educated guess. When a syndrome is identified or a specific diagnosis is made (such as Rett syndrome, Tay-Sachs disease, or trisomy 18), much more accurate predictions can be made, because these syndromes tend to follow a more predictable course. Cerebral palsy is not predictable in this way, because it is not a disease or due to a specific chromosomal abnormality. The symptoms depend on where the brain damage is, and this cannot always be seen even on the most sophisticated brain-imaging techniques like MRI.

Some parents have been prepared for a diagnosis of severely involved cerebral palsy, particularly when their newborn has been premature or has had intracerebral bleeding, only to find that at age 4 the child has mild hemiplegia. In contrast, some parents who have been told their child will be normal, or at most mildly affected, discover at an older age that the child is more severely involved. In cases such as these, the conclusion must be that the initial diagnosis involved an incorrect prediction; these outcomes should not be interpreted to mean that the initial brain injury has changed in any way. When a child is diagnosed at a later age, and with reliable criteria, predictions about abilities will be more accurate; parents should not be anxious that the prognosis will become worse over time.

As a parent, what early signs can I watch for?

If your child has very mild hemiplegia, there are usually no noticeable signs or symptoms, with the exception of early hand dominance. Left- or right-hand preference is usually not well established until 18 to 24 months of age in a normal child. Therefore, if your 5-month-old always reaches out with the same hand for toys or food, you should talk to your child's pediatrician. The normal hand is the one your child is using; the involved hand may be held in a fist most of the time, or you may notice that one arm or leg seems stronger or stiffer than the other. The fisted hand or the tightly held thumb is usually flexible and can be gently pulled out, but this is evidence of early spasticity in the involved limb, which gradually increases as the child grows. The position is sometimes referred to as a *contracture,* even though it is flexible.

If the arm appears weak or does not move normally, this may be a sign that the nerves in the infant's shoulder were stretched during birth. If your child has this condition (called Erb's palsy), you'll notice that he usually moves his fingers well but does not move his arm from the shoulder normally. Diagnosis of Erb's palsy requires a neurological evaluation. This condition should not be confused with cerebral palsy.

The child of 4 or 5 months who shows an unwillingness to use a hand or who consistently holds a fisted hand should be evaluated. However, a full-scale evaluation, which includes the appropriate scans, might not show a definable abnormality, even though the child clearly appears not to function normally. Scans taken at this early age do sometimes reveal cysts or other deformities in the brain, but these findings may have very little meaning in terms of the severity or pattern of involvement of cerebral palsy.

Between the ages of 5 and 8 months, children start sitting. Children with hemiplegia have a tendency to fall to the side affected by CP. They may realize that they are falling, but they may have trouble reaching out with their involved hand in order to stop themselves. As their balance improves, however, these children are able to sit very well. In the more severely involved child with hemiplegia, the ability to sit well may be delayed until 16 to 18 months. However, all children with classic hemiplegia eventually become good sitters.

As the child starts crawling "commando style," the involved side is often held in more rigidly at the hip, knee, and elbow. This position makes it look like the child is holding the affected side more closely to his body. It may even look as if the child is dragging this side.

Children with a mild hemiplegia may walk by 11 to 14 months of age. Many children with hemiplegia walk late, however, and many of them start walking on tiptoe. If your child walks late and continuously walks on his toes, these are two strong indications your child has CP. As he develops balance and confidence in walking, he may very well outgrow toe walking.

Are there any treatments available for children who show these signs?

For a child with these early symptoms, a thorough medical evaluation should take place, by the child's pediatrician or by a specialist such as a pediatric neurologist or developmental pediatrician. If the diagnosis of CP is made, then referral to a therapist is indicated. The primary treatment for the 5-month-old who shows an unwillingness to use a hand is to present the child with toys directed at the affected hand or with toys too large to hold with only one hand, such as a large ball. Finger foods can be presented in the same way. Some extra care may be necessary in opening and cleaning the fisted hand. Occupational therapists are the ones who will direct therapy for the child with an affected hand.

For the most part, however, your child should be treated like a normal child. One exception is a child with an extremely tightly fisted hand. In a child at this young age, an extremely tightly fisted hand occasionally requires a splint. Only in a child with severe CP do hand contractures occur at such a young age.

If your child is having problems crawling, this is a good time to start seeing a physical therapist. Advice from these experts can provide you with both direction and reassurance. Special braces or shoes are not needed at this age unless the child is trying to walk and is a persistent toe walker.

Is a walker recommended?

Some parents enjoy seeing their child moving about on her own in a sling-seat walker, but parents need to supervise the child very closely to prevent accidents. One safety guideline is to tie the walker to a post or piece of furniture, to limit the distance the child can travel. It is essential that a child in a walker stay away from stairs, as this is where most accidents occur. Also, the walker must be one that is engineered to be stable. Many physical therapists don't recommend walkers because they are concerned that bad movement patterns will be reinforced. Many pediatricians discourage use of such walkers for all children because of the danger that the child's mobility in the walker will lead them to fall off porches or down stairs, resulting in severe injuries.

The use of a sling-seat walker will not teach the child to walk sooner and can create dangerous situations. There is no evidence that the use of walkers does any long-term harm, however. The walker will not prevent a child from learning to fall, cause foot or hip problems, or delay the time when the child is able to walk independently.

Ages One to Three

During this period most children with mild hemiplegia are diagnosed, usually because they are toe walking and have not started to walk by age 15–18 months, or because they are more clearly not using one of their arms normally. If it hasn't been done before now, a full neurological evaluation is necessary, although it may not reveal any definable problem in the brain. The main reason this type of evaluation is recommended is not to find a cause of the cerebral palsy, but to be certain that no other condition is causing the child's symptoms. If there is a condition other than cerebral palsy, then it needs to be treated properly. Another reason for an evaluation at this age is if the parents are considering having another child and they want more information about the cause of their toddler's problems.

In many ways, caring for the child with hemiplegia at this age is not much different from caring for the child without a disability, except that it may be a little harder to determine the proper level of expectation. But parents can work with health care professionals to develop a level of expectation which is consistent with the individual child's ability. This is usually established by consulting with occupational and physical therapists, who often offer valuable counseling.

For example, it's not reasonable to expect any 6-month-old to eat with a spoon. Most parents know this from talking to other parents, consulting their child's pediatrician, or reading books. It is *just* as unreasonable to expect the child with severe hemiplegia to hold a cup in the midline (at the middle of the body) if the child is physically unable to hold a cup and bring it there, even at age 16 months. Parents need help from professional therapists to learn what to expect from their individual child at each stage of development, such as when the child might be expected to bring the cup to midline.

How should the affected hand be treated?

During this period it is important to present your child with toys that require two-handed manipulation and that stimulate your child to use the involved hand, even if only to assist the good hand. Give your child toys such as large stuffed animals or large balls and dolls too big to hold with one hand. Encourage her to hold a bottle or cup with both hands if she is able. Don't try to force your child to do anything that she is physically unable to do, however. If your child can't open her affected hand to hold a large bottle, then it is better for her continued development to get a bottle that she can hold with one hand, such as those that have an open split in the middle. A physical or an occupational therapist can make equipment recommendations.

At this age the development of fine motor skills can be encouraged by playing with your child in stacking blocks and putting pegs in holes. It's difficult to get your child to do these activities with the involved body part, especially if she is not motivated. It's best to encourage her in these activities but not to push her to the point of frustration. If your child refuses, the refusal is probably due to her impairment; it's not possible for her to do this task at this time. As your child continues to grow she may suddenly begin doing activities such as these with the involved hand, though much later than she did them with the normal hand.

Because each child is an individual and there are no tests that can define expectations for a specific child with CP, it's important to work with a therapist and a physician to help define these abilities. They may also be depended upon to make suggestions about hand braces.

When and how are braces used for the hand?

Generally, the fisted posture in which many children with hemiplegia hold the hand starts changing as they reach 2 or 3 years of age. This is also the time when muscles start tightening up, and it is the right time to consider bracing. The brace is used to prevent the muscles from becoming tighter.

There are a number of different braces for the hand. The two most frequently used are those that are designed to keep the thumb out of the palm and those that are designed to keep the fingers and wrist extended. The specific design used depends on the experience and philosophy of the therapist and physician, as well as on the needs of the specific child. Generally, hand braces are very well tolerated by children in this age group, but they usually do not improve the hand's functioning.

One drawback of the brace is that it reduces the feeling or sensation in the hand, which can make a child ignore the hand even more. At this age your child is developing use patterns, so it is not a good practice to keep the hand covered by a brace all the time, as this encourages the child to ignore it during play. At this age, too, muscles generally don't become tight quickly, and function often improves nicely if the child is encouraged and not restricted. For these reasons, the brace should be used only at night or for short periods during the day.

Is there any harm in not bracing?

The use of hand braces has great variation and not very well defined benefits or risks. Therefore, it is generally best to continue with whatever seems to provide the most benefit to your child, and to stop doing those things that don't seem to work. For example, if your child refuses to wear a brace and continually removes it, he does so because it hurts him or because it is in his way. This should be a sign to stop using the brace, or at least to try another one. The mainstay of treatment should be to encourage the use of the hand for functional activity, which in this age group means during play time. It is important not to try to force your child to do something that he physically is not able to do or that he does only with great difficulty.

What about my child's normal hand?

In the past, it was often recommended that the normal hand be restricted to encourage use of the affected hand. This philosophy was later abandoned in recognition of the stress this placed on the child. Until recently, parents were urged never to impair the normal hand, at the risk of causing negative consequences. Restricting the use of the normal hand has been shown sometimes to cause significant psychological distress, which can have long-term consequences. However, recent studies have demonstrated positive outcomes from a program of restricting normal hand use for a time. This program, "enforced use therapy," is not appropriate at this age level but will be addressed later in this chapter.

We recommend encouraging use of the impaired hand at this age (one to three) but not by restricting the normal hand.

What about walking?

A child who has not yet attained the developmental ability to walk cannot be made to walk. Consider this: no matter how hard a parent or therapist may try, it is impossible to make a 5-month-old normal infant walk by himself. Many moderate to severely involved children with hemiplegia at 15 months old are like a 5-month-old in that they do not have the developmental ability to walk—regardless of how hard people may work to help them learn to walk. Therefore, parents should not insist on their child walking but rather should focus on the things that the child *is* doing (such as crawling), expecting that in some months the child *will* walk.

Involvement of the leg becomes more noticeable at this age and is a significant factor in the delay in walking. But children with a typical hemiplegic pattern of cerebral palsy become good walkers if there are no other underlying problems. The child with mild hemiplegia typically walks within the same age range as a child without a disability. Children with moderate involvement are often delayed, however, beginning to walk between 18 and 24 months. The more severely involved child may not walk until between 24 and 30 months of age. Assistance from a physical therapist can be very helpful, especially for a child with significant developmental delay.

Each child has his individual schedule based on his development and level of involvement. Encouraging your child to stand and to take steps is fine, as long as it is approached with a healthy attitude—similar to the approach you would take with a normal child who is learning to walk. Always be sure your coaching is in line with what your child is physically capable of doing.

Does a child have to crawl before walking?

There are several therapy theories that suggest that all children have to crawl in a specific way before they go on to walk in order to develop a normal gait pattern. However, there are no empirical data to justify these theories. There are children who never learn to crawl but who just stand up and walk, and there is no harm in this.

There is great variation in crawling styles among children; most children with hemiplegia learn early on to do an asymmetrical "commando crawl" (similar to the low-to-the-ground crawl of the soldier under fire). Some can progress to a four-point crawl, but others cannot. The crawling pattern that works for the child should be encouraged, and there should not be too much emphasis placed on perfecting a particular type of crawl if the child does not seem comfortable with change. If a therapist insists on a specific crawling pattern, parents should consider switching therapists.

What problems do the feet present?

Foot problems in the child with hemiplegia are primarily due to a tight Achilles tendon ("heel cord"). The muscle that this tendon goes into, the *gastrocnemius,* seems to be the slowest to grow. It is the dominant muscle below the knee and the largest, and it is usually the most spastic. Problems with this muscle and this tendon are seen in the persistent toe walker.

Often when children begin walking they walk on tiptoe. This may in fact be normal in a child up to the age of 2 or 2¼, but a child should be walking flatfooted six months after he begins walking. Children with hemiplegia toe walk for a prolonged period, often for several years, and they toe walk on both feet, resulting in tightness on both the uninvolved and the involved sides.

The child with hemiplegia may also have a problem with his foot turning in, as do many normal children at this age. Although the foot may be flat, the whole foot appears to turn in. This pattern, which is due to a twist in the bones of the leg, often corrects itself as the child grows and develops better muscle control. Because the condition self-corrects, surgery, exercises, and braces are rarely necessary. If parents are very concerned, activities that require pointing the foot forward can be encouraged. These include roller skating, ice skating, and ballet—activities that are often preferable to physical therapy or home exercises because they involve the child in normal activities.

Can stretching or exercises help?

The usefulness of physical stretching as therapy is an issue about which a great variety of opinions exist. The child with spasticity is no different from anyone else in that she will benefit from stretching after being in one position for a long time: it feels good to get up and stretch after lengthy sitting. The child with spasticity needs help to stretch out the affected muscles. But the tightness that develops from the spasticity will not be overcome by physically stretching the child. It would actually require 8 to 12 hours of relaxed stretch each day in order to make a muscle grow. Clearly, it is impractical to spend 8 to 12 hours a day stretching a child!

It's good practice to stretch for short periods of time (5 to 10 minutes), twice a day, incorporating this into your child's daily routine like bathing and toothbrushing. But you must realize that your child's spasticity will be there forever. Although no exercise program has ever been shown to make a long-term difference in a child's disability, exercises prescribed by a therapist or physician should be considered. However, your role is that of parent, not therapist. It's important to consider the rest of the family, job obligations, and educational goals, as well as how the involved child is responding to other demands.

Exercise for the child with hemiplegia should be approached in the same way that physical exercise is approached for the nondisabled individual, the purpose being to keep fit and to feel and function better. There is room for flexibility, and no great harm is done by skipping a day or taking vacation time off. As with other exercise programs, the benefits are ultimately lost when the exercises are discontinued.

When are foot braces suggested?

The AFO (*ankle-foot orthosis*) or MAFO (*molded ankle-foot orthosis*) is a commonly used brace that is worn for the purpose of stretching the Achilles tendon. An AFO can be helpful to children with hemiplegic involvement who are walking on tiptoe, usually more so on the side affected by the spasticity. The brace is applied if the foot can be brought to a neutral position. If the foot cannot be brought to a neutral position, then surgery or another kind of treatment needs to be considered (see below).

Although there is no generally accepted routine for using an AFO, it's generally true that children who need to use the brace should wear it during the day in the same way that they wear shoes. There is no harm in the child's walking barefoot for periods of time in the evenings or after a bath. If the muscle is very tight, there may be some benefit to wearing the brace at night for an additional stretch.

A child will need time to get used to a new AFO just as most of us need time to break in a stiff new pair of shoes. The AFO must be adjusted if red areas of skin keep developing or if the foot does not stay down in its correct place. The AFO will feel very restrictive to the child, so even though the child looks better walking and standing, the AFO will not feel natural or comfortable to her. Once the child is used to the AFO, often several months later, it will feel very comfortable. Even then it is preferable for her to spend some time out of the brace. If a child is kept braced continuously, the foot may become hypersensitive and feel much like a limb feels after being in a cast for several months.

If the child continues to complain about the AFO, it should be carefully checked. To check an AFO, look for wrinkles in socks (a telltale sign that something is wrong); determine whether the foot has been fully placed in the correct position; and find out whether the toes are curled up inside the shoes, or whether the AFOs have been switched so that the right AFO has been accidentally placed on the left foot, and vice versa. If the AFO is applied by many different people (parents, siblings, daycare teachers, and so on), it is especially important to make sure that the AFOs are clearly marked as right or left. Applying the wrong AFO to a foot is a common error.

The type of AFO used depends on what is locally available. For the child who is running around, the best brace is a thin, light plastic, custom-molded brace, sometimes with a hinge at the ankle to prevent her from toe walking. It is imperative that the brace not be too restrictive on the calf area. As the child grows, braces are reevaluated for size, and new braces must be made. Generally braces are replaced yearly because of the child's growth. However, during rapid growth spurts it may be necessary to replace the brace more often. There are some orthotists who make AFOs that can be extended for length, but this feature adds very little to the length of time the brace will fit. Adjusting only the length of the AFO might be compared to attempting to make a pair of pants last a child for five years by making the legs longer each year.

Another problem with the hemiplegic foot involves a spastic *tibialis pos-*

terior muscle, which is located on the inside of the ankle and pulls the foot so that the toes point toward each other. This can cause the child to walk on the inside border of the foot. An AFO is a recommended treatment for this problem in a young child.

Are there any options other than surgery when braces aren't working out?

If the child's spasticity is the primary reason he cannot tolerate the brace and stretching has reached its limit, Botox injections may be used. Botox injections have become a very helpful treatment. Used appropriately, this medication can delay surgery for the very young child. Botox (generic name: botulinum toxin) is a chemical that significantly weakens a muscle when it is injected directly into that muscle. It is injected with a small needle, much like an immunization. Most children tolerate the injection well in the outpatient setting, although the injection may be administered after sedating the child, or numbing the skin with a local anesthetic. The chemical stays in the muscle where it is injected and its use is very safe. Unfortunately, the effect is temporary, lasting 3–6 months. Additionally, although Botox can be injected multiple times, in most children, each subsequent injection is less effective. This is because the body manufactures antibodies to the Botox, recognizing it as a foreign substance. For many children, after three to four injections over a period of 9–18 months, one sees little or no effect. But it is useful in delaying surgery for that amount of time.

If the child is not able to tolerate a brace because the tendon is contracted and spasticity is *not* a major component, Botox is unlikely to be helpful. Botox can also be used in the hamstrings and adductor muscles, as well as in the spastic upper extremity muscles.

Another possible option is serial casting. Serial casting (which involves placing the leg in casts that are changed every two weeks) is a method for lengthening the tendon that was popular in the past but now is seldom used. In cerebral palsy, this is almost always a temporary measure; that is, the foot returns to its former position within several months of removing the cast. Once in a while a child who has a very mild tightness and is not tolerating an AFO may benefit from serial casting for six to eight weeks. If serial casting fails, proceeding to surgical intervention allows the family to get back to normal functioning with fewer disruptions than repeated cast changes and long-term cast wear would mean.

When is surgery for the foot advisable?

When the foot can't be brought to a neutral or normal position despite the use of braces and/or Botox, then surgery to lengthen the Achilles tendon is indicated. Surgery is usually the best lengthening method. The younger the child is when the Achilles tendon is lengthened, however, the more likely he will need to have the procedure repeated as he grows. Ideally, one carefully planned surgery for lengthening suffices. Surgical correction is also possible for the foot that is turned in severely, but it is preferable to wait until a child is at least 6 years of age to do this procedure, to permit growth in the tendon.

The role of formal gait analysis has become an integral part of the evaluation of children who walk. It is a very involved procedure that takes the patient approximately 3 hours to complete. The child is first examined by a physical therapist, who records measurements of each of the muscles. The therapist then places sensors on the major muscles and the child is asked to ambulate on a specific walkway while computers register the changes occurring at the various muscle sites. These computer data are analyzed at a later date by a team consisting of an orthopedic surgeon and therapists. Their analysis includes recommendations for bracing, orthotics, therapy, and/or surgery, when any of these modalities are indicated. Typically, the gait analysis is ordered not on a routine basis, but when surgery is being considered. It is usually covered by insurance under those conditions.

What other muscle spasticity problems can children with hemiplegia have at this age?

Some moderate to severely involved children with hemiplegia may have tight hamstring muscles. Usually all that's needed at this age is exercise and stretching. Braces fitted to above the knee aren't helpful. The severely involved child may have some spasticity about the hip, although this is rare. Should it occur, it would be handled in the same way that spastic hip disease is treated in the child with diplegia (see Chapter 6).

Ages Four to Six

The problems of the child with hemiplegia in this age group are similar to those of the younger child. It is uncommon for children at this age to be self-conscious about bracing, and they seldom object to wearing a brace as long as it is comfortable and not too restrictive.

Therapy benefits the child most if she enjoys it. Most children resist therapy that consists of long periods of passive stretching or of being urged to pull the foot or wrist up. Again, it is not advisable to force a child to participate in an activity that she dislikes. At this age reluctance can also be due to the child's repeated failure or fear of failing. If a child is reluctant, parents may help to motivate the child by focusing on the result of the activity rather than on the activity itself—although choosing an alternate form of therapy is often the better solution.

What forms of therapy are most helpful at this age?

Therapy should now be focused on activities of daily living, such as learning to put on and take off shoes, use eating utensils, and ride a bicycle. The child can get stimulation from playing with large balls requiring two-handed play, and from reaching for and holding on to playground equipment such as jungle gyms. Bike riding, swimming, and ballet are activities that stimulate the development of coordination—and they're also fun. A basketball hoop placed at the appropriate height allows a child to play while shooting and dribbling the ball, both of which are beneficial activities.

Should I be concerned with hand function at this age?

A severely involved child can develop significant tightness at this age. It's very helpful for the child to wear a brace that lifts the wrist, extends the fingers, pulls the thumb out of the palm, and turns the palm upward. If your child is using his hand, it is crucial not to cover his palm, since this decreases sensation and will decrease function. Occupational therapy is usually best aimed at this age group, since this is the age for learning skills such as dressing, bathing, and using eating utensils. In addition, fine motor skills such as writing and coloring can be addressed more intensely. Hand surgery is only recommended for a small number of children, and then not until the age of 6.

What is enforced use therapy?

This is a structured program currently in use, with encouraging short-term results but without a great deal of long-term data. It is applicable to children with hemiplegia who have a potentially functional affected hand and arm but tend to totally ignore it. They appear to not be aware that the extremity "works." These are the children who are ideal candidates for this therapeutic treatment, because they actually have the ability to use the extremity.

The treatment involves a short period of casting the "normal" arm and hand (usually 4 weeks), forcing the use of the affected limb. A therapist is an essential part of the treatment. The therapist works intensively with the child during this period, guiding her to use the "ignored" limb with the restriction of the more functional limb. The goal is for the child to continue using the arm and hand after the cast is removed. In programs that have been working with this therapy, benefits have been reported in the months after cast removal, involving improved motor skills and increased unprompted use of the arm. It is, however, extremely important to only use this therapy with children who understand the purpose and who have agreed to the therapy. Restricting the "normal" extremity of a child without cooperation can produce significant distress and is not recommended.

How does spasticity affect my child now?

Problems relating to the arm and leg often become more noticeable as the child of this age begins learning an adult pattern of running. A normal running gait involves high lifting of the feet and reciprocating arm movements. As children with hemiplegia try to run, they tend to flex the affected elbow and wrist and turn the palm down. The arm tends to move away from the body. This arm patterning is typical and usually is quite noticeable. As the child's running gait matures this improves somewhat, but it never disappears. At this age a child is not generally very concerned with appearance, and parents should avoid focusing on appearance, as well.

As the child runs, the lower extremities also experience spasticity. The knee tends to be held in a stiffened position, which makes the affected leg swing out. The affected foot, if it is not braced or surgically corrected, has a tendency to trip the child. The foot may be dragging or turning in or out. Occasionally a severe flat foot develops.

What roles do casts, alcohol or phenol blocks, Botox, and surgery play?

Casting at this age has the same limited use as it does at younger ages. Casting is helpful only for spasticity that is not severe enough to need surgical treatment and yet interferes with the fitting of an AFO.

Alcohol and phenol blocks, used extensively in the past, consist of injections of medications into the spastic muscles. These injections must be administered under general anesthesia, since they are very painful. The decrease in spasticity that is achieved is temporary, lasting five to six months. Botox has replaced these blocks for children where temporary relief of spasticity is wanted.

Surgical lengthening of the Achilles tendon must also be done under general anesthesia. This procedure, if it is done at an appropriate age, can benefit the child for as long as five years. In many cases surgery can even result in permanent correction. The major risk for surgery is anesthesia. In our view, for the risk to be a reasonable one, the procedure must have a lasting result.

What is the role of the AFO at this age?

The AFO helps keep the Achilles tendon from becoming too tight and the foot from becoming flat. It can also help to control the foot that is rolling in. Heel cups and arch supports are usually less effective for this problem. This is an appropriate time in a child's life to consider preparing him to enter school with as normal a gait as possible, without the need for bracing, and this may be the appropriate age to consider surgery on the Achilles tendon.

What kind of surgery is usually recommended at this age?

The most common surgically correctable problem is the tight Achilles tendon that prevents the child from placing his foot flat on the ground. Lengthening this tendon involves a relatively simple procedure with few risks. Sometimes the procedure needs to be repeated as the child continues to grow, but often one lengthening is sufficient.

A foot that has a tendency to pull in while the child walks on the outside border can be corrected at the same time by a split transfer of the *posterior tibialis tendon.* Severe flat feet that roll in may need to be surgically corrected with a fusion (in which several bones are made to grow together). This procedure can often be postponed until the child is fully grown, however, and an AFO will usually take care of the problem in the meantime.

Tight hamstrings cause the child to walk with a crouched gait. This problem can be greatly improved by a lengthening, as well. Occasionally a child walks with his entire leg turning in. In this case the leg can be surgically derotated and realigned correctly.

Shortness of the involved leg generally becomes noticeable at this age. Interestingly enough, this shortness can be helpful for a time, as it prevents the child with a tight Achilles tendon from catching his toes when walking or running. A shoe lift on the involved side can actually cause the child to trip more. For some children, however—those who have a severe disparity in leg length (more than ¾ inch) just prior to or during the adolescent growth spurt—this leg length difference needs to be addressed. Special x-rays called *scanograms* accurately determine the difference in length between the two legs, and surgical options are available to equalize the leg lengths permanently.

The age of 5 to 6 years is an excellent time to consider surgical correction for a number of reasons. First, the child is now old enough to understand most of what is involved, and this lessens anxiety considerably. Second, when procedures are done and recovered from before school entry, the child won't need to miss valuable time from school. Additionally, improvements attained with surgery will most often be maintained for five or more years as the child undergoes a slow, steady growth until the adolescent growth spurt.

Planning for surgery ought to be coordinated to minimize disruption to the family's life. It is far more beneficial to the development of a child to keep his hospitalizations to a minimum than to have various minor surgical procedures every year or so. A team of physicians familiar with the multiple problems of children with cerebral palsy can be very effective in limiting the number of surgeries and hospitalizations, because they can predict and plan what a child might need. This approach allows for more than one corrective procedure to be done while the child is under anesthesia. In this way the child spends less time in the hospital and has less exposure to anesthesia risks. We want to stress the importance of consulting a surgeon who is experienced with cerebral palsy so that a practical, coordinated plan for all surgery can be formulated.

Ages Seven to Twelve

At this age children are developing a self-concept and so are becoming more aware of how they are different from their peers. To diminish those differences, it helps to direct therapies toward specific goals. In addition, it is preferable to use school vacation time for treatment or intensive therapy, so that time is not taken away from academic efforts. For example, if a child with moderate to severe hemiplegia is experiencing difficulty in self-dressing (handling buttons or tying shoes), the summer break can be the best time to work on improving this skill.

Almost all children with hemiplegia function well in normal age-appropriate classrooms. Teachers can easily be made aware of the specific child's special needs and can be called upon to help design and implement classroom adjustments. The teacher can also play a significant role in helping the other children in the class understand and be supportive of the child with the disability.

The goal at this age should be to place the child in the best situation for learning. A physical therapy program that detracts from this goal is not good for the long-term well-being of the child. Enrolling the child in after-school activities such as ballet, gymnastics, or karate provides the benefit of stretching along with the opportunity to function and interact with children without disabilities. There are many teachers who love to work with children to help them grow and enjoy sports without training them to become world-class athletes, and this type of teacher often welcomes the opportunity to work with a child with a disability. Thus, the child can concentrate on academics in school and can work out physically during extracurricular activities.

How are the hand and arm best treated at this age?

This is the age at which children begin to object to using arm splints or braces because wearing these devices makes them look different. If your child feels self-conscious and does not want to wear a brace, it is best not to force the issue, especially since arm braces provide little functional benefit at this age.

Mild arm involvement refers to the limb that is used almost normally but that has a tendency to flex at the elbow when the person is excited or running. This pattern continues throughout adulthood and is primarily a cosmetic concern. It is frequently handled by acquiring habits that control or conceal the movement in socially acceptable ways. For example, females may learn to carry a purse (and males a book bag), even purposely weighted, on the affected arm. Or they learn to place the hand in their pants pocket. When preadolescent children first become self-conscious about the arm, they often hold the affected hand with the nonaffected hand to cover up and control the deformity.

The moderately involved arm is one that is always flexed and pronated at the wrist and elbow, to some degree. *Pronation* refers to the rotation of the forearm and hand in which the palm of the hand is always turned away from the person's face. The hand may also have abnormal sensation, and the moderately involved arm is quite noticeable cosmetically. Although the arm can be used well as an assist, its pronated position prevents the child from being able to fully see what he is trying to pick up because he can only see the top of his fingers and hand.

This kind of involvement usually responds very well to surgical correction. The amount of *functional* improvement achieved varies depending on the presurgical status, but the *cosmetic* result is invariably excellent. If the child has been using the arm readily in most activities of daily living and also has fairly intact sensation, the surgery allows for easier use and the child will naturally use the arm more. The child is often more aware of the cosmetic result, while the parents notice improved function.

The severely involved arm is one that is used only to perform an activity that's impossible to execute with one hand. This hand usually has poor sensation as well as poor muscle control. Surgical treatment for this type of involvement is indicated purely for cosmetic improvement, because function is rarely improved, even though the hand may be better positioned. Poor brain control and poor sensation preclude significant functional improvement. Sometimes, if this is not well understood by parents prior to surgery, conflicts arise. Because the arm *looks* so much more normal, parents and teachers may inappropriately expect more function and even attempt to force a child to use an arm that he simply is incapable of using.

Age seven to twelve is the best age to correct the arm surgically, if indicated. Children are now old enough to understand a great deal in terms of the procedure and the recovery. They are also capable of fully participating in the rehabilitation process. Children at this age generally do not have well-formed or unrealistic expectations, which is an added benefit, since they are invariably pleased with the surgical result.

Delaying surgery until after age 12 can present some problems. As children go through the adolescent stage of development, they may become unrealistic in their expectations and are often self-deprecating. Though many adolescents may in fact breeze through this period as easily as they did childhood, those who are more upset over perceived, as well as real, deficiencies tend to be affected in two ways. First, they are more concerned about their appearance and are unhappy with braces or splints. Second, they have unrealistically high expectations about the outcome of corrective surgery and frequently are disappointed with the results. Good timing for surgery is essential. And the importance of making certain that the adolescent is fully prepared—that he has as complete an understanding as possible of various outcomes—cannot be overemphasized.

What are the specific surgical procedures?

The specific surgery is dependent on the level of involvement as well as on the function of the involved muscles. Surgery might be approached one way if there is a possibility of increasing function and another way if there is no such possibility, but in practice, function and cosmetics are generally approached similarly. A strict rule of medical treatment, of course, is to avoid doing harm, and in this case, surgery must be designed and carried out in a way that doesn't *decrease* function (with a few exceptions, as described below).

Before performing surgery, the surgeon will obtain a detailed history of the patterns of use and will give the child a careful physical examination. In some institutions, EMGs (studies that evaluate nerve/muscle connections) are performed before surgery in order to study muscle function in upper extremity analysis. This is not standard practice at the present time, however, since EMGs are used more in the area of research than in therapeutics.

Most surgery involves transferring muscle tendons, in order to achieve balance, or lengthening tendons, in order to relieve tightness. The flexed wrist is the most noticeable problem and is usually addressed by transferring to the top of the hand the tendon end of the *flexor carpi ulnaris* muscle, which then pulls the hand and wrist into the extended position. In this new position it is attached to a wrist extensor muscle tendon or to the finger extensor muscle tendons. If the fingers do not extend, the finger muscle tendons need to be lengthened. If the thumb is pulled into the palm, this is corrected by releasing the *adductor pollicis* muscle tendon in the palm or by moving a muscle tendon to help the thumb extend, or both.

The forearm is frequently in a pronated position, palm down. This can be addressed by transferring or releasing the *pronator teres* muscle tendon in the mid-forearm. Occasionally the forearm is flexed at the elbow and contracted. In this case the *biceps* muscle tendon is lengthened. Infrequently, a thumb joint fusion is indicated, and rarely, a wrist fusion is performed. Wrist fusions were popular in the past, but today they are only performed on a child who has a severely contracted hand or whose hand is completely without function. A fusion of this type should almost never be done at this young age because, although the cosmetic result is good, the procedure almost always reduces functional ability.

One guiding principle in this type of surgery should be to attempt to address as many problems as possible at the same time, taking advantage of *one* anesthesia exposure and *one* hospitalization. If they have any concerns about specific recommendations, parents should seek a second opinion, preferably from an orthopedist who is experienced in treating people with cerebral palsy. By taking these precautions a parent can hope to avoid bringing the child to surgery again.

What is the usual postoperative course?

If surgery involves the hand and wrist, the arm is placed in a cast extending from the fingers to the elbow. If the elbow has been surgically addressed during the same surgery, then the cast extends to the shoulder. The arm remains in the cast for four to six weeks. Analgesics (pain medication) may be necessary in the immediate postoperative period, but patients are generally quite comfortable in the supportive cast.

When the cast is removed, a short course (one to three times weekly for one to three months) of intense occupational therapy is very beneficial, and helps the child achieve the maximum benefit from the surgery. In addition, resting splints are often used full time for 6 to 12 weeks and often for a longer period at night, in order to maintain correction.

Generally, continued use of the night splint is most important for the growing child. There is little rationale for use of a night splint for more than 12 months with a child who has finished growing, since by this time the situation is unlikely to change, with or without splinting.

What is the role of bracing for the lower extremity?

The issues and problems of the lower extremities in this age group are much like those of younger children. The use of the AFO to help control the foot is often well tolerated. This is especially true if the child notices that the brace makes it easier to walk and run. In addition, the brace is fairly easy to hide with clothing, and peers may not even be aware that the child is wearing a brace. A good compromise for brace wear is to have the child wear the brace all day during school but allow him to remove it in the evening and on weekends. However, when an activity involves a great deal of walking, an exception needs to be made to include the brace.

During the summer children generally go without their braces much of the time, especially if they are doing a great deal of swimming. There is really no need for a child to wear braces in the water. One of the disadvantages of constant brace wear during childhood is the development of very small, thin calf muscles. A significant cause of the small calf is that spastic muscles don't develop normally, and using braces constantly or using braces that are too small serves to keep the muscle smaller (repeated surgical lengthenings of the Achilles tendon also cause thin calf muscles). Allowing the child not to wear his brace, as well as taking care to see that outgrown braces are replaced, can help minimize this problem.

What surgery is suggested for the lower extremity?

For most children of this age with hemiplegia, the goal should be to release them from the necessity of bracing. Doing so may include a weaning period as well as surgery. Early adolescence, when a child has begun the adolescent growth spurt but is not fully into puberty, is a good time for surgical corrections to be made. Surgery on the lower extremities can frequently be combined with upper extremity surgery.

The most commonly performed surgery is the lengthening of the Achilles tendon, which is appropriate for almost any child who is walking up on her toes. If this procedure was previously done when the child was 3 to 4 years old, this is often the age when it needs to be redone. This also is the age to correct a foot that turns in. If the entire foot is turning in, this is corrected by externally rotating either the *tibia,* in the lower leg, or the *femur,* in the upper leg. This is accomplished by an osteotomy, which involves surgically breaking the bone and realigning it in an appropriate position. If the foot tends to roll in as the child walks, causing her to walk on the outside border, a split *posterior tibialis* muscle tendon transfer may be indicated, which involves moving half of the tendon to the outside of the foot so the muscle will provide a balanced pull to the foot.

A severe flat-foot deformity is best treated at this age with a fusion procedure called a *triple arthrodesis,* which involves fusing bones around the heel bone. This procedure might also be indicated for a very stiff foot that is turning in. The advantage of the triple arthrodesis is that it lasts a lifetime, with a very low rate of complication.

Additionally, leg length discrepancies should be closely assessed and decisions concerning equalization should be made during this period. If the length discrepancy between the two legs is 1 centimeter or less, this may actually represent an advantage, because the child will trip less often. Even if the discrepancy is 2 centimeters (approximately ¾ inch), there may not be a significant problem. A larger difference is very easily surgically treated by stopping the growth in the longer leg. This procedure, called an *epiphysiodesis,* is timed to make the most of total growth while correcting length differences between the two legs.

What is the usual postoperative course?

The child who has had an Achilles tendon lengthening and split tibialis transfer procedures will go home with a leg cast, most commonly one that stops under the knee. This is usually a walking cast that will be worn for four to six weeks, followed by bracing for a short period in order to maintain correction. A child who has had an osteotomy (to correct a foot that points in) which involves the tibia is placed in either a short or a long leg cast for four to six weeks.

An osteotomy that involves the femur may include metal fixation, which means that a plate is inserted during the surgery. In this case, postoperative casting is not necessary. If a femoral osteotomy is performed without metal fixation, however, casting is necessary. The cast is either a *spica* cast (enclosing the hip as well as the leg) or a long leg cast (stopping at the hip).

A child who has a triple arthrodesis procedure will be in a cast (usually short leg) for a long time after the surgery. The first month after surgery he or she may be placed in a nonwalking cast, and for the next two months the foot is maintained in a walking cast.

After an epiphysiodesis procedure the knee is immobilized in a brace for approximately three to four weeks.

Ages Thirteen to Eighteen

This may be an extremely difficult time for the adolescent with a disability, or it may present few problems. The degree of involvement does not appear to have much bearing on the child's experience. Rather, the child's personality and temperament, and his family's and peers' acceptance of his disability, as well as the child's and family's goals, seem to have the most impact.

Children this age who have disabilities generally no longer enjoy participating in organized sports. They have usually accepted the fact that their success in this area will be limited, and they prefer to eliminate the stress of competing with their nondisabled peers. The adolescent who redirects his energies to areas where he is likely to have more success, such as music or academics, is often happier.

What is the role of physical therapy and exercise at this age?

Adolescence is the period in which children are actively working at separating from parents as they move toward adulthood and independence. Children with a hemiplegic disability usually enter into this process just like children without disabilities. For this reason exercise programs orchestrated by parents tend to be met with various forms of opposition. Rather than imposing an exercise program on the adolescent, parents should encourage him to exercise to maintain his flexibility in the same manner he is encouraged to accept responsibility for his personal hygiene and appearance. Parents may have to allow the maturing adolescent to suffer the consequences of his not having taken responsibility, but this often proves to be the best learning experience, a far more lasting and effective experience than parental harassment.

There is no reason for ongoing, or "chronic," therapy, which only tends to foster dependence and magnify the significance of the disability. Occupational therapy and physical therapy should be limited to short-term intervention either to help the child accomplish a specific activity or to provide postoperative rehabilitation. Whenever possible, everyone around the child should avoid connecting the concept of chronic illness with the disability.

What are the surgical considerations at this age? While some surgical procedures may have been done at an earlier age, parents should not preclude the possibility of making improvements, and the teenage years are certainly a time when the physical disability should be reevaluated. One patient who was a schoolteacher with a mild right hemiplegia had spent her entire teaching career being limited by significant walking difficulties because she could not place her foot flat on the floor. When she retired she hoped to travel, and she decided to find out whether something could be done for this problem. After a simple operation, her foot was flat and she could walk as much as she wanted to!

The positive aspect of surgery at this age is that whatever corrections are made are permanent—they will not be outgrown. However, this is a somewhat tumultuous period for many teenagers, who have unreasonable expectations. A child or a teenager who has psychological or behavioral problems should not have surgery until he or she becomes more stable and more mature.

The specific problems and possible surgical corrections for the affected arm are almost the same as for younger children. In some adolescents with severe involvement, there may be a great deal of stiffness. For some of these young people a wrist fusion is suggested, but the consensus among surgeons who treat individuals with cerebral palsy is that wrist fusion should be avoided unless there is no other way to deal with the problem.

Surgery on the affected leg and foot includes all the procedures outlined in the previous section for ages seven to twelve for all the same problems. If there has been no prior surgical treatment of the foot, the foot may be very stiff. In this situation, tendon transfers are not possible and a triple arthrodesis is indicated. An Achilles tendon lengthening procedure is often necessary with the increased growth at this age.

The correction of leg length discrepancies should be made with careful attention to keeping the affected leg slightly shorter to prevent the individual from catching his toes and tripping. In adults, generally a 2-centimeter (¾ inch) difference is well tolerated. If the problem must be addressed, the best approach is to shorten the longer leg surgically, either by arresting its growth or by removing a piece of bone. The first procedure is simpler but somewhat less predictable, since it involves estimating future growth. When a piece of bone is removed, it is usually taken from the hip or from the middle of the femur. The bone is then fixed with a plate or rod.

Another option is wearing a shoe lift that is fixed to every pair of shoes worn by the individual during her entire life. In view of the simplicity and excellent outcome of surgical correction, surgery is usually the preferred option.

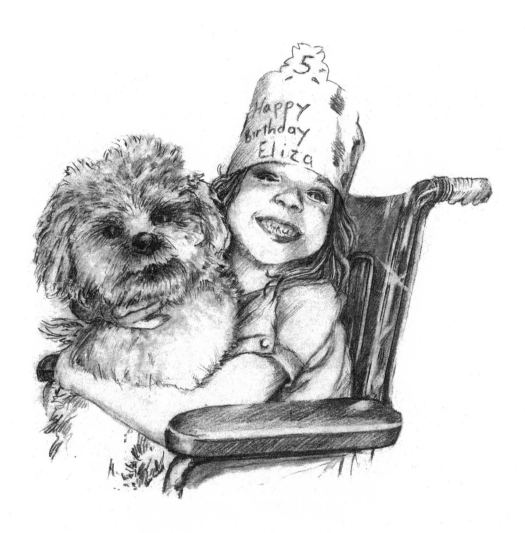

Diplegia

6

♦ D I P L E G I A is a form of cerebral palsy primarily affecting the legs. Most children with CP have some problems with their upper extremities, but for a child with diplegia, the upper extremities are clearly much less involved than the lower extremities. Almost all children with diplegia have spasticity, but they also have difficulty with balance and coordination. There is a good deal of variation among children with respect to involvement and severity of involvement.

If your child has as much involvement in his upper extremities as in his lower, then the chapter dealing with quadriplegia will probably be more appropriate for you to read, especially if your child has an athetoid component. If your child has asymmetrical involvement, with one side of the body clearly more affected than the other, almost normal, side, then the chapter on hemiplegia will be more relevant. A child whose primary motor dysfunction involves both legs and one arm is termed triplegic, and this child's challenges are addressed in this chapter.

What does diplegia look like?

The child with diplegia generally has nearly symmetrical involvement of both legs with only mild clumsiness in the arms. Spastic muscles and delayed growth of these muscles cause leg muscles to be short, and as a result the joints become stiff and the range of motion decreases as the child grows. For most children with diplegic involvement, the foot and ankle present more of a problem than the knee, and the hips may become dislocated (for this reason, the child's hips must be closely monitored).

Many children with diplegia were born prematurely and have had respiratory problems. Most of them have normal or near-normal learning ability. Mild eye problems, such as crossing, are common. For the majority of children with diplegia, growth and development are not a problem. Children with diplegia are eventually able to walk, although most of them begin walking late; they generally attend regular schools and become independently functioning adults.

Does diplegia have degrees of severity?

Diplegia is generally classified as mild, moderate, or severe. A child with mild diplegia is an excellent walker, walking without aids such as crutches.

Such a child has a normal tolerance for walking and can keep up with non-disabled children of similar age in activities requiring walking. With moderate involvement, a child is able to walk for most daily activities but may sometimes use an aid like crutches or a walker. A child with moderate involvement needs to use a wheelchair for activities involving extended walking, such as going to a shopping mall or an amusement park.

The child with severe diplegia requires an aid, such as a walker or crutches, for managing even small distances within a room, and walks only in level, uncrowded areas. To get around in public the child uses a wheelchair. Usually, even the most severely involved children are ambulatory enough to lift themselves into their wheelchairs independently and to move about their own rooms. A child who is not able to do this minimal amount of maneuvering should be diagnosed as quadriplegic, even if the upper extremities are not significantly involved.

Birth to One Year

Many infants who are born prematurely spend the first year trying to catch up with their age-matched peers. This first year sees the development of many milestones, such as head control, reaching out for a toy, sitting, starting to vocalize sounds, and finger feeding. Even though every infant has her own schedule and special circumstances, parents are often concerned about the rate at which these developments are taking place. There is a fairly wide range of normal development, and rates of catching up for premature infants vary; these circumstances make it very difficult to predict whether the infant who was born prematurely will eventually catch up completely or will have CP or some other developmental problem.

Can diplegia be diagnosed this early?

Making the diagnosis of cerebral palsy is difficult early on, although as a parent you may have been advised of the possibility because of your child's problems at birth. If your baby was born prematurely and has had significant medical problems, such as bleeding in the brain or breathing difficulties, he appears to be most at risk for developing diplegia. However, in order to know for certain whether your child has or will have cerebral palsy, you must wait for the child to grow and develop. Once her development starts to lag behind or is obviously abnormal, there is still very little anyone can say about how your child will eventually function. There are no specific tests or scans that can definitely prove that your child has or doesn't have CP, though there are several patterns of abnormality on CT or MRI (such as periventricular leukomalacia [PVL]) that are often seen in children who have CP (see Chapter 1). There are certainly no tests that will demonstrate how he or she will function at maturity.

Are there some warning signs?

The severity of involvement, even if diplegia is suspected, is extremely difficult to predict by any examination in the first year of life. The most common appearance of a child with a diplegic pattern is one of stiff lower extremities, with comparatively less than normal movement, and relatively normal upper extremities. Initially the child may appear to be exceedingly strong, but oftentimes this is a manifestation of spasticity.

Floppiness is also frequently seen at this young age. Some children are very floppy from birth and may appear to have no spasticity. They may eventually develop the same appearance of stiffness as the child who is initially stiff, however. There are some children with diplegia who appear completely normal, particularly in the first six months. Even examination by neurologists may not uncover an abnormality.

If your child was born prematurely, then normal development for him is counted from the day the child would have been born had he been born "on time" (at "term," which is 40 weeks' gestation). This means that if he was born at 36 weeks gestation (4 weeks early), we expect that his social smile should develop by 10 weeks of age, rather than the 6 weeks we usually expect. This "correction" for prematurity continues for the first 18 to 24 months of age.

By 6 months of age (corrected for prematurity if necessary) your child should roll over, start to develop a sitting balance, and move his legs in a fairly normal fashion. If this occurs, your child most certainly will not have severe involvement. At this age, children who have severe involvement will show significantly decreased movement, stiffness, or severe floppiness in the legs. If your child is sitting independently by 9 or 10 months and is pulling himself to standing, he is likely ultimately to have mild, or at most moderate, involvement. Even children who are not doing these things at this age may end up having mild involvement. It is simply too soon to be able to make an accurate prediction. Few children with even mild diplegia walk independently by 12 months of age.

What treatments are recommended at this age?

Although it is rare for a child younger than age 1 to have leg problems (and tightness or spasticity almost never require bracing, special shoes, or surgery at this age), exercise, especially gentle stretching, is good for the child who is not moving his legs on his own. It is best to incorporate this stretching into activities of daily living, such as diapering and bathing. The stretching should never be done so vigorously that it makes the child cry.

Infants generally respond well to infant stimulation programs, and these programs also put parents in touch with professionals who are comfortable with their infant and can tell parents about activities that will help stimulate the infant in a way that is appropriate for his level of development. These programs also offer reassurance that the parent's efforts are helping the child and assure parents that their child is developing at his maximum ability. Generally, involvement in a group program with other parents once a week or every other week is adequate.

Is a walker recommended?

Many parents enjoy seeing their child move about on her own in a sling-seat walker, but parents need to supervise the child very closely to prevent accidents. One safety guideline is to tie the walker to a post or piece of furniture, to limit the distance the child can travel. It is essential that a child in a walker stay away from stairs, as this is where most accidents occur. Also, the walker must be one that is engineered to be stable. Many physical therapists don't recommend walkers because they are concerned that bad movement patterns will result. The use of a sling-seat walker will not teach the child to walk sooner and can create dangerous situations. There is no evidence that the use of walkers does any long-term harm, however.

Ages One to Three

This is the age at which the characteristics of diplegia become more noticeable, mainly because, unlike other children at this age, the child with diplegia is not walking. This major developmental milestone becomes the focus for many parents. While the delay in walking is certainly important, it is much more important, at the age of 14 months, that the child be fairly healthy, eating well, growing normally, gaining weight, and developing hand function and speech.

By the age of three years, it is usually helpful for the child to be involved in a specialized school environment, such as a cerebral palsy center, which as a site of therapy is preferred by many medical professionals over the home. In a peer environment, focus can be placed on physical and occupational therapies, with emphasis on the child's disability. For children without brothers or sisters, the group environment is also helpful in developing interactive social skills.

What can I do to help my child walk?

A child cannot be made to walk before she is developmentally able to do so, and a child does not need to crawl in order to be able to walk. As a parent, you may work at offering the best possible environmental stimulation, within the scope of your personal schedule and the therapist's judgment. But you should never *force* your child to walk, or make her feel inadequate for not being able to accomplish this task. Providing a loving, supportive environment is the healthiest gift you can give her.

How can I tell if and when my child will walk?

Normal children start walking sometime between the ages of 8 and 18 months. Most children with diplegia are delayed in walking and do not walk until between 2 and 4 years of age. Children with mild involvement are usually learning to walk at age 2 to 2½. At this age they pull up along furniture and cruise like 10- and 11-month-old infants with normal development do. Some children with diplegia don't start walking until as late as age 8. Therefore, there are a good many years when it's possible that the child will begin walking. Once a child starts walking, she almost always continues to make progress in her gait. In general, by age 8 to 10 years the pattern of mobility has developed which will be the pattern that the child will have for life.

Are there special positions my child should avoid?

This is an area that sometimes generates conflict between therapists and physicians. Between 1 and 3 years of age, children with diplegia have a tendency to sit in a W position with their legs bent backward at the knee. This provides a very stable sitting posture and frees up the child's hands for play. It is also a very comfortable sitting position due to the rotational alignment of their legs.

Although there is no scientific evidence that this position is damaging or dangerous, there are those who think that this position causes hip and gait problems. In fact, however, children who sit in this position walk with their feet turned in only because the alignment of the legs, which allows them to sit this way comfortably, also causes them to walk toeing in. Most professionals recommend that parents allow children to sit in a comfortable position, particularly if they function well. Therapists may try to improve the child's sitting posture and utilize long sitting (sitting with the legs extended in front) and tailor-style positions. Size-appropriate chairs are important as well, as they can help the child to develop a good sitting posture.

As your child starts to move on the floor, she will probably use a commando type of crawl, dragging herself with her arms, her legs following. Allow your child to move and explore with whatever pattern of crawling works for her, bearing in mind that therapists will probably work to establish a four-point crawl. Although you may certainly work on the crawl at home, you should never restrict your child from using a crawl that works well for her.

What walking aids should my child use?

While children without diplegia start cruising at 9 months, children with mild involvement usually start to cruise at approximately age 2. The best walking aids are push toys such as small shopping carts and baby buggies, which work best when weighted down with sandbags because otherwise they tend to be very light. Children at this age seldom need walkers or crutches and usually do not like to use them.

If your child has moderate involvement and is just starting to pull to stand at age 2½, he will most likely be cruising at age 3. He will probably enjoy using a walker because of the freedom of movement it offers. Try letting your child use the walkers that push in front as well as the rear walkers. Experimentation allows the child, with the help of therapists, to determine which kind works best for him. Even at age 3, he will often enjoy pushing toys.

If your child has severe involvement, he will most likely be standing with support by age 3. If by age 2½ your child is not pulling to stand, a standing program should be initiated. Therapists usually recommend the use of ankle-foot braces (AFOs) to help with foot control, and a stander, usually the prone type. We also recommend one or two hours a day of standing if your child tolerates it. The use of a stander helps give children a sense of being upright, encourages head and trunk control and balance, and stimulates the normal development of bones and joints in the legs. Remember that most children with diplegia *will* be pulling up and standing early enough so that a standing program will not be necessary.

As children with diplegia start to stand, they usually go up on their toes. If they have good balance, they may walk around like little ballet dancers, but if balance is a problem, they frequently have difficulty walking. Ankle-foot braces (particularly molded ones) can help stabilize the child's feet and ankles. At this age, the goal of using these braces is to help the child get his feet flat and stable, eliminating the need for concentrating on controlling movement at the foot and ankle. Another condition that responds well to the brace is that of the very flat foot that tends to roll in; for this we recommend the use of a rigid brace, without hinges. It should extend to the tips of the toes to prevent the child from curling his toes over the end of the brace in a gripping fashion. It is more difficult to fit shoes over these longer braces, but generally a style of sneaker that opens far toward the front fits very well.

In the past, orthopedic shoes with attached braces were commonly used. While they may provide a benefit to a small number of children who react allergically to plastic, the vast majority of children are happier in plastic braces, concealed by clothes and worn with regular shoes. The cost, when one considers shoe wear, is comparable. There is almost never a need to use long leg braces or braces above the knee for children with cerebral palsy. Although children with disabilities such as spina bifida, polio, and spinal cord injuries benefit from using these braces, they tend to make walking more difficult. At this age, continuing to work with therapeutic exercises has the best effect. Surgery is seldom recommended at this age.

Is a wheelchair or a special stroller needed?

Between the ages of 1 and 3, most children with diplegia have good trunk control and sitting balance. Regular child or infant strollers are usually adequate for mobility. Special adaptive strollers or wheelchairs are not needed at this stage, unless your child doesn't have good trunk control and needs additional support.

What are the concerns regarding the hips?

By the time a child with diplegia reaches the age of 2, there is a need to begin close and regular examination of the hips for possible spastic hip disease. The spasticity in the muscles around the hip joint puts the child at significant risk for hip dislocation. This dislocation occurs very slowly and is a gradual phenomenon in which the head of the femur (which is round like a ball) moves out of the socket of the hip joint. The most serious consequence occurs when the hip becomes completely dislocated, eventually causing early arthritis and pain as the child grows. Pain sometimes occurs as the hip is dislocating, too. This process of gradual dislocation is called *subluxation of the hip.* Spastic hip disease can be detected by close observation and appropriate x-rays; a hip examination is necessary every six months, and x-rays need to be done periodically. At this young age, muscle release surgery can usually prevent the hips from becoming completely dislocated.

What problems do the feet present?

As we pointed out earlier, at this age it is very common for children to be walking up on their toes or, alternatively, to be noticeably rolling their feet in. Both of these problems are best controlled with foot braces (AFOs) and very rarely need surgical correction at this young age. These braces must be replaced as the child grows.

Some children will have an excessive amount of turning in from the foot or leg, causing them to trip a good deal. Heavy braces to try to correct this should be avoided. Rather, the child should work with therapeutic exercises. If necessary, the problem can be dealt with at an older age with surgery.

Ages Four to Six

This is the age range at which the child with diplegia makes the most significant physical improvement in motor function. By the time your child reaches age 6, he or she should be ready to devote time and energy to school. Once the child reaches kindergarten or first grade, the focus should be on cognitive issues. If at all possible, therapy should now be deemphasized, even discontinued, and children who are able to should be in regular school settings.

How much and what kind of therapy might my child need at this age?

The frequency and specific type of therapy is dependent on your child's severity of involvement, the individual response to therapy, the availability of services, and the parents' ability to provide services. The child who is more severely involved will probably benefit most from therapy because he is less able to stimulate himself. The child with mild involvement moves about and plays fairly readily, thus providing a good deal of his own therapy.

There is agreement, professionally, that the period from age 4 to just entering kindergarten or first grade is the best time to focus on therapy. However, there is no absolute agreement on the ideal number of sessions. Most children at this age will not tolerate more than five half-hour sessions a week. Some children will tolerate considerably less. If your child is resisting, back off and give him time to explore on his own. If you are involved in the therapy, it should be a pleasant experience for both parent and child. Your role is not that of physical therapist but that of parent, a role that includes many things more important than exercises. Doing some exercises at home is better than not doing any, but you should not feel guilty if other necessary activities at home prevent supervising your child's exercising.

There is very little evidence that physical or occupational therapy is directly related to a child's long-term functioning. Therapy *does* provide benefits to the child, and the therapist can be of significant benefit to the parents with direction and suggestions. The benefit of therapy is somewhat similar to that of reading to a child of this age. Most children enjoy being read to, and this does appear to stimulate a later interest in reading and, possibly, in school. It is hard to prove, however, that reading to a child two hours a day is better than two hours a week or two hours a month.

What type of walking aids are now appropriate?

There are no hard-and-fast answers to this question, as each child will choose the walking aid that best suits her needs and her social situation. It helps to keep in mind, however, that this is the age for assessing and working out the child's mobility status. The goal is for the child to be as mobile as her peers by the time she is ready to begin school. The focus should be on mobility and not entirely on walking. A child who can walk very fast with a walker in almost every situation and on any terrain, but who is quite slow with crutches, should not use crutches for school. The crutches should be used at home and in the context of therapy, allowing her time to become more proficient with their use, with school use as a goal.

For the more severely involved child, there may still be the question of whether he will *ever* walk. This is impossible to answer until the child is in fact walking or has reached the age of 7 or 8. Even at that point, walking is not an all-or-none issue. Many children are able to walk short distances around the house but never walk independently outside for longer distances. It then becomes a question of which means of mobility works best for the child. In home situations he may hold on to walls and furniture; in school he may use a walker or crutches; for an all-day excursion to an amusement park, he may choose a wheelchair. This is similar in concept to the individual without a disability who walks at home, rides a bike to go short distances, takes a car for longer rides, and gets on an airplane for great distances.

Could my child need a wheelchair? What type of stroller or wheelchair is best?

Most children at this age who still need to be pushed in a stroller have outgrown standard-size strollers. Families need to evaluate their need for a replacement in terms of how it will be used, where it will be used, whether the child will be able to manipulate it, and how it will be transported in the car. Large strollers are generally quite light and appear less medical than wheelchairs, in addition to being easy to fold up and transport. Their wheels are small, however, and this makes them difficult to push on rough ground. The child can't push herself in a stroller, and she may be concerned about its appearance because it resembles a baby stroller.

The standard wheelchair is certainly more costly as well as clearly medical in appearance. However, children often prefer it because they don't want to look like a baby in a stroller. They can also help choose the color. Most children with diplegia can independently manipulate a chair (power wheelchairs are discussed in Chapter 7 and in Part 2); clearly, the family's environment, as well as the individual child's needs, must be considered when a choice of chair is made.

My child isn't walking at all. Can I do anything to encourage her?

Problems with balance, muscle coordination, spasticity, and leg alignment are the four general causes of *delayed* walking. Any of these problems may also *prevent* a child from walking. Some children may have only one factor affecting them, while others may have several. Generally at this age it's possible to begin to identify and address the specific problems that are preventing the child from walking.

Difficulty with balance (*ataxia*) is a common problem that prevents a child from being able to walk. Even children who walk well with a walker may not be able to progress to crutches, because of balance problems. Typically these are children who cannot stand without holding on to furniture or another person. The balancing mechanism, located in the brain, continues to develop and mature until a child reaches the ages of 8 to 10.

Physical therapy can be very helpful in maximizing your child's balance. Therapists help children exercise and practice falling in much the same way that gymnasts and dancers learn to perfect maneuvers with good balance. Many children between the ages of 4 and 6 develop a protective fear of falling. It is important during this stage not to force them to use crutches. It is better to work in a therapeutic environment where falls will be cushioned by mats, allowing the child to develop a sense of safety. Some therapists suggest heavy shoes to help with balance. Braces are not usually helpful, and there is no surgical treatment that will improve a child's balance.

Lack of muscle coordination makes it difficult for the child to place his feet in the proper position for walking. At an early age, this phenomenon shows up as the inability to initiate steps. The process of taking steps involves the co-contraction of two muscles successfully working in harmony. If muscles are working against each other, the child cannot take any steps. Again, therapy can be helpful in working with the child to develop strategies to control his muscles. Usually by ages 8 to 10 the combination of maturity and therapy yields significant improvement with respect to this problem.

Surgery can be helpful in improving the balance between different muscles. This is accomplished by transferring the overpowering muscle in a way that increases the ability of the weaker muscle. Sometimes the knee is prevented from bending because of muscles pulling excessively in the front; this is improved when part of the muscle is transferred to the back of the knee. Sometimes a child's foot rolls in or out excessively. This imbalance can often be corrected in a brace, but if it is severe, it can also be addressed surgically with transfers or lengthenings of muscles about the ankle.

Spasticity is another problem that contributes to a child's difficulty in walking. Spasticity causes the stretched muscle to pull back and other muscles to become tight as the child attempts to move. Spasticity varies with the child's activity, state of health, growth, and mood, as well as with the time of day. Stretching the muscle and putting it through its range of motion helps to keep it loose but has no effect on the underlying spasticity. Spasticity also prevents muscles from growing normally. As children grow, the very spastic muscle becomes shortened, resulting in a joint that cannot move normally.

There are a number of oral medications that are helpful in reducing spasticity (see table 6). However, for most children the side effects and compli-

Table 6   Medications for Spasticity

Name (Generic/Trade)	How Given	Possible Side Effects[a]
Diazepam/Valium	By mouth Via G- or J-tube Rectally	Sedation; fatigue; weakness; memory disturbance; ataxia; depression
Dantrolene/Dantrium	By mouth Via G- or J-tube	Weakness; drowsiness; lethargy; dizziness; nausea; diarrhea; can also cause liver damage
Baclofen/Lioresal	By mouth Via G- or J-tube Intrathecally (injected into spinal fluid in back via a pump)	Sedation; weakness; fatigue; abrupt withdrawal can cause hallucinations Dizziness; light-headedness; drowsiness; nausea; vomiting; decreased blood pressure; respiratory depression
Botulinum A toxin/ Botox	Injected into spastic muscle	Localized pain; generalized fatigue; transient weakness

[a]One or more of these side effects may occur.

cations of these medications outweigh the benefits. The decrease in spasticity is often short-lived, and withdrawal of the medication typically leads to a temporary increase in spasticity.

In addition to the oral medications, two surgical procedures involving the brain or spinal cord are in use today as treatment for spasticity. The *dorsal rhizotomy* involves cutting the nerves coming from the spinal cord. The second procedure, which is less invasive, involves placing a pump under the skin of the abdomen which feeds an antispasticity medication, Baclofen, via a catheter to the fluid surrounding the spinal cord. The physician can adjust the level of medication as needed. This procedure is reversible, and little post-surgical rehabilitation is necessary. Neither procedure has had long-term studies.

The best results from rhizotomies seem to be in children who have excellent balance and few muscle coordination problems, and who are walking fairly well despite severe spasticity. Children between the ages of 3 and 7 have the best results. A child who is making good progress in walking would not be a candidate for surgery until he has reached a point where he cannot progress because of the spasticity. Also, problems with balance can actually be increased with a dorsal rhizotomy. The use of dorsal rhizotomy peaked in the early and mid-1990s. Since then, many facilities have moved away from doing rhizotomies because the outcomes are not clearly better and there is definitely a higher complication rate than with standard treatment. There is also very little long-term experience with Baclofen pumps in ambulatory children with diplegia, although this approach may have a more defined role in years to come.

Bone and muscle malalignment is another problem that interferes with walking, and most frequently children have difficulty with their feet turning too far in, causing them to trip as they walk. Feet that are rolling in or out and mild tiptoe walking can usually be corrected with an AFO. A hinged AFO should be worn if possible. If the turning in is coming from the hip, thigh, or lower leg, no brace or cable can be applied that will result in better function for the child, although the cosmetic appearance may improve. Children without spasticity often show an improvement in malalignment as they grow. However, children with spasticity seldom improve as they grow, and surgical correction of the problem is necessary, usually before the child begins first grade. This timing prepares the child to enter school in the best possible condition.

Bone malalignment is corrected by surgically cutting the bone (*osteotomy*) and resetting it in a corrected position. Muscle lengthenings involve cutting the tendon. The entire muscle system must be evaluated so that lengthening one muscle does not create an imbalance. Typically, a child who needs his Achilles tendon lengthened has tight hip and knee muscles as well. If only the Achilles tendon were lengthened on a child who is toe walking and has tight hamstrings, the child would walk flatfooted but with a crouched gait. Thus, the timing of muscle lengthenings is crucial, because as a child grows the muscles retighten.

I've heard about surgery to help children walk better. When is the best time for this?

Determining when to perform surgery to make a child walk better requires a highly individualized and often subjective evaluation. There must be careful consideration given to not impeding a child's progress by holding back necessary corrective surgery, while also attempting to time surgeries so that a child has a minimum number of operations in his lifetime. The younger a child is when muscle lengthenings are done, the more likely it is that the child will need to undergo additional lengthenings as he or she grows. On the other hand, delaying necessary surgery will often impede a child's progress in walking.

Minimizing the number of surgeries a child has is essential in attempting to prevent the child from seeing himself as "sick." Operating on a child at an age when he can understand some of his experience and cooperate with postoperative therapy is also beneficial to the child. Generally, just before a child enters first grade is an appropriate time for the first surgery. Most children with diplegia can be treated surgically at this age, with the final adjustment made at the end of adolescence.

With good planning, including grouping procedures, the majority of children will undergo only two orthopedic surgeries in the pre-adult years. This ought to be the goal, and it certainly is the ideal situation. Even if this goal can't be met, there is no reason for a child with diplegia to have an operation every year, for four or five years, as was typical 15 or 20 years ago.

To avoid repeated surgeries and recoveries, it's essential for the child to be evaluated by an orthopedist who is experienced with cerebral palsy and who can perform several necessary procedures while the child is under one dose of anesthesia. The orthopedist must be highly skilled and able to predict the impact of one procedure on another.

Should I be worried that my child might have a hip dislocation at this age?

Hip subluxation and dislocation are certainly significant concerns. Your child must be examined at least every six months and x-rayed as necessary. At this age children are generally x-rayed every two years, unless the examination demonstrates excellent hip motion with very little spasticity. The risk of developing hip problems is related to the severity of involvement. Children with very mild involvement are at low risk for developing hip problems, but as many as 50 to 75 percent of children with severe diplegia develop hip abnormalities that require surgical intervention. Releasing the muscles in the groin (the adductors) which are applying abnormal forces to the hip is the simplest surgical procedure, and should be done as soon as recommended because of its simplicity and generally excellent outcome.

Should I be concerned about my child's back?

Although back problems are a concern, they do not need to be monitored as closely as other areas at this age. There may be the appearance of a *scoliosis* (curvature to the side) or *kyphosis* (round shoulders), but these are almost always flexible deformities. X-rays and treatment are generally not considered at this age because the deformity is not fixed. These conditions do require periodic evaluations by a physician, however.

Are there any upper extremity problems?

The child with typical diplegia by definition has no significant problem with her upper extremities. However, children with diplegia do frequently have difficulty with fine motor coordination, like that required for coloring and writing. Some children do have a significant problem with one arm or hand, despite the fact that they have a diplegic pattern. Refer to the discussion of the upper extremities in Chapter 5 if your child has such a problem.

Ages Seven to Twelve

The early school years usually bring about significant changes for children, including children with a disability. By the time a child reaches this age, the rate of physical improvement has leveled off in areas such as balance and coordination, and it's a good idea to refocus the child's attention away from additional physical improvement and toward intellectual learning. Children without a disability are also being encouraged to concentrate more on academics and less on play at this age, but for the child with a disability these years usually involve coming to terms with a decreased level of physical function.

What school environment is best for my child?

The choice of school environment is often difficult. In some districts parents are not given reasonable options, and this of course complicates the process of placing a child with special needs. The current trend is for inclusion of most children with diplegia, meaning that they are placed in regular classes. This tends to work well for the mildly affected child, as the child can be integrated into most normal activities. Children who have more significant cognitive disabilities are sometimes included only for classes such as music and art, allowing for some interaction with peers. Children with a significant physical disability need to attend school in buildings that are accessible to wheelchairs, walkers, or crutches. An appropriate and accessible toileting facility must also be available.

It is important to consider many factors when choosing a learning environment for your child. You must consider that children need to be in an environment where they can feel successful while learning, without constantly being frustrated. Children clearly benefit from interacting with other children who don't have disabilities, but they need to be placed in an appropriate learning environment, as well. Make certain that properly trained staff are available to meet the needs of your child and to manage interactions with the other children. It is often uncomfortable for the child to be identified as different from the other children, so it's important for you to strike a balance when choosing the appropriate school environment.

What is the role of adaptive physical education?

Many children with mild to moderate diplegia can enjoy normal activities of physical education until they are approximately 10 or 11 years old, when sports tend to become more competitive and the child cannot compete effectively. Alternative physical education (PE) activities, such as adaptive PE, are beneficial. Adaptive PE can be structured by a physical education teacher, providing good physical activity while enhancing the child's self-esteem. If it is desirable and available, informal physical and occupational therapy may also be provided for the child with cerebral palsy while children without disabilities are engaged in routine PE.

How much therapy is necessary now?

For the child with mild diplegia, the start of first grade is a good time to discontinue formal physical and occupational therapy. These therapies should be replaced by physical activities such as swimming, dance class, karate, or horseback riding lessons. Children are often involved in these activities at an even younger age, usually because the parent has identified an interest and located a capable teacher.

Formal therapy at this age has no long-term impact and is similar to an athlete's daily training routine, in that when the training is discontinued, the athlete's ability starts to regress. Because a child cannot be expected to continue physical therapy indefinitely, cultivating her interest and ability in an activity that she can continue throughout her lifetime is a healthier option.

Additionally, formal therapy takes time away from the child's schooling, study time, and possible interaction with other children. An exception should be made for therapy that focuses on teaching specific activities of daily living, such as dressing, and postoperative rehabilitation therapy. These types of therapy are recommended as needed.

The child with severe diplegia may not be able to participate in extracurricular physical activities. Again, it is extremely important to make sure that therapy, especially for children with normal intelligence, doesn't interfere with academic learning. Academic subjects and knowledge are most beneficial for the child in the long term. Certainly, a routine home exercise program has many benefits, and parents can stress the importance of such a program just as they do the importance of daily hygiene.

Will my child's walking continue to improve?

A child reaches his maximum physical ability to walk by 8 to 10 years of age. The child who has limitations in terms of endurance and distance when he is 8 to 10 will almost certainly not do better when he is 16. In fact, the adolescent growth spurt typically adds 12 inches and 50 to 75 pounds to the child's frame. Because his muscle control and coordination do not improve, this extra height and weight make walking more difficult. This period of adjusting to new body dimensions, often referred to as the clumsy period, is experienced by normal adolescents as well.

The 8-year-old with diplegia who is using all his ability to walk at age 8 is not going to walk as well when he ages and has extra height and weight. This does not mean that a child who walks well at age 8 will need a wheelchair at age 16. It is likely, however, that a child who is worn out from a shopping trip at age 10 will need crutches for a shopping trip at age 16. The child with severe involvement who has to struggle with a walker at age 8 will probably be a full-time wheelchair user, except possibly in his own home. In short, parents should not expect major regression, but they can anticipate that their child's walking skills will plateau, with some mild decreases in function.

For both child and parent, frustration can easily result if these changes are not anticipated or haven't been planned for. Up until the age of 8, continuous gains are being made and it is easy, though incorrect, to anticipate that these gains will continue. Frequently, the parents or the child will want to increase the amount of physical therapy, under the false assumption that even more therapy will result in greater gains. As mentioned previously, a far more rewarding approach is to increase the focus on academics.

At this time, both parents and child should be working to accept the reality of the child's level of function; often this is easier for the child than for the parent. Clearly the child will be at a distinct disadvantage if her parents have not been able to deal with their expectations, particularly as the child enters the difficult period of puberty.

What is the best type of walking aid?

The specific aid will most likely vary with the walking environment. A child may hold on to walls in his home, use crutches at school, and prefer a wheelchair for the amusement park. What the child finds works best for him is what he should be allowed to use. Generally children want to use the least obtrusive assistive device that they are comfortable with. Therefore, a child who wants to use crutches usually needs them; the child who does not want to use them is probably stable without them. Parents and therapists should help the child find what works best for him and not force their preferences on the child.

Some children need an assistive device but are not able to understand the need because of a moderate to severe mental disability. Some children who have not developed a healthy fear of falling don't understand this, either, and the child may need to wear a helmet to avoid injury.

Children with severe involvement are at risk for becoming less interested in walking as they get bigger and walking becomes harder. A similar phenomenon occurs in children without disabilities; as they gain weight they watch more TV, eat more food, and get less exercise. Because obesity poses a significant problem for children with diplegia, parents and others need to work with these children to help them avoid obesity. As a parent you should establish firm guidelines requiring your child to get some exercise appropriate to her ability. Your child needs to learn that exercise and good eating habits are the cornerstones to good health, and that it is especially important for her to work on these areas.

What braces are indicated at this age?

The use of braces is usually limited to molded foot braces (MAFOs) or, occasionally, smaller shoe inserts for children who may need them. Usually foot deformities can be corrected with surgery. However, delay of surgery for optimum effect may make it necessary for the child to wear a brace for one to two years. Most children will not object to wearing braces when they are young, but any objections can be dealt with by adjusting the brace or clothing so that the brace is covered up. When the child's reluctance to wear the brace involves other children's reactions, the teacher may find that explaining the use of the brace provides both an excellent lesson for other children and a solution for the wearer.

What shoes should my child wear?

Usually an athletic shoe is the best choice for the child with diplegia, with or without a MAFO. Today, athletic shoes are well constructed and well accepted in almost any social setting. Since the MAFO is providing almost all of the foot support, it is certainly not necessary to purchase an expensive shoe. There is no harm in a child wearing more formal dress shoes on special occasions, with or without braces. Even if a child does not walk as well without braces, occasionally wearing dress shoes can provide a psychological boost without causing any long-term physical damage.

Will surgery improve walking at this age?

At this stage of development, improvement in walking has reached a plateau. If a child is walking without difficulty but has some mild problems, it is best to address these after puberty. On the other hand, if a child has significant problems that can be improved with surgery but were not dealt with before the child started school, they should be addressed now. There is almost no doubt that existing difficulties will increase in severity with the adolescent growth spurt in puberty. Not confronting significant problems also puts the child at risk for additional psychological stress.

My child walks with her knees bent. What can be done?

Walking with bent knees is referred to as a crouched gait and is the most common gait problem in children with diplegia in this age group. If the crouched gait is severe it should be treated, since it can prevent a child from getting around. Once a child has become wheelchair bound due to this problem, it is extremely difficult for her to return to her prior level of walking ability.

The crouching is caused by tight muscles, specifically the hamstrings and *iliopsoas* muscles. It can be treated by surgical lengthenings and, occasionally, using a MAFO to help the child to stand straighter. There are some other, less common causes for the crouching, such as overlengthened Achilles tendons or severe flat feet, and these have their own treatments. The child who has increased crouching will tire out earlier and want to walk shorter distances. During rapid growth spurts crouching usually gets worse, because the muscles aren't growing as fast as the bone.

The cause of the crouched walking pattern is often complex. The primary problem is increased contracture of the hamstring, but there are usually significant secondary problems, such as feet that turn out or that are severely flat. A gait analysis is often required to determine all the causes of crouched walking and to plan a correction of these various components of the problem. After surgery, intense physical therapy is recommended to improve the gait pattern, and the child will need to wear special AFOs that help to support the knee when the child is standing. Usually some crouching persists, but this outcome is preferable to one in which the child develops a gait pattern in which the knee snaps back into hyperextension (also known as back-kneeing). This complex problem should usually be addressed by an orthopedist who has experience with children who have gait problems secondary to cerebral palsy.

What's the treatment for severe flat feet?

Wearing an AFO is the preferred treatment for severe flat feet at this age, if the position of the child's foot can be adequately corrected this way. There are surgical procedures that stabilize the foot—the deformity can be permanently corrected with a triple arthrodesis, for example, which involves fusing together the bones around the heel bone (*calcaneus*). But it's best to delay this surgery until the child's growth is almost completed, since the procedure will stop most of the growth in the foot. As always, the child should undergo the fewest possible surgical procedures, to minimize disruptions. If the child cannot function well, of course, then surgery must be considered.

Is there any treatment for spasticity?

Spasticity may be treated at this age with a dorsal rhizotomy, which involves cutting nerves close to the spinal cord, although this is now done only on rare occasions. Intrathecal Baclofen pumps are being used for some children with this level of disability, but the long-term outcome is still largely unclear. Muscle releases and lengthenings are well-established procedures that predictably work well, though they do not directly decrease spasticity.

Should I still have concerns about hip subluxation and dislocation?

Hip subluxation does continue to be a concern, although the child with diplegia who walks well and has had no hip problems by this age is unlikely to develop problems later. Children whose hips show mild to moderate subluxation must continue to be watched closely, with x-rays every two years throughout the teenage years. By this age, any child with severely subluxed or dislocated hips should have been treated. If a child with severe hip problems has not been treated, then the child should have bone surgery, usually involving additional reconstruction of the hip socket.

Are there back problems that I need to monitor?

As a child approaches puberty, she needs to be watched more closely for scoliosis, since the adolescent growth spurt can produce a larger curve and, eventually, a stiffer curve. Back curvature can be monitored by physical examination, and with x-rays when necessary. The severity and pattern of increase of the curve will dictate how often x-rays will be needed. The risk of developing scoliosis caused by cerebral palsy is fairly low for children who are walking. If scoliosis does develop and become severe, however, professionals usually recommend surgical correction.

Ages Thirteen to Eighteen

During this period of a child's development, a major issue is separating from the family. Adolescents with mild to moderate diplegia and normal intelligence often cope with this issue similarly to the way children without disabilities do. It's not uncommon for young people to feel as if their parents are trying to control their lives. It is, in fact, often difficult for parents to allow a child who has a disability to be independent, and to separate from them. This is especially true for children with more significant disabilities—children whom parents feel a need to protect.

What can I do to help my child develop independence?

As they enter the adult world, a world in which they will interact mostly with individuals who don't have disabilities, teenagers will as a matter of course experience failures and disappointments. But these experiences will help them to develop a sense of self, something that all children need to do.

It is important to allow the teenager to make reasonable decisions and to give him choices in the decisions being made for him. Adolescents often resist having anything to do with outward signs of disability, for example. They may not want to see doctors or therapists, and they may be opposed to wearing braces or exercising. As they mature, teenagers must be allowed whenever possible to make decisions about such things for themselves, even when the outcome of those decisions is likely not to be as good as the outcome would be if the teenager followed parental advice (see the next question, below).

The teen with moderate to severe involvement who is handicapped will probably experience more difficulty separating from his parents and developing independence. A person who needs assistance in the activities of daily living, such as dressing, will of course have a more difficult time. Such teens should be offered as many choices as possible, and should be allowed the freedom and distance from their parents that makes it possible for them to interact with other caregivers. Children who aren't able to get out of a wheelchair by themselves can develop a sense of independence by being permitted to give instruction to the people who assist them.

Using service dogs for the handicapped is a relatively new concept, similar to the guide dogs used by people who are visually impaired. These dogs can be very helpful in fostering independent living. They are taught to retrieve needed items and to help with such tasks as opening doors, and they can be trained to assist the individual who has specialized needs. It goes almost without saying that "man's best friend" can be a wonderful companion.

My child refuses medical care. What should I do?

Although the adolescent should continue to have yearly general medical checkups and orthopedic evaluations every six months to two years, the severity of the diplegia will of course dictate the frequency of medical visits. If the teenager resists this type of routine medical care, parents should first attempt to address any objections: might the teen be more comfortable with a different doctor, for example? Clearly, if a teen who needs care is not able to respond reasonably to a parent's attempt to help, then parents must assume more responsibility for seeing that he or she receives proper medical attention.

Suppose that the young person recognizes that wearing a brace improves the function of his limb but resists wearing it anyway, because the issues of self-image and peer acceptance are more important to him than limb function. A flexible approach by the parents would be best. In this case, they can recognize that doing without the brace at this age will not have a long-term negative effect. On the other hand, a significant advantage of MAFOs is that they are easy to conceal under clothes, so a compromise with a resistant teen may still be a possibility.

What can I do to help my teenager deal with diplegia?

Adolescents frequently have a difficult time as they go through puberty and attempt to develop a personal value system. The teen with diplegia is certainly no exception. What's interesting is that there does not seem to be a significant correlation between the severity of a teen's involvement and her response to the involvement. In fact, it is not uncommon to find a teen with a very mild disability having more trouble accepting the disability than another child who has a severe involvement.

Much of what goes into coping style is derived from the individual's personality. The teen with very mild involvement may have difficulty because she is "almost normal," as opposed to a teen who has severe limitations and knows that she will never be in a situation that is physically similar to that of individuals without disabilities.

Many adolescents with moderate diplegia go through puberty and develop a healthy self-concept with more ease than a child who has no health problems at all. There are other children who need extra help in accepting their disability, and this help can be obtained from licensed, trained counselors. There are psychologists, social workers, and psychiatrists who specialize in helping children deal with disabilities, and the child who is having significant behavioral difficulties should be referred for professional counseling.

My teenager used to walk better a few years ago. What happened?

There is no further improvement in walking after a child has reached the age of 8, 9, or 10, unless he undergoes surgery for a correctable deformity. Adolescent growth leads to a decrease in endurance and coordination that is related to adjusting to the increase in body size. This is rarely a serious problem, unless it is not anticipated or understood. There is a tendency, at times, for a parent to assume his or her child is getting lazy or is less motivated, and this often fosters conflict. Instead, parents must balance the need to encourage a teenager to stay active with the need to allow her to accept a comfortable level of mobility, as determined by her disability.

There is a normal decrease in mobility as individuals mature. The 16-year-old certainly spends less time running around than the 6-year-old. For the individual with a disability, the frequent side effect of less activity—weight gain—can make walking more difficult, which in turn can mean more weight gain as a result of less walking. This cycle can be a lifelong concern for some individuals.

Why is my daughter starting to walk with her knees bent again?

The most common recurrent problem for the adolescent with diplegia who has had previous surgery is an increase in the crouched gait and flat feet. The crouch is most likely a result of hamstrings that have not been able to accommodate to the increase in height. The crouched gait can be a significant problem if left untreated. If it becomes severe, it is harder to treat and puts the teen at significant risk for no longer being able to walk, so it should be addressed immediately. A moderate degree of crouching which does not seem to be getting worse is best dealt with when the teen stops growing. Then there can be a final surgical correction.

The fact is that, for a number of reasons, surgery to correct a crouched gait frequently does not result in a 100 percent correction. Because teenagers often have unrealistic expectations concerning surgery—even after the surgeon has provided a thorough explanation of the anticipated outcome—it's often beneficial to the whole family for the teen to be involved in making decisions about surgery. The physician or surgeon should allow ample time to explain the procedures and answer questions. Taking these steps preoperatively often leads to better cooperation by the teen in the postoperative therapy program. The teen needs to understand that, while no surgery can completely take care of the problem, he has some influence over the outcome.

After surgery to lengthen the appropriate muscles, short-term intensive physical therapy is usually necessary. Once the teen has good correction, it is important for her to keep active doing things to maintain the correction. A therapist can suggest appropriate activities.

What can be done to treat increasing flatfoot deformity?

As a child gains weight, the feet become increasingly flat and pronate more. MAFOs, which are usually effective when a child weighs 50 pounds, generally can't be used when the adolescent reaches 150 pounds. Then there is simply too much weight, causing painful skin pressure as the MAFO holds the foot in position. Surgical correction may involve fusions of the small joints in the foot or different kinds of osteotomies (bone cuts) to correct the flat foot. Different degrees of severity and different surgeons' experience determine the specific procedure that is likely to be recommended.

It is often not easy to decide when feet need to be surgically corrected, though a general rule is that the foot that is causing problems for a person as an adolescent will most likely cause problems for him as an adult. When foot pain is not relieved by adjustments in shoes and inserts, there is definitely a need for treatment. Problems with foot position and shoe wear provide less clear guidelines. Keep in mind that this surgery can easily be done at any time from age 10 to age 40 with little difference in outcome; of course, delaying surgery may also mean delaying relief of symptoms.

What about toe problems that cause pain and calluses?

During adolescence the toes often begin causing problems. The big toe may develop a painful bunion (a large bump on the side of the toe that rubs on the inside of the shoe). The toe with the bunion may begin to bend toward the second toe and even overlap it, causing more discomfort. The easiest solution is to wear soft shoes that are not tight.

If the foot with the bunion continues to be painful, experts recommend surgical correction. There are many different bunion operations that are performed on individuals who don't have cerebral palsy, but most of these approaches will not work well for individuals with CP. Again, it is important to consult a physician who has expertise in treating cerebral palsy before having surgery.

Other toe deformities, such as hammer or claw toes, can cause calluses and be very uncomfortable. They often make walking more difficult for the individual who is already stressed, and may make it difficult to wear shoes. These problems are easily treated with surgery, when necessary.

Are there other leg and foot problems that can be corrected at this age?

In most cases leg and foot alignment has been corrected by this age, but adolescence is certainly an excellent time to make a correction, particularly after the growth spurt. Bone procedures can be combined with muscle lengthening, making it necessary to expose the child to anesthesia only once.

These alignment corrections range from the straightforward to the complex. Most professionals recommend that a gait analysis be performed to help make decisions about proper treatment. Such analyses are conducted in a laboratory specializing in analyzing the gait problems of children with cerebral palsy. This evaluation can provide excellent information prior to surgery.

Should I be concerned about hip development?

For some individuals, the problem of hip subluxation needs to be monitored through adolescence. If the teen has a mild to moderate involvement and his hips have been normal up to this age, it is very unlikely that any problems will develop. X-rays are generally not needed in this group of teens after the ages of 8 to 10.

Children who have had hip problems or subluxation need to be followed closely by physical examination and x-rays through the adolescent growth spurt and into the teen years. Any change in the hips during the adolescent growth spurt usually needs to be treated with surgery, with both bone procedures and muscle lengthenings. At this age, too, it is often necessary to address the hip socket surgically.

Continued monitoring and treatment as necessary will help the child reach adolescence and adulthood with hips that are as near to normal as possible. This is the child's best hope of avoiding the early development of arthritis, which can cause significant walking problems and pain.

What about scoliosis?

Scoliosis, or side-bending curvature of the spine, as a result of cerebral palsy is not a common problem in children with a mild to moderate pattern, but when it does occur it becomes severe during the adolescent growth spurt. It must be carefully monitored with physical exams and x-rays. This type of scoliosis should not be confused with *idiopathic scoliosis* (spinal curvature), which can occur in adolescents, usually girls, who are otherwise normal.

The spinal curve in the teen with cerebral palsy is usually not helped by brace wear, and doctors often suggest surgery if the curve progresses to 45 to 50 degrees. A spinal fusion prevents any further progression and corrects a significant portion of the curve. (Scoliosis is discussed in more detail in the next chapter.)

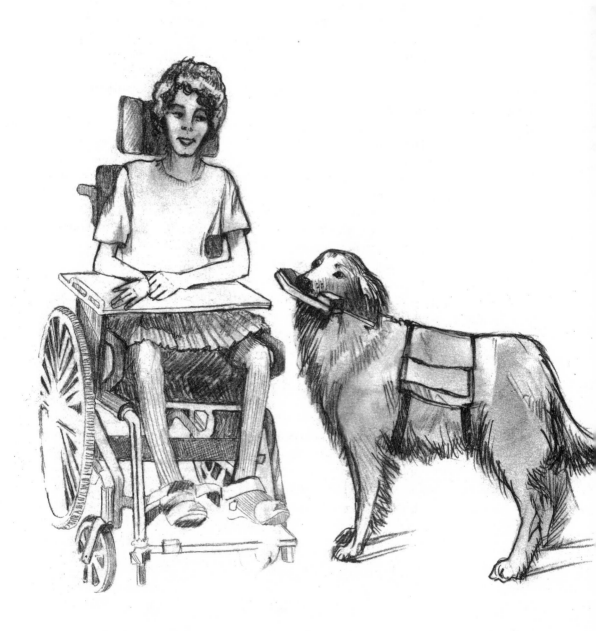

Quadriplegia

7

♦ QUADRIPLEGIA is a form of cerebral palsy in which both arms and both legs are affected. Severe diplegia is often mistaken for mild quadriplegia, primarily because almost everyone who has diplegia has some involvement of their arms as well as their legs. For people with diplegia and for those with mild quadriplegia, there is mild dysfunction of the arms, but it is not a significant disability. The terminology used to describe the degree of involvement can vary greatly, even among specialists, because it is so difficult to fit a great number of individuals with differing functional factors into any specific category. There are always overlaps, and there are differences of opinion about what the proper diagnosis is.

There are many people whose degree of cerebral palsy is not properly described by a broad term like *quadriplegia*. For this reason, several different kinds of quadriplegia have been identified and named.

What do the different kinds of quadriplegia look like?

The child with *moderate spastic quadriplegia* sits quite well, can lift himself into a wheelchair independently or with assistance, may be able to do very limited walking with a walker, and has enough hand function to feed himself. (Someone who primarily has spasticity and can walk well has diplegia. The needs of such a person are addressed in Chapter 6.) A child with *severe spastic quadriplegia* can't walk, even with assistive devices, is not able to move to and from a wheelchair independently, usually isn't able to feed herself, and has difficulty sitting.

Athetosis (making large, uncontrollable movements) usually affects the upper extremities more than the lower. Most individuals with athetosis have a quadriplegic pattern, although the degree of involvement varies widely. Children with *moderate athetosis* are able to walk and can use their extremities well enough to take care of most activities of daily living on their own. Children with *severe athetosis* are not able to walk independently and often are not able to transfer (move into and out of a wheelchair) by themselves. Some children with severe athetosis are unable to feed themselves and have speech problems, as well. Many children with severe athetosis have difficulty sitting and need special seating support.

Other terms that are often confused with the terms described above are *pentaplegia, tetraplegia,* and *triplegia.* Pentaplegia describes a child with poor head control and four-limb involvement. Tetraplegia is essentially another term for quadriplegia. Triplegia refers to involvement of three limbs: both legs and one arm. Children with poor head control and quadriplegia are discussed in this chapter, in the context of severe spastic quadriplegia or severe athetoid quadriplegia. Parents whose children have triplegia, are mildly affected, and can walk will find the most relevant information in Chapter 5, on hemiplegia. Parents whose children have moderate leg involvement but walk with assistive devices will find the most relevant information in Chapter 6, on diplegia. The child with triplegia who can't walk is considered in this chapter, in the context of moderate spastic quadriplegia.

Birth to One Year

The first year of life is one of rapid changes. The infant learns to control the movement of her head, reach for a toy, roll over, and sit by herself without support. A delay in the development of these abilities is often the first sign of a problem in children who have quadriplegic pattern involvement. An experienced mother or grandmother often will notice that the infant does not "feel normal" when she holds him in her arms. She may say that the infant doesn't move normally, or is either stiffer or more floppy than expected. But such signs of problems may be subtle and hard to put a finger on.

Can quadriplegia be diagnosed at this age?

The early diagnosis of quadriplegia is difficult, as is the early diagnosis of diplegia and hemiplegia. However, children who had certain kinds of medical problems at an early age are at higher risk of later being diagnosed with spastic quadriplegia. Certain complications in the early development of the infant are associated with quadriplegia. These complications include extreme prematurity (less than 28 weeks gestation), very low birth weight (less than 1,500 grams), bleeding in the brain, severe asphyxia (lack of oxygen), bacterial meningitis, and shaken baby syndrome (see Chapter 1). Children who survive these complications may have mild, moderate, or severe involvement, or they may be normal. As mentioned in Chapter 1, other disorders can look like CP, especially quadriplegia. Particular suspicion should be raised in the infant without any risk factors for CP. These infants should have appropriate testing done for other neurological diagnoses.

Although many children with traumatic beginnings grow and develop normally, parents' and physicians' suspicion and concern is raised when children have a history of early significant problems. A definitive diagnosis is rare during infancy, but parents are often given an idea of what might be ahead for them and their child. However, it is important to remember how tentative these predictions are.

What can be done for the high-risk infant during the first year of life?

For the infant who is considered high risk because of medical problems in infancy or because of early signs of developmental delay, an infant stimulation program is often recommended (this is addressed further on the next page). In addition, any ongoing medical issues need to be addressed, and the infant's growth and development should be optimized.

Nutrition is one of the most important issues. A child who is not growing either is not getting adequate nourishment or is having severe medical problems that are inhibiting growth. The brain needs energy to grow and develop, and it uses the same energy as the muscles and bones. Therefore, if the muscles and bones are not growing, it's likely that the brain is not growing, either. Medical problems can drain a lot of energy from a child or can be part of the reason a child does not want to eat.

Children with quadriplegia may have hydrocephalus, a condition that makes it necessary to place a shunt, a surgically implanted device that prevents fluid from building up in the brain. Shunts must be checked periodically, and a child who has frequent infections should be checked carefully and often. Infection around a shunt—or any other infection—must be treated aggressively, and attempts must be made to prevent such infections by treating their cause.

Do children with quadriplegia often have seizures?

Seizures are frequently associated with cerebral palsy. Because seizures can have a significant effect on the growing child, careful attention to seizures, and treatment to achieve maximum control of them, is strongly advised. (Seizures are discussed in Chapter 3.)

What kind of feeding problems might a child with quadriplegia have?

Feeding problems caused by oral motor dysfunction are commonly associated with quadriplegia. This dysfunction of the muscles of the tongue and mouth can make chewing and swallowing difficult. Feeding problems can affect the child's nutrition and can also lead to chronic aspiration and pneumonia.

Gastric reflux, in which food comes back up the esophagus, can cause spitting up or vomiting. Sometimes the child coughs when this happens, and then food particles are introduced into the lungs, causing bronchitis and pneumonia. Some children have a poor gag reflex, and they, too, are susceptible to respiratory infections. It is often helpful to sit the child up after feeding him or her. Several medications may be used to help control these problems. In the most severe situations surgical options may be recommended, ranging from placement of a gastrostomy tube to a fundoplication. (See Chapter 3 for a full discussion of feeding problems and their treatment.)

What causes irritability?

Some babies are irritable for no apparent reason, and this includes some babies with cerebral palsy. But children with spastic quadriplegia may be irritable for reasons associated with their condition. These babies may be experiencing gastric reflux, not necessarily vomiting; they may be having seizures, but not necessarily seizures that parents easily recognize. It is unlikely at this age that their irritability is due to pain, although reflux can certainly be accompanied by discomfort.

Should I start my child in therapy at such a young age?

Although no absolute proof exists that early therapy changes the functional outcome of the child, most children benefit from early developmental stimulation therapy that is provided by physical and occupational therapists. Early exposure to a therapist is also often an invaluable resource and support for parents. Therapy should be delayed until the baby is medically stable, however, and until it can be handled without putting too much stress on the heart and lungs. Premature babies usually need to gain at least enough weight to be at approximately normal newborn weight. After a severe brain trauma, such as a near-drowning, therapy should not be started until the blood pressure and heart rate are stabilized and do not change when the child is handled. The therapy, when initiated, must be administered gently so that the child isn't agitated. Agitation can cause blood pressure to rise, and if severe this may cause further brain damage.

Ages One to Three

Abnormal development in a child becomes more clearly recognized and defined as the child approaches his first birthday. Most children at this age are rolling over, sitting, pulling to stand, starting to say words, and even walking independently. Of all these developmental milestones, walking is usually of greatest concern to parents of a child with a developmental delay. Parents naturally become concerned about the long-term prognosis if their child has not achieved head control when other children his age are walking. It is at this time that a diagnosis of quadriplegia is often made.

Some parents adopt the mistaken notion that more therapy or use of a special brace or a walker will make it possible for their child to walk. This notion is often fostered by a combination of factors, most importantly, by a lack of understanding of the child's problem or difficulty in accepting how severe the problems are. Anxiety also plays a role. Physicians need to spend time with parents, to help them gain some perspective and understanding of the complex problems facing them and their child. Parents should be encouraged to focus on the developmental skills that can be addressed now, and to set aside, for the time being, their concern about developments that will only become clear with the passage of time.

What are the most important health issues at this age?

The most important issue at this age is whether the child is thriving, gaining weight, and growing in height and head circumference. The long-term best outcome for any child requires that he get adequate nourishment in order to grow and develop. The child's actual weight is less important than whether the child is gaining, staying the same, or losing weight over time. The child who is not getting enough nourishment and not growing is also not going to develop optimally. The child's overall nutrition and health are much more important than any therapy, brace, or other device. Good nutrition is essential to normal growth and maximum development.

Another health issue at this age is constipation. The child who cannot get around on her own may become constipated and uncomfortable, and may express this discomfort by becoming irritable. An appropriately designed bowel program can be a great help in this area (see Part 2, on caregiving techniques, for a description of such a program).

Are physical and occupational therapy beneficial? Physical and occupational therapy are important for the child's stimulation and to help the family develop realistic expectations. The therapist is a great resource for the parent in gaining information about future equipment needs and can assist in being a "doorway" to the medical community. Therapists can also teach parents how to touch and hold their child. However, it is important to understand the limitations of what the therapist can do. A physical therapist, no matter how experienced and knowledgeable, can't *make* a child walk. He or she can work to keep the child's joint range of motion at its maximum and can provide valuable strategies for helping with balance, so that the child has the best possible chance of walking if she is capable of doing so. The actual ability to walk and to balance are functions of the brain. At present, no one knows how to overcome the damage the brain has suffered and get it to function normally.

In the same way, occupational therapists can help enormously with activities of daily living such as self-feeding. But they can't make a child who has quadriplegia have normally functioning hands and fingers. The goal of any of the therapies should be to help the child. Therapy itself should not be the goal. Therefore, therapy should not consume the child's life; nor should anyone suggest or believe that therapy will satisfy unrealistic expectations. The child can receive therapy in various ways, some of them of benefit to both the child and the parent; for example, there are infant stimulation day care centers where the child can be placed for both day care and therapy.

Parents need to maintain contact with the therapist. In this way, the therapist can answer many of the parents' questions as well as provide suggestions for home activities that would help the child and family. Many of these suggestions will be practical, while others will be fun and stimulating.

In terms of when therapy ought to begin, the situation is somewhat different for the child who sustains a brain injury at age 2 up to age 5. After an injury, a child may very quickly develop severe muscle tightness and contractures. Parents may believe that this possibility should have been addressed earlier by therapy, but the safe time for starting therapy varies with each child. Just after an injury the brain swells, and everything possible must be done to reduce this swelling and prevent additional swelling, including avoiding agitating the child and raising his or her blood pressure. At some point, from several days to a month after the injury, the swelling diminishes and the brain begins to heal. This is the time to start therapy.

How many doctors does my child need?

Generally, by age 1 or a year after brain injury, a child can be followed by a family pediatrician. Specialists can then be consulted as the need arises, thereby limiting the time spent by child and parent in doctors' offices. Not only is this helpful in a practical sense, but it is also psychologically beneficial. Most children with cerebral palsy need to be seen by specialists at times—a pediatrician can't provide for *all* the child's needs. What the pediatrician can do is refer the child for dental, orthopedic, neurological, and other consultations when necessary. Chapter 9 defines various medical specialties and suggests guidelines for obtaining proper medical care for your child.

Are children with quadriplegia often mentally retarded?

Children with quadriplegia may have mental retardation, but many children are thought to have mental retardation when in fact they are only very limited in their ability to communicate. Having a child tested by appropriately trained individuals is essential in order to evaluate his or her potential. (Mental retardation is further discussed in Chapter 3.)

What about self-injurious behavior?

Self-injurious behavior, or SIB, often begins at this time and is usually seen in children with spastic or hypotonic quadriplegia with some degree of mental retardation. It is very rarely seen in children with athetosis. (During the adolescent period, athetoid movements can become strong enough to cause injury accidentally. The treatment of this problem is different from the treatment for voluntary self-abuse.)

The most common self-abusive behaviors are hand biting, hand hitting, head banging, and eye scratching. The behavior generally is worse when the child is left alone or is not involved in some activity. Treatment should focus on finding ways to keep the child occupied and distracted. Other methods, such as rewarding desired behaviors, may be tried but may not be successful because of the child's cognitive limitations.

Restraints, such as elbow extension splints, helmets, and face guards are occasionally used, but they may only frustrate the child and make matters worse when the restraints are not in place. Clearly, if the self-abusive behavior is causing significant bodily harm, such as risking blindness or the loss of fingers, the child must be protected from himself. (See Chapter 3 for a more complete discussion of self-injurious behavior.)

What type of seating is best?

Most children with quadriplegia are not sitting well by age 1, although many of them eventually develop the ability to sit. At this age parents should concentrate on supporting the child's upper body, encouraging head control and providing head control as needed. This is especially important to improve the child's feeding, communication, and interaction with the environment. Between the ages of 1 and 2, the child should be fed while seated in a seat facing the person feeding him. The seat may be a chair with special trunk (upper torso) supports or with a special contour (plastic contoured seats, such as the tumble form, are one alternative). For best results, the child's needs should be assessed frequently by an occupational therapist, who can recommend the best seat for the individual child.

In choosing a seat, it's important to consider whether only a feeding chair is desired or if a combined stroller and feeding seat would be more useful. These combination devices are popular, and there are a number of them on the market. Generally, they have a nice appearance and resemble a standard baby stroller rather than a medical wheelchair. Some seats can be used as car seats, although these tend to be a bit heavy and bulky. Most parents do not find them convenient for routine use, though they may come in handy as a car seat when traveling extensively. The chair should be ordered with a lap tray. Toys can be placed on the tray in front of the child, and the chair can be used as a desk, as well.

There are also a large variety of positioning and play chairs available, which the child may use in school or therapy. If one of these seems especially well suited to the individual child, the parents may want to order one or make one for use at home. These chairs include corner chairs, saddle chairs, benches, cylinders, and swing chairs.

Is a walker recommended?

The use of a child walker is controversial. Some therapists believe that walkers are detrimental to development, and others see them as useful. Many parents prefer to use them because children seem to enjoy the increased freedom of movement, though sometimes the movements consist of stiffening or flailing rather than being purposeful. The walker will not prevent a child from walking independently if he is capable of doing so. Nor will the walker make a child who cannot walk do so.

There is no scientific evidence that a short period of time spent in a walker is either harmful or beneficial, but the walker may represent an emotional issue for parents. Children without disabilities use this type of seated walker, and when a child with cerebral palsy uses a walker he may appear more like a normal child. This is in contrast to the child's use of a stander, which a child without disabilities would not use. Our position, simply stated, is that using a walker is not going to harm the child as long as safety precautions are taken with regard to staircases and objects that can tip the device over. This is crucially important, because many children have been seriously injured when left unattended in a walker.

Is standing important?

We believe that there are many benefits to standing, although most of these have not yet been documented scientifically. One benefit is the strengthening of bone; standing improves both the quality and the size of bones. This has been proven in studies of children with spina bifida who stand and walk with braces. They have fewer fractures, even as adults, than children who constantly sit in wheelchairs. This has been shown as well for adults with cerebral palsy who no longer walk but continue to have better bone mass, apparently from having been standers as children. Cerebral palsy and spina bifida are different conditions, but it is reasonable to assume that the benefits of weight bearing should be at least similar, if not the same for children with either condition.

Another benefit of standing is in the area of development. Many therapists and doctors believe that standing helps the development of balance, head control, and spatial conceptualization. Thus the child who may later be able to use a power chair gains a better sense of the three-dimensional space that he will eventually move around in. These beliefs of doctors are difficult to prove, but we do know that nondisabled children develop these concepts in just this way. It seems logical that children with cerebral palsy need the same stimulation to develop their abilities to the greatest extent possible.

How can I tell whether a stander would be helpful for my child?

Between 18 and 24 months of age is usually a practical time to start considering a stander, because by then the child's acute medical issues are mostly resolved and parents and doctors have a good sense of the rate of gain in development. By this time, many children with quadriplegia are able to move by crawling or rolling on the floor. Some are able to scoot in the sitting position, and some are able to pull to a standing position. If a child is able to pull to stand by 24 months, she can bear her weight and most likely will progress with time to a walker. If a child has not reached this milestone at 24 months, she should be started in a standing program with a stander.

There are three types of standers: prone, supine, and freedom, or parapodium, standers. The freedom or parapodium stander is most useful for children with spina bifida who have normal upper bodies. It has almost no usefulness for children with cerebral palsy, because most children with CP have poor upper body control, and will end up falling forward in this type of stander. Those children with CP who have very little upper body involvement usually are able to pull to stand or are able to use a walker.

Children with poor or no head control should be started in a supine stander. The disadvantage of this type of stander is that the child leans backward, and therefore his field of vision is limited to the ceiling. A good thing to do is to hang interesting objects above the child's head to provide stimulation, or to position a mirror to reflect the activity that's going on in the room.

For children with some head control, the prone stander is better because it stimulates them to hold up their heads. In addition, a lap tray placed in front of them can allow them to play while they are standing. The tilt of both the supine and the prone stander can be adjusted so that the child is as upright as possible and yet comfortable (see Part 2 for more complete discussion of standers).

How much time should my child spend in the stander?

It is usually best to start with a short period of time, say 10 to 15 minutes. As the child becomes accustomed to the stander, a parent should try to work the child up to a one-hour stretch twice a day, if the child tolerates it. Standing should not be a period of great difficulty for the child, however. By working with different positions and involving the child in activities, the parent can make time spent in the stander more enjoyable for the child. Physical therapists can help parents design a successful program for their child.

If the child develops a severe aversion to the stander, it may be better to stop working with it for several months and come back to it with a new approach. For the child who is not walking, the goal should be to stay with a standing program into and through adolescence. There are many adults who still find it useful.

Are motorized wheelchairs appropriate at this age?

No, they are not. Motorized wheelchairs are often very appealing because they are "state of the art" and for many parents may represent the best that they can provide for their child with a disability. However, a motorized chair for a child with cerebral palsy should not be considered until the child is approximately 6 years old.

A child with cerebral palsy who would be able to drive a motorized chair at age 3 would most likely be capable of cruising (walking around by holding on to furniture), and that child will be a very functional walker within a year or two. An expensive motorized wheelchair will provide little benefit to such a child. On the other hand, the child who will eventually need a chair is not likely to be able to drive a motorized chair at age 2 or 3, because of other impairments (such as visual difficulties, attention deficits, fine motor dysfunction, or cognitive impairments). There are a few exceptions, mainly children with various conditions that have no intellectual impairment associated with them. These children might appropriately and effectively use a motorized chair at this age.

Are there other pieces of equipment that might be helpful?

For the child who is not able to sit independently, a bathing chair can be very helpful. There are several different types available commercially, or they can be constructed using PVC pipes and cloth or netting. Purchasing these devices puts a financial strain on some parents. It's usually easier to obtain funding for seats and wheelchairs than for standers and bathing chairs. Sending letters of medical necessity (provided by the physician's office; see Part 2) and being persistent are often the best ways for parents to approach insurance carriers. Community service organizations may also provide financial assistance for such purchases.

What are the predominant bone and joint problems at this age?

Up until a child reaches the age of 1, there are almost never any cerebral palsy–related problems with the bones and joints which need to be addressed by anything other than evaluation and observation. Starting at 1 year of age, however, close follow-up is important. The most severe problems, which often start to become evident at this age, are hip subluxation and hip dislocation.

The hip is a ball-and-socket joint. *Subluxation* refers to the condition in which the ball slowly pulls partially out of its appropriate position in the socket; *dislocation* is the condition in which the ball has come completely out of the socket. Both conditions are called *spastic hip disease* and are caused by tight or spastic muscles about the hip. Spastic hip disease is a common problem for children with quadriplegia; as many as 80 percent of children with severe involvement are affected. Pain is sometimes associated with spastic hip disease and can cause a child to be irritable.

With proper monitoring, follow-up, and treatment by an orthopedist familiar with spastic hip disease, hip dislocation can be avoided. Monitoring begins with a physical examination. If the examination reveals a limitation of motion in the hip so the legs cannot be spread apart to a total of 90 degrees, an x-ray needs to be taken and repeated every six months. The x-ray indicates whether the hip is properly located within the socket. If the hip starts to move out of the joint, the tight muscles need to be treated. Nonsurgical treatment has proven unsuccessful in preventing hip subluxation. Braces, casts, and exercises have been extensively used without much success, and so these approaches have been almost completely abandoned by most orthopedists treating children with cerebral palsy. To date, there is no proof that botulinum toxin prevents hip subluxation.

The medical community agrees that spastic hip muscles need to be treated, although there's a good deal of difference concerning exactly which muscles should be released and how the child should be treated after surgery. Some surgeons prefer the use of casts or braces postoperatively to maintain correction, while others prefer to use only therapy or exercises. Finding a surgeon who is thoroughly familiar with spastic hip disease becomes crucial, because of the variety of treatment possibilities.

If muscle-release surgery is not successful, *varus osteotomy* of the femur bone may need to be done at an older age. In addition, an *acetabular osteotomy* (reshaping the socket) is sometimes also necessary. Both surgeries are very successful if done at a young age. Occasionally with severe spastic hip disease, a muscle release that initially was successful ends up needing to be followed by the varus osteotomy. The key to the successful treatment of spastic hip disease is close observation and early treatment. The greatest problems arise from late recognition of the problem. Bones in a hip that has been out of place for a period of time undergo changes in shape, making the best treatment outcome far more difficult for even the most highly skilled surgeon. All children with quadriplegia should be evaluated every six months by a physician who understands these issues.

Scoliosis, which is side bending of the spine, and *kyphosis,* which is bending forward, are also common problems. At this age, these are only symptoms of the child's poor upper body control, and they should be observed over time by the physician. The child must be provided with adequate support in seats and standers. This curvature is not related to the structural spinal curves that develop later, frequently at adolescence.

Feet can also present problems. Because of poor muscle control, they are often very flat, or if there is spasticity, they may point down so that the child only bears weight on her toes. As the child is started in the stander, small braces on the feet are often needed either for support or for position. These AFOs (ankle-foot orthoses) may be made by a therapist or an orthotist, and at this age are used mostly when standing. Some children will have less spasticity or will be able to move more easily when sitting in the chair with their braces on. The braces inhibit spasticity and may be worn most of the day for comfort. If the child has severe spasticity and the foot cannot be positioned properly in a brace, botulinum toxin injection of the gastrocnemius muscle (calf muscle) may be helpful in controlling foot placement within the brace. Surgery for foot problems is rarely recommended at this age.

The use of hand and upper extremity bracing at this age may or may not be recommended. It is most useful for the child who is developing severe *contractures*, in which the fingers or limbs assume a fixed position. Braces are usually made by an occupational therapist and are worn by the child for anywhere from one to six hours a day, in an attempt to keep the muscle stretched. If a child tolerates the braces well, they may be left on during the night. Splints made from a neoprene material allow for more functional hand mobility during daytime use. Rigid braces are less functional but have the advantage of controlling more severe contractures. Children who are using their hands for reaching or manipulating objects should not have the hand covered for prolonged periods of time. This is extremely important, because the brace will decrease sensation in the hand and may discourage children from exploring with and using their hands.

Ages Four to Six

Children in this age group continue to develop rapidly, both mentally and physically, and patterns and potential abilities become much more clearly defined. By the time the child reaches the age of 6, his or her basic pattern of involvement and abilities can be determined, although neurological development will continue at a significant rate for at least several more years. The child who is not able to sit independently by age 5 will almost certainly never walk independently, but will continue to improve in head and upper body control. The cognitive abilities of the child can also be much better defined as he or she gets older.

The primary goal for children in this age group is preparation for school, although by this age children with disabilities should already be in a program with other children and therefore should be somewhat accustomed to separating from their parents and interacting with peers in a structured setting. A major concern should be that the child continue to grow physically, because the brain can only develop if it has enough nourishment. The best indication of adequate nutrition is good overall growth in the child.

What role does physical and occupational therapy play at this age?

As the child approaches school age, education should be the predominant concern, and therapy that contributes to this goal should be stressed. Occupational and speech therapy, as well as communication efforts that make the most of the child's learning potential, are most important. Therapy that is focused on physical gains can be incorporated into the school program or even accomplished through play. An appropriate balance prevents the child from regressing physically while making it possible for him to grow intellectually.

Can drooling be controlled?

Drooling is a symptom of oral motor dysfunction involving the muscles of the mouth and throat, similar to the problems the child may be having in controlling the muscles in her legs and arms. Various medical and social consequences are associated with drooling. Mild drooling can usually be managed with small bibs or bandanas. At this age, it is possible to teach the mild or moderately involved child to try to keep his mouth closed and to swallow. As children get older, drooling often significantly improves. However, drooling can become a problem when the child gets into a school environment, where it may damage books or computer keyboards as well as interfere with the child's social life. Severe drooling may cause skin irritation around the mouth and face. Medications or surgical procedures can be used if necessary (see Chapter 3).

What about seizures?

Seizures continue to be a problem for the child with quadriplegia. When there are changes in the child's behavior, or when a new, different movement pattern develops and the child is not able to control it, seizures should be suspected. As the child grows, seizure patterns may change. It should not be assumed that the child is not having any seizure activity just because the usual seizure pattern is absent. Also as the child grows, the dosage of medication often needs to be adjusted, and it's important to monitor drug levels. The side effects of medications also need to be monitored. (For a fuller discussion of seizures, see Chapter 3.)

What is necessary in terms of vision and hearing screening?

It is vitally important to evaluate vision and hearing as part of preparing your child for school. If your child was tested at an earlier age, then a simple checkup is appropriate. A child who has never been fully evaluated, however, should be examined within the limits of her functioning level. That is, the examining physician, audiologist, or optometrist must know whether the child is unable to respond to questions because of deficits in her sight or hearing, or whether the problem is due to mental retardation; in the latter case, the child may see and hear perfectly but may not perform well on a vision or hearing test because of cognitive limitations.

An accurate assessment of the child's visual and auditory capacity will help to place her in the appropriate school or classroom and to develop a communication system for her to use. Eyeglasses and hearing aids, if indicated, may make a significant difference in the child's interest in her environment, as well as in her ability to learn.

My child has communication problems. What can be done for him?

This is a good age to begin teaching simple nonverbal communication skills to children who aren't able to talk. If your child can use his hands, he may begin on his own to develop a sign language that works for him and his caregivers. Around age 3, many children can begin to learn formal sign language, although the ability to learn formal sign language, like the ability to learn any language, depends on the child's cognitive level. For children who have limited hand function, eye signing and facial expressions make communication possible.

At this age, communication allows the child to understand that she can influence and, to some extent, control her environment. Another way for the child to learn this is for her to play with toys, record players, and TVs that she can control by using electrical switches or joysticks. Becoming proficient at manipulating these devices is a skill that will be valuable later, when the child uses computers, communication systems, and motorized mobility devices. Many electric toys can be very easily adapted for the child with a disability; sometimes all that's needed is an on-off switch that the child can control by touching it. (Communication systems are discussed more fully later in this chapter.)

What concerns should I have about my child's teeth?

Spasticity in the mouth muscles prevents the parent from being able to properly clean the teeth, and because the teeth are constantly bathed in food particles, the child has a much higher risk of developing tooth decay. The lack of proper brushing also causes gum hypertrophy, a condition in which the gums overgrow and may almost cover the teeth. Some medications used to control seizures, such as Dilantin, may aggravate gum hypertrophy, and in some children the overgrown gums need to be surgically trimmed back. A dentist can help prevent tooth decay and gum hypertrophy, and can treat these conditions if they occur.

What decisions need to be made about seating?

Appropriate seating continues to be important for feeding, transportation, and positioning for maximum hand use. All these functions can often be accomplished with one wheelchair that is fitted with a lap tray and good chest supports and, if needed, a headrest. Hip guides and hip abductors are sometimes necessary for proper lower extremity alignment. Some parents prefer to use one chair for feeding, a stroller for mobility, and a separate seat with a lap tray for play activities. One reason parents like this arrangement is that it looks less medical or it makes the child appear less disabled.

As the child grows older and begins riding the bus to school, multiple seating arrangements become more difficult to manage. The problems arise not only in terms of providing all these different seating arrangements in different settings (at home, at school, and elsewhere), but also in maintaining two, three, or four seats with proper adjustments for support. If the family goes to a restaurant, for example, and the child has a properly fitted wheelchair adapted for feeding, all his needs—transportation, the freedom of mobility, and the assurance of a proper feeding position—can be met with one chair.

Strollers have the advantage of not looking like a medical device and of being more easily transportable, but they have the disadvantage of providing poor trunk support for the child. The older child may also object to the appearance of the stroller because she associates it with babies. And it's impossible for a child who is sitting in a stroller to push the stroller. For these reasons, using a wheelchair can be a significant symbol of growing up and independence. A child with some limited ability to use her arms may be able to push a regular wheelchair quite well, if it fits her properly. Wheelchairs come in a variety of colors, and children generally enjoy having a say in choosing a color.

Is this the right age to introduce a motorized wheelchair?

It's often difficult to decide whether to provide a child with a motorized chair, and the decision is usually complicated by the fact that not everyone involved in the decision agrees. There has been much debate about fitting power chairs to 2- or 3-year-olds, for example, but this is almost always appropriate only for children with *osteogenesis imperfecta* (very brittle bones) and *arthrogryposis* (very stiff joints). Children with these conditions are cognitively normal and have normal balance and motor control. If they aren't walking by the age of 2, they aren't likely to become fully functional walkers and will be dependent on the chair for long-term use.

Children with cerebral palsy, however, are very different in that most of the children who would be capable of using a motorized chair at age 3 are already cruising and will be very functional walkers within the next year or two. Getting a motorized wheelchair for such a child would be counterproductive. Conversely, most of the children who will eventually need a chair are not able to handle the controls at a younger age, so a motorized wheelchair would be of no use to them. Thus, it seldom makes sense to introduce a young child to a motorized wheelchair.

The most appropriate age at which to introduce a power chair is around 6 years. As with other things, this is an average, and some children who will be able to handle a chair later, after they have grown and developed, will not be ready for a power chair at age 6. Some children get around pretty well with a walker from the age of 6 through age 8 or 9, while they are small and in the lower grades. However, as time passes, the child's need for motorized transportation will probably have to be reevaluated. For one thing, as children move into the upper grades the schools get larger, and the long hallways may be tiring to manage with a walker. Another consideration is the child's increasing weight, which may also make it difficult for her to use a walker.

There are two areas of controversy regarding motorized chairs. Some parents want their child to have a power chair even though it would not be appropriate for her. These parents are often motivated by a desire to provide everything possible for their child, and in their eagerness to provide for her, they sometimes overlook the fact that her functioning level and safety awareness must be considered with respect to handling the chair.

On the other extreme are parents whose child does some walking but is too slow and unsteady to be a functional walker in a busy school environment. These parents sometimes worry that the child will stop walking and regress if he has a motorized chair. This fear is unfounded. The situation is similar to that of a 16-year-old who gets his first car. Initially, certainly, he wants to drive everywhere, and he does walk less often. But he doesn't forget how to walk, run, or ride his bicycle. It soon becomes apparent to the 16-year-old that it is easier to walk to his friend's house down the street than to open the garage door, back the car out, and drive 100 yards. In the same way, the child with some walking ability soon learns that it is easier to walk around the house than to try to maneuver the wheelchair in close spaces.

Just as the teenaged driver must demonstrate competence before she can get a driver's license, the child with a disability must demonstrate competence before being allowed to operate a power chair. She must be able to understand that pushing forward on a stick causes her to move forward (playing with a video joystick is good practice for this). She must also understand about danger areas, so that she doesn't drive over curbs or down stairs. If she should drive into a corner, she must be able to back up and turn around to get herself out. She must be able to see in order to drive a chair, but she doesn't have to be able to use her hand or fingers to control the chair. There are joystick controllers for power chairs (like the ones in videogames) as well as head, mouth, leg, and foot controllers. The sensitivity of the controller and the speed of the chair must be adjusted according to the child's age and abilities.

When children with cerebral palsy start to use power chairs, they may have trouble with spatial perception at first. For many children, this is because they have never moved around on the floor independently, and they lack experience. Some children have vision problems, as well, or their balance may be poor, and this can further limit their ability to move appropriately in space. The bottom line is that any child who is using a power chair for the first time needs training and guidance.

It is usually best to work in confined spaces, such as a room in which objects are arranged closely together. This type of close maneuvering is usually easiest for the child to learn because he or she has more experience manipulating objects in a small environment. The best way to provide training for the child is to walk in front of him, providing a focus of attention. It may take some children months or even several years to learn to drive in a relatively open area, and to stay on a sidewalk.

Parents should choose their child's chair and controller, as well as seating support systems, only after getting advice from school therapists and their child's doctor. The home environment and transportation systems must be taken into account in making this decision, and parents should be prepared to describe any limitations posed by either or both of these. For children who are easy to fit, selecting a chair can often be done within the school system, where the child may even be able to take several different kinds of chairs for a test drive. For other children, it may be best to make these decisions based on a short-term admission to a hospital's rehabilitation unit, where the child can be evaluated on several systems, and the parent's home and the available transportation system, as well as the school environment, are carefully considered.

It is usually not a good idea to select a chair in the salesroom of a wheelchair dealer. Typically, the dealer will carry only one or two brands and may be motivated to encourage you to choose one of them. It's possible that the salesperson won't even be well trained in satisfying the mobility goals of a child with a disability. Our recommendation is to choose a chair in a setting that provides both an unbiased opportunity for choice and the help of trained personnel, as described in the preceding paragraph, and then purchase the chair through a dealer with a reputation for good service.

For more information about different styles of chairs, you might consult the section on wheelchairs in Part 2 of this book. Another good source of information is other owners of motorized chairs, who can provide valuable advice about the reliability of local sales people and repair shops. Motorized chairs generally require more repair and service than cars, so before you buy a chair, it's essential to know how and where you are going to get good service. Some hospitals have wheelchair clinics staffed with persons who can service the chairs.

What about walking?

You may have ongoing concerns about how or if your child will walk. As your child grows older, predictions become more reliable, so by this age things are certainly becoming clearer. Again, it's important to remember that a child must have head control before he can sit independently, and he must be able to sit before he can walk.

Can standers, braces, and walkers help?

By this age, almost all children should be in a standing program for weight bearing to help with bone development, body control, coordination, and balance. Children who have difficulty controlling their ankles, either because they go up on tiptoe or because their foot turns or rolls into a flat-footed position, should have plastic ankle-foot braces made to help them stand. Only children with the most severely affected feet need ankle surgery, and even then it is usually only a minor lengthening of the Achilles tendon or transfer of half of the tibialis posterior tendon. Either of these procedures will allow the foot to fit properly into a brace. (Surgery for flat feet is discussed in the next section.) Braces above the knee have no benefit, and children who can't control their knees need to be placed in a stander that provides knee control.

Walkers in which the child sits (gait trainer) continue to be controversial. Some therapists believe that the posture and movements of the child in the gait trainer have a detrimental impact on development of balance and upper body control. However, we know of no scientific evidence to support this. Positioning devices (e.g., ankle prompts) can be added or subtracted from the device to assist with controlling upper extremity, trunk, and lower extremity positioning. The biggest concern with walkers is safety. It is our opinion that if the child enjoys being in the walker, and his parents want the child in a walker and can watch the child very closely to keep him safe while he's in it, there is probably no harm in using a walker for short periods of time, about one hour daily.

What hip problems can occur at this age?

Spastic hip disease, or hip subluxation or dislocation, continues to be a big problem at this age. Children with severe quadriplegia have an 80 percent chance of developing hip subluxation, and children with moderate quadriplegia and those with athetosis have a slightly lower, but still very high, risk for this problem.

Hip dislocation, the end result of subluxation, can only be avoided if it is detected and dealt with early. The surgical release of the tight, spastic hip muscles is a relatively simple procedure and can often prevent dislocation. Many children with severe cerebral palsy need bone surgery to place the hip in a more stable position, however. If the dislocated hip remains untreated, the surgical procedures for correcting the problem become much more complex, placing the child at an increased risk for complications. To avoid extensive surgery and the possibility of complications, it is essential to continue close monitoring, with a physical examination every six months and x-rays as needed.

Should I be concerned about my child's spine?

Generally spinal deformities are less of a problem at this age than is spastic hip disease. Many parents are concerned about scoliosis, although at this age it is still mostly due to poor upper body control and is best managed by good seating support and by a standing program. Kyphosis (forward slumping) is also due to poor upper body control, but it may be more difficult to manage than scoliosis. A harness or a reclining, tilting seat can be helpful. For some children a body brace is useful for postural control, although this can create feeding and breathing problems. Only rarely does kyphosis become stiff and permanent. Your child's spine should be routinely examined as part of his scheduled medical care.

What about my child's upper body?

Some children with severe athetosis may dislocate a shoulder because their posture is abnormal—for example, they may keep their arms above their head and behind them. Lifting the child by the arms may also result in a dislocated shoulder. The best treatment for dislocation is avoiding the activity that caused the dislocation in the first place, which may mean using a splint that restrains the arm in a position down at the child's side. This is especially helpful at night.

Elbow tightness may cause a problem for dressing and bathing, but the elbow is usually flexible at this age. Short-term splinting is helpful. Splinting may also be suggested as treatment for wrist flexion and to keep the thumb out of the palm. The advantage of a splint is that it keeps the tight wrist, elbow, or thumb stretched out. The disadvantage is that the splint can decrease hand function. While it may be true that the contracted upper extremity becomes useless, it is also true that a continuously splinted upper extremity doesn't have a chance of learning to function. For this reason, we only recommend short-term splinting—usually just at night. Botulinum toxin injection into spastic muscles can often be helpful with or without the combination of splinting.

Could my child have knee problems?

The child with very tight hamstrings will not be able to extend his leg at the knee. At this age tight hamstrings, though a common problem, are not likely to be as troublesome as they may become in adolescence. Physical therapy stretching exercises are generally all that is needed, and splinting is only occasionally used. The child may get stiff knees, but they are usually due to spasticity; again, stretching exercises are usually sufficient treatment. Botulinum toxin injections into the hamstring or quadriceps muscles for tightness may be helpful if a contracture of the tendon has not occurred.

Do the feet pose specific problems at this age?

The most common concern for parents is the tight Achilles tendon (heel cord), and this often can be managed with stretching exercises, Botox, and the use of a molded ankle-foot brace. A severe tightness that cannot be modified by these methods may need to be lengthened surgically. If your child cannot be fitted with any type of acceptable footwear, or if the position of his or her feet causes difficulty with standing, surgery is recommended.

Flat feet or feet that tend to roll out are also problems, and are most easily noticed when the child is standing. Using an AFO or a shoe insert, such as a heel cup, is a good idea if it helps your child stand, but some braces try to create an ideal arch and may cause your child discomfort. If the brace is painful it must be repaired or removed permanently.

There is no scientific evidence that these braces make any permanent change in the shape of the foot, particularly in shaping an arch. Sometimes feet get better as the child grows and muscle control improves, and sometimes they get worse. The braces probably don't have any effect on this.

Comfortable braces often do make it easier for the child to stand, however, and in this case they are helpful.

At this age, surgery should only be considered in the most severe flat-foot deformity, when bracing has proven to be completely unsuccessful. Those who do have surgery have a fairly high recurrence rate and may need to have repeat surgery at an older age. There continues to be a large spectrum of opinion concerning flat feet in cerebral palsy, and there aren't many scientific studies to back up any one opinion. The best thing to do, generally, is to weigh all other options before turning to surgery for this problem at this age.

What about my child's toes? For the child with overlapping and cocked toes caused by spasticity, it is usually difficult to wear shoes. At this age, the best treatment is to provide your child with soft and roomy shoes. Soft silicone toe spacers that can be placed between the toes may also be helpful in preventing callouses. If his toe condition worsens, simple surgical treatment is available and often provides good correction.

Ages Seven to Twelve

This is the age range when a child's physical and cognitive potential can usually be determined. By ages 8 to 10, children reach their maximum physical capabilities—their ability to sit, walk, and use their arms has fully developed. They may learn to function more effectively, but significant new abilities do not emerge, as they did during their younger years.

As a parent, this may be an especially hard time for you as you continue to work hard with your child and hope for gains while seeing less progress. In addition, you may be receiving a good deal of input from your child's teachers and therapists, as well as medical personnel. Your child has now been in the school system long enough, and therapists have worked with your child often enough, to be able to define your child's abilities with a fair degree of accuracy.

Certainly, your child will continue to learn and will improve in some physical abilities, as all growing children do. However, the pattern will now be clearly established. This means that if your child is not walking by age 10, he or she will never be an independent walker. If your child has not learned to recognize any words by age 10, he or she clearly has a cognitive impairment and will never learn to be a functional reader (unless the cause of the reading problem is an untreated visual problem).

You can prepare yourself for this stage of development by accepting the difference between the rapid developmental gains of the period from birth to age 6 and the much slower rate of gain after age 6, and by understanding that this contrast in development exists in normal children, as well. Your child's slowed development after age 6 may, however, affect you psychologically and emotionally more than their child's slowed development affects the parents of a child without disabilities. This is to be expected.

What kind of therapy is most important?

When adults with cerebral palsy are asked this question, their response is speech or communication therapy. These skills are especially important for children who have a high cognitive level. If the oral speech is too difficult for strangers to understand or the child's ability to speak is very limited, augmentative communication should be provided.

What is augmentative communication?

Augmentative communication refers to a method of communication other than speech. Signing, a method of communicating with hand signals used by people who are hearing impaired, may be useful, although children with quadriplegic cerebral palsy have too much upper extremity involvement to sign efficiently, except for a few basic signs. The simplest augmentative communication device is a communication board that displays pictures or words appropriate to the child's functioning level and current situation. These can be hooked up to computers with speech synthesizers.

For the child who is severely involved physically and who has difficulty using his hands, the use of eye signs is a good, simple way to communicate. This form of communication is slow, however, because it essentially limits responses to either a yes or a no answer. Head pointing sticks with computer attachments are another option.

Developing an efficient communication system should be a major part of your child's early education. Hospital centers with augmentative communication clinics can use a number of different systems to evaluate your child, usually on an inpatient basis. But you need to keep in mind that this process is much like buying a wheelchair, in that there are many different options and prices, and it's not wise to go to a dealer who may be influenced by what he sells.

Parents may find that paying for these devices is difficult, since Medicaid coverage varies from state to state, and insurance coverage may vary, as well. In regard to insurance, it is important not to accept an initial rejection, but to continue to resubmit until you are satisfied with the result. Organizations such as local variety clubs, the Easter Seal Society, and churches may provide assistance with funding. (See Chapter 10 for more information about finding sources of funding.)

Is speech therapy helpful for the child whose cognitive abilities are severely affected?

Yes. Most speech therapy for children with quadriplegia and severe cognitive disability, where communication is not a goal, focuses on teaching swallowing and feeding techniques. The therapist will evaluate swallowing function, if this has not already been done, and provide pointers to parents for preparing food and feeding their child (see Chapter 3 for more details).

What is the role of an occupational therapist?

An occupational therapist works with your child to develop functional skills involving his or her hands. At this age, the focus should be on becoming independent with activities of daily living. For children who can write, improving handwriting is a goal. For those who may have more upper extremity involvement, an occupational therapist helps the child develop skill in using a keyboard. The occupational therapist also focuses on improving function with the tasks of daily living, as well as finding positions in seating and hand use that allow for optimum function. This becomes increasingly important as children grow. Again, the therapy should be much more function oriented; focusing on stretching and exercising at this age is inappropriate. If stretching is needed, passive stretching with the use of nighttime splints is more time efficient and cost effective.

The amount of time the therapist spends may vary from three times a week with the child who is working on learning a specific new task, to a monthly evaluation for the child who seems to be functioning well. If your child is doing well in the classroom and functions well during play, it's best not to take time away from those things for therapy.

How much physical therapy is needed?

This depends a good deal on the individual child's needs and on the availability of therapy. As with occupational therapy, physical therapy should be balanced with school and play time. The child who is doing well academically should not be removed from the classroom for therapy unless there is a specific short-term goal he or she is trying to achieve. In general though, therapy gradually takes on the role of *maintaining* function rather than stimulating *new* function.

For the child who is moderately affected by CP and who is cognitively normal, therapy should be functionally oriented, offering as little interference as possible in the child's education. Such a child will be able to become a contributing adult member of society by virtue of her cognitive abilities, and her physical limitations will not be significantly changed by hours of therapy in late childhood. She needs to learn early on that her time and energy are more effectively used in developing her intellectual abilities, and she should be encouraged to succeed in this area.

As parents, you need to ensure that therapy time is spent on functional skills and not on hours of preventive stretching exercises. These exercises may temporarily prevent some stiffness, but they take valuable time from the child's educational development or from opportunity for socializing with peers in play. Parents need to strive for a balance, keeping in mind that a little knee stiffness is much less important than the development of a child's intellectual potential.

Children who are wheelchair dependent should not remain in a seated position all day. They need to be given an opportunity for some exercise, and the best way is by having them take part in an enjoyable activity, preferably one that they can participate in for a lifetime. Swimming and adapted horse-back riding are excellent options.

The child with severe physical involvement may find it difficult to get exercise and may need continued therapy provided by a physical therapist, or an exercise program prearranged by a physical therapist and executed by school personnel. Children with severe cognitive and physical involvement should have routines worked out for positioning changes, adequate seating with support, and a regularly scheduled standing program. The therapist may also help the self-abusive child by describing methods of prevention and protection to caretakers.

Determining how much physical therapy is appropriate for a specific child depends upon many variables. At this age, the child who is doing well in school and is not having specific new problems may touch base with his therapist once a month or every six months, if he is in a program designed by the therapist and carried out by school personnel. By contrast, the child who has a specific problem that the therapist is currently working on with him may need to be seen three times a week.

What kinds of problems are there with therapy in school?

There are two basic conflicts here. The first is an issue of cost versus gain in terms of the child's development. Not every child with cerebral palsy, even those with moderate to severe quadriplegia, needs therapy. In fact, taking some children out of the classroom for therapy might actually be harmful in terms of intellectual growth. Second, in many schools therapists' time is quite limited, so that choices must be made about which children will benefit most from the available services. The Individualized Education Plan (IEP) process provides the opportunity to evaluate the child in terms of his best interests, but the parent who does not feel comfortable with the outcome of that process may have to pursue the issue further.

Sometimes the child's doctor prescribes therapy. If the child has had surgery and postsurgical therapy is indicated, it is not necessarily the responsibility of the school to provide this kind of therapy. Postsurgical therapy is medically indicated and most likely is covered by medical insurance.

Separating therapy as part of education from therapy as a medical treatment can be difficult and may be complicated by the fact that schools often don't have enough therapists to meet their students' needs. In addition, there are no absolute criteria by which decisions can be made about which children need therapy in school. The parent or caretaker is usually the child's strongest advocate, but the parent also needs to weigh carefully the issue of cost of time lost in the classroom for the purpose of therapy. If the school's lack of therapists poses a significant problem, parents may consider forming parent groups and becoming active at school board meetings to insist that the number of therapists in the school system be increased.

Should my child be placed in a special school, or would he benefit from "inclusion"?

The answer to this complex question depends on what's available within the educational system in the particular geographical area, as well as on the cognitive, physical, and psychological needs of the individual child. The purpose of the IEP is to evaluate the child in terms of his or her educational best interests, but if parents or caretakers are not in agreement with the recommendation of the IEP, they should be willing to take on an advocacy role and try to get the recommendation changed. (See Chapter 11 for more details on dealing with the educational system.)

What can I do about my child's drooling?

At this age excessive drooling can cause significant physical problems, such as wetting books, papers, and computer keyboards. Occasionally if drooling is severe, skin irritation can develop around the mouth and face. It is also cosmetically unappealing, of course, and has the potential of being emotionally disturbing to the cognitively aware child. There are several options for treatment, including therapy (with a speech therapist), medication, and surgery. (Drooling is covered in more depth in Chapter 3.)

Are there respiratory problems at this age?

If the child has had recurrent bronchitis or pneumonia over the years, he should be evaluated for aspiration of food or saliva. These problems tend to occur in children with more severe physical involvement. (This topic is discussed in Chapter 3.)

What dental care is needed?

The severely involved child who has difficulty brushing her teeth and gums often develops an overgrowth of the gums, sometimes covering the teeth (gum hypertrophy). Some medications also cause gum problems. Gum hypertrophy can lead to infections and tooth decay, so good oral care and regular checkups are essential. In some situations, gum disease must be treated surgically.

What about my child's hearing?

By this age, your child's hearing should have been thoroughly evaluated. Even if your child had many ear infections earlier in life, the frequency should be diminishing by the time he reaches this age. A child who continues to have infections needs to be thoroughly evaluated, as does a child who has trouble breathing. Abnormal palate, infection or enlargement of the adenoids, gastroesophageal reflux, and allergy may all contribute to ongoing otitis media.

What about eye problems?

Any treatable eye problems should have been addressed by the time your child has reached school age. Children with moderate to severe involvement, especially children with athetosis, often have difficulty tracking a moving object or focusing. These difficulties are often combined with dyslexia (a reading disorder that causes letters or words to appear backwards), though it may be difficult to separate the problems from each other. One area of controversy involves determining the appropriate eye therapy for these problems, with techniques varying in different regions of the country.

What about feeding problems?

Feeding problems encountered when your child was younger continue at this age. (Problems related to swallowing, reflux, regurgitation, and constipation are all addressed in depth in Chapter 3.)

Should my child be in a wheelchair?

Concerns about wheelchair use are essentially the same as those encountered in the previous age group. However, there are several issues that now become more important and need to be addressed for the 7- to 12-year-old. The child of school age usually has started to become aware and concerned about appearance. By age 6 or 7, strollers should not be used, especially for children who want to start feeling grown up. An adult-type wheelchair, particularly in a color that the child has chosen, is usually far more appealing.

Children who are dressed neatly and are seated in a good-looking chair are attractive, and often people who come into contact with them will react more positively toward them than toward a child whose physical appearance has been neglected. This is especially true in public areas and in schools. For the child who is aware, an attractive appearance also instills self-esteem. But even when the child is not aware, parents will feel better if the child looks comfortable and well cared for. Discussion about the use of a power wheelchair ought to be ongoing, especially for the child who is not quite able to keep up pushing a manual chair, and for the child who is making cognitive progress and is able to use power responsibly.

Is my child likely to break bones?

Osteoporosis (weak bones) occurs most commonly in the quadriplegic child over 9 years of age who is unable to bear weight. The causes of this problem appear to be multiple. They include the lack of weight bearing, poor nutritional intake, and the use of some seizure medications. Poor bone strength may predispose the child to fractures of the long bones and, less frequently, to compression fractures in the spine. The most common fractures are seen in the lower extremities, especially above or below the knee. Most broken bones occur from very minor trauma such as while moving the child or during a physical therapy session. Many such fractures may go unrecognized at first, with the child having pain and crying for an unknown cause for several days before the diagnosis is made. Initial x-rays may even appear normal if the fracture is nondisplaced. In such cases a special imaging study called a bone scan is helpful. Nonambulatory children who are at risk for weak bones or who have had more than one broken bone should be monitored with a bone density test (DXA). Children with low bone density measurements should have their diets assessed for mineral and vitamin content, and their diets should be supplemented if some or all of these nutrients are deficient compared with the recommended dietary intake (RDI). More severe cases may require treatment with a medication (called a bisphosphonate) that helps to improve bone strength. Treatment of a fracture is usually nonsurgical and involves a very well padded cast. Surgical treatment is only necessary in some severely displaced fractures (see Chapter 3 for more details on the evaluation and treatment of low bone density).

What ankle and foot problems might my child encounter?

This is the age when the severe flat foot causes problems with standing. If the foot cannot be held in good position with a molded AFO, then surgical intervention is recommended. A lengthening of the heel bone (calcaneal lengthening) or realignment of the heel (calcaneal osteotomy) can be performed in some patients with the proper indications. These procedures avoid fusion of the joints. Surgical treatment usually requires *subtalar fusion* (the fusing together of two bones in the heel). The *triple arthrodesis,* in which four bones are fused, is a procedure that yields a more predictably permanent result. A lengthening of the Achilles tendon may also be recommended at this age; it rarely needs to be redone at a later age.

Ankle deformities in children at this age usually make it difficult for the child to wear shoes or to stand properly. Addressing these problems is usually deferred until the child is older. For a full discussion, see "Ages Thirteen to Eighteen" in this chapter, below. There are some minor toe problems at this age which will become more prominent in adolescence. (These are addressed in the next section as well.)

What about my child's knees?

Tight hamstrings cause difficulties in standing, and may also cause problems with sitting or lying down. When the child with tight hamstrings sits down, the pelvis tends to roll back, causing the child to sit bent forward. As before, physical therapy stretching is usually adequate. When the problem interferes with activities of daily living like standing and sitting, however, then surgical release or lengthening is recommended. Tight rectus muscles cause the knee to be held straight all the time and make sitting difficult. Surgical release of these muscles is very helpful if this is a significant problem.

Will my child's hips still cause problems?

Yes, the hips still need to be watched, especially hips that are borderline normal or that have been surgically treated for dislocation. This is especially true as the child approaches the adolescent growth spurt, when the hips may again start dislocating after having been stable for a number of years. Hips that are changing must be x-rayed every six months until they are treated or are again stable for two years. As the child gets older, simple muscle releases are less reliable as treatment and usually need to be accompanied by varus osteotomy of the femur and often a pelvic osteotomy, as well. These surgeries correct the problem. Again, with close follow-up and appropriate treatment, a child will not end up with a hip dislocation.

Sometimes longstanding, neglected hip dislocations become very painful. The first step in addressing this difficult situation is to decrease the activity to the hip, stop physical therapy exercises, and start anti-inflammatory medications, like aspirin or ibuprofen (Advil). If this doesn't work, then reducing the hip surgically may help, or the hip may be totally replaced with an artificial joint. Excision of the femur (castle or girdlestone operation) is almost always ineffective at this age, because the child continues to grow and the hips become painful again.

Are there any problems with the arms?

During childhood the function of the arms becomes fully developed and contractures also start to develop. Occupational therapists will be working to help the child use his or her arms as much as possible, and especially for activities such as self-feeding, manipulating switches, and using joysticks and keyboards.

Some children with severe functional motor involvement develop contractures that make dressing and bathing difficult. Surgical release of arm contractures may be considered, but surgery is usually not performed until early adolescence. (This is discussed in the next section.) Splinting should continue as long as it does not interfere with the child's functioning.

Is spinal curvature a problem now?

As the child gets older and taller, especially as puberty begins, scoliosis usually starts getting worse, and the child may bend more and get stiffer. The best way of dealing with spinal curvature at this age is to make sure that the wheelchair has good lateral chest supports. A brace is one way of helping the child sit better, but usually the problems caused by the brace outweigh the benefits. Also, the brace does not have any impact on the eventual outcome of the scoliosis. (For a full discussion of scoliosis, see the next section.)

Kyphosis, or forward bending of the spine, is usually at its worst at this age. Even positioning a child in a chair may prove difficult, because the children tend to roll forward into a ball. Using a soft plastic body brace can help correct this problem and make seating easier. Many children outgrow this deformity, although there are a few who don't, and these children may need to undergo a spinal fusion, usually in early adolescence.

Ages Thirteen to Eighteen

At this age independence is the primary goal, but how it is achieved varies greatly depending upon the child's physical involvement and cognitive ability. Normally during adolescence, children start to separate from their parents and make plans for the future. The process of achieving independence, though necessarily modified, should be encouraged in the child with cerebral palsy. The level of CP involvement clearly must be considered, but the disability should not be considered to be inconsistent with independent living. From a psychological perspective, it's crucial to communicate this conviction to the adolescent.

Some adolescent personalities develop rather abruptly, whereas other adolescent personalities undergo a long period of developing maturation.

Either way, adolescence is often a stressful time, whether or not the child has a disability. It may be difficult for parents of a child with cerebral palsy to separate the normal turmoil of adolescence from the problems related to the disability. One thing to keep in mind is that the growth spurt and hormonal changes of adolescence can affect seizure patterns and otherwise affect behavior in a child with CP.

After addressing some specific questions about problems that develop or become more severe in the adolescent years, the remainder of this chapter discusses issues of independence. In this discussion, we group individuals according to their predominant disability. Although categorizing children this way is far from ideal, it does make it easier to take differences into account. (Chapter 4 discusses many of these issues from a developmental perspective.)

At this age, what problems occur in the upper extremities?

Adolescents with an athetoid pattern may develop shoulder dislocation that produces some discomfort, though the shoulder rarely remains out of the joint. The best treatment is for the teen to learn to avoid the positions that cause the dislocation. Sometimes this means avoiding putting the arm in a certain position while sleeping (using a splint at night to keep the arm positioned at the side may solve this problem). Shoulder dislocation can be surgically addressed with soft tissue repair. However, it may recur. Shoulder fusion can be used to treat recurrent dislocations. Fortunately, surgery is rarely necessary.

People with severe spasticity sometimes develop elbow contractures that make it difficult to clean in the elbow crease and that can make dressing difficult, too. To address this problem, the biceps and brachialis muscles in the elbow may be lengthened or released; the surgeon is careful to retain enough muscle to keep the arm flexible. In a similar fashion, the thumb can become contracted (fixed to the palm), making it difficult to clean the hand. This, too, is best addressed with surgery, which fixes the thumb in a straight position, permanently allowing easier dressing and cleansing.

Contracture is also common in the wrist, with severe flexion to the palm side. A minor surgical procedure, in which a tendon is transferred in order to keep the wrist extended, can be very helpful. Small joint fusions in the hand are sometimes helpful, but these should only be performed by surgeons experienced in the particular problems associated with cerebral palsy.

Some people gain significant functional improvement, along with improved cosmetic appearance, following upper extremity muscle release or tendon surgery. Improved hygiene and cosmetic appearance are the most likely results, with improved function a pleasing but uncommon result of surgery. The hand of the individual with athetosis is problematic. Surgery in these children is frequently complicated by a return of the hand to its former position. For this reason, surgery is best avoided in the child with athetosis.

What treatment is available for scoliosis?

Scoliosis, or side bending of the spine, occurs in children with hemiplegia and diplegia, but it occurs most commonly in children with quadriplegia. Scoliosis is caused by poor muscle control. There is no known method of prevention, nor any form of nonsurgical treatment.

This scoliosis is very different from the scoliosis that nondisabled children, most often girls, develop and that can be treated with braces. Unfortunately, there continues to be a great deal of confusion among physicians and therapists who are unaware of the intrinsic difference between the scoliosis related to cerebral palsy and the scoliosis of normal teenagers. The treatments that are somewhat effective for normal individuals have no effect on the individuals with cerebral palsy, because their scoliosis is directly related to the cerebral palsy.

Braces may be temporarily helpful for the child with cerebral palsy for position, particularly sitting, but it is often easier to use wheelchair modifications to help the child sit upright, because these don't have to be applied to the child. But neither wheelchair modifications nor wearing a brace will have any effect on the development of scoliosis. In other words, by age 20 the spine will be curved the same amount whether a brace has been worn full time for 10 years or has never been used.

Braces give some children gastrointestinal, as well as respiratory, problems, and need to be remade as the child grows. Rigid braces can cause pressure sores. When a brace is used, we prefer a soft brace made from a more flexible synthetic material. This type of brace is better tolerated by the child. One advantage of the brace, however, is that it is worn under clothing and therefore does not interfere with wheelchair support positioning as seasons change and bulky coats are added and removed. Another advantage of the brace is that it gives better support because it fits more securely. There is no harm in using both wheelchair modifications and a body brace.

In making the decision to modify a wheelchair or apply a brace, the possible risks and complications must be considered, with the overriding understanding that neither will have any impact on the continued development of the spinal deformity. Some doctors think that the development of the scoliosis may be slowed, but there really is no evidence for this, and the consensus among orthopedic surgeons who care for children with CP is that there is no impact.

For the child who is severely physically affected, there is a 75 to 90 percent risk of developing scoliosis, and the only effective treatment is a spinal fusion. This surgery involves straightening the spine, placing steel rods along the spine, and implanting bone graft so that the spine and the rods heal together as one bone. There have been great advances in this area of surgery, and even children with severe curves can be adequately straightened so that they can sit in a straight-backed chair.

This is a major operation, usually lasting three or four hours, and must be performed by a surgeon who has experience with surgery for scoliosis associated with cerebral palsy. The surgery for this scoliosis is different, and uses different rods, from the surgery for scoliosis in normal adolescents. Most children recover rapidly and are sitting up in a chair three or four days after surgery, without the need for casting or bracing. And most of them are ready to go home two to three weeks after surgery.

For children with very severe and stiff curves, it is sometimes necessary to do an additional, smaller surgical procedure before approaching the back, in order to remove some of the discs that become deformed and stiff between the bony blocks (vertebrae). Although this adds approximately one more week to the average hospital stay, it allows the surgeon to achieve a far better result in the correction of the curvature.

Once the spinal fusion is complete, growth is no longer possible in the spine, although the legs and arms continue to grow. Therefore, the ideal situation is to have the child grow as much as possible before the surgery without the curvature becoming stiff and fixed. This usually means delaying surgery until the child is between 12 and 16 years old, but then only one surgical procedure is necessary and usually provides excellent correction.

Sometimes a curve has become so severe by the time the child reaches age 8 or 9 that surgery must take place, sacrificing some growth. This is a rare occurrence and is much more likely in a child who begins to develop scoliosis at age 2, 3, 4, or 5.

What other spinal deformities might occur?

Kyphosis is a curvature of the spine in which the child bends forward and has an appearance similar to that of an elderly individual. Kyphosis is very common when children are young, but most children with cerebral palsy outgrow this condition as they achieve better upper body control. A few children develop stiffness and become fixed in this position, however, which may make sitting very difficult. For these children, surgery can correct the deformity by fusing the spine using bone graft and metal rods, similar to the procedure described above for scoliosis.

Lordosis, the least common spinal problem in persons with CP, refers to the curve in the spine which makes the arch in the lower back. This, too, becomes severely exaggerated in some children with cerebral palsy and causes problems with sitting and often back pain. The only treatment is to perform the surgery described above.

Spine surgery sounds frightening. What complications can occur?

No surgery is without risk of possible complications. The parent and surgeon should spend time together discussing the risks and benefits of surgery. Clear and realistic goals and expectations must also be discussed. If the child is medically involved, the parent must be prepared for a higher risk of complications after spine surgery. The most frequent complications include gastrointestinal problems, respiratory problems, and wound infection. The child's surgery should be performed at a hospital with an experienced pediatric intensive care and medical staff, as all these complications are treatable.

In addition, intraoperative bleeding that requires blood transfusion should be expected. An experienced pediatric anesthesia staff is critical during the surgery to help manage this potential problem. It is important to keep in mind that although complications can occur, the long-term benefits of spinal deformity surgery and keeping a child in a well-balanced upright position outweigh the risks in the majority of children with CP. The decision to proceed with surgery is ultimately up to the parent and the benefits should be carefully weighed against the potential risks.

Do adolescents generally have hip problems?

Children who have had problems with subluxating hips earlier in life need to continue to be watched, but not quite as closely as when they were younger. Now x-rays only need to be done every one to two years, and if the hips are normal, only a physical examination may be necessary. Sometimes the hips start to sublux again at the same time that the scoliosis is developing. If the hips are dislocating at this age, surgery involving the bone rather than just muscle usually needs to be done. Often, a pelvic osteotomy is also needed to reshape the acetabulum, or cup of the hip.

All efforts should be made to prevent the hips from dislocating, because dislocated hips often become painful later, and then they are very hard to work with. Orthopedic surgeons experienced in dealing with CP are able to keep the hip in the socket, and, with good treatment, to keep the hips almost normal. It's essential for the child to be checked regularly by a surgeon who is experienced in the treatment of spastic hip disease.

This is the age at which the problems associated with the neglected dislocated hip start becoming most painful. The first course of treatment involves avoiding activity that irritates the hip and using arthritis medications like aspirin or ibuprofen (Advil, Motrin) to decrease the inflammation. Acetaminophen (Tylenol) is effective for the relief of pain, but it is not effective for the treatment of inflammation, which is thought to be a major source of pain in a condition such as this. If taking medications and avoiding certain activities does not effectively manage the pain, then surgery is the next option. There are a number of available procedures, but unfortunately none of them has a high rate of success.

Putting the hip back into the joint is the first step, if the arthritis is not too severe. If this is possible, it has the best long-term results, although sometimes persistent stiffness or pain makes a second surgical procedure necessary. The real advantage to this surgery is that there are good second choices. Total hip replacement is another choice, but it is often technically difficult and potentially problematic. When it is successful, however, it gives an excellent result. *Proximal femoral excision* is yet another alternative. This surgery involves removing the top portion of the femur (upper leg bone). This surgery is used fairly frequently but can often result in a hip almost as painful and occasionally as stiff. It is important to keep the child in traction for six weeks following a proximal femoral excision to allow a scar to form.

Unfortunately, the high failure rate of the proximal femoral excision leaves only the alternative of removing more bone. Each successive removal of bone makes seating more difficult, as the legs become shorter. This operation is the procedure of last resort. Another option may be to fuse the hip joint, but this makes the child completely stiff. *By far the best course of action in terms of hip dislocation is prevention.* Some children who have had dislocated hips for several years have no pain and, in this case, we would recommend leaving the hip dislocated. It would certainly cause the child pain to make a surgical attempt to put the hip back in place.

As teenagers grow and hip muscles become tighter, diapering and perineal care can become difficult, particularly for menstruating females. When the condition has reached the point where one person must hold the child's knees apart while another washes the child or changes the diaper, then some surgical muscle releases should be considered. Osteotomy of the bones at the hip, or relocating dislocated hips if they are recent dislocations with little associated arthritis, are possibilities. Without surgery, this difficulty with personal care will only become worse as the child gets older, stiffer, and stronger.

Another common hip problem is the so-called windswept hips. This occurs when one hip is contracted inward (adducted) and the opposite hip is contracted outward (abducted). The primary problem is with positioning the child in a sitting and lying position. The adducted hip may be dislocated, requiring both muscle release (adductor release) and bone reconstruction (varus osteotomy and acetabular osteotomy) whereas the abducted hip usually requires varus osteotomy only. The goal of the surgery is to realign the legs to point them straight ahead as well as to treat the dislocated side (if a dislocation is present).

What if my child has both scoliosis and a dislocated hip? Should one be treated before the other?

It is not uncommon for both scoliosis and hip dislocation to occur together. If both are equally severe, the spine is usually treated first, followed six months later by treatment of the hips. Some children with severe hip pain and a mild to moderate scoliosis must have their dislocated hip treated first, to alleviate hip pain, before the scoliosis is treated. Both treatments have been previously discussed.

What are some common knee problems at this age?

Tight muscles behind the knees (the hamstrings) that prevent the knees from straightening out is the most common problem in children who don't stand. These muscles sometimes become so tight that the child has a problem settling her feet comfortably on the footrest of the wheelchair. It may also be difficult for the child to lie down if she can't straighten out her knees. Children with this problem often position themselves so that one leg is turned out and the other in, or they lie and sit with both knees spread far apart. This makes sitting difficult and is also not cosmetically appealing, especially for females.

If the child is able to stand and these muscles become tight, they should be surgically lengthened in a procedure that will allow the child to stand as straight as possible. Occasionally, though rarely, the hamstring contractures can be severe enough that they can't be released sufficiently to correct the problem. When this occurs, a distal femoral osteotomy, in which the femur bone is cut and extended just above the knee joint, often produces good results.

In contrast to hamstring tightness, which causes the knee to be fixed in a flexed position, is the knee that can't bend. This is usually caused by spasticity or contracture in the rectus muscle, which is located in the front of the upper leg. This situation makes it very difficult for the child to sit in a wheelchair, and sometimes the muscle is so tight that the child's feet become sore from being kept forcibly secured to the wheelchair.

Mild cases of rectus tightness can be treated with stretching exercises that are done when the child is being dressed or transferred. The surgical release of the rectus muscle is a fairly simple procedure that should be considered if seating is a problem. Knee problems that are more of an impediment to walking or standing are covered more fully in Chapter 6.

Could my child have problems with his feet?

Two common types of foot problems occur in older children, feet that point down and in (equinovarus foot) and feet that point down and out (equinovalgus or planovalgus foot). A good foot position is necessary to allow for proper standing and shoe wear. Treatment options include (1) accepting the deformity and accommodating the deformed foot with soft comfortable shoe wear, (2) controlling the foot deformity with bracing, and (3) correcting the deformity with surgery.

Although standing is recommended, there are children who do not stand. If these children have foot position problems, it is preferable not to force their feet into shoes or braces. Rather, their feet can be kept protected and warm with slipper socks, slippers, or soft moccasins. There are many readily available options that are both inexpensive and comfortable.

The child who weight bears with a less severe (flexible) foot deformity can usually be held in a brace with the foot in a good position. It must be remembered, however, that bracing has not been shown to prevent or permanently change any foot problems. When a child's foot deformity is severe, causing difficulty with standing in a child who weight bears, or the child's skin is breaking down because of rubbing against shoes or braces, the problem needs to be addressed surgically. Equinovarus foot deformity may be due to spasticity or contractures. Releasing or lengthening the Achilles tendon and lengthening or transferring part of the *posterior tibial tendon* are helpful procedures when there is minimal bone deformity in the foot. Equinovarus deformity with deformity in the bone and most severe equinovalgus deformities do well with a triple arthrodesis or subtalar fusion, in which joints that are causing the problem are fused. Most children who do not stand do very well in soft shoes and do not require surgery.

What about the toes?

A common toe problem is the severely cocked-up, or flexed, big toe. This occurs most commonly in adolescents with athetosis. Wearing shoes is often difficult and painful, because sores develop. Two options are available. First, the child can wear very large, soft shoes with a large toe box. Or the deformity can be corrected surgically, by fusing the big toe joint. The first option offers the easiest solution, although the surgical procedure is relatively simple and usually gives an excellent result that lasts the rest of the child's life.

Cocked-up toes or overlapping toes may be a problem in the small toes and may also cause sores when the toes rub against a shoe. They can be dealt with surgically, by a minor procedure in which a small joint is excised and the toes are fused straight, or the adolescent can wear large shoes to prevent the formation of sores. None of these toe problems should be seen as an emergency. The surgeries can be done with the same success at age 10 or age 80.

Similar problems may occur from severe bunions, and these, too, are best treated with correction and fusion. A person with cerebral palsy has a different kind of bunion from the bunion deformities that other people get, and this bunion should not be treated in the same way that those other deformities are treated. If the person with cerebral palsy has a standard bunion operation, the bunion will recur. It is generally best not to have the same surgeon who did a good job on grandmother's bunions operate on the adolescent with cerebral palsy, unless that surgeon is familiar with the essential differences between these deformities.

Ingrown toenails can also be a problem and are usually caused by trimming the nail back too far at the edges or by the nail rubbing against the shoe, causing the shoe to dig into the flesh of the toe. If the toe becomes inflamed, it can be treated initially with warm water soaks twice daily. Continued irritation from wearing shoes should be avoided. For severe inflammation, antibiotics may be needed, and some people develop an abscess that needs to be drained. Nails should be trimmed frequently, and straight across, not rounded. Recurrent ingrown toenails may require partial toenail excision.

What methods can be used to control my child's spasticity?

Increased muscle tone or spasticity may cause difficulty with positioning, problems with proper hygiene, or sometimes pain. The role of muscle surgery in treating tight muscles has already been discussed. Other methods that are used to help control high muscle tone include oral medications, medication that can be injected directly into the tight muscle, and surgical implantation of a pump to reduce muscle tone.

Oral medications can be used to help control muscle tone. However, their use is usually limited. Although many people generally feel that these drugs are noninvasive, this is a misconception. These drugs all act at numerous sites in the brain and spinal cord and can therefore alter or depress many functions including alertness, mood, cognition, and personality. The physician prescribing the medication should carefully monitor for these side effects. Two commonly used drugs are Valium and oral Baclofen. Valium is best used for a short time such as to help control postsurgical muscle spasm. Long-term use frequently results in tolerance with the drug becoming less effective. Drowsiness is another common problem. Oral Baclofen has been shown to have better efficacy in head injured children and spinal cord injured children with spasticity. Its use in the child with CP is limited. It may cause difficulty with seizure control in children with seizures. It also must be weaned slowly when being discontinued.

Botulinum Toxin A and B are available for off-label use (the medication is approved by the FDA, but not for this purpose) to control spasticity in some tight muscles. Botulinum Toxin is best used when there are specific muscles (six or fewer) that are spastic. It is a relatively safe drug without known systemic effects if it is not injected into the bloodstream. It acts locally within the injected muscle to block the release of some of the nerve signals to the muscle. There are very few side effects, which may include some temporary soreness within the injected muscle.

In children with generalized spasticity (increased muscle tone involving arms, legs, and the trunk muscles), Baclofen can be given directly into the spinal canal by a small pump surgically implanted under the skin (called intrathecal Baclofen). This method allows the Baclofen to be given in much smaller doses than the oral medication because it is acting directly on the nerves in the spinal cord to control the high muscle tone. The pump is about the size of a hockey puck and is surgically placed under the skin in the lower abdomen. A small plastic catheter is tunneled under the skin around to the back and then inserted into the spinal canal, where it infuses a very small but constant dosage of Baclofen. It can help to relax high muscle tone in the legs, trunk, and arms. Parents must be willing to bring the child in to the physician who manages the pump every 4 to 12 weeks to refill the medication inside the pump. This is done with a small needle stick through the skin into a port on the pump. Intrathecal Baclofen has been extremely helpful in managing high muscle tone in the quadriplegic patient. The pump is best placed and managed at a medical center that is set up to do a preoperative assessment and trial to test the effects of the medication in the child before the pump is actually surgically implanted, as well as follow-up care after implantation.

What are the issues of independence for adolescents with various degrees of involvement?

Adolescents who are cognitively normal and mildly involved physically. For adolescents who have normal intellectual function and are able to walk with assistive devices, the issues are essentially the same as for normal teenagers—allowing for a great deal of variation with respect to individual response. All teenagers want to be "normal," but their idea of normal is often based not on reality but on perceptions acquired from the media and on their personal fantasies. They may form unrealistic goals about their weight, their skin, and their muscle strength. Ultimately, most children in this group will be incorporated into society and will have jobs and families.

Some children with disabilities focus so intently and exclusively on overcoming the disability that they require psychological counseling to help them gain perspective. Some children in this age group have unrealistic expectations about the outcome of surgical procedures, too, and they may perceive surgery as unsuccessful. This is primarily due to the child's unrealistic hope for a cure. That expectation may persist even when the treating physician gives the child a detailed explanation of the procedure and its expected outcome.

Adolescents who are cognitively normal and moderately involved physically. Children with more severe involvement, and especially those with speech and movement disorders, often find adolescent socialization, including dating, difficult. Most teens are initially awkward with members of the opposite sex. As a coping mechanism, they often strive for conformity in dress and values. The adolescent with a physical disability clearly has more to deal with in terms of socialization. It is therefore not unusual for teens with disabilities to have limited sexual and socialization experience.

Adolescents who are not able to walk and need some assistance with activities of daily living, such as bathing or dressing, can be fairly independent most of the time and usually have adequate communication skills. Their problems are very similar to those of the previous group, but they have obvious limitations and they need help in areas where normal children have outgrown the need for help. Teenagers typically become secretive and self-conscious about their bodies at this age. A teen who requires assistance with bathing or dressing is likely to experience some conflict about this.

At this age, it may become apparent to the child that total independence is not a realistic goal. If a child has not achieved this by the age of 16, it's unrealistic to expect that he will be capable of independent self-care in the future. Accepting his limitations may take considerable psychological work. Parents and therapists should focus on helping the adolescent learn how to direct his own care, providing both realistic goals and a sense of control.

One way to foster maximum independence is through independent living training, which is often available in rehabilitation facilities. The goal is for the child to learn to do all he can for himself, as well as to learn how to direct untrained individuals to help him do the remaining things. The best age for the adolescent to work on this training is between 12 and 16 years.

Independent living training in a rehabilitation facility is also an excellent method of working on separation issues. The training usually takes place over a period of weeks at a residential facility. It may be the first time the parent and child have been separated for an extended time. It may actually be as hard for the parent as for the child, if not harder. However, this is an essential part of growth and maturity, and the child should be provided the opportunity and freedom to develop his independence. Parents need to let go with the understanding and realization that they will not always be around to provide for their child. Additionally, the important planning for the possibility of college or work cannot be effectively accomplished if the issue of separation has not been addressed.

It is important to respect the maturing child's right to privacy, though this may be somewhat difficult for a teen who needs help with toileting. Closing doors and respecting the teen's requests for privacy whenever possible is essential. Adolescents in this group often have little opportunity to work on issues of sexual socialization, primarily because they are still working on issues of separation. These teens need to be offered opportunities to be involved with their peer group within the community.

Adolescents who are cognitively normal and severely involved physically. All the issues that apply to adolescents with moderate involvement also apply to adolescents with severe physical involvement. But the adolescent with a severe disability also needs help with all activities of daily living and usually requires an alternative means of communicating. Difficulties in the areas of daily living and communication can be very frustrating and energy consuming. It is understandably upsetting for the adolescent when people don't take the time to try to understand her and assume that she is retarded. Every effort should be made to plan for the future; adolescents in this group eventually need to become self-sufficient with the help of a full-time trained aide.

A child who is severely involved is usually not able to direct an untrained individual in her own care, and plans should be in place to ensure that trained caregivers with whom the child is comfortable are always available. This is especially important in the event the child needs to go to the hospital or to be cared for by a caretaker other than the one to whom she is accustomed. For a child who is unable to communicate orally, it's imperative to seek medical treatment at a facility whose staff are familiar with the needs of individuals with severe disabilities, or to make certain that knowledgeable, trained caretakers are present to be sure that the child receives adequate care.

A teenager in this group almost never has an opportunity for sexual socialization as a teenager and only occasionally as an adult. He or she has sexual feelings and desires, though they may be difficult to address. (This aspect of development is discussed further in Chapter 4.) The teen's difficulty in communicating, as well as the attempt to cope with normal maturation issues, often leads to withdrawal and depression, and this may not be recognized or addressed properly because of the communication difficulties. Priority should be given to providing communication systems for these adolescents. This is probably the single most important service that the medical care system can provide. (See earlier sections for information about communication systems.)

Adolescents with mild cognitive and physical involvement. Adolescents with mild cognitive impairment who are able to walk, with or without the use of assistive devices, face issues that are very similar to the issues facing children without disabilities. However, they need additional structure and guidance concerning schooling, training, and, ultimately, job opportunities. They also need to be given the same opportunities to fail that parents give to normal teenagers, although achieving a balance of help, guidance, and letting go is never easy.

Adolescents in this group may have significant difficulty dealing with social interactions, and their difficulty may show up as depression or anger. Parents should make it possible for these teens to discuss their feelings with a professional counselor before the feelings become overwhelming. With proper guidance and within the appropriate environment, most of these youngsters become fully self-sufficient members of society.

Adolescents with moderate cognitive and physical involvement. Although many of them are able to walk with assistive devices, these adolescents need to be in a structured and supervised living and working environment because of their cognitive limitations. If the adolescent is presently cared for at home, the main issue of concern for the family is to plan for the future, when the current primary caregiver will not be able to care for the child. These plans should be recorded in writing, and they should be described to the teen's next of kin.

If institutional care is likely to be needed in the future, facilities should be investigated in advance. One of the very attractive alternatives to institutionalized living is the structured group home, in which the person is able to move away from home but still lives in the same community and is able to go home on weekends and holidays. This arrangement closely parallels the situation of the child who leaves home when he finds a job but continues to be involved with his family in the same community.

Adolescents with severe cognitive and physical impairment. Adolescents in this group need full-time trained custodial care. They don't have all the psychological problems that beset adolescents with milder involvement, however. The main issue for this group is the need for good planning for the future. If the parent is the sole full-time care provider, then plans must be made for alternative caregivers. The parents of severely involved children often have the misconception that their child has a short life expectancy. However, the vast majority of individuals who reach their teenage years will probably outlive their parents. Thus, long-range planning really is a necessity. Additionally, unexpected events such as an accident or illness sometimes make it impossible for the primary caregiver to continue to provide care.

If no alternative plans have been made, the state social service agency will assume responsibility for the child, who will be placed in whatever facility is available, often without regard to what the parents may have wanted. Rather than let this happen, it is far better to make arrangements with a facility or with other individuals willing to provide the necessary care before something interferes with the present arrangements. Ideally, an alternative caregiver will previously have provided some care, perhaps as respite care, and will be familiar with the teenager and his needs. Having some familiarity beforehand with the new caregivers also provides the child with comfort and security in a new environment, if the need should arise for a move.

Parents must allow themselves the opportunity to ask how much longer they can continue to care for their child. This is a difficult issue and one that can lead to conflict between parents. Divorce, unfortunately, is a fairly common result of the strains and conflicts that prevail in the family of a child with a severe disorder. Some parents are poorly equipped to handle the extra stress, and some are not willing to give up a previously pursued career in order to provide full-time care of the child. Once a parent has psychologically come to terms with the extent of care that he or she is willing personally to provide, there are various alternatives to consider.

After taking into account many factors—such as the home environment, schools, siblings, availability of respite care, and financial resources—parents may decide that it's better for the child to be in another environment. They may choose to relinquish parental rights and never see the child again, or they may place the child in a group home or chronic care facility and visit the child there or bring the child home for weekend and holiday visits.

Another option is foster care, in which the child is placed with another family for care. In this arrangement, the parents retain their rights and have the opportunity to take the child on weekends, special occasions, or whenever they want to spend time with the child. There are some caregivers, mostly women, whose occupation as foster parents is to care for children with disabilities. Many of these persons provide excellent care, although their services are in great demand and they are hard to find. Some individuals providing foster care, however, lack either the appropriate skills or other options for work, and they may be motivated by selfish needs not always leading to the best care for the individual. So, this choice may provide the child either with the best of care or with very poor care, primarily because there is little supervision over the care provided. Parents need to thoroughly investigate any situation that they are considering for their child.

There should also be some discussion about the level of medical care which parents want to provide in life-threatening situations. This is an emotionally charged subject in which religious, ethical, and practical factors are intricately interwoven. Parents need to reach an understanding in advance about their wishes for their child's care so that they aren't faced with making a difficult decision without having first given this issue serious consideration and discussion. Parents should also make sure that any doctor treating their child is well aware in advance of their wishes regarding medical treatment in a life-threatening situation. Discussing these decisions allows the parents and the physicians to become comfortable with them. Many parents decide to provide all the care necessary to ensure the child's comfort (such as correcting scoliosis) but not to take heroic measures to prolong life (such as permanently putting the child on a ventilator). This includes doing everything possible to improve the ability of caregivers to care for the child.

Often there are difficult decisions to make, and it seems as if a fine line is being drawn between providing medical care to improve the child's quality of life and providing care to prolong life. If, for example, a child's kidneys fail, a plan to transplant a kidney in order to prolong the child's life might well be decided against fairly readily. A decision regarding gastric surgery for a child who experiences frequent pneumonias related to reflux and aspiration may be more difficult to make, particularly if the pneumonias respond well to antibiotic treatment.

The decision to operate on a severely involved child can be very difficult. Scoliosis is usually treated with surgery, because, although it is major surgery, the result allows for better seating and more comfort. But if a child develops a severe bowel obstruction, the parents may elect not to have surgery because a bowel obstruction usually brings on death quickly, without much pain, whereas the surgery for bowel obstruction may involve a very long recovery period with a great deal of discomfort.

Clearly, such decisions must be made on an individual basis. They are easier if parents and physicians have established a compatible working relationship before an acute situation arises. Then parents can be more comfortable with their decisions and can be confident that the physician is prepared to abide by those decisions.

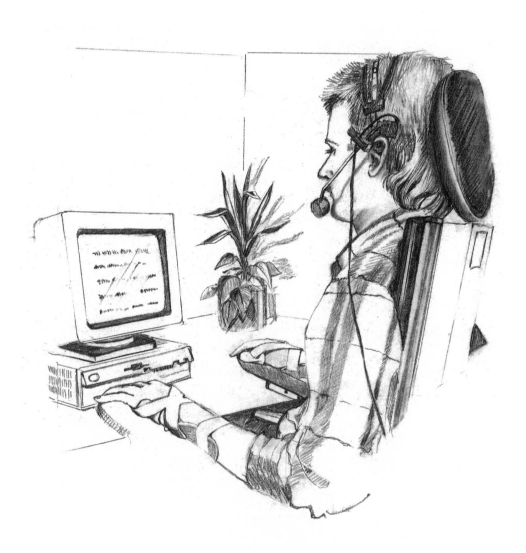

The Adult with Cerebral Palsy

8

♦ CHILDREN with cerebral palsy become young adults, middle-aged adults, and older adults. They live in a community and relate to their families. In fact, they deal with many of the same issues that nondisabled people do. The purpose of this chapter is to provide some insight into how the adult with cerebral palsy deals with the process of aging.

Aging can be considered the counterpart of growth and development in the child, the main difference being that aging takes place over a longer time and with more variation from one individual to another. The person with a disability attempts to meet all the challenges of the nondisabled person, with some additional challenges thrown in. Concerns usually center on independence, intimate relationships, and employment. There may be significant psychological issues as well, and the adult with cerebral palsy may find it more difficult than the child to obtain medical care.

The degree of difficulty a person encounters in establishing independence depends on the individual person and his or her family, as well as on the severity of the disability. This transition is much harder for adults who need the most care. Generally, children who have functioned well in a regular school environment can be expected to meet the challenge of transition to adulthood and independence in much the same way that their classmates or siblings handle this process. For some teenagers or young adults, however, having a disability makes it psychologically difficult to establish a positive and healthy self-image. For those who have previously functioned well in a regular school setting, this is most likely an adjustment reaction to the transition process (similar to the difficulty the child without a disability has in adjusting to going off to college or breaking up with a boyfriend or girlfriend). Whenever problems such as depression or behavioral changes emerge, they should be taken seriously and psychological counseling should be obtained.

What are the important issues for the person with cerebral palsy during the transition to adulthood?

The important skills learned at this stage are socialization skills, especially the development of intimate relationships. Dating and trying to gain acceptance from peers can be very traumatic for any young adult, but the effort required of people with CP can be draining. They may have to use 100 percent of their energy just to keep up with their peers who are only giving 25 percent. As they move into the adult environment, with more competition and without the buffered environment of school and a supportive home environment, individuals with CP often experience fatigue, both from the increased psychological stress of dealing with a less receptive environment and from the physical stress of the increased physical demands present in a college or work environment. They may get worn down from the fight to keep up.

Another source of stress that may not be fully encountered until the person leaves school and tries to enter the job market is prejudice against people with a disability or handicap. If she is a woman or a member of a racial minority, this can compound the prejudice that she may experience. Understanding their rights, forming alliances with others in minority groups, and being willing to openly confront discrimination are important mechanisms for people with disabilities who are dealing with prejudice.

Young adults are quite self-conscious and concerned about their personal image, and their partner is often seen as an extension of themselves. A young man often tries to enhance his self-image by being seen with a beautiful young woman, and vice versa. The stresses generated by the cultural focus on physical appearance are present not only for the person with cerebral palsy, but for many people who are not considered perfect. However, this is also a stage in life when individuals are learning that there is more to a person than appearance. It becomes clear that a relationship is much more dependent on communication, understanding, mutual care, and concern.

This lesson can be fostered in group environments, which allow individuals with disabilities to learn socialization and intimacy skills and to meet suitable marriage partners. Many group environments are organized around special interests, social activities, and spiritual concerns. This type of socialization certainly provides an advantage over the generally accepted norm of meeting the ideal partner in an environment filled with strangers. Meeting people under traditional dating circumstances is especially hard for people with a disability because of the very real physical and psychological barriers present between themselves and the nondisabled population. People living in areas where they are having problems meeting others for friendships or romantic relationships might consider using a dating service, either one found on-line or in periodicals that serve people with disabilities.

Adults with Impairments

Adults with impairments due to cerebral palsy are typically people who can manage all activities of daily living without needing to expend significantly more effort than the nondisabled population. This includes most people with hemiplegia and many with diplegia who have normal cognitive function. By definition, an impairment is an abnormality of body structure or function, such as spasticity or contractures, that does not actually cause any limitation in the performance of one's usual activities.

Howard is a 39-year-old man with mild to moderate right side hemiplegia who currently works as a computer program systems analyst. He has been married for 10 years and has three healthy, active boys, ages 2, 5, and 8. Howard and his wife, Joan, have always had open communication concerning his impairment. The only problem cerebral palsy caused him in terms of parenting was learning to carry and care for his newborn infants. Due to his affected right arm and hand Howard was afraid that he might drop them. But this was easily solved with a little practice.

Having children made Howard think about how he would feel or how he would deal with the situation if one of his children had a disability. He had no answers to this question, except to want to pass on to his own children some of the same lessons he learned while growing up, specifically that it is important to find your own way of making things work. The children know that their father types with one hand very effectively and that he had a high school teacher who helped him learn to type.

Howard has not had any medical problems since a foot operation at age 17. He can't quite extend his right elbow all the way, and he does have a slight limp. These are so well integrated into Howard's movements that very few of his co-workers even know that he has cerebral palsy. He golfs, swims, water skis, snow skis, and goes sailboating. He does not have a special exercise program, but when he notices some tightness or stiffness, he knows he needs some physical activity. He does sometimes worry about developing a neurological or orthopedic problem that would significantly alter his activity or functional level.

Howard started as a physical therapy major in college, but in his third year he switched to nursing. After graduation he trained as a rehabilitation nurse specialist and worked for 10 years, until he felt a need for a change. By working evenings, he earned a degree in business administration and changed his career from nursing to computer systems analysis.

What are the usual living arrangements for adults with impairments?

These adults generally get married and have children and enjoy a lifestyle that is very similar to that of the general population. Specific problems related to cerebral palsy are usually minor from a medical perspective, but they may be more significant in relation to occupational choices.

Howard has experienced some discrimination, especially when he wanted to enlist in the Air Force Reserves for extra income as a rehabilitation nurse and was told that he could not apply because he had cerebral palsy. This was tough to hear, especially when he wasn't even evaluated with respect to how much his impairment affected him. Another time he was asked if he had a physical disability while renewing his driver's license. When he said yes, he had to repeat the entire driving test, even though he had been driving for six years with no change in his condition. This almost resulted in his having to pay higher insurance premiums. He later realized that he should have said no, since he is impaired, not disabled. He learned quickly that using the right terminology is important in many situations.

The Americans with Disabilities Act makes employment discrimination in the private and government sectors illegal. If you think that you're being discriminated against, check with legal counsel and learn what your rights are.

What about discrimination? Job discrimination against individuals with an impairment still goes on, although with the extension of equal opportunity rights to people with disabilities, the incidence of discrimination should decrease. The largest area of overt discrimination continues to be with health, disability, and life insurance. Obtaining insurance coverage usually is possible only if the person can join a group plan carried by an employer. The health insurance system is changing rapidly, and there is increasing public recognition of discrimination in these areas. Educating lawmakers about the needs of people with disabilities has had a very positive impact. You can participate by contacting your representatives and expressing your concerns.

Adults with Functional Limitations

Adults with functional limitations are primarily those with moderate to severe diplegia or mild to moderate quadriplegia. Such adults are able to be independent, but their impairment significantly restricts their ability to perform certain activities of daily living. Their occupational choices and relationships may be influenced by their impairment. Most people in this category have normal cognitive function, although some people with mild mental retardation could also fit into this group. People with only physical impairments have somewhat different problems from those encountered by people who also have cognitive difficulties. The discussion in this section focuses on the issues faced by people who have only physical limitations.

Sam is 46 years old and works as a mechanical engineer in the research division of a major company. He has athetoid patterned cerebral palsy with a moderate degree of involvement in his hands and arms. He is able to walk without using any aids, but he has speech difficulty, especially when communicating with people who don't know him. He grew up in a very supportive family with a mother who he feels protected him too much but with a father who pushed him with appropriate expectations. Because he loved to build things, his father encouraged him, never pressuring him about time. His father's patience fostered an early interest in engineering. In grade school he was thought by several teachers to be retarded because of his speech difficulty, especially when they met him for the first time and did not have the patience to listen to him and understand him. Because of this difficulty and at the insistence of his father, he was placed in a special education class where the teachers took the needed time and interest in his abilities. In the special education classes he excelled academically.

After Sam graduated from high school, his vocational rehabilitation adviser thought Sam's interest in going to college was a waste of time and money, and he discouraged Sam from applying to schools. Sam feels this was in part due to the fact that the state vocational rehabilitation system was always short of money and tried to find the cheapest thing to do for clients, sometimes without thoroughly considering their interests and abilities. Initially, too, he was told that he could not pursue a major in engineering because he could not draw. By devising his own mechanical aids for drawing, he managed to draw so well that his instructors told him he had the best mechanical drawings they had seen in a master's degree thesis. Ironically, then, Sam graduated from college with a master's degree in mechanical engineering.

Ellen and Sam met through personal advertisements placed with a dating service for people with disabilities and were subsequently married. Ellen is 44 years old with a moderate to severe spastic quadriplegic pattern involvement of cerebral palsy. She has normal speech but is not able to walk. She uses a wheelchair, which she can push for short distances. She can do most activities of daily living by herself. Ellen also grew up in a very supportive family, and both her parents encouraged her to be all she could be, within the scope of her limitations. She entered a regular kindergarten and remained in mainstream educational classes all through high school. She completed four years of college and works as a travel agent. Ellen remembers her educational experience differently than Sam, since she did not receive the "retarded" label, largely because her speech wasn't affected.

Because of these different experiences, Sam and Ellen have somewhat different feelings about the current push to mainstream children in school. Sam feels it may at times be a way for the system to save money and may not be in the child's best interests, especially a child with significant speech problems. Both Ellen and Sam, however, support inclusion whenever it works for the child, as it clearly did for Ellen. They both worry that the attempt to have the child in a "normal" environment may dominate and that, as a consequence, the child may receive less than the best education. Sam recently decided to get involved with his local district's school board because of his strong feelings.

What are the usual living arrangements for adults with functional limitations? Many young adults with functional limitations and normal intelligence get married, although often somewhat later than adults without such limitations. However, fewer adults with disabilities marry than the age-matched nondisabled population. Most of these adults live either independently or in close proximity to their families.

If mobility is a major problem, their independence hinges on public transportation or on the possibility of obtaining adapted transportation, such as a chair lift–equipped van. Funding for this type of vehicle is often limited, and obtaining one frequently requires coming up with innovative approaches to fundraising. A number of volunteer community agencies, such as the United Cerebral Palsy Associations and the Easter Seal Society, are interested in helping people with disabilities. These agencies, even if they can't provide funds themselves, usually know where to turn for help. Obtaining a driver's license and a personal motor vehicle provides a large measure of independence, and anyone who is capable of accomplishing these things ought to try very hard to do so.

What special medical considerations are there for those with impairments and functional limitations?

There are a number of issues that are more common to people with impairments and functional limitations, although the issues are by and large the same ones the general population faces. Good general medical care continues to be important but also may be neglected because of difficulty in finding physicians who are willing to provide care for the adult with CP. Many adults with CP get good care for acute problems but do not get good **preventive care,** such as periodic general health evaluations, Pap smears, breast exams, and rectal exams. The best way to find a physician is not to wait until you are ill but to obtain the names of two to four physicians and visit their offices and interview them. This lets you know how comfortable the physician is with you and lets you see whether the office is accessible to you. **Dental care** is also a problem for many adults with CP. Many have poor dental hygiene and caries ("cavities"), and finding a dentist who has the skills and is willing to devote the time necessary may be difficult. Many of those with CP also have problems with drooling, which may be treatable with medication or surgery (see Chapter 3).

Adults with impairments and functional limitations due to spasticity must get adequate exercise to avoid stiffness. This need often conflicts with increasingly busy lifestyles, just as a full schedule interferes with the nondisabled person's ability to exercise. The same discipline is required to set up a routine in which the individual does get exercise and stretching. If the activity is one that the person enjoys doing, such as swimming, the person is more likely to stick with it. Many young adults give up walking by age 25, for reasons of fatigue and inefficiency of walking, and because wheelchairs provide greater mobility and independence.

Musculoskeletal problems are very common as these young adults get older. Cervical neck pain (especially in those with athetosis), back pain, and pain in the weight-bearing joints (hips, knees, and ankles) can be found in a high percentage of adults with CP, especially after age 40. Of those who are still walking at age 40, many give it up at this point because of this pain. Contractures of the lower extremities are also common, especially among those who have stopped walking. Another common complaint is carpal tunnel syndrome, a type of overuse syndrome, which develops because of chronic, repetitive, and atypical uses of muscles or joints. This can be seen in those who are working at computer keyboards over many hours a day, or in those who use crutches or push manual wheelchairs over many years.

Adults with functional limitations are also vulnerable to chronic **dehydration** as a result of decreasing, by choice, their fluid intake to avoid difficulties in public toileting. This can contribute to **constipation.** Constipation is a common complaint of aging adults, as well as those with functional limitations. Attention should be paid to this problem by changing the diet, using stool softeners, and having bowel movements on a regular schedule. Regularity can be achieved with improved toilet accessibility in the workplace and, sometimes, attendant help. Adequate water intake is also essential.

Sam recognizes that his disability places him at increased risk for developing arthritis in his neck, and for falling. At the same time, he argues, he is not going to break his leg snow skiing or playing basketball, as a coworker of equal age might. This argument has not helped Sam with the insurance company, and he is presently without medical coverage. Because Ellen uses a wheelchair, she finds it impossible to use many public bathrooms, which are not large enough for wheelchairs to maneuver in. She finds the Unisex wheelchair bathrooms best, when available, because then Sam can also enter and help her.

Finding physicians has also been difficult. Ellen has had an especially difficult time finding a gynecologist who will take the time to deal with her spasticity, which is always a problem. On one occasion, she tried to tell a new gynecologist which positioning and speculum size would work best and found that he felt offended. Sam has had similar problems finding a dentist because of his difficulty in controlling his mouth movements. He suggested a clamp to hold his mouth open, but several dentists ignored his suggestions.

As adults neither Sam nor Ellen has had serious medical problems, although both have to deal with chronic constipation. Sam has also had some problems with arthritis in his neck, although it has resolved with rest, therapy, and medication; so far, there hasn't been a need for surgery. Sam and Ellen do both worry about maintaining their current level of functioning and remaining independent.

What are the prospects for employment?

In the 1980s, studies showed that only a small percentage (from 12 to 17 percent) of adults with CP were employed. More recently, published reports have shown far more adults with CP (as high as 50 percent) achieving competitive employment and independent living. People with milder involvement, good family support, and proper medical treatment had the highest rate of employment. People whose speech impairment was a major part of their disability had lower rates of employment.

A common misperception in the general population about people with functional limitations is that the person is retarded. This should be confronted immediately with a discussion of the person's abilities. As an example, if the person with a functional limitation is seeing a physician who ignores the person and only talks to the sponsor, the person being examined should openly say "I have a college education. I know that I'm occasionally hard to understand when I speak, but I can understand very well what you're talking about."

Sam and Ellen were married 16 years ago, and both have continued to work. During their adult years, they have experienced discrimination due to their functional limitations. For both, finding jobs has always been difficult. Ellen had 54 interviews before finding a job as a travel agent. Sam sent out 107 resumes and received only two offers for interviews. Many large international companies would not even consider them because of their disabilities. Obtaining health, life, and disability insurance has been extremely difficult. With passage of the Americans with Disabilities Act, these kinds of difficulties have been eased significantly.

Many people obtain jobs through a network of friends and professional associations. This route is advantageous, especially for the person with a functional limitation. Individuals with severe physical limitations but normal cognitive function may find that getting a job in the private sector is almost impossible. These individuals should push state agencies to help set up or find jobs. Employment is an important aspect of an adult's psychological health. Volunteer organizations can help with special circumstances, especially when being employed prevents the person from getting assistance from government agencies.

Sam and Ellen bought a house that was in a price range appropriate for their income. However, the house needed to have a ramp built for Ellen's wheelchair, the bathroom had to be made wheelchair accessible, and the laundry area had to be moved upstairs, all of which created significant added expenses for which there was no help available. If they were not working, the county welfare agency would have provided wheelchair-accessible transportation. However, because they were earning money, this was not available. Their income was not large enough to allow them to purchase a hand-controlled, wheelchair-accessible van, which Ellen needs for transportation. Assistance in buying this type of vehicle is often available through volunteer organizations, but obtaining funds requires some initiative on the part of the person who needs help. Modifications to the house may also be tax deductible if the modifications are needed because of a person's disability. A tax adviser can help you determine which of these expenses can legally be claimed for tax purposes.

Adults with Disabilities

This group, adults with disabilities, varies greatly, from those who need assistance because of mental retardation to those who have normal cognitive function but severe physical disabilities. This group also includes individuals with both severe mental and physical disabilities. By definition, these are the people whose disability is severe enough to interfere with their ability to participate in a typical societal role.

John was cared for from birth by a foster mother whose five older children were all in school. Mary was a secondary school teacher and writer who felt the need to adopt a special child. Because adoption would have removed all state assistance, John legally remained a foster child so the family could obtain state assistance for medical expenses and other special needs. But he was raised as one of Mary's own.

John started walking at age 5 with poor balance and is considered to have moderate spastic quadriplegic CP with moderate speech impairment and a moderate degree of mental retardation. John has an outgoing personality, endless good spirits, and an obsessive will. His mental disability affects his judgment, impairs his perceptions, and causes perseverations (persistent repetition of a word, gesture, or act). He is happy to be with his family, his closely knit local community, and his church, and he is never moody or persistently angry. In general, he has unquenchable optimism and a totally positive outlook on life.

Although John needs supervision for daily living activities, as well as direction to maintain appropriate behavior, he has become a full member of the extended family. Although he was never adopted, the state agency "forgot" him, expecting that he would be cared for by the foster family. When John turned 18, Mary successfully applied to become his legal guardian. Even if he had been adopted, this step would have been necessary at age 18 if Mary was to continue to have any legal responsibility for John.

By the time John was 26, Mary had retired and was in her seventies. She started to plan for John's future care and arrived at a decision with the rest of her children. When Mary died, John would be cared for by Hal, the oldest son, who had four children of his own in grade school. At this time, there was discussion about building several group homes for adults with disabilities in the community. The family felt this might be an even better option for John, since the people building these homes were members of the church to which John belonged. Two homes were built, one for men and one for women. Application was made, but the family felt the chances were very slim that John would be chosen, because other families seemed to have a much greater need for custodial care.

The group directing this effort wanted this home to work, however, and they believed things would be easier if they started with adults who were well known in the community and who were not too difficult for caretakers to manage. Because of John's good nature and community ties, he was chosen. After the choice was made there was only one month until moving day. During the transition John stayed at his new home but every other weekend came back home to stay for the night. Since the new home was only several blocks from his old one, it was easy for John to come home when any special occasions such as a birthday occurred. John quickly adapted to his new environment and was happy.

Things did not go well for Mary. Her friends would typically greet her with statements like, "How wonderful that you're free now, with John in the group home," and would not hear her sadness. Although John's father seemed to welcome the new freedom to come and go with friends without looking out for John, for Mary things were very different. She now awakened in the morning without anyone to care for, for the first time since her oldest son was born 46 years before. Mary had enjoyed caring for John and had not seen him as a burden, but instead appreciated his humor and lively engagement as a conversational partner. With John gone and her husband focusing more on his hobbies, Mary became depressed. After several sessions with a psychologist, Mary learned that the kind of sadness she experienced when John moved was a natural consequence of loss. It was also a reasonable cause for grieving, even if others around her could not appreciate it. With time, Mary found peace in her new life.

What are the usual living arrangements for adults with disabilities?

Care and housing arrangements for the disabled adult vary greatly from one community to another. The environment of a small group home, with full-time house parents, is probably ideal, although it is not available in many communities. There are some adults who require too much care for the usual small group home. Larger group homes with staff rotating by shifts are another alternative that works well in some communities. Adult foster homes are yet another possibility. Options that many parents find least desirable are nursing homes or state hospitals. Although these are not ideal environments, there may be no other alternative for some adults requiring very intensive or skilled care. These options should not be immediately dismissed as poor choices, since there are many nursing homes and state hospitals that are well run and staffed by very competent and caring personnel.

Parents of adults should find out what is available in their community long before they expect to use these facilities. If adequate facilities are not available, parents may want to consider forming a church or community group and look into establishing group homes. This is how most good small group homes are developed. In many ways the transition from parental home care to outside care for the adult with a disability should follow a pattern similar to the normal child who eventually leaves the parental home to live independently. Many adults with disabilities continue to live with their families until circumstances necessitate a change in living arrangements. Planning for the time when a change may become necessary is extremely important for the adult with a disability as well as for the family. Planning seriously and over a long time for any change can make the transition much easier for everyone when the change occurs. Making a change in an emergency situation, such as when there is serious illness or death of the principal caretaker, can be traumatic for everyone involved.

What special medical problems do adults with disabilities have?

The adult with a disability continues to have the same medical problems that were present earlier, if they haven't yet been adequately addressed. Pain from dislocated hips or scoliosis, for example, may continue to be present in the adult if they have not been fully corrected in childhood.

As was mentioned for those with functional limitations, this population also lacks adequate preventive medical and dental care. Hearing and vision impairments, epilepsy, and gastroesophageal reflux are fairly common in this population (these problems are discussed in Chapter 3) and may worsen in the adult even if they were adequately dealt with in childhood.

The young adult with disability is also prone to some special medical problems. One set of problems is **urinary tract infections and incontinence.** Infections are often associated with poor perineal hygiene and/or the use of a urinary collecting device or Foley catheter. Bladder incontinence is a particular problem among the nonambulatory (those who spend most of the day in a wheelchair or bed) and can be improved by following a regular toileting schedule. Incontinence often occurs late in the day after not voiding all day, and frequently during transfer activities. As mentioned earlier in this chapter, deliberate restriction of fluids to avoid this problem often leads to **constipation.**

As discussed in Chapter 3, **osteopenia (low bone density)** and **osteoporosis** are a significant problem for many adolescents with CP. This problem only gets worse as they become adults, especially because many of them give up walking as they get older. Fractures after minimal trauma, or after a fall in those who are ambulatory, may be fairly common. Those who have had one such fracture are at an even greater risk for recurrence. Osteoporosis is a concern for the elderly population at large, especially postmenopausal women. In the disabled population, this problem is present among both men and women, and at much younger ages than in the rest of the population. Consideration needs to be given to early evaluation of bone density (usually with a DXA scan) and to possible treatment with medications (such as vitamin D and/or bisphosphonates).

Postural back pain is often associated with inadequate wheelchair equipment. Crutches, canes, braces, and wheelchairs need to be reevaluated periodically to be sure they are still appropriate for the individual and still fit his or her needs.

The Young Adult with Cerebral Palsy

Some of the problems people with cerebral palsy have are specifically related to the person's age. One common problem that develops in this group is loss of motivation and desire to pursue goals, when the person is no longer in the school system. Some mentally high-functioning but severely physically involved individuals become disheartened when they can't go to college or find employment. For those who have been able to attend college, facing unemployment related to their disability is profoundly disturbing and can seriously affect their motivation.

Some of these challenges are well described by Josh and by his mother, who submitted the following about his life during adolescence and young adulthood.

A YOUNG MAN'S VIEW

I'm Josh. I'm 24 years old and I have cerebral palsy. I have been living on my own for the past three years. Now that may not seem like much, but when I was born they didn't know if I was going to survive. I'm a fighter. I've had twelve surgeries and spent the first five years of my life seeing one doctor after another and physical therapists for hours at a time. It's been a long and winding road for me to get where I am, but I think I am going in the right direction. I've decided to tell you about the time of my life between 13 and now. It was a very traumatic and changing time for me. I guess the best way to start this narrative is with one word, nothing. Nothing is what I did between the ages of 13 and 18. I mean I went to school, graduated with a 2.96 gpa, and the only reason it was that high was because of my test-taking abilities. I never did any homework or studied. I got the grades that I got by paying attention in class. Now that I look back on it I think it was a mistake. If I had done my homework, I would have graduated on the honor roll.

The events that have gotten me where I am started before I graduated. High school was mostly about being pushed around and called names by the other kids, dodging being thrown into lockers, and being called "tard." But my freshman year of high school I had a teacher for World Civ by the name of George M. Mr. M is a very unique teacher. He has since become the principal of that high school. He made me want to be in his class. I will never forget the day I decided I wanted to be a teacher. It was the day before my very last orthopedic surgery. Mr. M decided that before he would start class we would have a party for me. So we're sitting there talking and eating snacks and I said to myself, "This is what I want to do. I want to make other people feel the same way I do right now." I can say that is the exact moment that I wanted to be a teacher.

Let's flash forward to my first year of college. I had just gotten accepted to a five year program that would end with me having a masters in education. I wasn't ready for college. I decided I'd rather smoke pot than go to class. So I failed out. Then I thought that I wanted to be an artist so I applied to the School of Visual Arts for photography. I was accepted. When school started I became very depressed. There were days when I didn't get out of bed until five in the afternoon. I didn't want to do anything. So needless to say, after two semesters I failed out again. That was the end of my college days. My parents brought me home. I continued to be depressed and didn't know what to do with my life.

When I got home that's when it got hard. My parents and I were not getting along, I wasn't doing anything, and I was just wasting away. At first I tried to work at a convenience store, but I wasn't able to stock the shelves or clean fast enough. Then I worked as a computer consultant, and I kept that job for a total of five months when they told me they wanted someone with more graphic design abilities. I think that was just a nice way of firing me. My parents decided that I had to do something. So they insisted that I enroll in the local community college and I did stay there and received computer certification. My mother drove me to and from school every day and I did complete that certification. I was somewhat proud. But I still had not become my dream of being a teacher.

That was when my parents and I decided that I couldn't live with them anymore.

I decided to move into Center City. I come from a very fortunate family and my parents were nice enough to help me with my rent. They have been helping me for the past 3 years. It seemed that the only way I was going to be able to find a job in such a big city was with some help, so I went to OVR, the Office of Vocational Rehab. Through OVR I was introduced to Liberty Resources.

Liberty Resources is a CIL (Center for Independent Living). At Liberty Resources, adults with physical and neurological disabilities are given opportunities that would otherwise be difficult to get—specifically job training. A very large portion of Liberty Resources is called the Workplace Academy. It is a group of classes specializing in workplace skills and etiquette. Through OVR I was enrolled in a few of these classes. While I was waiting for these classes to start I went in and talked to the director about what I can do to keep myself busy until I start my classes. She and I decided that I could do some volunteer work. I decided to ask her if I could teach. I explained to her that I have computer certification and that I would have no problem helping teach the computer classes they offered there. I've been volunteering at Liberty for the past seven months. There has been talk of a permanent teacher's aide position.

It may have taken me a while, and I've taken many different roads, but I think I am on the verge of reaching my goal of being a teacher and fulfilling my ambitions. I can only tell you that I think I've learned that it is important to take a risk in life. I have been fortunate to be exposed to many different people and things in my life. I guess you can say we grow when we grow up. I now work and help many people with many challenging disabilities. Sometimes I still get angry with people for not seeming to accept my cerebral palsy, but I now realize that is their issue, not mine. Again, I say take a risk and reach for your dreams. I'm still reaching.

A MOTHER'S VIEW

When Josh started middle school at the age of thirteen, he was full of hope and so were we. He was totally mainstreamed, which we had fought for because we felt he belonged in that situation. He was smart, intelligent, and very eager to learn. I should say that throughout his entire school years he was thrown in and out of special ed, mainly because of behavior and insubordination. When he liked a subject, his star shone brightly. When he liked a teacher, he did the same. He was a very sociable guy and loved to talk . . . and debate. He was small for his size, so he was constantly being challenged by bigger boys. He was a bully's dream. Because of his limp and his somewhat bent over appearance, he was constantly the target and butt end of jokes and taunts. He came home every day after school either crying or complaining about something or someone. His grades began to slip and he stopped doing his work. All he wanted was to be accepted by his peers and it was a very sad time for him and us. His usual gregarious personality became sullen, he never smiled any more, and we became worried about him. He was seeing a psychologist, which took the pressure off of us, but to no avail. Right before his thirteenth birthday and bar mitzvah, he had an emotional breakdown and was placed at Child Guidance Hospital for thirty days. That time caused much stress and fighting in our lives, for Joshua, his parents and siblings. After coming out of Child Guidance, he went back to middle school and again was taunted by the children. He was tripped in gym class, broke his knee, and needed to be in a cast for eight weeks. The day his cast came off, he was tripped again and that was the last straw. I went to his school with my "dukes up" prepared for a big fight. We got no cooperation from the public school and my husband and I decided to take him out of public middle school. He was in the eighth grade. We searched for all types of schools and finally made the decision to send him to a private school about twenty minutes away. The only compromise we had to make is that they insisted he repeat the seventh grade as he really hadn't done much work. We agreed. He really liked the school and started out doing very well. He was being academically challenged, but he was still acting out because he so desperately wanted to be accepted. But he was liked at this school and we loved their philosophy. He was treated kindly and with respect and accepted for his differences. He was even on the school basketball team. He suited up and played sometimes. It was a great boost to his morale. He made friends and flourished. He was happy. And so were we.

Then he decided that he wanted to go to a public high school and I feel it was the beginning of a great depression. He barely did any work the entire four years of high school. If he liked the teacher, he was fine. He battled kids every day who called him names and taunted him. He was thrown into lockers, bullied and at times would act out in school. He did have some teachers who protected him; a few students too. After graduating he tried college, but failed out because of not going to class. We brought him home and he signed up for computer certification. Loving computers, he succeeded and flourished. He had several jobs, but they didn't last because he had a problem with authority. Finally his cousin found out about a place called Liberty Resources, which is a nonprofit organization that helps people with disabilities function in the real world. It was a wonderful experience for Josh, as he loved the people there and they were willing to give him a chance. He took more computer classes and also classes to help him look for, get, and keep a job. At this point, he is teaching computers to other disabled adults and loves his role as a teacher's assistant. He is waiting to hear whether they will hire him permanently. A great lesson was learned here. If you persist and try hard, you can turn your life around and do something productive with your life, no matter what . . . we are very proud of the wonderful job and effort our son is providing for himself and others. Growing up for anyone has its bumps and peaks and valleys, but growing up challenged can also provide the person with a desire to succeed. Our son, Joshua has done just that.

What can be done for the person who is no longer motivated?

When an adult is no longer motivated, it is important to determine if he or she is clinically depressed. Depression can affect the young adult just like anyone else, and should be treated with psychological counseling and, when appropriate, medication. The person who loses interest in his normal activities, is not interested in interpersonal relationships, and becomes withdrawn should not be ignored for long periods of time. These bouts of depression are easier to treat if they are addressed early by referral to a clinical social worker, psychologist, or psychiatrist.

How can the person with a disability overcome barriers to employment?

Although current laws are designed to protect individuals with disabilities from discrimination, in reality there are both physical and psychological barriers to overcome. In the past, many employers made their workplaces physically accessible only when economically motivated to do so. However, providing physical access in the workplace is now legally required by the Americans with Disability Act.

Typically there is a good deal more acceptance of people with disabilities in the educational community (students as well as teachers) than in the free market. Certainly, individuals who have attained a college education, and particularly those with a graduate degree, have less difficulty finding a job than those without degrees.

The first step in dealing with barriers to employment is understanding that they exist and anticipating them. Networking with known contacts when looking for employment often yields better results than trying to enter the open market where no one knows you. This style of job hunting is usually the most fruitful style for anyone, regardless of education, skills, or other capabilities: if you have access to a network in the area in which you would like to work, use it.

What problems are encountered by people with disabilities who have never functioned independently?

There are really two groups, broadly speaking, within this category. First is the group with severe physical involvement but adequate cognitive function. It is important for these people to have a say in their life plans and goals. For this group of people, a major problem in gaining maximum independence is the need for attendant care to help them in activities of daily living. Parents need to be very careful not to impose their desires unilaterally, just because the person can't physically live independently. It is also often very difficult for them to obtain financial backing. Limited resources can be a source of frustration for the person and his or her family, because there are many ways to make environments less restrictive if more resources were available.

This difficult fact of life needs to be addressed politically. It is necessary to educate local and national politicians, as well as to lobby for the needs of individuals with disabilities. Again, it is important to express your needs to volunteer organizations like the United Cerebral Palsy Associations and the Easter Seal Society, whose main purpose is to provide help to individuals with disabilities.

Social interactions have always been difficult for both Sam and Ellen. Sam has had problems because of his speech difficulty. Ellen was pushed at a young age to play by herself, and she learned to be very content alone. Social interactions were especially difficult during junior and senior high school. Both Sam and Ellen had the feeling that nondisabled teenagers did not want to be caught dead with a "cripple" and as a consequence avoided them. Even now, social relationships are difficult because co-workers and neighbors find Sam's communication problem and Ellen's wheelchair just too much trouble to deal with. Others frequently do not include them in social activities. This difficulty with inclusion can be overcome by focusing on developing deeper friendships with a few, as opposed to superficial relationships with many people.

The other group is composed of those who are disabled to the point of needing total custodial care. It is important for parents or other caretakers to have plans for moving such individuals to a structured environment at some point, where adequate care can be given. This should not be seen as a failure on the parent's part but as one aspect of the normal process of maturing and making the transition to adult life. Most of these children will outlive their parents. The most beneficial contribution a parent can make is to formulate good long-term plans. This does not mean that the children are being "put away," any more than sending another child off to college is "putting them away." These children usually come home to visit on vacations, weekends, and holidays, just like children who are away at college.

Often group homes in the local community provide a more socially stimulating environment than living at home with aging parents. This is not to say there haven't been situations in which severely involved children who were doing well at home (because of the excellent care the parents were providing) deteriorated when they were placed in a custodial facility. But it may be very hard for parents to accept the fact that the time has come when their child will be better off living away from home. Focusing on the years when they were able to provide care may be helpful for these parents, who may also benefit from psychological counseling.

What sexual issues need to be addressed in young adulthood?

There needs to be a sufficient discussion of birth control with those who might be sexually active. Often, even cognitively normal but physically involved men and women have a limited understanding of birth control issues, primarily because they have less opportunity to learn. The general population contributes to this by believing erroneously that the individual with a disability lacks interest in sexual activity. This bias may even be seen within the medical profession. The adult with a disability should not be embarrassed to bring up this issue with caregivers and certainly with his or her doctor.

An example of this problem is illustrated by the comment of a young adult man who was asked how he managed to deal psychologically with the need for therapy and bracing to allow for his difficulty in walking. He replied that he spent much more time and concern thinking about sex as a teenager than he did about how he was walking; however, the doctors and therapists only wanted to talk about his walking. Birth control issues can be especially difficult for people with mental retardation, especially for females who may be taken advantage of because of their lack of judgment or their naiveté. There is frequently a desire to give adults as much freedom in their community as possible, which may bring with it the risk of unwanted or unprepared-for sexual activity. This is a difficult moral and social issue that the adult's guardians must carefully consider (see Chapter 3).

To whom does the adult turn with medical problems related to his CP?

The child with a disability usually has medical care available to him. The same specialists may not treat adults, however. While it is true that growing children undergo many changes and thus need close medical monitoring, the adult must have specialists available, as well. Sadly, many people with disabilities endure physical problems that may in fact be treatable, but lack of the appropriate medical or surgical care makes treatment unavailable. Finding a good and trusted general physician is critical to good health, and when things do not seem quite right, do not hesitate to consult him.

Some people struggle through life with correctable foot deformities and only at retirement finally decide to see if something can be done to improve the situation. The person needs to find an informed and interested orthopedist who is familiar with that kind of problem. Many individuals with disabilities get used to putting up with pain and discomfort and in fact are counseled "just to live with" their problems. Certainly, there is a limit to what modern medicine can do. However, new discoveries are being made all the time, and all efforts, within reason, should be made to relieve any discomfort.

What specific problems might the young adult female have?

Adequate fluid intake is necessary to maintain good health. Young women (and less frequently young men) sometimes restrict their fluid intake so that they do not have to deal with toileting problems. This is a very dangerous habit, because it can contribute to chronic constipation and lead to kidney failure.

Young women who are interested in childbearing are concerned with the impact their disability may have. There is no known reason why a woman with cerebral palsy should not have her own children (see Chapter 3). It's a good idea to consult a genetic counselor before conceiving a child if there are any concerns about the cause of their disability and the possibility that it may be genetic. Most women, even with significant spasticity, can have a vaginal delivery, although a cesarean delivery may be necessary for a woman with significant hip deformities. Even a completely paralyzed woman may have a vaginal delivery, although her blood pressure needs to be closely monitored to avoid stroke, which can occur if the blood pressure rises extremely rapidly to high levels.

What are the stresses of child-rearing for the parent with cerebral palsy?

The anxiety that all new parents have may be magnified for the parent with CP, but this usually subsides as the parent finds special ways to adapt baby care to fit his or her abilities. Being a parent is a great equalizer. One man whose disability required him to use a wheelchair said that caring for his infant son made him feel like a full person because his son did not care that it was difficult for him to get out of bed in the middle of the night. When the baby was hungry, he cried until he was fed.

The responsibility of parenting can add significantly to the difficulties of daily living, whether a person is disabled or not. Having children should always involve advance planning, with consideration given to the cost and effort involved.

The Person with Cerebral Palsy at Midlife

For most of the population, the most significant aspect of midlife is experiencing and coming to terms with the physical problems associated with aging. For the person with cerebral palsy, the effects of aging are noticeable at a younger age. Adults in their twenties and thirties start to notice that they are getting stiffer and weaker, particularly if they have not stayed active and done their stretching exercises. Many adults with CP also commonly report significant physical fatigue, associated with bodily pain, deterioration of functional skills, and low life satisfaction. Although the normal process of aging tends to come on prematurely for the person with CP, otherwise it is no different from the process for individuals without cerebral palsy. Aging does not directly change the level or degree of spasticity; however, the slowly increasing stiffness and weakness contributes to decreased function.

Adults in the general population must make an ongoing effort to counteract the effects of aging, but again, this is substantially the same effort that individuals with cerebral palsy must make, beginning at a slightly younger age. Good exercise habits should be learned early, but it is never too late to start. Water activities such as swimming or stretching in warm water are often the easiest and best-tolerated exercises for people with spasticity. Strength training for adolescents and young adults with CP has been shown to improve muscle strength and walking ability without increasing spasticity. Participants in such programs also report psychological benefits such as a feeling of increased well-being.

Do people get weaker as they get older?

To some extent getting weaker is a normal part of aging, but it happens at a different rate and level for the person with CP. For adults with a disability who often push their bodies to the maximum for activities of daily living, the muscles may wear out prematurely from overuse. This doesn't mean that the muscle stops working; rather, there may be increasing weakness as the muscle is continually stressed. This condition has been identified in people who have had polio, but probably also exists to some extent with cerebral palsy. The main treatment consists of modifying activity—for example, by using power wheelchairs for long distances, such as shopping at the mall. As noted above, strength training, especially for the lower limbs, may also be of benefit in improving strength and walking ability without increasing spasticity.

What are overuse syndromes?

Overuse syndromes are conditions in which pain or disability results from repetitive activity. The most common problem of this kind in the general population is carpal tunnel syndrome, in which there is irritation of a nerve in the wrist caused by repeated wrist motion such as typing. People who use crutches or push manual wheelchairs are at high risk for developing carpal tunnel syndrome. The symptoms include numbness in the thumb and index and long fingers. The sensation can cause individuals to awaken from sleep and often is relieved by hanging the hand over the edge of the bed.

The initial treatment for carpal tunnel syndrome is the use of anti-inflammatory medication such as salicylic acid (aspirin) or ibuprofen (Advil) and a splint worn at night. If this does not give relief, a very simple operation to relieve the pressure on the nerve is usually done under local anesthesia, often on an outpatient basis. The results are usually quite satisfactory.

Tendinitis of the wrist is another condition that commonly results from using crutches and pushing manual wheelchairs. It is usually treated with anti-inflammatory medication and splinting. If this treatment does not provide relief, a minor surgical release may be necessary.

Are individuals with cerebral palsy more likely to have arthritis?

Adults with two conditions related to cerebral palsy are at significantly higher risk for developing arthritis: the person who has athetosis and the person who has a subluxated or dislocated hip. The person with athetoid cerebral palsy has frequent movements of the neck, which cause increased wear and early arthritis. Despite this, many adults with athetosis don't develop neck problems.

Sometimes arthritis begins when the person is in his twenties but more commonly it occurs in the 30- to 50-year age range. Usually it is noticed as neck pain, but it can also be associated with arm or shoulder pain. The primary treatment for arthritis in the neck caused by athetosis is wearing a soft neck collar to try to decrease the movement slightly. Muscle relaxants (such as valium) are sometimes helpful in decreasing movement, too, but most muscle relaxants can cause drowsiness, which may interfere with an individual's lifestyle.

Taking anti-inflammatory medications is helpful in decreasing the soreness caused by arthritis. The use of such physical therapy approaches as traction, heat, massage, ultrasound, and electrical stimulation may also help. Often, over a period of several weeks to two months this discomfort settles down and the pain goes away. Rarely does the arthritis become severe enough to necessitate a cervical spinal fusion.

The other cause of early arthritis and pain is hip dislocation and subluxation. This problem can now be completely prevented by proper treatment in childhood. Many adults weren't properly treated for this problem in childhood, however, because they grew up at a time when there was not a good understanding of how to treat or prevent it. If the affected hips become painful, decreasing activity and using anti-inflammatory medications is the first line of treatment, but painful hips usually require surgery. For the alert and walking patient, a total hip replacement usually gives the best result, although this operation doesn't always work. Removing the arthritic ball of the hip joint is another option, but often this does not completely remove the pain, and it typically leaves the limb very short, which may make sitting difficult.

The Older Person with CP

The age-associated problems of stiffness and arthritis tend to continue as a person gets older. This typically is a time, too, when it becomes increasingly difficult to continue certain activities, especially walking. The older adult should be encouraged to reassess and make necessary adaptations. A change in lifestyle may give rise to depression, which, if it continues, requires professional counseling.

Friends and relatives may make comments such as "Don't give up," "Keep fighting," or "If you don't keep going, you'll never walk again," which, although well intended, demonstrate insensitivity and do little to boost the spirits. Whenever possible, these types of comments should be addressed directly by the person with CP by explaining that slowing down is a known medical part of aging in any person, although it's slightly different in magnitude for the person with CP. Society doesn't expect the 20-year-old, 40-year-old, and 80-year-old to each have the same endurance and ambulating abilities; so we need to allow the same for the maturing person with cerebral palsy.

A person needs to find a balance between overdoing and underdoing activity. Usually the person who has the best concept of the right level of activity is the person with the disability, and this person must learn to tell other people gently that he or she is managing the problem with medical supervision.

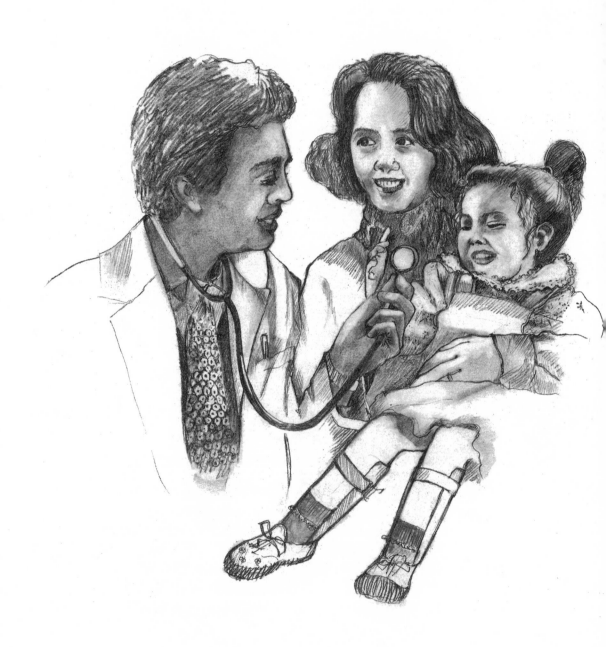

How the
Health
Care
System
Works

9

♦ WHEN PARENTS seek professional help in caring for their child with significant long-term disabilities secondary to cerebral palsy, they will encounter several different systems. One of these, the health care system, exists to provide for the physical and psychological needs of the child with cerebral palsy, and to address problems, whether these problems are acute or ongoing. Dental care, nutritional support, immunizations, and surgical procedures to maximize function are all provided by the health care system.

Two other professional systems for supporting the child with significant long-term disabilities are the educational system and the legal system. The function of the educational system is to teach the child to use his cognitive abilities as fully as possible. Legal, social, and community service systems help families to manage the day-to-day financial and emotional needs of the child and the rest of the family. These two systems, which interact with each other and with the health care system, are discussed in chapters 11 and 12. Financial aspects of health care, such as insurance, are discussed in Chapter 10.

In the first part of this chapter, we describe the various components of the health care system and how they work. The second part of the chapter describes the various health care providers whom you and your child may encounter.

How many and what kinds of doctors does my child need to see?

Many families with children who have multiple disabilities find it difficult to determine how much and what kind of health care is right for their child. As it turns out, some children receive insufficient health care while other families are burdened with care for the child that is excessive or redundant. In the latter case, taking the child to see specialists and trying to keep up with all their recommendations can become a full-time job. There was one family whose 2-year-old child over time developed ongoing relationships and appointments with 24 health care providers. This is clearly excessive, and yet for a parent it is sometimes difficult to know which health care services provide exactly what they need.

What kind of doctor is best for my child?

First and foremost the child needs a primary care physician. This provider, who may be a physician (generally a pediatrician or a family practitioner), nurse practitioner, or a physician assistant, will direct the family's use of other health care specialists whose services are needed by the child. For children with complicated medical problems, a pediatrician is the preferred health care coordinator or director, since the pediatrician is likely to have had specialized training as well as experience in managing these problems. It is this primary care provider who will provide a "medical home" to the disabled child.

What is a medical home?

The medical home is an approach to providing care that is accessible, continuous, comprehensive, family centered, compassionate, culturally effective, and coordinated. There are many advantages to having such a "medical home." Children with a medical home are less likely to experience delayed or foregone care, less likely to have unmet health care needs, and less likely to have unmet needs for family support than children without a medical home. Families with a medical home have significantly fewer parents' missed workdays and hospitalizations for the children.

In addition to coordinating chronic and acute medical needs, the primary care provider provides preventive care, including immunizations. Having a regular source of care was found to be the most important factor associated with receiving preventive care services.

What do I do if my primary care doctor is unfamiliar with CP?

Not all primary care providers are familiar with the health care needs of the child with cerebral palsy. They may be slow to make referrals to appropriate specialists, for example. When this occurs, it may be difficult for the family to know how to proceed. One point to remember is that as your child's parents, you are her or his best advocate. Never fail to make your observations and recommendations known to the physician. If you believe that a more timely referral to a specialist is in order, tell your child's physician. You and the physician must forge a collaborative relationship on your child's behalf, and open, direct communication is important to successful health care management.

How can I improve communications among my child's health care providers?

Whenever you begin a new relationship with a physician, take with you on the first appointment the names and addresses of the other specialists involved in your child's care. At each visit, ask that copies of all relevant dictations be sent to the specialists you designate.

Due to HIPAA regulations, such requests must be put in writing and signed by you. In your request, include the following information: your child's name, birth date, and address; parents' names and address(es); a statement indicating that you want information from today's visit to be sent to "so-and-so," with the names and addresses of the person or persons. Most facilities have their own Release of Information Authorization forms for your use, but anticipating this need and bringing with you the names and addresses of the appropriate physicians and others who should receive this information will make it easier to fill out completely.

You also have a right to obtain a copy of the records for yourself. You will, however, need to put that request in writing, too; add your name to the list of people you want to receive records. Be aware that there may be a fee attached to all these requests. Bring copies of all recent records in your possession each time you visit a specialist. The specialist needs to know what's going on, and by sharing these records, you will help to enhance communication.

How can I make the best use of information from my child's doctors?

Some children with cerebral palsy have a relationship with a different medical specialist for each body system, as well as relationships with a variety of other professionals such as physical therapists, occupational therapists, nurses, and social workers. For a child to benefit from the evaluations of these various health care professionals, all of the information they generate must be coordinated. This serves the dual purpose of keeping all of the child's medical caregivers informed about the child's condition and progress and preventing redundancy in care (for example, the unknowing repetition of expensive and sometimes painful diagnostic tests).

As noted above, the parent must make certain that information from each visit with a specialist is sent to the primary care provider (PCP) and to other specialists by way of the medical records. The PCP will help the parent understand the findings of the other specialists, and these specialists' reports will assist the PCP in managing the child's care.

Another helpful professional is a case manager, who may be employed by an insurance company or a state agency. Case managers can help coordinate your access to care, help you understand the recommendations of various specialists, and help provide direction for the care of your child.

What is a patient case manager?

Because children with complex medical problems have so many health professionals involved in their care, the concept of a patient case manager (also called a patient care manager) has evolved. Most case managers are nurses or social workers who provide excellent support to the family and assist in coordinating the child's many health care providers. The case manager may make recommendations regarding specific health care specialists.

Government agencies or specialty clinics may assign a case manager to a child, and such a person will generally have the family's and the patient's best interests at heart. But insurance companies have also begun to employ patient case managers, and the primary goal of case managers hired by insurance companies is to avoid duplication and the redundant use of resources. In this situation, parents will need to be especially strong advocates for their child (see Chapter 12, "Being an Advocate for Your Child," as well as "Managing the System" in Part 2).

What if I do not receive public assistance, do not have access to a case manager, and do not meet eligibility criteria for various programs of public support?

If you are living just above the poverty level, you may be ineligible for many social service programs. If you have no medical insurance for your child, you may have difficulty finding a doctor to see your child for regular care. Contact your local Department of Public Health, as many states operate primary care health clinics for just such families. In addition, many states have a program known as CHIP or SCHIP which will provide medical insurance coverage for children who are not eligible for Medicaid and are uninsured.

Parents who are in a difficult financial situation often take their acutely ill child to an emergency room. Each time a child comes to the emergency department, she may be seen by a different physician, who most likely will be unaware of the child's specific health issues and therefore may not be able to provide the best care for the child. A series of visits to the emergency room is not a good way to provide medical care for any child, in part because it makes it impossible to coordinate care. Instead of relying on the emergency room, parents should find out where the local public health clinics are located.

State and local agencies such as the public health, social services, and health and social services departments can provide this information. Call the clinic to find out who manages the clinic and whether you would be required to pay for any service (there may or may not be fees associated with the service). It's very possible that you and your child could receive primary health care through a clinic program.

What can I expect my child's primary care provider to do?

The primary care provider may be a doctor, a physician assistant, or a nurse practitioner. The primary care provider (PCP) should get to know your child and your family, so that he or she is able to integrate the child's care with the family's needs. He or she should specifically be interested in observing the growth and development of your child and making certain that routine physicals are performed and immunizations are up to date. Usual childhood illnesses such as viral illnesses, ear infections, and rashes should all be treated by the primary provider. Questions about specific problems should also be addressed first to the primary care provider. If your child has an illness that is very rare or very complex, the primary care provider may choose to consult with other specialists.

What should I do if my child's primary provider is uncomfortable with my child's condition?

Children with multiple or complex medical problems can be a challenge for a primary care provider (PCP), who is often under stress because he sees many patients and may have very limited time. Providing health care for your child should be a cooperative effort, in which both the family and the PCP share what they have learned about the child, and the PCP continues to support the family and help them sort out complex and confusing issues. If the PCP is not willing to take the time to help the child or appears intimidated in dealing with the child who has a disability, it may be necessary to find another provider with whom you and your child can develop good rapport.

Who should be my child's primary care provider—a pediatrician, a family physician, a physician assistant, or nurse practitioner?

Family physicians have medical training that includes children and adults, though usually their experience with children, especially children with disabilities, is limited. The advantage of the family physician is that he or she will have a broader view, one that includes all the members of the family. In this way, a family doctor may be more helpful to parents, because he or she can incorporate and deal with general family dynamics and can monitor the effect of the disability on the different members of the family, especially the parents. In addition, the family physician will be able to continue as primary care doctor for the disabled child as he or she grows to adulthood, whereas many pediatricians stop seeing patients after a certain age (often, but not always, at age 21).

The advantage the pediatrician brings is more specialized training and experience in the problems of children, and especially, more training and experience in the problems of children with disabilities. If the family develops a comfortable relationship with the pediatrician, one that allows for free and comprehensive exchange of information, then this is the person who ought to provide primary care for your child.

There are also physicians trained and certified in both pediatrics and internal medicine (called Med-Peds training), who combine the advantages of the pediatrician and the family physician. Their training in pediatrics is far more extensive than that of the family physician, and they have an advantage over the pediatrician in that they can treat the entire family and continue to treat the disabled child into adulthood.

There are also nurse practitioners and physician's assistants (PAs) who may work with any one of these physicians as part of their practice and can function as the primary care provider for your child. These nurses and PAs may also specialize in the care of children, and they often have a bit more time than the physician to answer questions and help provide training around procedures or specific care techniques.

In the end, parents have to find the physician or practice that best meets their needs. They must balance the medical knowledge and skills that the nurse or doctor brings, with the willingness of the doctor or nurse or PA to spend the extra time that is needed in providing care to the disabled child and answering the family's questions.

How often does my child need to see the primary care provider?

This depends on the problems and the nature of the child's disability. As a minimum, your child should be seen by his or her primary provider at least as often as the schedule recommended by the American Academy of Pediatrics for well child care. It is very important for children with disabilities to have a complete routine physical examination periodically, and not to ignore check-up visits. Immunizations are often delayed and common childhood problems such as hernias and undescended testicles may be missed in children who visit the physician's office for acute problems but never undergo a full physical examination.

Which specialists does my newborn need?

The newborn intensive care nursery is usually managed by a neonatologist, who is a pediatrician specializing in the care of ill newborn children. These specialists generally care for the infant with special needs until the infant leaves the intensive care nursery and goes home. They are the primary attending physicians during this period and consult other specialists as needed.

Upon discharge, the neonatologist generally transfers care to a primary care physician of the parent's choice in the community, although the neonatologist may also see the infant after discharge to follow up on any outstanding medical problems. Neonatologists are generally not involved in the child's care after the child reaches the age of 1 or 2.

When first discharged from the hospital, what physician does my child need to see?

When the child is discharged you should follow up with your primary care provider. If there are specific problems that were identified and evaluated in the intensive care nursery, such as breathing problems from prematurity, your child may need to be followed up by other physicians, as well. As your child grows and his or her needs change, referrals to other health care specialists may be needed. As noted earlier, the PCP and the family need to work together in making decisions about calling in specialists.

Who should check my child's eyes, and how often?

If the child was in intensive care as a newborn and exposed to oxygen, as many premature babies are, his or her eyes should be checked by an ophthalmologist before discharge to home. For the infant who has no such history, assessing a child's vision is part of a routine physical examination performed by the primary physician. It may be difficult to get young children to cooperate during an eye examination, especially children who have spasticity or a variety of disabilities. If the extent of the child's visual abilities cannot be conclusively determined by the physical exam, then your child may need to visit an ophthalmologist or a neurology specialist to determine whether using more sophisticated vision tests would be helpful.

Follow-up eye visits may be necessary, depending on what the examination or specialized tests reveal about visual function. If the child is found to have normal eye function, then visual screening at school age is the usual next step. If significant disability is present, then follow-up as indicated by the specialist is appropriate. Ask your PCP about making a referral to an eye specialist if you are concerned that your child cannot see properly.

When should my child's hearing be tested?

Routine screening of hearing in the newborn is now done in most newborn nurseries in the United States. As is true for vision, routine health visits to the primary care provider should include an assessment of hearing. If there is any question about the child's hearing, various tests can be done to clarify the level of function. Audiometric tests can be performed by an audiologist, for example, often in coordination with an ear, nose, and throat surgeon. If this isn't helpful, then a brainstem auditory evoked response (BAER) can be done. This is a special test that can be used even for a very young child. Discuss your concerns and questions with your PCP or case manager.

Which specialist should treat seizures in a child?

Some PCPs are comfortable testing and treating children who have seizures, while others will want to refer your child to a specialist. Children with new seizures would be referred to a pediatric neurologist, a physician who specializes in treating illnesses of the nervous system in children. Seizures that are easy to control and for which no specific cause has been found might continue to be treated and followed up by the child's family doctor or pediatrician. Seizures caused by fevers (called febrile seizures) are limited to one or a few episodes and do not need treatment. These can be evaluated and followed up by your primary care provider. (For more information about seizures, see Chapter 3.)

Does my child need to see a specialist to follow up on a cerebral shunt?

The surgery to place a shunt in the brain to drain excess fluid from the ventricles of the brain is performed by a neurosurgeon. There are pediatric neurosurgeons who specialize in treating children, but many neurosurgeons treat both adults and children. The child with a shunt may be followed by a pediatric neurologist or a pediatrician, and if there are no problems a neurosurgical evaluation every one to two years is a good course of treatment. If the shunt functions well, more frequent follow-up is not necessary.

My child has problems with swallowing and poor weight gain. What kind of doctor do we need?

The primary care physician should be the first to evaluate this type of problem. He or she may make a referral to a specialist—a developmental pediatrician, for example, who specializes in the evaluation of these problems—to help evaluate swallowing function and poor weight gain. The developmental pediatrician often works with a team, who participates in the evaluation. The team may include a nutritionist, who can evaluate how much nourishment your child is actually getting and how much he needs; a speech pathologist or an occupational therapist, who is trained to do swallowing evaluations; the staff of an x-ray department, who can perform special tests, such as x-ray swallowing tests; and a pediatric gastroenterologist, who can evaluate your child's gastrointestinal system. Swallowing and weight gain problems can be very complicated to treat, but treatment is exceedingly important to the child's growth, and therefore it is important to make use of a full team of specialists (see Chapter 3 for more details of this problem).

Who should my child see if he vomits frequently?

This is another situation that should first be brought to the attention of your child's primary care provider. If referral is needed, the PCP will probably recommend that your child see a gastroenterologist. Chronic or recurrent vomiting is best evaluated by a pediatric gastroenterologist, who specializes in caring for the gastrointestinal system and may utilize tests such as endoscopy (looking into the stomach) and a pH probe. If a problem such as gastrointestinal reflux is identified and medicine can't control it, then a pediatric general surgeon may be called to do a surgical procedure to correct it. Pediatric radiology specialists are also called upon to perform sophisticated x-ray tests and to evaluate the function of the stomach and intestines (see Chapter 3 for more details of this problem).

Who should clean my child's teeth and how often?

Dental examinations every six months starting at age 18 months are especially important for the child with CP because normal saliva flow, chewing, and swallowing are frequently disrupted. Good professional cleaning and evaluation for gum overgrowth and development of cavities is important. If your family dentist is not comfortable dealing with a child with a disability, then seek the services of a pediatric dentist, called a *pedodontist.* These specialists are familiar with and specialize in caring for the teeth of children, especially of children with disabilities. If your child has significant gum overgrowth, he or she may be referred to a dental surgeon who can surgically reduce the overgrowth.

Who can help me with my child's severe constipation?

Severe constipation can be a difficult problem, and one seen frequently in children with CP. It is important to bring this problem to the attention of your primary care provider so he or she can monitor and treat your child. If your PCP is not comfortable treating this problem in children with CP, your child should be referred to a developmental pediatrician specializing in the care of such children, or to a pediatric gastroenterologist who will be able to set up a program to help with this problem.

Who can help with toilet training?

Special education teachers and school nurses and therapists frequently have routines that can be used in toilet training children with disabilities, and they can describe a routine for you or provide a written explanation of what's involved. You can also request information from your primary care provider or a developmental pediatrician. (See also the description of toileting routines in "Toilet Training," in Part 2.)

If your child resists behavioral attempts at toilet training for urine and is believed to be cognitively able, then an evaluation by a pediatric urologist may be suggested. He or she can test your child's bladder function and abilities to make certain that there is not a physical problem with your child that is causing problems with incontinence.

Who should I see concerning my child's difficulty with her arms, legs, or back?

The problems related to the bones and muscles are addressed by pediatric orthopedists. The pediatric orthopedist generally addresses deformities and problems with the functioning of the hands, arms, legs, and feet, as well as deformities of the spine such as scoliosis and kyphosis. This health care specialist attempts to improve alignments that can make the child function better and works to *prevent* deformities insofar as is possible.

After a consultation or treatment with a pediatric orthopedist, it is generally best to schedule routine follow-up examinations, because a child's deformities change as the child grows. Follow-up with an orthopedist every six to twelve months is usually indicated, and it is preferable to follow up with a pediatric orthopedist who is interested in the child with cerebral palsy.

Who will tell me what kind of bracing my child needs?

Recommendations for bracing vary, depending on the child's problems and on the specialist making the recommendation. A physical therapist frequently assesses a child for the possible benefits of bracing the legs, and an occupational therapist evaluates and makes braces for the child's hands and arms. The orthopedist or physiatrist (physical medicine specialist) usually evaluates the child and writes the prescriptions for bracing. In some communities, pediatric physiatrists routinely follow children with cerebral palsy and prescribe braces. In many other communities, pediatric orthopedists routinely follow patients and provide brace prescriptions.

Generally, routine follow-up with both an orthopedist and a physiatrist is not necessary. If the child is followed only by a physiatrist, however, the physiatrist must be a pediatric physiatrist who is familiar with all types of deformities and will actively monitor the child for the development of problems that will need an orthopedic surgeon, such as hip dislocation and scoliosis. If the child is followed by a pediatric orthopedist, then the pediatric orthopedist should pay attention to the child's bracing and seating needs. There are some circumstances where therapists recommend braces and primary care physicians write the orders. This situation is less than ideal, because few primary care physicians fully understand the appropriateness of the brace.

Who should evaluate my child's seating and recommend an appropriate chair?

Seating is much like bracing, in that it involves the disciplines of physical therapy, occupational therapy, orthopedics, and physiatry. In ordering a chair it is important to take into consideration the family's, as well as the child's, needs. (For a detailed description of the appropriateness of wheelchairs, refer to Chapters 6 and 7 and the wheelchair section of Part 2.)

Medical Care Providers

The following medical providers have specialty training and expertise that allows them to provide specialized care for the child—and for the entire family. Your family may encounter many of the following medical specialists as your child grows and develops. One way to determine whether a physician or other health care provider is competent in the special area in which they practice is to ask if they are "Board Certified" in this specialty.

What is Board Certification?

Board Certification—For a physician to be recognized as one of the specialists listed below, they need a certain number of years of specialized training (called residency or fellowship training), and then they must pass a certification examination administered by an appropriate specialty board. Most of the pediatric specialty boards are administered by the American Board of Pediatrics, though some medical specialties such as neurology and psychiatry (American Board of Psychiatry and Neurology) and physical medicine and rehabilitation (American Board of Physical Medicine and Rehabilitation) have their own board. The surgical specialties (such as general surgery, orthopedics, and neurosurgery) also have their own board, and accredit surgeons in these specialty areas. Although there is special fellowship training to be a pediatric surgeon, there is no board certification in pediatric surgery or in the surgical subspecialties at the present time.

To remain board certified, physicians must stay up to date and must be retested periodically by their specialty board. If a physician is board certified, it means he is believed to be competent by a group of peers in the specialty area.

Adolescent specialist.   Physicians with this specialty training may first have trained in pediatrics or in internal medicine (or both) and then done specialized training in adolescent medicine. They have training and experience in treating the unique emotional and physical problems of adolescents, including drug abuse, adolescent pregnancy, and hormonal dysfunction. They may also be the physicians who perform a teenager's first pelvic exam and prescribe forms of birth control, which for the disabled youngster can be vitally important but also medically complicated.

Audiologist.   An audiologist is a professional who specializes in testing hearing, and evaluating the degree of hearing impairment. An audiologist also specializes in the maintenance, prescription, and development of hearing aid devices.

Cardiac surgeon.   Primarily involved in performing surgical procedures on the heart and chest, the pediatric cardiac surgeon is trained in general surgery as well as in the specialties of pediatric cardiac surgery and chest surgery.

Cardiologist.   A cardiologist addresses problems of the heart. The pediatric cardiologist is a medical physician who is trained in pediatrics and in the specialty of cardiology.

Chiropractor.   The chiropractor has graduated from chiropractic school, where the main emphasis is on manipulative therapy. The theories and perceptions of chiropractors differ significantly from the theories and perceptions held by medical physicians. Some of the techniques employed by chiropractors are similar to those used by physical therapists, although the rationale for treatment and healing is very different. For children with CP, there seems to be little gained by frequent or long-term chiropractic treatments. Although the chiropractic treatments are generally not harmful, they place another burden on the family's finances and time.

Dentist. This practitioner has graduated from dental school. Some dentists then take subsequent specialization training in pediatrics. The specialist most likely to be encountered by the parent of a child with cerebral palsy is the *pedodontist,* a dentist who specializes in the care of children. An oral surgeon is often consulted for mouth and tooth surgery.

Developmental pediatrician. A developmental pediatrician is a medical physician who has trained in pediatrics and has extra training and experience in the developmental problems of children. There are two types of specialized training (and certification) in this field: neurodevelopmental disabilities and developmental-behavioral pediatrics. Certification in neurodevelopmental disabilities means the physician has expertise in treating children with physical and neurological disabilities, often in many aspects of their care, ranging from treating seizures to constipation. Physicians certified in developmental-behavioral pediatrics have special expertise in treating behavioral issues of children, whether they have disabilities or not, and often treat children with ADHD. There is a great deal of overlap between these two types of developmental pediatricians, as well as with child neurologists, child psychiatrists, and pediatric physiatrists.

Endocrinologist. A pediatric endocrinologist is a medical physician with expertise (and certification) in the diagnosis and treatment of medical problems associated with the various hormonal systems of children. These may include dysfunction of the thyroid or parathyroid glands, growth hormone deficiency, diabetes mellitus, and delayed or precocious sexual maturity. Pediatric endocrinologists have training in general pediatrics and then extra training and experience in endocrinology.

Gastroenterologist. A pediatric gastroenterologist specializes in the care of stomach and intestinal problems of children. Such problems might include poor weight gain, swallowing difficulties, frequent vomiting, and severe constipation, diarrhea, or other gastrointestinal problems. Pediatric gastroenterologists have training in general pediatrics and subspecialty training in gastroenterology. They also perform a variety of procedures, from looking into the intestinal system with a lighted tube called an *endoscope* to doing special tests, such as a pH probe, which measures acid in the esophagus as a sign of reflux. These specialists also perform some minor surgical procedures, such as placement of feeding tubes.

General pediatrician. A pediatrician is a medical doctor with specialty training in pediatrics, which is the care of infants and children, usually until age 21. These practitioners specialize in caring for the routine illnesses of children, giving immunizations, and preventing disease in children. They are concerned with the child's general growth and development. Based on their evaluation of the child, pediatricians will make referrals to any specialist and collaborate with that specialist in the care of the child. Usually parents should turn to their general pediatrician first when their child has a new problem.

Med-Peds.   Physicians with this training have usually had training for two years in pediatrics and two years of internal medicine, thus making them eligible to be board certified in both specialties. They provide primary care to children and adults, and are often the ideal physician to provide care to a disabled adolescent who will need ongoing care into adulthood.

Nephrologist.   A pediatric nephrologist has training in general pediatrics and subspecialty training in nephrology (diseases of the kidneys). The nephrologist is responsible for treating children with chronic renal failure, including performing renal dialysis (maintaining patients on the kidney machine). There are also many chemical (electrolyte) imbalances that can occur due to problems in the kidney, which the nephrologist addresses.

Neurologist.   Some neurologists work with both adults and children, but the pediatric neurologist is most commonly involved in the care of children with cerebral palsy and seizures. This medical physician has training in general pediatrics and intensive training in neurology (diseases of the brain and nerves). Their certification includes neurology and psychiatry, with special competence in child neurology. Neurologists are the physicians who interpret EEGs (brain wave tests) looking for seizures, and they often are the ones who diagnose a neurological condition such as CP.

Neurosurgeon.   The primary role of a neurosurgeon is to operate on the brain and spinal cord. A neurosurgeon is a surgeon whose specialty training is in neurosurgery (surgery on the brain and nerves). A pediatric neurosurgeon also has training in performing surgery on children. For the child with CP, neurosurgeons might be consulted to place a brain shunt for hydrocephalus or to do a dorsal rhizotomy.

Nurse.   Most nurses have a bachelor's degree in nursing, and many have master's degrees. There are many specialty areas of nursing, each with its own certification. If the child is a patient in the hospital, he may see nurses specializing in operating room care, recovery room care, intensive care, and bedside care within the hospital.

Pediatric Nurse Practitioners (PNPs) and Clinical Nurse Specialists (CNSs) are Advanced Practice Nurses (APNs) with a master's degree. They work under the direction of a pediatrician or specialist and assist the physician in providing primary care, specialty care, case management, and coordination of care to children with cerebral palsy, children with other special needs, and healthy children. They are also excellent resources for families of children with special needs. Nurse Practitioners and many Clinical Nurse Specialists are able to perform a full physical examination, and comanage, along with their physician colleague, new or chronic health issues. Depending on the state in which they practice, they may have authority to write prescriptions. In addition to their RN license, PNPs and CNSs must have an Advanced Practice Nurse license and they must be professionally and legally certified in the state where they practice.

A parent with a child with cerebral palsy will most likely encounter the school nurse, who is a pediatric nurse. School nurses are also an excellent resource for ongoing care and the various problems that a child with CP may encounter.

Nutritionist. A nutritionist may have a bachelor's or a master's degree in nutrition and may be found in a variety of health care settings, including schools, public health departments, hospitals, and doctors' offices. The role of the nutritionist is to ensure that the child is well nourished. To do this, the nutritionist may monitor how a specific child compares to what is considered normal height and weight for a certain age. The nutritionist assesses feeding history, dietary intake, and blood tests that reflect nutritional status in order to determine whether the child has nutritional deficiencies. For the child with CP, the nutritionist advises parents about methods and specific food types that will provide proper nutrition and meet requirements for caloric intake.

Occupational therapist. An occupational therapist has a bachelor's or a master's degree in occupational therapy. There are a number of subspecialties within occupational therapy. The therapists primarily encountered in the treatment of children with cerebral palsy, are pediatric occupational therapists. The primary issues they address are fine motor skills, improving the functioning of the upper extremities, and, especially, the child's skills in activities of daily living, in order to maximize the child's independence. They also make hand splints and provide recommendations for seating.

Ophthalmologist. An ophthalmologist is a medical doctor and a surgeon specializing in problems of the eye and eye musculature. Areas of specialization include determining a child's ability to see, performing surgery to correct crossed eyes, and diagnosing and treating eye diseases.

Optometrist. Although not a medical physician, an optometrist has a doctoral degree in optometry. Optometrists specialize in evaluating sight and prescribing eyeglasses. They generally do not prescribe medications except for some limited topical medications. They can examine the eye for problems of refraction and can write prescriptions for exercises and corrective lenses. They do not do surgery. For the child with CP, they may be involved in evaluating a child's visual ability, in addition to fitting eyeglasses.

Orthopedist. The pediatric orthopedist is a surgical physician trained in general orthopedics with specialty training in pediatrics. For the child with CP, routine follow-up with an orthopedist if the child is significantly involved is important both to prevent deformity and to help maximize the child's function. There are many different subspecialties in orthopedics; generally the child should be treated by a pediatric orthopedist who has expertise in the area of specific concern. Within pediatric orthopedics, there is a group of physicians who are interested in cerebral palsy.

The orthopedist does surgery on the musculoskeletal system. There are some pediatric orthopedists who follow children with cerebral palsy who do surgery only on the lower extremities and then refer the child when needed to an orthopedic spine surgeon or a hand surgeon with a subspecialty in this area. Your specific community arrangement dictates how these referrals are handled, but many pediatric orthopedists specializing in the care of children with cerebral palsy are able to address all of the surgical needs of the child related to the musculoskeletal system.

Orthotist. An orthotist makes and fits braces for the legs and arms. This is the specialist who usually makes the AFOs worn by children with CP. Most orthotists have had special training, have served an apprenticeship, and were certified by passing a national examination. They use the most modern materials—very strong plastics, which often require special equipment to mold and shape—to construct AFOs and other braces. (Some simple braces for the legs may be made by physical therapists, but the materials they use are often weak and tend to break easily.)

Osteopathic doctor. An osteopath is a medical physician who has graduated from osteopathic school, a school whose curriculum is identical to that of most medical schools. Osteopaths specialize, just as medical doctors do. Upon graduation the osteopathic physician receives a degree called a Doctor of Osteopathy (D.O.), whereas upon graduation from medical school a medical doctor receives a Doctor of Medicine (M.D.). D.O.'s and M.D.'s practice similarly and may train at some of the same institutions. Once in practice, it would be hard to distinguish these two types of physicians in terms of their practice or knowledge.

Otolaryngologist (ENT). This is a surgical physician who after medical school primarily trains in ear, nose, and throat surgery, and subsequently specializes in one of many different areas. Pediatric ear, nose, and throat (ENT) specialists are the otolaryngologists most often encountered by families with children with cerebral palsy. These physicians address severe ear problems such as hearing problems and may be involved in the identification of the cause of the hearing problem, and in its treatment, such as placement of a cochlear implant or of a hearing aid. They are also involved in placing ear tubes, addressing some swallowing problems that originate in the throat, performing tracheostomies, providing care for tracheal tubes, and doing surgery on the upper airway and on the salivary glands if there is excessive drooling.

Physiatrist. A physiatrist is a medical physician whose training is in physical medicine and rehabilitation (PM&R), a specialty devoted to care of people with physical disabilities. The physiatrist tests the patient's functioning, sets up goals for the patient, and manages rehabilitation to reach the goals that have been set. Some physiatrists specialize in the care of children. They have done extra fellowship training in pediatric rehabilitation, and in addition to being certified in PM&R, they can also be certified in Pediatric Rehabilitation Medicine. In some communities, the pediatric physiatrists run the cerebral palsy clinic and provide excellent services for prescription of wheelchairs and braces. Recommendations for therapy and educational programs are also within their specialty. Physiatrists do not perform surgery, but rather refer the child to an appropriate orthopedist if surgery is indicated.

Physical therapist. The physical therapist has a bachelor's or a master's degree in physical therapy. P.T.'s are interested in improving a patient's muscle tone, movement patterns, gross motor skills, range of motion, posture, and balance. They often use exercise and whirlpools, and help their patients practice walking and standing. Their goal is to improve as far as possible the child's gross motor skills such as walking, sitting, and transfers from one place or position to another. There are many subspecialties in physical therapy. Generally for the child with cerebral palsy the pediatric physical therapist is recommended. Most physical therapists working in school systems are pediatric P.T.'s. There are also a great variety of therapy techniques, and any therapist may have individual certification in one or a number of these techniques, such as NDT (neurodevelopmental therapy). The P.T. is frequently the first to spot problems such as hip deformities or scoliosis which may need orthopedic care.

P.T.'s can also be an excellent resource for providing suggestions for medical care providers, especially for specialty care for children with CP. In fact, the P.T. who is treating many other children with CP may be the best source of this information.

In addition to physical therapists, there are P.T. assistants who have associate degrees and can provide therapy under the direction of a P.T. P.T. aides have on-the-job training and may do therapy as prescribed directly by the P.T.

Physician's assistant. A physician's assistant generally has a bachelor's or a master's degree as a midlevel practitioner, and may also have extra training in an area of specialization. The physician's assistant may work directly with the physician in examining and treating the child, and may assist in the operating room. The physician's assistant in the cerebral palsy clinic can be a valuable source of suggestions on care and treatment for the child with CP, and can provide useful general and specific information about cerebral palsy. Many physician's assistants develop in-depth knowledge because they devote their efforts to helping patients who have specific kinds of medical problems.

Podiatrist.   After finishing podiatry school, the podiatrist specializes in the care of foot problems. Generally podiatrists are focused on the front of the foot and are not trained in treating the whole body system. Few podiatrists have special training in the care of children with cerebral palsy. For the child with cerebral palsy, questions related to foot deformities are best addressed by the pediatric orthopedist.

Psychiatrist.   A psychiatrist is a medical physician who specializes in behavioral problems, emotional disorders, and mental illness. The psychiatrist prescribes and is the recognized medical expert on the effects of medication on behavior. Pediatric psychiatrists have subspecialty training in the psychiatric problems of children. They may also provide counseling in addition to prescribing medications.

A question parents frequently ask is whether their child should see a psychiatrist or a psychologist. The answer for any one child depends in part on how the child and the family relate to the specific therapist. The major distinction between the two is that the psychologist is able to provide sophisticated testing, whereas the psychiatrist is able to prescribe medications. Both can counsel patients and their families, as can social workers.

Psychologist.   The psychologist has earned a Ph.D. in issues relating to behavior. Some psychologists have special training in child development; they may use standardized tests to determine the child's intellectual potential and current level of functioning. Other psychologists have special training in counseling families and children, and they may help families and children to address behavioral problems. A psychologist also makes recommendations for the best educational setting for the child. Psychologists are often associated with schools in providing testing. Psychologists do not prescribe medications.

Pulmonary specialist.   A pediatric pulmonary specialist is trained in general pediatrics and has completed subspecialty training in pulmonary diseases (diseases of the lungs). He or she evaluates and treats difficult problems related to the lungs and may perform procedures such as a bronchoscopy, a procedure that involves the use of a lighted tube to look at the airways of the lung (trachea and bronchi) from within. For children with cerebral palsy, common lung problems include frequent pneumonia and bronchitis secondary to aspiration. Severe asthma is another common problem addressed by the pulmonary specialist.

Social worker.   The social worker has a bachelor's or master's degree in social work and is trained to help families cope with their needs. Social workers are found in a variety of settings—the community, school, hospital—and are associated with a variety of private organizations such as the United Cerebral Palsy Associations (UCPA). Social workers help with the social part of living with a disability, such as family and financial aspects. Social workers provide counseling, may be case managers, and advise families on how to gain access to community services. They help investigate social situations. Medical social workers tend to work in hospitals to help families deal with the problems of an acute medical illness. They can address behavioral problems and help parents investigate resources. Psychiatric social workers may provide counseling and help families with behavioral issues. General social workers work for the state and help identify and secure child welfare services and housing as needed.

Speech therapist. The speech therapist works with language, speech, swallowing, and hearing, and specializes in developing techniques to teach children to talk. These practitioners may help the child who has a speech or hearing problem to speak properly or to use sign language. They may also be involved in developing augmentative communication devices, from simple picture boards to sophisticated electronic devices. They are especially important to the child who is cognitively able to communicate but has a communication disability. Another major area addressed by the speech therapist for the child with CP is swallowing problems. The speech therapist may be involved in evaluating, via the barium swallow test, the child's ability to eat safely. They may also be involved in trying to improve the child's ability to chew and swallow safely through various therapeutic methods.

Surgeon. A pediatric surgeon is a surgical physician who has undergone training in general surgery, as well as subspecialty training in pediatric surgery. For most problems requiring surgery on the gastrointestinal system, the liver, or the abdomen, the general surgeon is consulted. Many pediatric surgeons also perform limited specialty surgeries, such as needed to treat undescended testicles. They also remove skin lesions.

Urologist. A pediatric urologist is a surgical physician whose training is in urology with subspecialty training in pediatric urology. This specialist performs tests on and investigates problems of the urinary tract and male genital system, primarily looking at its mechanical functions and making surgical corrections.

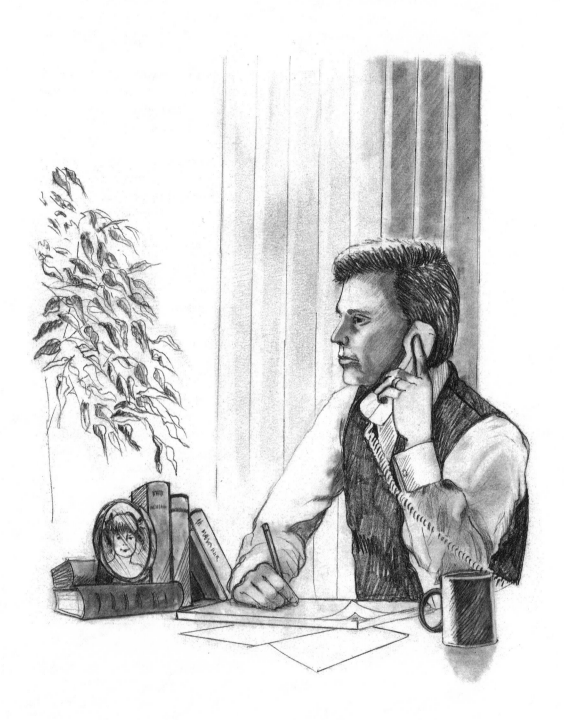

Financing Care for the Child with Cerebral Palsy

♦ HEALTH CARE EXPENSES for a child or adult with a chronic condition can be very high and can impose a financial burden on families, the extent of which is highly dependent on the nature and severity of the condition. Many families with a member who has a chronic illness can expect to incur high health care expenses year after year. While the needs of individuals vary, most children or adults with cerebral palsy require hospital care, ambulatory care, and case management services—and the cost of all this health care adds up.

This chapter describes various ways in which families and individuals can pay for health care. Health insurance has been undergoing intense scrutiny, however, and it is possible that there will be extensive changes in what we now know as the health care system in the future. What is presented in this chapter is an overview that is intended to provide a starting place for families and individuals seeking information about paying the high costs of health care. A list of providers of specific services may be found at the end of the chapter.

How is health care financed?

Funds come from a variety of sources. The most common sources are a family's own funds, private health insurance, government programs, and private philanthropic sources.

How much of the cost does the family cover?

It is estimated that families of children with a disabling condition pay about one-fifth of their children's medical care bills directly out of pocket. Some pay more, some pay less. The adult, on the other hand, pays according to their employment status. If the adult is employed, health insurance usually supplements the adult's expenditures for health care. If the adult is dependent and is without private health insurance or other resources, Medicaid may cover the cost of medical care. Many private insurance policies do not provide chronic care coverage; Medicaid pays medical bills for some low-income people who meet eligibility requirements as determined by the state.

What is private health insurance?

Private health insurance is insurance that is provided for by private individual or group funds (such as from an employer), rather than insurance that is offered by public funding through a government unit or agency (Medicare, for example). For the most part, private health insurance that covers a dependent child's medical expenses is group coverage that is part of the parent's work benefits package. Group coverage private insurance of this type can be a fee-for-service plan that pays for the service after the service is provided or a managed care type of insurance. Typically, a group insurance program obtained through employment is more generous with benefits, but this must be evaluated by the family. Individually purchased policies tend to contain restrictions on services covered and frequently exclude preexisting conditions. It is unlikely that a family will be able to get private insurance for their child with CP, nor would private insurance companies issue individual policies to an adult with CP.

Another well-known form of private insurance is managed care. This form of insurance came into existence to deal with rising health care costs, and their primary purpose is to contain costs (this is known as "cost containment"). Currently, many policies are administered through a primary care physician who then makes necessary referrals to other health care professionals. Many policies include specific physicians within the "network" of the plan, and patient-subscribers are fully covered only if they are treated by those physicians. Some policies allow for treatment by other physicians who are considered "out of the network," or privately chosen, but the patient bears an additional expense for consulting these physicians. Children with CP and other developmental disabilities may continue coverage as a dependent on their parents' private or employer-sponsored group medical plans even after the child leaves the school system. Parents can be 60 years old with a child who is 40 and still have coverage for their disabled child as a dependent. Be sure to confirm this with your employer and insurance company. If an employer is changing group insurance companies, it would be wise to check on continued dependent coverage prior to the plan change. If a person with CP is a full-time employee of a company providing group benefits, she cannot be discriminated against and must be offered *all* of the programs (medical, dental, pensions, and short- and long-term disability) that are available to other employees.

The scope of coverage and the benefits available in private health insurance vary significantly from policy to policy and from group to group, and can often be confusing. It is critically important for parents to check policy provisions. There are policies that exclude benefits for specific conditions, such as mental retardation or autism. Parents seeking employment should carefully check on the benefits offered. Employers who self-insure can make their own plan provisions.

What services are covered under private insurance, and what are the limitations?

Each policy must be read carefully and judged separately. No assumptions can be made about the extent of coverage. The family must investigate their own coverage and become knowledgeable about their benefits before they incur large costs. The employee should consult with the personnel office, or the office that oversees administration of the health insurance plan, for assistance in understanding benefits and gaining access to them. Commonly covered expenses include such things as a hospital room, surgeons' and physicians' services provided in a hospital, and outpatient diagnostic tests, such as x-rays.

Private health insurance may be adequate when a child's needs are limited to basic physicians' services and basic hospital services. When the child with a disability has multiple needs consisting of both community and home service and care, however, private insurance may not provide the financial protection needed for access to all health care needs.

What do I need to know about any health insurance policy I'm considering?

Deductible clauses, co-insurance, maximum benefit levels, and limits on out-of-pocket liability are the four parts of any health insurance policy that require close scrutiny. A deductible is the amount of money a family must pay before the insurance company will pay anything. When considering an insurance policy, evaluate what the deductible will mean to you in terms of out-of-pocket costs. Co-insurance is the portion of charges that must be paid by the family after the deductible portion has been met. It is not uncommon for the family to bear 20 percent of hospital, physician, and related fees, even after the deductibles have been met. Maximum benefits are the dollar maximum, or ceiling, that the insurance company agrees to pay in a given period of time or for a given illness. For a specific illness, the insurance company will pay a specific amount. Or, the insurance company will pay a certain amount for each insured person every year, or the insurance company will specify a maximum lifetime ceiling for the cost of treatment.

The limit on out-of-pocket liability, or a "stop-loss clause," is the limit the insurance company imposes on the family's out-of-pocket expenses for a given calendar year before the insurance company pays 100 percent of further covered charges. Covered charges vary from policy to policy, and the family must not assume that a specific treatment is subject to this limit without first verifying this with the insurance company.

If my insurance will not cover all my expenses, can I purchase more?

Yes, but insurance policies covering a broad range of catastrophic problems are very expensive. If you can afford the price, you can probably buy almost any type of coverage you desire. These policies carry a hefty premium and very large deductibles and co-insurance requirements.

Are there limitations to the fee-for-service policies?

While group policies tend to be more generous in their coverage, this is not *always* the case. Preexisting clauses may exist in the policy, limiting access for children with chronic conditions. Insurance may not pay for preexisting conditions. This is an important issue to evaluate when changing jobs and employers—and therefore health insurance carriers.

Routine dental care, eyeglasses, hearing aids, and routine physical examinations may also be excluded from policies. Mental health services and home adaptations to allow the child to be cared for at home are frequently not covered.

What limitations can the insurance company impose on care or treatment?

The insurance company may recommend that you seek treatment with one of its preferred providers, usually within its network, who agree to provide service at a predetermined cost. If you agree to utilize a preferred provider, the insurance company pays the physician a higher percentage of covered charges—approximately 90 percent instead of 80 percent.

Insurance companies often utilize a second surgical opinion. In certain types of surgical cases, a second opinion must be obtained or the insurance company will not pay the full benefit. Often, the second opinion must come from one of the company's preferred providers.

What do HMOs provide?

Health maintenance organizations (HMOs) are a form of managed care. They can be both insurers and providers of care; they offer prepaid health plans. Employers may provide HMOs as part of their benefits package, in which case a monthly premium is paid by the employer, with the employee usually contributing a specific dollar amount to the premium, as well. HMOs usually provide preventive services as a benefit, while most fee-for-service programs do not. Families select a primary care physician within the plan who then authorizes care required from any other physician or hospital within the plan or network. The approach is used to keep all needed services within the network in order to keep costs under control. If a referral is made to a physician outside of the plan or network, there is no way of controlling charges, because the plan does not have a contract with that physician.

What government assistance is available?

Medicaid is a program of federal grants to states that pays for certain health services for eligible people. The eligibility criteria are specific to each state but are based on financial need. Each state may add services over and above those required by the federal law.

Medicaid (known by different names in different states, such as TennCare in Tennessee and TEFRA in South Carolina) is a program run by the states; a percentage of the costs is funded by the federal government. It is not available in all states for children under 18, unless the child qualifies for SSI. If a child under 18 applies for SSI, eligibility is based on the parents' income and assets (less than $2,000 in assets, less than $2,100/month income). For most of those states that provide Medicaid without SSI, eligibility is not typically based on parents' assets or income, but rather on the child's assets. If assets do not exceed $2,000 and the child meets the medical criteria, he would normally be eligible. However, it is important that you check with the state in which your child is residing. At age 18, the income and assets of the person with CP (but not of his or her parents) become the critical factor in determining eligibility.

What kinds of services are covered by Medicaid?

Generally inpatient hospital care, physicians' and other outpatient services, skilled nursing services, and lab tests are covered. Coverage of things such as medications, home health care, eyeglasses, and dental care are determined by the individual state. Investigate limits of Medicaid coverage in your state. Medicaid regulations change from time to time because of budgetary constraints and use of resources, and Congress continues to reform laws with respect to eligibility, reimbursement, and benefits.

For children who are highly dependent on technology, who might otherwise remain in the hospital to receive skilled nursing care, Medicaid has a program for those seeking greater independence that is aimed at reducing the costs of hospitalization and decreasing unnecessary hospital stays. Referred to as the Medicaid Home and Community Based Waiver, the program pays for the needed care, but the care is given in the home or a community-based program certified to provide such services, such as a group home. Because eligibility requirements vary from state to state, you'll need to call your Medicaid office or social services department for assistance in evaluating whether or not you can benefit from this program.

Medicaid also covers long-term care. However, benefits vary among the states, and assets of the individual must be below $2,000. Some people try to rid themselves (or spend down) their assets to qualify. This "spend down" can be avoided by creating a "Payback Special Needs Trust" and transferring the person's assets to this trust. The money is available to the person but is not considered a "countable resource" for Medicaid eligibility. Medicaid may invoke a "three-year look back provision" in the case where assets are transferred. This means that the person would have to wait three years for Medicaid benefits to begin. To avoid this situation, you may want to consult with a special needs planner.

What is nursing home insurance?

This is insurance that would cover basic care in a nursing home or other long-term care (LTC) environment. Some policies may include coverage for long-term skilled care, but the operating word is "skilled." Skilled care means that the individual requires nursing care, under the policy definition of nursing. The cost of long-term care for individuals who require custodial care rather than nursing care will not be covered. Custodial care is rarely covered by insurance policies. LTC is getting more expensive as elderly citizens continue to live longer. This coverage is far more affordable if parents have the foresight to purchase this type of policy prior to age 65. In addition, it is important that those buying LTC are willing to go to a nursing home. Anyone who would not live in a nursing home would be wasting their money. An alternative is an "at home care policy." These policies typically are less expensive. Many provide for both professional services and those given by a family member or friend.

Are there other programs for children with special needs?

Yes. What used to be called Services for Crippled and Handicapped Children is now called Programs for Children with Special Health Care Needs. These are included under the Maternal and Child Health (MCH) Block Grant and provide case management and other health services such as nursing, social work, and physical and other therapies to eligible children with chronic illness. Each state sets its own eligibility criteria and its own list of services covered. Currently, there is an income requirement; that is, families must earn less than a certain level before services are offered. Information on Programs for Children with Special Health Care Needs may be found at the local office of the state health department, or you can get information from a health care provider or the state health department responsible for the MCH Block Grant programs.

What is SSI?

Supplemental Security Income (SSI) is an income support program for aged, blind, and disabled adults, and for children with disabilities. Eligible children live in low-income households (less than $2,000 in assets, less than $2,100 per month in income) and must meet the SSI criteria of disability. If a child is eligible to receive SSI, health care services are received through Medicaid. Contact the local office of the Social Security Administration (SSA) to determine eligibility. The SSA requires documentation regarding your assets, income, and age, and the child's age. The adult with a disability is reviewed independently of the family. Adults with CP who have limited assets or who are unemployed may qualify for SSI funding.

SSI eligibility for children under 18 is based on parents' income and assets as well as the child's. After age 18 it is based solely on the child's income and assets and medical eligibility requirements. Parents face the problem of how to keep their child eligible throughout his lifetime. This is where certified special needs planners should be consulted for assistance. Most financial planners, insurance agents, and attorneys are not familiar with or qualified to advise on the proper way to protect assets for a person with a developmental disability. By proper special needs planning, parents will be able to pass assets on for their child's care and have these assets protected from being used to reimburse the government for Medicaid services received by the child. Without proper planning, it is possible that the child will become ineligible for Medicaid when receiving assets from family members. In addition, if a proper will has not been prepared by parents, at their death the state of residence for the person with CP will appoint his or her guardian and trustees and decide who gets the parents' assets. Medicaid could immediately take assets received by the person with special needs for reimbursement. Grandparents also need to be part of this planning, because their will can negate a properly prepared plan by parents.

What is SCHIP?

The Balanced Budget Act of 1997 established the State Children's Health Insurance Program (SCHIP), which gives grants to states to provide health insurance coverage to uninsured children up to 200% of the federal poverty level (FPL). States may provide this coverage by expanding Medicaid or by expanding or creating a state children's health insurance program. However, states do not have to participate, and they can also choose to wait up to three years to implement the program without losing any funds. The legislation sets eligibility criteria. States can decide to cover all of those children or to target coverage to a narrower group of children. The eligibility criteria are to cover uninsured children who are:

- not eligible for Medicaid
- under age 19; and
- at or below 200% of the federal poverty level.

Where can I get information on these and other programs?

For the most part, it is up to you to pursue support that may be available to your child. Some people who may be helpful include your child's primary physician, community and public health nurses and social workers, teachers, members of voluntary organizations, and members of your local Developmental Disabilities Council. You can also contact the various departments listed within the appropriate chapters of this book, and the organizations listed in the Resources section, at the end of the book. The section on "Managing the System" in Part 2 may also provide useful information.

What about getting help?

Professionals who work with children and adults with disabilities are very helpful. If they do not have an answer for you, they can usually refer you to someone else who does. An easy way to begin is by calling your public health agency and explaining what it is that you want. That phone call will give you many contacts. As you'll soon discover, there are many ways to gather information on resources and programs, services, and agencies, but it is mostly up to you to do the investigating. There is no "one-stop shopping."

One good agency to contact is the National Dissemination Center for Children and Youth with Disabilities (NICHCY) (see Resources section). Ask NICHCY to send you information on the topic that concerns you. The information is free, and you'll receive it fairly quickly. Ask in particular for the resource sheet for your state, which lists the names and addresses of key agencies that are involved with individuals with a variety of disabilities. You can also ask for lists of national resources on a particular topic. NICHCY exists to provide "free information to assist parents, educators, caregivers, advocates, and others in helping children and youth with disabilities become participating members of the community." (They encourage duplication of their materials, too.)

Many associations can provide a list of resources that are available for people with cerebral palsy. One of these, the United Cerebral Palsy Associations (UCPA), is listed in the phone book under United Cerebral Palsy; each region has a local chapter that can provide information on local resources. One thing to remember is that the agencies you are calling within a specific community usually know the services offered in that community. If you require a broader range of information, you will have to contact federal agencies or the national headquarters of UCPA.

It is often helpful to contact your state senator, assemblyperson, and federal congressperson, and the offices of other politicians for assistance in locating the proper government office to help you gain access to services. It's a good practice to keep a log of all contacts. Record the names, phone numbers, addresses, and the day and time you called. Indicate whether the office was helpful to you, and what your conversations were about. You may not need the agency at the present time, but you should tuck the information away for future reference.

Group activities and support groups are valuable for a number of reasons. For one thing, the people who attend can share resource information with you. While getting out of the house one night a week to attend a support group may not seem like the most exciting use of your time, it is a good way to find out from other parents what kind of help they are getting and how they are getting it. Additionally, the emotional support, both given and received, can be of great value. The UCPA frequently organizes support groups or parents' groups related to CP. If you can't attend all of them, at least try to attend a few. Get to know other parents. You may learn a lot from them.

What organizations in the private sector provide help for families?

Organizations included in the private sector are groups and agencies such as the United Cerebral Palsy Associations, the Easter Seal Society, the Epilepsy Foundation of America, the Arc: National Organization on Mental Retardation, and the American Foundation for the Blind. A great range of services and assistance is offered by private agencies—for example, residential day programs, recreation services, home case management, and respite services. Call these agencies to evaluate the scope of services and to find out whether you would benefit from them.

From time to time while you're exploring for services you may come across a fund that is made available for specific purposes. This may be a scholarship fund or a fund for vacations for people with special needs, for example. Finding these opportunities requires persistence. Ask your librarian to direct you to resources or directories on philanthropic foundations.

You may also want to consider fundraising on your own. If you are interested in fundraising, the sky seems to be the limit in terms of what people will do for you and offer to you. Parents and friends of children with cerebral palsy have organized all sorts of community activities, from car washes, school dances, and marathons, to direct solicitation of donations in containers at local convenience stores. Parents have mailed out letters to every organization imaginable in an attempt to obtain donations for equipment, health care, special schooling, and communication devices. An effort of this magnitude requires a good deal of work and persistence. Furthermore, it is critical for individual fundraisers to work only within the legal guidelines established by the federal and state governments. You needn't be dissuaded by these guidelines; you only need to be aware of them, and to follow them.

Are there social service agencies I can call for assistance?

There are many agencies in your community that you can contact for a variety of purposes, though there is no *one* specific place to go for help. Many agencies provide a variety of services, some of which overlap, some of them with great gaps in service. Your state or local department of social services can offer a great deal of guidance about how to proceed with a variety of issues. Many, but not all, states have a book that lists available services and agency offices which is available to the public for a price. It gives an excellent accounting of all the human service agencies involved in the care of individuals in a particular state or region.

Contact the Developmental Disabilities Council in your area for information. To locate the one nearest you, contact the National Association of Developmental Disabilities Councils (see Resources section). Groups like the United Cerebral Palsy Associations, the Easter Seal Society, and the March of Dimes Birth Defects Foundation can help by directing you to appropriate local services. All social service agencies are community specific, meaning that the organization and administration of the services and the channeling of funds are unique to each region. Contact your local agencies for help.

Where can I get the services I need?

In the following list, the need or service is listed in the left-hand column, and various groups that provide the service are listed in the right-hand column. Contact these groups for help, or ask these groups to direct you to other groups that may be able to help you.

Food	Religious groups; government-funded programs like school meals and food stamps
Shelter	Red Cross; homeless shelters; foster care; emergency housing (state or local department of social services); Salvation Army; private organizations (UCPA)
Clothing	Salvation Army; religious organizations; Goodwill agencies
Legal advice	American Bar Association; Legal Aid Services; the courts; local legal organizations or agencies
Financial support	Religious and volunteer organizations; United Way; service clubs; city or state department of social services; philanthropic foundations
Emotional and physical	Disease-oriented groups; friends and family; religious organizations; private and government organizations; community outreach programs; support groups

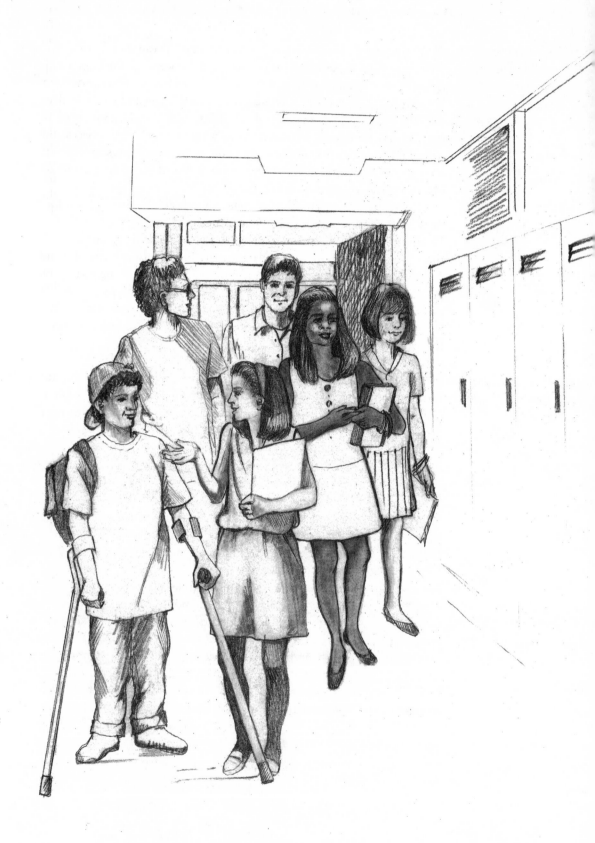

Navigating
the
Educational
System

II

♦ THIS CHAPTER discusses issues related to the education of children with disabilities. Much of the material in this chapter comes from federal public laws and regulations, which can be accessed from a number of resources, some of which are identified at the end of this chapter, and in the Resources section at the end of this book. Among the most helpful to parents is the National Dissemination Center for Children with Disabilities (NICHCY) and UCP, both located in Washington, D.C. These agencies provide information to parents, often in English and Spanish, which will help them help their child.

The inclusion of children with disabilities in public schools or the opportunity to participate in publicly supported education, currently assured under the Individuals with Disabilities Education Act (IDEA), is a relatively recent phenomenon. Federal laws requiring public schools to provide free appropriate public education to children with disabilities originated in 1970 with the passage of the Education of the Handicapped Act (EHA). This act established minimum requirements with which states had to comply to receive federal financial assistance. The amendment of the EHA in 1975 as the Education of All Handicapped Children Act (EAHCA, Public Law 94-142) marked a watershed in providing many important legal protections that remain intact today. These protections have been carried into its subsequent revisions and renaming as the Individuals with Disabilities Education Act, IDEA, first in 1990, then again in 1997, and most recently in 2004.

Core principles of Public Law 94-142 that survive through IDEA and its reauthorization assure that students who are determined to be eligible for special education are provided an appropriate educational program. It also assures that parents participate in the decision making about their child's education with full due process guarantees. In the IDEA 1997 update, goals of reauthorization included: strengthening the role of parents, ensuring access to the general education curriculum with the participation of students with disabilities in statewide assessments, encouraging use of mediation to settle disagreements between parents and educators, increasing the focus on effectiveness of teaching and learning, and reducing paperwork requirements.

Important highlights of the reauthorization of IDEA in 2004 included emphasis on the importance of positive behavioral supports and the use of behavioral reinforcement as a component in a student's individualized education program plan (IEP). It also provides funds for teacher training in this area. The bill for the first time includes consequences for schools that fail to comply with IDEA, with the possible loss of some federal funding for schools found to be in noncompliance with the law for more than two years. Another provision prohibits school officials from forcing parents to medicate their children as a condition for attending school. Schools will be required to evaluate many components of a student's life, rather than just focusing on test scores, when considering whether a student is eligible for special education services.

States are required to have in place policies and procedures that guarantee certain procedural safeguards. These ensure that parents be provided with the information they need to make decisions about the provision of a free appropriate public education, and that there be procedures in place to resolve disagreements between parties. Congress recognized that families should have "meaningful opportunities to participate in the education of their children at school and at home."

The process of determining whether a child is eligible to receive special education services begins with a full and individual evaluation that may be the result of a parent's or school's request. If the school initiates the request, parents must be asked for their written approval to evaluate their child, and they must be given notice of their right to object. Similarly, if a parent requests the evaluation, the school may deny the evaluation, but it must assure the parents of their due process rights to continue to pursue evaluation and possible eligibility for special education services. In certain circumstances, an additional evaluation by an independent evaluator may be warranted, in which case there will be no charge to parents. The purpose of this evaluation is to gather information related to the child's progress in the general education curriculum, to determine the educational needs of the child, and to determine whether the child needs special education and related services.

The term "special education" in the context of the law and entitlement to services means specially designed instruction, at no cost to parents, to meet the unique needs of the child with a disability. This can include: (1) instruction conducted in the classroom, in the home, in hospitals and institutions, and in other settings; and (2) instruction in physical education.

Children who are eligible for special education services have the right to a clearly written IEP. The IEP is the keystone of the process that assures an appropriate education for each child. It is the document that describes the child's needs for specific instruction or teaching, annual goals, and how progress toward those goals will be measured and reported to parents, the related services and aids that will be provided, the extent of participation in programs for students without disabilities, what, if any, modifications will be necessary in the administration of statewide assessment of student achievement, and, beginning at age 14, the inclusion of transition planning as a part of the process. The IEP is developed jointly with parents and school personnel at a meeting convened at a mutually convenient time. Parents have the right to be included and approve the educational plans for their child, or if there is not agreement, they also have the right, through a due process procedure, to appeal any decisions made about identification, evaluation, and placement of their child.

Children with disabilities also have the right to receive a variety of related educational services that make access to education possible. These related services may include transportation and such developmental, corrective, and other supportive services as may be required to assist a child with a disability to benefit from special education. Such supportive services include speech-language pathology and audiology services; psychological services; physical and occupational therapy; recreation, including therapeutic recreation; social work services; counseling services, including rehabilitation counseling; orientation and mobility services; and medical services (where the medical services are for diagnostic and evaluation purposes only).

Specific health-related services may be included as a school district obligation under IDEA according to the findings of two U.S. Supreme Court cases. In 1984 the Tatro case established that the medical service exclusion of IDEA did not apply when "clean intermittent catheterization" was necessary for the student to benefit from the special education program, and could be performed by a nurse or other qualified person, not necessarily a physician. More recently, in 1999, the court, in the case of Garret F. who was a special education student and also ventilator-dependent, determined that the school district was responsible for providing full-time nursing services at school, citing justifications similar to the Tatro case. Specifically, because someone other than a physician could administer the services needed by this young man, this qualified them as related services, not subject to the medical exclusion of the IDEA.

The IDEA requires that states provide public education for children with disabilities, ages 3 to 21, no matter how severe the disabilities, unless state law or practice does not provide these public school services for any children ages 3 to 5 or 18 to 21. This law, like its earlier version, Public Law 94-142, requires that children with disabilities be educated in the least restrictive environment (LRE), which means in the setting most like the local school that he or she would have attended if not for the disability (see table 7).

Services provided under Part C of IDEA, the Infants and Toddlers with Disabilities program, serving children ages birth to 3, must be provided in natural environments which include the home and community settings in which children without disabilities participate. The law also requires that early intervention services necessary to meet the unique needs of the infant

Table 7　Features of the Individuals with Disabilities Education Act (IDEA)

Free and appropriate education is to be provided to all children, regardless of how severely they are disabled
As much as possible, children with disabilities must be educated in settings with children who do not have disabilities
Age limits are established for children to receive educational services
Services the child will receive must be defined
Mechanisms by which this program must be carried out are stipulated
Mechanisms for conflict resolution between parent and professional are in place

or toddler and the family, including frequency, intensity, and the method of delivering services also be included in the statement of natural environments in which early intervention services shall be provided.

What is the definition in these laws of a child with a disability?

The regulations for IDEA identify these disabling conditions:

　1. "mental retardation, hearing impairment (including deafness), speech or language impairments, visual impairments (including blindness), serious emotional disturbance, orthopedic impairments, autism, traumatic brain injury, other health impairments, or specific learning disabilities **and**

　2. who, by reason thereof, need special education and related services."

What are the confidentiality protections that must be provided to my child and family?

The Buckley Amendment (Public Law 93-380), also known as the Family Educational Rights and Privacy Act (FERPA), gives parents of students under the age of 18 and students 18 and older access to the student's educational record. This law also provides parents and students with the right to review the record and to receive a copy of it. They have the right to a full explanation of the contents of the record. If they believe the record is inaccurate or misleading, they can ask that it be changed. School personnel may not destroy any part of the record if there is a pending request to review its contents. If there is a disagreement about the record, then the parents must be advised of their rights to a due process hearing. This might happen if the parents requested that the record be changed and the school objected to changing it: in this case, the school must tell the parents that they have the right to a due process hearing.

The schools have the right to release part of the record to certain other education and social service agencies without parental permission. A record of all requests and a listing of the parts of the record that were released are included in the student's record. The schools are obligated under law to communicate with parents and students in their primary language, even if that language is not English.

Certain school activities involving a special education student's health information are required to be carried out in ways that protect confidentiality and comply with the Health Insurance Portability and Accountability Act (HIPAA) of 1996. The extension of HIPAA to students requires schools to ensure that safeguards are in place for the disclosure and electronic transmission of "protected health information." However, a student's health information that is considered part of the official education record of that student and covered by the Family Education Rights and Privacy Act (FERPA) is not "covered" by HIPAA. The U.S. Supreme Court decision in Falvo (2002) provides further guidance by narrowing the definition of educational records to those maintained by the school district or other school entity, extending FERPA protections only to those records. The confidentiality rules will vary based on whether the records are "educational" or not.

What other education laws apply to children with CP?

One other such law is the Carl D. Perkins Vocational and Technical Education Act of 1998, which provides funding for secondary and postsecondary vocational training while the students are still in school. Its purpose is to develop more fully the academic, vocational, and technical skills of secondary students and postsecondary students.

In accordance with this law, vocational education programs and activities must be organized in the least restrictive environment, and this activity must be part of the Individualized Education Plan. This law gives students equal access to a full range of programs available to nondisabled students, including apprenticeship programs, career guidance and counseling, cooperative education programs, and occupationally oriented courses of study.

What are the provisions of the Early Intervention Act of 1986?

This law (Public Law 99-457) provides services and related activities for children of all ages with disabilities. Section 619 extends the law to ensure that beginning at age 3, all children with disabilities receive a free, appropriate public education, including an Individualized Education Program plan, due process, confidentiality, and provision of services in the least restrictive environment. The services may be offered in the home, or they may be center-based. The child should have access to the same related services that are provided by IDEA: occupational therapy, physical therapy, speech therapy, school health services, social work, and so on.

Check with your state department of education to learn about the programs available in your state. It may also be useful to contact other relevant departments (public instruction, education, health, and social services) in your state to find out which agency is primarily responsible for implementing the law.

Part H of Public Law 99-457 provides for early intervention services for eligible infants and toddlers and their families. Eligible children will be those from birth through age 2 who are developmentally delayed as defined by an individual state, who are at risk of developmental delay, or who have conditions that frequently result in developmental delay. Contact your state's departments of education, public instruction, health, or social services to determine what services in your state can be accessed under Part H of Public Law 99-457.

What does the "Lawyer's Fees" Bill of 1986 provide?

In 1986 Congress addressed the issue of parents' recovery of attorney's fees for successful special education claims made under the IDEA. The "Lawyer's Fees" Bill of the Handicapped Children's Protection Act provides that, in a legal dispute brought by the parents over special education placement, if the parents win the suit, the courts may order the school district or the state to pay the parents' legal fees.

What about the Rehabilitation Act of 1973 (section 504) and the Americans with Disabilities Act of 1990?

These two compatible federal laws exist to prohibit discrimination against individuals with disabilities in employment programs or services if that individual is otherwise qualified to participate. Section 504 provides that "no . . . qualified individual [with a disability] . . . shall, solely by reason of his [disability], be excluded from participation in, be denied the benefits of, or be subjected to discrimination under any program or activity receiving . . . federal financial assistance." Under both acts, a person with a disability is defined as any person with a physical or mental impairment which substantially limits one or more major life activities. Discrimination against such a person is prohibited by any group or activities receiving federal funds. These include programs and activities that provide vocational training or education, public and private colleges, public and private day care centers, preschool programs, public and private elementary schools, and public and private adult programs. Employers and service providers must make an effort to make their services, facilities, and programs accessible to individuals with disabilities.

The Americans with Disabilities Act guarantees equal access to individuals with disabilities in transportation, public accommodations, state and local government services, employment, and telecommunications. Employers must provide reasonable accommodations to individuals with disabilities, such as restructuring or modifying jobs or equipment, as long as those accommodations do not impose undue hardship on the company. Public transportation must be accessible to people with disabilities. Special transportation services must be made available to those who cannot use fixed route bus transit, unless this poses an undue burden for public transportation.

Private establishments like restaurants, stores, and hotels cannot discriminate. Physical barriers to access must be removed or another means of access must be arranged. (This means that these establishments must install ramps for wheelchairs, doors wide enough to accommodate wheelchairs, bathrooms that can accommodate wheelchairs, elevators with buttons in Braille, and so on, unless to do so imposes an unusual economic hardship.) All new construction must be accessible.

What are the implications of the "No Child Left Behind Act" for children in special education?

Although not specifically designed for special education, the federal No Child Left Behind Law (NCLB) of 2001 contains several items that are relevant to children with cerebral palsy who are in need of adapted or specialized instruction. No Child Left Behind represents comprehensive national education legislation that intends to improve school accountability for achievement and safety, and to provide school performance information and some increased control to parents. It directs states to create grade-level standards for what students should know, and requires testing of that progress annually in grades three to eight, and again in grade ten. Consistent with requirements of IDEA reauthorized in 1997, states are required to include students with disabilities in regular assessments. Beginning in July 2000, students unable to take part in a state's regular assessment with accommodations are to be provided alternative assessments. NCLB builds on IDEA 1997 and requires that the assessment scores of all students with disabilities be included in the state accountability system, including the scores of alternate assessments.

Current law allows students with disabilities to be assessed in several ways. They may take part in the regular testing, with or without accommodations. They may also take an alternate assessment that is aligned either with grade level achievement standards or with alternate achievement standards. Determination of whether a special education student participates in the standard or alternative testing rests with the student's IEP team. Without the demonstration of "Adequate Yearly Progress" at the local school level, funding will be adjusted and in some cases, parents may be given the opportunity to change schools or access tutoring assistance for underachieving students.

What types of schools do children with special needs attend?

Children with special needs attend many different kinds of schools. Some schools have a typical 9-month program, while others offer an extended school year (ESY) program to eligible students. There are schools specific to the child's disability, such as schools for the hearing impaired or orthopedically handicapped. Many children attend regular schools, where they are "included or mainstreamed" in a classroom with children who don't have special needs. The child with a disability may or may not have an aide in the regular classroom.

There are also regular schools where children receive their instruction in a self-contained classroom for children with disabilities. Alternatively, some children are instructed part-time in the learning-disabled classroom and receive various necessary therapies during the school day, but are included for selected learning situations, such as music or social studies. Children with very mild physical disability may only be separated from their peers for an adaptive physical education class.

The type of school situation in which a child does best is dependent on many factors, including the child's disability, the available services, the child's IEP, and, in some circumstances, the parent's advocacy. In order to determine where your child will go to school and what kind of services he or she will have access to, an assessment of your child's development and abilities must be made.

What should I do if I think my child has special needs?

You will need to arrange to have your child assessed to determine what kind of help she or he needs. Sometimes the parents aren't aware of their child's needs, or they don't realize that the school system can provide special services; in these cases the school, or an individual teacher at the school, may ask that the child have an assessment.

In short, there are three ways that a child can be identified for an assessment:

1. Parents can request an assessment.
2. If your child is in school, the school may ask parental permission to assess a child based on a screening.
3. An individual teacher who knows your child well may ask for an assessment.

What is an assessment?

An assessment involves gathering information about your child and his development. It generally includes determining what kind of help your child needs. Information comes from a variety of sources: parents, the assessment team, the child's doctors and medical history, and reports and results from developmental tests. This assessment forms the basis for the Individualized Education Plan, the written document describing the child's needs, as well as the services that are to be provided to the child.

Who does the assessment?

An assessment may be performed by a team of professionals that includes a special education teacher, an occupational therapist, a physical therapist, a speech and language specialist, medical specialists, and a psychologist. Individual state policies determine what types of professionals make up the team. To perform the assessment, these professionals observe and test the child, and determine her strengths and weaknesses.

Who should I contact for information on early intervention programs and special education programs?

You can call your local elementary school or school district office and ask for the contact person who is in charge of these services. Or you can obtain a copy of the resource sheet for your state that is available through the National Dissemination Center for Children with Disabilities. This document will tell you who the appropriate contact person is in your state's education department. Write to NICHCY at P.O. Box 1492, Washington, D.C. 20013-1492, or call 1-800-695-0285.

What is Child Find?

Child Find is a service, offered by many states, under the direction of the state's education department. (In some states, it exists under other names.) Its mission is to identify and diagnose unserved children with disabilities. Child Find makes a special effort to identify children from birth to 6 years, but they are interested in identifying all unserved children. Anyone residing in a school district can request Child Find screening. Criteria for determining who is screened and at what age are determined by each district.

What are early intervention services?

These are programs designed to identify and treat a developmental problem as soon as possible. Once it has been determined that your child is eligible for early intervention services, you will be assigned a case manager who will help develop an Individualized Family Service Plan (IFSP). The IFSP describes the services the child will receive, when and where he will receive these services, and how his progress will be evaluated. The case manager is involved with your family until your child reaches 2 years of age. The case manager then helps you move on to programs for children ages 3 through 5.

What does free and appropriate public education mean?

This provision, originally from Public Law 99-142 and now in IDEA, means that special and related services are provided at all educational levels: preschool, elementary, and secondary. These services are offered free to children because they are provided under the state education agency and are funded with public monies. This education must meet the needs of the child as identified by the IEP.

How are related services obtained?

Related service needs are identified during the evaluation process of the child with special needs. The IEP will identify the related services needed for the student. The IEP serves as a written commitment for the delivery of services to the child with special needs.

What happens if I don't agree with my child's IEP?

If the school determines that your child does not need certain services and you think she does, you can appeal the decision of the team. If you choose to appeal the IEP, be certain to get some professional advice on how to proceed.

Who should I contact for help?

Get in touch with NICHCY and ask for information on the Parent Training and Information (PTI) centers in your state. The Parent Training and Information Center is a federally funded agency that provides parents with the knowledge and know-how needed to become partners in their child's education. It can provide you with the information you need to go through the appeal process if that becomes necessary.

Can I get an independent evaluation of my child's abilities and strengths?

You can always obtain an independent evaluation of your child. Sometimes the school agrees that there is a need for a second opinion and sets up the evaluation. If the arrangements are made through the school, the school pays for the independent evaluation. If you wish to make the appointment and seek the second opinion independently, you will be required to pay for it.

In any case, the school district must provide you with names of other professionals who can provide the assessment. Parent groups are good resources for information and for recommending specialists, too. Local hospitals often have specialists on staff who get together as a team to provide assessments.

What happens at an IEP meeting? The people who evaluated your child explain their findings, what tests they used, and the scores your child achieved. You share your observations about your child with these specialists. You may want to ask for the testing results before the meeting to give you time to review them and plan ahead. On the basis of this meeting the IEP is developed, and you are asked to sign it. The plan lays out exactly what the school intends to do during the school year. And every year after that, the school must schedule a meeting with you to review your child's progress and to develop the next year's IEP.

What is included in the IEP? Included in the IEP are statements of annual goals, short-term objectives, and specific special education and related services, in addition to an explanation of who will provide the services. Additional statements about what percentage of time the child will participate in regular educational programs, target dates for the initiation and duration of special services, and criteria for evaluation, which will measure progress, are included.

What if I'm not able to attend the IEP meeting? The law and regulations governing the development of the IEP require that a meeting of the parents and professionals be held at a mutually convenient time. Every effort should be made to work out a schedule. Sometimes meetings are planned for after school hours, but typically a meeting can be planned during school hours at a mutually agreed-upon time.

Is there anyone who can help me understand all of this? There are federally supported programs in each state that support parent-to-parent information and training activities for parents of children with special needs. The Parent Training and Information Projects conduct workshops, publish newsletters, and answer questions by phone or mail about parent-to-parent activities. They are very helpful in evaluating the educational system in your state. Contact NICHCY and ask for the listing of the Parent Training and Information Centers' federally funded parent programs.

Will these laws and rules change over time? To a great extent, the basic emphases of these laws have stayed the same for the past 20 years, though the laws may be interpreted differently from state to state. However, because IDEA needs to be periodically reauthorized, various groups lobby lawmakers for changes in these laws. Specific provisions requested by school districts or others advocated by parent groups may be introduced at these times, and parent support groups will likely know which of these provisions might weaken the law to the detriment of children. Since these groups cannot lobby lawmakers, it is up to parents and other individual citizens to do so.

What can I do to keep abreast of issues?

Keep in touch. Join parent support groups, where information is shared. Get on the mailing list for NICHCY and the United Cerebral Palsy Associations (UCPA). Contact NICHCY for information on Federally Funded Parent Programs. These programs provide information and training to enable parents of children with disabling conditions to participate more knowledgeably in their child's care. Phone the school districts and the Developmental Disabilities Council in your area and ask for information.

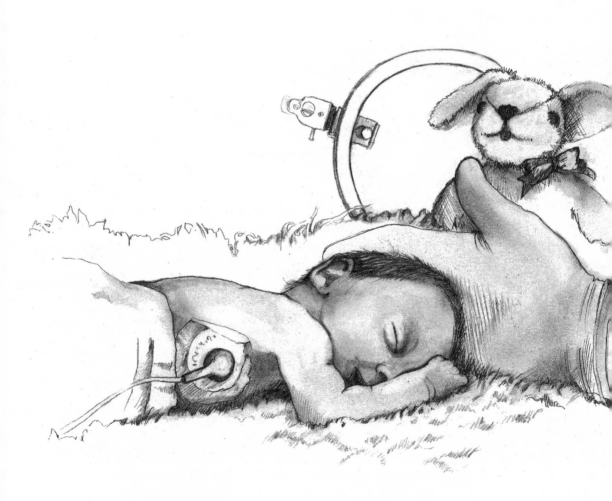

Being an Advocate for Your Child: Using the Legal System

12

◆ FOR MANY PEOPLE, any discussion of the legal system evokes images of complicated procedures and tense courtroom scenes. High costs also come immediately to mind. Although it's true that the legal system can be confusing and even intimidating, this is not necessarily so in the area of the rights of the disabled. People with disabilities, their family members, and their advocates can effectively, inexpensively, and easily use the law to obtain services and benefits.

A series of lawsuits in recent years has served to raise society's level of awareness about the lack of services available to people with disabilities. Legislatures, both state and federal, have responded by passing broad-ranging laws recognizing that people with disabilities have the right to be fully integrated into U.S. society. These laws, which are administered by federal, state, and local agencies, go a long way toward ensuring fair and equal treatment, and they make it easier for people with disabilities and their advocates to obtain services. The people who staff these agencies are generally conscientious; nevertheless, bureaucracy and budget concerns sometimes interfere with the process. As a result, some individuals with disabilities are wrongly denied services to which they are entitled. For this reason, it is important for people with disabilities and those who advocate for them to understand what the law requires as well as how to go about obtaining rights under the law.

To be an advocate, or champion, for the rights of the individual with disabilities, a person must be willing to learn what the individual's rights are, understand how the system works, and use the system to obtain maximum benefits. Although most people think only of lawyers when they think of advocates, there are in fact many different types of advocates. We begin this chapter with a description of the various kinds of advocates who may be helpful to you and your child. The rest of the chapter then takes up specific issues pertaining to the law as it applies to people with disabilities. Other legal assistance agencies are listed in the Resources section at the end of this book.

The legal advocate, or lawyer.   We usually think of a lawyer when we think of a professional advocate representing the child or parent in litigation, and there's no question that employing a lawyer trained in handling disability cases is generally a wise decision. Whether it is or is not *essential* to obtain the services of a lawyer is often determined by the specific problem that needs to be addressed. If there are complicated legal issues with respect to educational requirements, or if parents need to write a will that provides for the survivor with a disability, then parents need to consult a lawyer specialized in these areas. Your family's general practice lawyer can usually refer you to a lawyer who specializes in disability cases. In addition, agencies such as the United Cerebral Palsy Associations (UCPA), school districts, legal service agencies, and social workers can provide referrals to lawyers who specialize in this area of the law. Bar associations also offer lawyer referral services to the public.

The legal system overall is moving toward alternative disposition resolution (ADR), in which mediation and arbitration are commonplace options. For example, the IDEA regulations require states to offer mediation to resolve special education disputes. Such alternatives may be less expensive and intimidating options for parents to pursue.

Protection & advocacy (P&A) agencies.   Every state has a P&A agency which provides advocacy and legal services to persons with disabilities, usually for free. The National Association of Protection and Advocacy Systems (NAPAS) has background information and links to all state P&As on its Web site at www.napas.org. The P&A system has been expanding since its inception in the mid-1970s to include a number of discrete programs. The primary programs that would be of most interest to persons with CP would be those earmarked for developmental disabilities (PADD) and assistive technology (PAAT). P&As engage in a wide variety of advocacy, including systemic litigation, individual litigation, legislative and regulatory advocacy, and provision of information and referral services.

The parent as advocate.   As noted above, a lawyer is not the only advocate who can benefit your child. It is a fact that the most important advocates for most children are their parents. To be an effective advocate, a parent needs to become very well informed about the laws pertaining to disability as well as about how the system works. A good place to begin is to obtain a set of your state's regulations, copies of which are usually available at no or low cost. You should also read publications on self-advocacy, which are available in bookstores and libraries. It is virtually impossible to be an effective advocate without knowing the rules of the game. The scope of benefits parents obtain from the government and insurance companies may be directly related to how aggressively the parents advocate on behalf of their child.

Because the parent is not only the child's advocate but also the child's caregiver, the parent must be aware of two risks involved in serving as the child's advocate. First, advocacy can become a full-time occupation in its own right. Second, parents can become overwhelmed with the time commitment and begin to feel that more gains could be made if more time was spent—and their commitment, though well intentioned, may eat into the time they have available to spend in their other role, parenting their child (or children). Parents should only spend as much time in their role as advocates as they are comfortable with, and then accept that they do not have to do everything.

Being an assertive advocate also requires a certain personality, someone who is willing to confront others and to be in the public eye. Parents who simply cannot manage this type of advocacy should seek help from other advocates and not feel guilty about doing so. Joining local councils (such as developmental disabilities councils and special educational councils) and local branches of national organizations (such as UCPA), can be very helpful for parents who cannot serve as their own child's primary advocate but who can nevertheless contribute time and effort to advocacy groups. Each state has a DD council that serves as a systemic advocate for persons with developmental disabilities. Check the National Association of Councils on Developmental Disabilities Web site at www.nacdd.org, which has a link to councils in individual states. A list of councils in all 50 states is provided. Special education councils are required by the IDEA regulations. Participation in such councils provides an opportunity to network and receive free training. Such organizations provide valuable information, and the collective power they wield is often impressive.

The citizen advocate.   A citizen advocate is someone with experience or training who is willing to become a child's advocate on a voluntary basis. Many communities have a citizen's advocacy board, often organized by parents to help provide this type of service. Alternatively, the local chapters of nonprofit organizations, such as UCPA or the Epilepsy Foundation of America, may offer citizen advocacy. Many of these volunteers have gained a great deal of experience by working with other children with disabilities and can be very effective in obtaining services and providing parents with a sense that the right services are being provided for their child.

The press as advocate.   Newscasters and columnists are often interested in "human interest" stories and can be very effective in helping to obtain services for a child. It is important to provide members of the press with your story in a manner that gives them the facts but also conveys the emotional impact of your situation. It is not a good idea to write a letter to the newspaper that consists solely of a personal attack on those who have thwarted your attempts to get help for your child. Instead, provide a documented history of your phone calls, the responses or lack of responses, and the effect of the problem on your family. Do not lie or exaggerate. Consider whether it is a good idea to include personal names; the better approach is generally to use generic terms, and to identify the person only by a position or title ("a staff member," for example). Let the press know that you are available for a personal interview. Make copies of the letter you send to the press and send them to all the individuals who have been giving you the runaround. Consider writing a letter to the editor of your local newspaper or organizing a group of parents to write to the editor about an issue of broad interest that affects many children or adults with disabilities.

The case manager advocate.   A case manager is usually a trained nurse or social worker who is employed by an agency or an insurance company. State social service agencies may provide a case manager to help a parent negotiate a complicated medical problem. Nonprofit organizations such as UCPA and the Easter Seal Society, as well as many private charities, will also fund case managers to provide these same benefits to the child and the parents. There are also volunteer case managers with specialized training in this area. In order to assess how effective the case manager will be—how strong an advocate he or she will be for your child—you must first know who the case manager's employer is and the reason the case manager was assigned to your child.

Case manager advocates employed by insurance companies are becoming much more popular. These individuals can coordinate care and make sure that resources are used effectively. It is important to remember, however, that these individuals are employed by insurance companies whose underlying goal is to minimize the cost of care and thereby improve the profit margin. In spite of this potential conflict of interest, these individuals can be very helpful to parents, especially in directing them in methods of using the complicated and often fragmented medical care system.

Parents may want to obtain the written standards that describe the case manager's duties. This should be public information if the case manager is a government employee or contractor. Since caseloads are often excessive, case managers may not uniformly offer all services to which the parent may be entitled. If the parent has the policy in hand, he will be able to "prompt" the case manager to offer the entire range of authorized services. The parent may also wish to diplomatically request information on the availability of grievance systems. Almost all social services agencies and insurers have at least internal grievance systems, which may or may not be well advertised. If the case manager knows that the parent is aware of the grievance system, the case manager has an incentive to "aim to please."

Child protection advocates.   The government has a mandate to protect children from harm, including possible harm or neglect caused by parents. All states have child protection laws requiring certain professionals (such as doctors and teachers) and other individuals to report suspected abuse. This suspected abuse is then investigated by child protection advocates who issue a report announcing their findings in the case. A child protection advocate may be assigned to monitor a child over a long period; in this sit-uation, the advocate is usually a court-assigned individual. Such advocates are for the most part dedicated and interested in the child's welfare, and many of them are well-trained professionals with extensive experience. Bud-get concerns in many states have resulted in low pay for these individuals, however, as well as extremely heavy caseloads. In some areas, poorly trained individuals may be working in this capacity.

It's important for parents to understand that if they are involved with child protective service advocates, those advocates will primarily be consid-ering the interests of the child; if there are allegations that the parents have abused the child, then the parents may need their own advocate. This may be one situation in which the parents' attempt to advocate for the child may need to be delegated to a professional.

Overall, federal law is clear on the point that these agencies should at-tempt to prevent unnecessary separation of families. The goal of most child protection advocates is not to remove children from the care of their parents or to punish the parents, but to look out for the child's best interests. Fami-lies should be assertive about asking for support services that will benefit the child within the family unit. One method of guarding the child's best inter-ests is to identify problems or stress areas and help the family deal with these. The goal, whenever possible, is to help the family solve problems and stay together. If parents understand this as the primary goal and accept that the child protection advocate is in fact attempting to look out for the child's best interests, then the alleged problems can often be resolved in a positive way.

Legislative advocate. Industry and large special interest groups have long hired professional lobbyists to advocate for their interests. For people with disabilities, however, the most effective advocacy is usually done by parents whose efforts are directed to members of the legislature. For a par-ent advocate to become an effective legislative advocate, he or she must spend some time learning the system. It is important not to be intimidated by position and titles, since legislators are people like you who are looking to please you and who are often very touched by personal stories. Most people serving in government really *do* want to make life better for the people who elected them and whom they are serving, and you should operate under the assumption that they are interested in helping you.

You may directly contact either a state or a federal legislator and request an appointment or opportunity to speak with him or her. Inviting a legisla-tor to parents' groups, to special school events, or to a camp for children with disabilities may present an opportunity for advocacy in which the par-ents and children don't have to travel to where the legislature meets. And leg-islators often welcome the chance to learn from seeing people in their own environment and to have direct contact with those who make use of the ser-vices of government agencies.

When you approach the legislator, present a specific problem that can be addressed. It is very difficult for a legislator to be helpful when he or she is approached with general anger and frustration and comments such as "Life is hard" and "No one is willing to help." If this is how you feel, you should first work on defusing your anger and focusing your general frustration by talking with other parents or professionals. Try to understand what your specific problems are. Then, when you address your legislator, you can be concise and thereby more effective.

For example, suppose that your insurance company from your place of employment claimed that they would cover the cost of medical goods and orthotics, but when you went to purchase such items you were told they would only cover one pair of braces in the child's lifetime. Naturally, you are frustrated. Upon further investigation you discover that although the insurance company advertised that it would pay for braces, the small print of the contract limited coverage to one pair during the child's lifetime. Such a ploy unfortunately is common. It is clear to everyone that one pair of braces suitable for a child at 2 years of age is not going to last for a lifetime. You may take this specific frustration to your legislator and ask him or her to introduce a bill that would make it illegal for insurance companies to use this type of deceptive advertising. Legislators are likely to be receptive to this type of specific request, and they can, in fact, initiate legislation to bring about a change in the law. This mechanism has been utilized to pass many laws—those providing access to public buildings, preventing discrimination against people with disabilities in the workplace, and providing for special education.

The Partners in Policymaking program originated in 1987 and is now available in almost all states. It is an innovative leadership training program for adults with disabilities and for parents of young children with developmental disabilities. The program trains people to serve as effective advocates, including legislative advocates. There is an on-line course on how to communicate with public officials. An example of recent training topics in one state included the following: (1) local, state, and federal policy and legislative issues; (2) how to meet public officials and give legislative testimony; (3) community organizing; and (4) working with the media. Thus, the skills one needs to advocate effectively with elected officials can be learned through this program or others like it.

Self-advocate. Probably the most effective advocate, especially in the legislative arena, is the self-advocate. Teaching the child, as he grows, to be able to advocate for himself within his capability will provide him with a powerful tool to carry throughout his life. You can begin by teaching your child that he needs to be verbal about his needs and his abilities. For example, an intelligent child with a speech disability needs to be taught that he should be direct with strangers, explaining that having a speech disability does not equal having mental retardation. As children become older and start driving, they can learn to advocate for their rights to disabled parking; and they can advocate for access to public buildings.

Many adults with disabilities find that they have periods in which they grow tired of constantly having to advocate for themselves and for other people with disabilities. But this is almost universally recognized as a necessary part of functioning in society. Teaching children this lesson in a gentle and socially acceptable way is important. An increasing number of programs teach children and young adults with disabilities to be self-advocates. Some DD councils offer such programs, as do local chapters of private agencies, such as UCP. The Partners in Policymaking program mentioned earlier also teaches self-advocacy skills.

What is guardianship? Guardianship is the legal means by which a person is appointed to act on behalf of an individual who is incompetent, and to protect that person. Guardianship is regulated by state law, which varies from state to state. In all states, however, guardianship of a minor child is automatically given to the birth parents until the child is legally considered an adult, at either age 18 or age 21, depending on the state. At the age of adulthood, the person automatically becomes his own guardian unless guardianship is specifically assigned to another person.

An adult needs to have a guardian appointed if he or she is unable to manage financial affairs, make decisions concerning medical care, or direct or plan activities of daily living. Because the birth parents' guardianship is automatically terminated at the age of adulthood, they must petition the court to continue in that role. Even in situations where an adult is obviously unable to participate in or manage his or her own affairs, and guardianship assignment is fairly straightforward, the court must still be petitioned. Specific local mechanisms are different; ask a social service professional or your family lawyer for information about how to proceed.

Often the level of competency of the child or young adult is not clear-cut, and in these situations a guardian should be appointed with care. Appointing a guardian removes significant civil rights from the individual. Although this varies from state to state, guardianship often severely restricts an individual's ability to manage his own money, makes marriage illegal without the consent of the guardian, and eliminates voting rights. For these reasons, the appointment of a guardian in a borderline situation should involve careful consultation with the social service professionals and lawyers familiar with this issue. Because of the serious implications of guardianship, the court often appoints an attorney to represent the individual independently of parents and others.

A person with a mental disability or mild mental retardation does not automatically need guardianship. The issue of mental competence also varies with situations and circumstances and can change over time. States have increasingly recognized that there are gradations of competency, and most states have assigned three levels of competency: full competence, partial competence in specific areas, and complete incompetence. In the past, individuals were considered to be either fully competent or fully incompetent. Now, in situations in which the level of competence is uncertain, a full evaluation by a professional with expertise in this area is strongly recommended.

There are also alternatives to guardianship. For example, in lieu of appointment of a guardian of the property, there are corporate bill-paying services that will, for a small fee, manage a consumer's funds. Another option available in approximately half the states is an AARP-sponsored money management assistance program. States may also offer bill-paying assistance as part of an attendant services program. Finally, if the individual with a disability has the capacity to sign a power of attorney, the individual may appoint a relative or friend to deal with financial matters.

What types of guardianships are there?

There are different types of guardianship in most states, with the major types being either *plenary guardianship,* which involves complete and full control of the individual, or *limited guardianship,* which only applies under specific circumstances. The birth parent is a plenary guardian who can in many situations continue to serve in the same role even after the child has reached the age of maturity.

For individuals who may be able to manage some of their affairs, limited guardianship in specific areas should be considered. Financial and estate guardians are examples of limited guardianships.

A financial guardian may be appointed to help an individual manage his or her funds, which includes paying rent and dispersing income, such as SSI or SSDI payments. A guardianship of the estate is usually appointed for individuals who have significant resources, such as property or income-producing investments. The guardian of the estate is also appointed by the court, which usually requires the guardian to be bonded and to operate under strict rules, limiting the types of investments that may be made to only low-risk investments.

There are also different mechanisms of guardianship (table 8). The most common way for someone to become a guardian is to file a petition. For example, a parent may petition to be named guardian for an adult son or daughter.

Table 8   How Do You Become a Guardian?

By filing a petition with the court asking to be named guardian
By being named guardian in a person's will (testamentary guardian) and having it approved by the court
By being appointed by the court
By assuming collective corporate guardianship
By being appointed by the state as a public guardian

Because of the significant powers a guardian may have, parents may wish to name someone who will become their child's guardian after their death. This provision can be made in the parents' wills, when the parents specify a desired guardian. Court approval will still be needed, but the court will generally defer to the "nomination" of the guardian, though it can reject the recommendation for cause. We suggest that parents give this matter considerable thought and discuss with the proposed guardian the concept of a guardianship and what actions the parents would like to see taken. If a guardian was not named in a parent's will, the court may select a consenting relative, or even an unrelated person or agency as guardian. Because of the potential for a conflict of interest, and because different people have different strengths, parents may wish to consider naming one person as guardian of the individual and another person as guardian of the estate.

The collective corporate guardianship is a mechanism by which a nonprofit organization is established to be guardian of a number of people. This is often set up by parents of individuals with disabilities and allows individuals with limited financial resources to have a financial guardian with some professional training appointed for them. Regional associations for people with mental retardation have established a number of these collective corporate guardianships.

Typically, public guardians are appointed by the state in the event of a parent's or parents' death that leaves the child or incompetent adult without a caretaker. These public guardians are usually social workers or a state or local agency. The individual may reside in a foster home or other supported living arrangement. Public guardians are professional individuals with training who have a keen interest in doing what is best for the person in question; however, they deal with a very large caseload and consequently have extremely limited opportunities to get to know any one individual.

Who will make the best guardian if one is needed?

People who serve as guardians take on a very serious and large responsibility. To handle it well, they need to be personally familiar with the individual they are overseeing, understand the individual's condition and medical problems, understand the individual's family values, and be aware of all special needs. Parents, as long as they are able, usually serve this function best. Because of the large responsibility, if parents are no longer able to be an individual's guardian, it may be better to split guardianship into one guardian for the person and another for the estate, or to use a structure such as a collective corporate guardianship. These concerns need to be discussed with professionals familiar with the family and the individual in need.

What is the role of a guardian?

Guardians can do almost anything for the person with a disability that that person would do for herself, if she could. The plenary guardian exercises full rights for the individual and all of the individual's assets as outlined by the law of the state. Once a guardian is appointed, he or she must file a report with the state at some predetermined frequency. Some states require that guardians be bonded. One of the important areas of guardianship is to give consent for care, education, and medical treatment for the individual over whom they are placed. There are three types of consent.

Direct consent is that consent given by the individual who will be treated. *Substitute consent* is given by the guardian of the individual. *Concurrent consent* is a combination of consent by the guardian and consent by the patient. Professionals may use concurrent consent in a situation in which an individual's mental competency is uncertain or hasn't been determined. For example, when an individual with moderate mental retardation wishes to take birth control pills, the individual may be asked to give her consent, and the parents may also be asked to give their consent, before a prescription is written. If the parent has been given legal guardianship of the individual, then the individual may not give consent but can still give assent. (*Assent* is the legal term by which a person who has been determined to be incompetent by the court or who is not of an age of competency agrees to a treatment or a procedure in addition to the consent of the legal guardian. This approach may also be used for treatment given to teenagers who are not of legal age to give consent, but who are certainly very involved in their own treatment plan.)

Giving consent for medical treatment, especially for surgical procedures, is often a very difficult and serious concern for parents. Guardians of adults have the same concerns, since it may be very difficult to determine what is in the individual's best interests. This is especially true for procedures that involve significant risks or procedures that make significant changes in the person's body.

The courts have placed limitations on a guardian's ability to give consent for another individual, especially in the area of birth control. In general, guardians may not give consent for irreversible birth control methods, such as tubal ligation, removal of ovaries, or hysterectomies, unless that treatment is needed to correct a pathological process and is not being done for birth control purposes only. Guardians *can* give consent for reversible birth control mechanisms such as birth control pills or injections.

What are the caretaking options when parents cannot care for the child at home?

There was a time when placement in an institution such as a nursing home was the only alternative to living at home for disabled children and adults. Today, however, most persons (especially children) with chronic disabilities are not in institutions. The Supreme Court's *Olmstead* decision in 1999 accelerated the movement toward community placements. Based on the Americans with Disabilities Act (ADA) of 1990, this decision mandates that individuals with disabilities live in the most integrated setting that is appropriate for their needs. Under the court's decision, states are required to provide community-based services for persons with disabilities.

Based on this ruling, states have moved to expand home- and community-based services, including small group homes and family support. Funding for community-based service is available to states under the Medicaid home- and community-based services waiver. The waiver, which refers to "waiving" Medicaid's previous requirement of funding care only in institutions, is designed to provide services in the community as an alternative to institutionalization. Typically, the individual must have a qualifying disability, meet a level of care standard, and require certain support services. Such services can include case management, homemaker assistance, home health aides, personal care, respite care, transportation, physical or occupational therapy, and others.

Specific to children is the "Katie Beckett" waiver, adopted by Medicaid programs in most states. Essentially, states have the option of providing Medicaid to children (up to their 19th birthday) with significant disabilities regardless of parental income and resources. Children must meet an SSI standard of disability and level of care standards. The parents can then tap home health, private duty nursing, therapy services, and so on to support the child at home.

Another alternative to institutional placement is placement with another family. This could be placement with extended family members, such as grandparents, or with an adoptive or foster family. In most situations, the parent continues to be the personal guardian, which means that the parent has to give consent for medical treatment, such as surgical procedures. Children who are in foster care may go to the parental home on weekends, holidays, or special occasions, depending on the parent's ability and willingness to be involved. This type of complicated caretaker arrangement needs to be carefully worked out among the various parties, with everyone, including the involved parent, understanding what's involved.

Permanency is the philosophy and practice of securing permanent family placement for all children, including those with special needs. Healthy People 2010 (published by the U.S. Department of Health and Human Services) includes a goal of having no child or young adult (up to age 21) with special health care needs living in congregate or institutional care by 2010. Statistically, the number of children living with grandparents and other non-parent caregivers has been increasing. Federally funded programs are available in all states, which may provide support services to such caregivers.

When it comes to foster care, in addition to legal and financial considerations, there are often significant psychological and emotional implications for the parents. When another family is able to take their child into their home, the parents may feel that they have failed in caring for their own child. This is one of the reasons many parents resist foster care placement and often prefer to see the child placed in a group home or institution. Counseling for the parents may help them understand that foster care placement does not mean that they are failures, but that each person and family has certain strengths. It sometimes helps parents when they recognize that foster care parents are paid a salary, and it is therefore their job to care for children with disabilities.

Are guardianship issues different for adoptive parents than for birth parents?

Adoption is a legal procedure in which an adult becomes a legal parent and has the same relationship to a minor child as do birth parents. The adoption laws with respect to children with disabilities may, however, differ somewhat from the laws pertaining to children without disabilities. Because the laws vary significantly from state to state, we strongly recommend that you consult a general practice lawyer or a professional with expertise in this area if you are considering adopting or have recently become the adoptive parent of a child with a disability.

Prospective adoptive parents and their lawyer need to look into what benefits the child will receive before and after adoption. In the past, it was common for the adopted child, regardless of disability, to be treated exactly as a biological child, so that the parents' income had to be included in all means-testing federal and state programs, such as SSI and Medicaid. ("Means testing" is a system of determining eligibility for financial assistance that is based on parental income and other financial resources.) Because of this law and the costs involved in raising children with disabilities, in the past many children with disabilities were not adopted and remained wards of the state.

The trend in many states recently has been to change the laws so that children with disabilities continue to be eligible for all the programs they were eligible for prior to the adoption, such as SSI and Medicaid, without means testing based on the adoptive parents' income. This area should be investigated and considered prior to going through with an adoption. As noted, because of the laws in some states, it's possible that a person may be better able to provide care for a child with a disability if he or she remains in the foster parent role, rather than becoming an adoptive parent. However, the disadvantage is that the child could be taken out of her foster home by the state agency, even if a strong emotional bond has developed between the child and the foster family, whereas an adopted child is part of her family permanently.

There are also adoption assistance programs, which vary from state to state, whereby individuals are given cash benefits as well as medical assistance and social services when adopting a child with special needs.

For instance, adoptive parents of a special needs child may be eligible for a one-time payment of adoption expenses incurred in connection with adoption of the child, such as attorney fees, court costs, and other expenses directly related to the adoption. A portion of adoption expenses may be tax deductible.

There are also federal and state subsidy programs, in addition to tax incentives, for special needs adoptions. The federal Title IV-E adoption assistance program provides monthly financial assistance to parents of eligible children to help meet any of the child's needs. The automatic Medicaid coverage available through this program is "worth its weight in gold," since medical costs may be extremely burdensome and most private health insurance is oriented toward acute care and not toward treating developmental disabilities. To be eligible for this program, the child needs to have been eligible for SSI before adoption. Adoptive parents do not have to meet any financial eligibility criteria to receive assistance through this program. For children who are not eligible for Title IV-E assistance, there are state adoption subsidy programs. These may cover medical expenses, living expenses, and special or extraordinary expenses incurred by the adopted child. See the Resources section for more information.

How do guardianship concerns relate to foster parents?

There may be an option for a long-term foster parent to obtain complete guardianship of a child. Most foster parents, especially those with short-term placement, are given only custodial rights over the person with a disability; these rights enable them to provide care for the child or older person, usually in conjunction with a state-assigned professional child care worker or child advocate. But, because the role and rights of the foster parent can range from complete guardianship to short-term physical care of the person, the prospective foster parent must fully understand the extent of his or her rights regarding the child's care.

The specific level of responsibility should be put in writing, so that when the child is brought for medical care or other emergencies, health care professionals are aware of the legal custody situation of the child. It is not sufficient for the foster parent to say that he or she has complete guardianship; the foster parent must present a court-authorized document. Like foster parents, older siblings, grandparents, and aunts or uncles who care for a child with CP must obtain guardianship through a court order. Documentation of this order should always be available when guardians other than the birth parents are securing medical care. If children receive most of their medical attention at one facility, a copy of this authorization should be included in the child's medical chart.

Is adult foster care different from foster care of a minor child?

The trend recently has been toward encouraging adult foster care, in which a family takes one or two adults with disabilities into their home and cares for them in the same way that another family does foster children. The issues of guardianship in this situation, however, are not changed from those of other adult situations. What's essential is for the areas of guardianship to be defined and assigned by the court—and then recorded in a legal document.

What other living arrangements are being developed?

The current view is that individuals with disabilities, just like all other people, prefer autonomy and self-directed services. This view is reflected in attendant services programs in which the disabled person is given public funds to hire support workers, who they can then hire and fire. There is also a growing "home of your own" movement in which parents may join to purchase a group home for 3 to 4 adult children with disabilities. The state provides support services but does not own the home.

What other legal concerns do people with cerebral palsy have?

Over the past few decades, laws have been passed that significantly affect people with major disabilities. These laws have for the most part arisen from an increased awareness by the general population that people with disabilities should be incorporated into the community as fully as other citizens. Many laws have been passed regulating the educational setting for children with disabilities, and similar laws have been passed for adults regulating their access to public facilities and preventing discrimination in the workplace.

How do the laws affect education for the child with cerebral palsy?

Although it is hard to believe, until the early 1950s, children with major disabilities were often completely excluded from public education. In the 1950s and 1960s there was a resurgence of interest in establishing special schools that were locally operated exclusively for children with disabilities. Many of these schools were segregated, so that children with visual handicaps, orthopedic handicaps, or major cognitive disabilities, for example, were taught in schools that were separate even from each other. Many of these schools were very large facilities, often understaffed and with few resources. Some of these "schools" were, in fact, full-time boarding institutions, and little education took place there.

This situation was dramatically changed in 1975 with the adoption of Public Law 94-142, also known as the Education for All Handicapped Children Act. This federal law (and state laws that have been patterned after it) is based on the dual principles of inclusion and integration of all children. In terms of inclusion, the law requires that a free and appropriate education be provided for all children, no matter how severe their disabling condition. In terms of integration, the law requires that children with disabilities be educated in settings where they are integrated with children who do not have disabilities to the maximum extent possible. This aspect of the law is known as placing the child in the least restrictive setting and has resulted in removing many children from special schools and returning them to regular classroom education.

The Education for All Handicapped Children Act (renamed the Individuals with Disabilities Education Act) is an extensive and detailed law that defines many of the aspects of the education to which children with cerebral palsy are entitled. (Children with CP are not automatically eligible but must meet specific criteria.) The law sets age limits for children who must receive educational services; it defines which services the children must receive; it defines a specific mechanism by which this program must be carried out, including evaluations and written responses of which the parent must be aware (the Individualized Education Program, or IEP); and it states what related services are required. There are also specific mechanisms for resolving conflicts between parents and professionals, or between professionals who hold differing views. The full details of this act are discussed in Chapter 11.

What laws apply to adults with cerebral palsy?

For adults, the workplace replaces the school as the main setting in which a person interacts with others and society in general. Just as children with disabilities formerly were segregated in the school setting, historically people with disabilities were almost entirely excluded from employment opportunities. Congress took the lead in prohibiting job discrimination against persons with disabilities with the passage of Section 504 of the Rehabilitation Act of 1973, which makes it illegal for agencies and institutions that receive federal funding to discriminate against persons with disabilities. After extensive publicity and lobbying by numerous advocacy groups for individuals with disabilities, the job-related rights of these people were greatly expanded with passage in 1990 of the Americans with Disabilities Act (ADA) (table 9).

The employer cannot discriminate even in its advertisements. For example, an employer may not advertise for "able-bodied" persons. Moreover, the employer may be required to provide accommodations in the interview and assessment process. For example, if a typing test were required for a secretarial position and an applicant asked to use his adaptive keyboard, this would be a reasonable accommodation. The employer could not insist that the applicant use the standard keyboard used by all other applicants. While in general terms, the laws relating to the workplace are primarily composed of commands telling the employer what it *may not* do, there are exceptions. For instance, Section 503 of the Rehabilitation Act includes an affirmative action obligation for employers with contracts with the federal government of $10,000 or more. It requires that such companies contracting with the government "shall take affirmative action to employ and advance in employment qualified individuals with disabilities." Many large employers have such contracts, and persons with disabilities may wish to focus efforts on soliciting employment with such firms.

What specific restrictions are provided for by the Americans with Disabilities Act?

Part of the Americans with Disabilities Act incorporates concepts from Section 504 of the Rehabilitation Act and specifically prohibits employment discrimination against qualified people with disabilities in federally funded

Table 9   *Features of the Americans with Disabilities Act*

An employer must assess an individual with a disability applying for a job by the same criteria used to evaluate an individual without a disability

An employer must make reasonable accommodation for the hired person

Employers must provide access to all public places

There can be no discrimination in public accommodations against persons with disabilities by employers or businesses, or in public buildings

Life and health insurance companies cannot deny coverage based on an individual's or a family member's disability programs. Specifically, the act states that "no otherwise qualified individual with disabilities in the United States shall solely by reason of his disability be excluded from the participation in, be denied the benefits of, or be subjected to discrimination under any program or activity receiving federal financial assistance." Disabilities are fairly widely defined as any limits an individual has that impact on his or her "major life activities"—which include caring for himself or herself, or performing tasks such as walking, seeing, hearing, speaking, breathing, or learning.

The Americans with Disabilities Act extended this prohibition against discrimination to all private and public employers, though this was later modified by the U.S. Supreme Court. The court decided in the Garrett decision in 2001 that state employees who sue their employer in federal court cannot receive monetary damages under the ADA. They also decided in a different case that the assessment of whether a person has a qualifying disability is undertaken with full consideration of ameliorating supports (like taking medicine or using an assistive device). Thus, if a person uses such a device and therefore is no longer limited in a major life activity, they would no longer be eligible as a person with a disability under the ADA.

The law states that "no employer shall discriminate against a qualified individual with a disability because of the disability of such individual in regard to job application procedures, the hiring or discharge of employees, employee compensation, advancement, job training, and other terms, conditions, and privileges of employment." In other words, the employer must appraise an individual with a disability who is applying for a job using the same criteria that would be used to appraise an individual without a disability. The employer is required to make reasonable accommodation for the person with a disability who is qualified for the job. This "reasonable accommodation" has been interpreted to mean removing job obstacles that would prevent the otherwise qualified person with a disability from working. This may mean removing physical obstacles, providing for movement in the workplace, modifying equipment so that it can be used by a person with a disability, and restructuring the job setting and schedules as well as training and policies to accommodate the person's disability. Failing to make these accommodations is a violation of the law; however, the employer is not required to hire the person with a disability if doing so would impose "undue hardship" on the employer. Undue hardship is determined based on the net cost to the employer. An employer should determine whether funding is available from an outside source, such as a state rehabilitation agency, to help pay for all or part of the accommodation. In addition, employers should determine whether they are eligible for certain tax credits or deductions to offset the cost of the accommodations.

Another part of the ADA provides access to all public places by prohibiting discrimination against people with disabilities. This means that all forms of public transportation, such as trains, subways, and city buses, must gradually become accessible to those with disabilities. This means "phasing in" accessible buses, etc., though there are still some older vehicles that may not be accessible. Architectural barriers such as stairs in buildings and narrow doors must also be removed or bypassed to the maximum extent feasible, and all new buildings and facilities must be constructed without these physical limitations. This aspect of the ADA also applies to private companies providing transportation services, such as bus companies, airlines, and taxi companies.

Another important aspect of the ADA is its prohibition of all discrimination in public accommodations against people with disabilities. This applies to almost every business or place frequented by the public, including restaurants, bars, theaters, stadiums, concert halls, hotels, inns, bakeries, grocery stores, gas stations, professional offices such as those of doctors and lawyers, bus and airport terminals, libraries, galleries, and physical exercising facilities, such as gyms and bowling alleys. Businesses are required to make reasonable accommodations, for example by making doorways passable for someone in a wheelchair. Again, the law allows the business to plead unreasonable cost and thereby avoid making the structural changes necessary to provide access. Nevertheless, this aspect of the ADA should provide greater overall access and freedom of movement and opportunity for people with cerebral palsy to move in the public sector.

How does the ADA affect life or health insurance?

Another part of the ADA prohibits discrimination by life and health insurance companies, which are not permitted to deny coverage based on an individual's or a family member's disability. The practical effect of this provision, however, is uncertain because it continues to allow insurance companies to deny coverage if the denial is based on "sound actuarial principles" or "reasonable anticipated experience." This means that an insurance company is not allowed to reject an applicant for insurance based on the disability; however, it may reject the applicant based on experience which shows that a similar person utilizes more services than the average person applying for insurance. Because of this uncertainty, many individuals and families find it very difficult to obtain life or health insurance unless it is in the context of a mandated group plan through employment. Some states are attempting to further tighten the prohibitions against discrimination by insurance companies with respect to people with disabilities.

Can someone with cerebral palsy get a driver's license?

For individuals who are able, one of the major opportunities for developing independence is the ability to drive a motor vehicle. The individual state laws regarding the specific driving requirements for persons with disabilities vary widely, but all have four general rules. *First,* the individual's eyesight must be good enough to allow him or her to read road signs. The level of corrected vision must be well defined and documented before a person can obtain a driver's license. *Second,* individuals with a physical disability must document their ability to manage the controls of the vehicle they plan to drive. All states provide for limited licenses that prescribe modifications to the vehicle the individual will drive (hand controls and specific mirrors are examples). Some automobile companies or dealers will modify a vehicle to make it possible for the person with a disability to drive. *Third,* individuals must have sufficient cognitive function to be able to understand the laws, to read signs, and to be able to plan and understand the use of a motor vehicle. *Fourth,* all states have specific laws regulating the circumstances under which a person with seizures may obtain a driver's license. These laws vary widely, so if you have seizures, you'll need to obtain a copy of the law in your state before proceeding. Some states require doctors to report all seizures in a patient with a driver's license. If the patient has well-controlled seizures, the state will issue a driver's license. The individual needs to work with the state licensing board and the physician treating the seizures.

All states have special driver's education classes in which a person's individual disability is evaluated and driver's training is given in a specifically modified vehicle. The trained driving instructor then assesses whether the individual is skillful enough to continue with the training. A license is usually only granted after the person has demonstrated driving competence for a state officer. Special education specialists or vocational rehabilitation professionals can provide further information about driver's education classes for people with special needs.

What are the legal provisions for financial care for a person with cerebral palsy?

All parents must consider the subject of providing financial protection for their dependent children, but financial considerations for parents who have a child with cerebral palsy may be more complicated than those for parents of a child without a disability. It is crucial for these parents to consult a professional who has a strong background in financial planning, accounting, and law, and who understands how these areas apply to the family's specific situation. In planning both for the family's financial security and for the financial care of the child, many areas should be examined, such as family assets, expected retirement income, the appropriate amount of life and disability insurance, and the amount of federal funds for which an individual is eligible.

The last area—identifying and obtaining federal funds—is complex, and parents should certainly obtain professional advice and assistance from a financial adviser and an attorney. We will briefly describe several of the federal programs administered by the Social Security Administration below. Also see Chapter 10, "Financing Care for the Child with Cerebral Palsy."

When is an individual with cerebral palsy eligible for Social Security and Medicare?

If an employed person becomes disabled, he is eligible for disability insurance, and his spouse and children are also eligible for SSDI. Eligibility for Social Security Disability Insurance (SSDI) is determined by the amount of the individual's prior Social Security contribution and by the length of service of the employed person. Those eligible for SSDI are the spouse, minor children, and adult children whose disability occurred before age 22. Those eligible for survivor's insurance include the same group: widow or widower, minor children, and adult children whose disability occurred before age 22. The benefit received (either by the adult or the child with a disability) is not determined by assets or income level, but is determined solely on the basis of whether the person has met the federal standard for disability. The National Organization of Social Security Claimants Representatives (NOSSCR) is an organization comprised of attorneys who specialize in Social Security. It provides a resource to persons seeking expert assistance on Social Security issues.

Medicare is a medical insurance program that uses the same criteria for eligibility as SSDI. Minor children of workers who have paid into the Social Security system, as well as adult children whose disability occurred before age 22, are eligible for Medicare. This health insurance is for acute health management, but also covers costs of wheelchairs and other assistive technology. Recent amendments have now added a drug benefit as well.

The other major federal program administered by the Social Security Administration is Supplemental Security Income (SSI), which is available to individuals based on their financial need. SSI is available to children with significant disabilities if their parents' income and resources are low enough. SSI benefits can be paid even to parents of infants and toddlers. Some individuals start receiving SSI at age 18 because the law stops "imputing" parental income and resources to a person once he turns 18. In other words, children of "poor" parents may receive SSI from an early age. Children of more affluent parents will probably not qualify (due to deeming of parental income and resources) until their 18th birthday. If the beneficiary is over the countable resource limit (generally $2,000), he is simply not eligible for SSI. Certain types of homes, household furniture, and clothing are excluded, up to certain limits, from the calculation of a person's assets.

There are many provisions for how assets and the living situation are considered. For example, SSI benefits are generally reduced by one-third if the person lives with someone else. Also, SSI benefits are reduced to a minimal amount, if the person lives in a facility paid for by Medicaid, the medical insurance program associated with SSI. The benefit amount is also affected (and may be reduced) by countable income.

The rules of eligibility for Medicaid are generally similar to those for SSI. The major benefit of Medicaid is that, in addition to acute health care, it provides for long-term chronic care. Medicaid will pay ongoing long-term nursing home or institutional placement care for an individual.

In addition to these federal programs, there may be other programs administered by other federal agencies, such as the Bureau of Indian Affairs and Armed Forces Retirement Benefits programs, as well as Private Pension Survivor's Benefits, which need to be investigated. Any and all appropriate assistance for which a person is eligible should be pursued.

Do parents of children with cerebral palsy need wills?

In addition to considering the issues of guardianship and financial planning, parents should also provide for the distribution of their estate, whether they have children with cerebral palsy or not. If parents die intestate—without a will—the estate will be distributed as required by the state code. If parents want to make specific provisions for their child with disabilities which are different from those for any of their children without disabilities, they can only do this through a will. Parents should seriously consider how they want to divide funds between healthy children and children with disabilities so that the child with a severe disability will be protected. A special needs trust or a group trust is often the best way.

Under certain circumstances, it may be necessary to consider disinheriting a child with a disability (discussed in detail below). This may be the best provision for the whole family, because it allows the state to assume responsibility for the child's care. This is certainly a very important consideration in future financial planning, and especially in preparing a will where the needs of the whole family are considered and not just those of the individual with the disability. Because of the complexity of the circumstances, it is advisable to consult an expert in the field of estate planning for people with disabilities.

For parents of a child with cerebral palsy, what considerations are important in drawing up a will?

If the extent of the disability or the age of the child is such that the parents are complete guardians of the child, then they should state whom they wish to have as the ongoing guardian of the minor child over whom they have guardianship. This is called *assigning a testamentary guardian*. The guardian named in the parents' will must also be formally appointed by the courts. Courts usually give great weight to the parents' choice of guardian as stated in their will, and often the testamentary guardian named in the will is appointed by the court to be guardian. When making these provisions, parents should seriously consider the different levels and types of guardianship that are most appropriate. This part of the will must be reviewed periodically, since individuals and their circumstances change over time. These provisions of testamentary guardianship are true for both minor children and for adults over whom an individual holds guardianship.

What are the advantages of disinheriting a child with a severe disability?

Though it sounds cruel, there are several reasons why disinheriting the child with a disability might be in the child's best financial interests. A child with a severe disability, especially one who also requires guardianship, usually is eligible for all the means-tested government programs such as SSI and Medicaid. As soon as this individual acquires a certain level of assets or income, these means-tested program benefits are reduced as the government's way of allocating scarce resources to those most in need. This means that it will simply be used to replace government benefits. In essence, when the child receives the inheritance, his government benefits will be cut off until all the inheritance is spent, at which time the benefits will begin again. This has the same net result as if all the inheritance were given to the government and the means-tested benefits to the individual were continued. Therefore, instead of allowing the individual with a disability to inherit equally and by the same unrestricted mechanism that a child without disabilities inherits, a parent may consider several other options, including completely disinheriting the child, establishing a trust fund with specific allocations of how the money may be spent, or leaving the child a significantly reduced sum at a level that will not diminish the means-tested government benefit.

Another possible reason to disinherit your child is that the guardianship requirements change significantly for a person with a disability to the point where the state often requires a guardian of the estate to be bonded. This increases the cost to the assets of the incompetent person, and if those assets are not very large, they will quickly be depleted. Another consideration is that if individuals who are incompetent or only marginally competent inherit funds, this often makes them targets of unscrupulous people who will try to take advantage of them. Providing the funds in the context of a trust fund may, in fact, be a better method of protecting the individual.

Finally, most states do not allow an incompetent person to make a will, which means that the estate of this person upon his or her death will be distributed according to state laws. Although a competent person can bequeath assets to a specific charity or to specific persons, an incompetent individual cannot.

All the above are reasons you might consider for disinheriting a person with a disability, but before taking this step it should be carefully discussed with lawyers, accountants, and financial advisers familiar with this area of planning.

What are the disadvantages of disinheriting the child with a severe disability?

It is important to consider the feelings of the person with a disability. The concept of disinheritance may make the individual feel unloved or uncared for. This feeling may be prevented by bequesting the person an amount that will not have an impact on means-tested income. Parents may also wish to explain the reasons for the specific inheritance and to include with the will letters that express love and concern and explain the special care that the person will receive.

What is a trust?

Trusts hold money or property that the grantor (the person who sets up the trust) leaves for the beneficiary's economic benefit. Unlike an outright gift or inheritance through a will, trusts usually contain carefully written instructions on when and how to use the trust's contents. Parents (or others) can set up a trust while they are alive or as part of a will. If parents set up a trust while still alive, they can be the trustees (the persons who manage the trust). They can also assign someone else to be the trustee. A trustee can be a person or a financial institution.

There are many different types of trusts that serve different purposes. Laws that affect trusts differ from state to state. An attorney who specializes in special needs trusts should be consulted in developing a trust in this context. For example, each state may have separate standards that determine whether a trust is a "Medicaid qualifying trust" so as to authorize disregard of income and principal. These standards may be quite complex.

What kind of trusts are most commonly used for children with special needs?

Most states offer some form of supplemental, discretionary, or cooperative master trust. These are the types of trusts usually recommended when parents want to protect their child's governmental benefits.

Supplemental trusts.   These are designed so that the principal and its earnings supplement the beneficiary's care but do not replace the funds required to pay for this care. This kind of trust is good for the recipient of SSI and Medicaid whose assets cannot exceed certain levels. The trust grantor can carefully direct the trust not to replace the cost of services covered by Medicaid. Instead, the trust would require the trustee to only provide funds for certain items, services, or expenses not covered by SSI or Medicaid. As an example, a supplementary trust could be established providing income that allows a certain individual to spend money on entertainment, such as going to the movies, traveling to visit friends and relatives, and purchasing small gifts for loved ones. Because this money is restricted to specific uses, the income from such a trust, if it is not too large, will not be considered as income in a means-tested program. Because the principal of the trust is not an asset of the individual beneficiary, it also cannot be considered in means testing for federally funded programs.

Discretionary trusts.   Some states allow the grantor to give the trustee full discretion in how much or how little of the trust to distribute. This kind of trust can also contain provisions that limit distributions so that the person remains eligible for government benefits. The trustee must be very careful not to distribute money from the trust for goods and services or outright to the beneficiary in a manner that will disqualify the beneficiary from receiving government benefits. There are drawbacks to this kind of trust. The trustee must be very knowledgeable about the type of benefits a person is receiving and the related eligibility requirements. Also, the trustee has total power over distribution of funds and may hold back trust distributions to the detriment of the beneficiary.

Some other potential dangers exist in establishing a trust in which the trustee is given full discretion on how to spend the funds. For example, the government may attempt, through legislation or the courts, to direct the trustee to fund or reimburse public outlays such as Medicaid, or count the full amount available for trustee disposition as a resource. The problem is that a trust established under today's legal standards must anticipate changes in the law 20 to 40 or more years from now. It has been suggested that an "in terrorem" provision be inserted in trusts such that, if the government successfully "breaks/invades" the trust, the principal and proceeds revert to other relatives. This would be a disincentive to the government trying to "break/invade" the trust.

Master cooperative trust.   Also called "pooled trusts," these are special trusts established and managed by a nonprofit organization and created to help disabled individuals and their families. Instead of setting up an individual trust account, these types of trusts allow families to pool their resources with other families. A group trust allows a parent to fund a trust for a child without affecting eligibility for public benefits, while specifying support services and allowable uses. Such trusts are available in many states. Because the funds are pooled, the potential for higher returns is enhanced. Another advantage of this form of trust is that individual parents may lack sufficient funds to meet minimum requirements of a commercial financial institution, but can do so by pooling their funds with other parents. The group trusts often have lower minimum trust amounts. In addition, because the pooled account is usually managed and invested as one large account, administrative fees are less. Beneficiaries of these trusts usually receive earnings based on their share of the principal.

How do I set up a trust?   There are basically two ways to set up a trust: It can be testamentary (as part of a will) or inter vivos (living).

A testamentary trust is part of a will and does not take effect until after the person who drew up the will dies. Such a trust could be funded by life insurance proceeds, which do not normally pass through the will. This is a way to fund a fairly large trust if a parent lacks significant assets to leave through a will. Parents can change the trust's terms any time the will is changed. So if the intended beneficiary should die first, the will and trust can be changed.

A living will means the person sets up a trust before dying. In doing so, parents and others can make regular gifts to such a trust. Grandparents could make testamentary bequests from their will to such a trust. Parents can be the trustee and manage it at their own discretion, or they could assign someone else to be trustee to see how that person would manage the trust. Living trusts are either revocable or irrevocable. A revocable trust can be changed or ended by parents before they die. With an irrevocable trust, parents set up the trust and give up most power to change or end it. Each way has different tax advantages, depending on the size of the parents' estate, family situation, and other factors. Remember to consult with an attorney who specializes in special needs trusts.

What happens when the beneficiary dies?

The trust must spell out what happens to the trust when the primary beneficiary dies. For example, a $50,000 trust may be established, with a specific bank as the trustee, with instructions to distribute income to a child with a disability as the beneficiary. The beneficiary may use this income for a specifically defined purpose as listed in the will. When the beneficiary dies, the trust may provide that the money will be divided among relatives of the beneficiary or the grantor. In this way, parents are setting aside money that benefits the child with a disability and that is then passed on to their other children or grandchildren, for example, upon the death of their child with a disability.

In establishing a trust, it is important to consider who will be the trustee. A large trust should probably have a corporate trustee, usually a bank. Although an individual trustee can be established, many states require a bond in those circumstances. The trust may also be established as a mandatory trust that requires the trustee to pay a fixed amount of money to the beneficiary at predetermined intervals.

How do I obtain legal help to collect damages from an injury that may be the cause of my child's cerebral palsy?

It is your legal right to bring a lawsuit to collect for damages due to medical malpractice or other injuries that the child incurred because of the actions of someone else. There are many scenarios in which injuries to children occur, such as falls, near-drownings, smoke inhalation, overdosages of a substance, or adverse effects of drugs or surgery before, during, or after birth, which may cause cerebral palsy and permanent disability. Injury during birth as a cause of cerebral palsy has been a major concern for many years, but is now understood to be a cause in only a small percentage of cases of cerebral palsy.

There are lawyers whose specialty is evaluating injuries and preparing suits for medical malpractice. The best reference for finding such a lawyer is usually your family lawyer or a general practice lawyer. Also, bar associations, referral services, or parent groups may be good sources for recommendations. A competent lawyer will evaluate the evidence and then discuss with you whether he or she feels there is legal evidence sufficient to pursue a malpractice claim. These lawyers usually work on a contingency fee, which means that they will receive a specific percentage, varying from 25 to 50 percent, of the amount recovered. Therefore, they will probably tell you if they feel you do not have a good case, because they do not want to spend their time and money unnecessarily. Some attorneys will ask the parents to pay their out-of-pocket expenses.

If my child has cerebral palsy due to a birth injury, doesn't that mean that I am entitled to a malpractice insurance settlement?

Medical malpractice, especially with respect to a birth injury, may be very difficult to prove. A malpractice claim requires proof that the medical care your child received was in some way below the ordinary standard of care in the community. The occurrence of even significant injury in the course of medical treatment does not automatically establish that malpractice has occurred if that medical treatment is deemed to meet the community standard of practice.

In addition, there must be harm or damage suffered by the individual as a direct result of this deficient practice. As an example, if your child was accidentally given a drug dose that was ten times higher than the recommended amount, this clearly falls below the community standard of practice. However, if this error did not lead to any harm or damage to your child, then there may be no malpractice recovery.

Just because your child has cerebral palsy does not mean that there has been some kind of medical negligence. Most children have cerebral palsy because of damage suffered in their mother's womb unrelated to any issues of medical care. On the other hand, there are certainly incidents where inadequate medical care during pregnancy, delivery, or shortly afterwards was responsible for the child's cerebral palsy. For most children, cerebral palsy caused by such injuries does not become apparent until the child is at least 6 months old.

What's the best thing to do with a large settlement resulting from a malpractice lawsuit?

It is often a good idea to place large settlements from medical malpractice lawsuits into a trust fund for the child. Sometimes the trustee can be the parent, but often the trustee is a corporate entity, such as a bank. The court may define how the trust is to be used—say, for medical care or perhaps setting aside a specific amount for housing. Spending money from the trust for certain items, such as specially modified vans, is usually allowed. Parents may receive a certain amount every month to help them care for the child.

Another, more simple option for protecting funds from a malpractice case is an annuity. This is an insurance policy that can be structured to pay out at varying amounts over the course of the child's life with the principal to be distributed to designated persons in the event of the child's death. Because annuities generally earn tax-free interest, they can grow substantially during the early years when needed payments may be small. Then by the time the child requires greater funding for housing or supportive services, the annuity can be structured to pay out at a higher level. The terms of an annuity are usually determined by the parents and the attorneys involved. The earlier information on structuring funds so as to not displace public program (SSI, Medicaid) eligibility applies here as well. Malpractice attorneys are sometimes not expert in this context and may need to consult colleagues who specialize in this field to structure the settlement in a way most beneficial to the injured child.

Are there special programs that pay damages for medically caused injuries?

Some states, such as Florida, have established birth injury programs in which benefits may be obtained outside of the malpractice legal system. The federal government has also established a program for children sustaining injuries due to vaccinations in which the insurer is the federal government.

Benefits are paid out of this program if it is shown that the immunization caused the child's injury without having to go through a lawsuit.

How can I use the law to help my family member who has a disability?

The legal system exists to provide protection for individuals, including people with disabilities. Recent legal developments have provided much more opportunity for individuals with disabilities. To take advantage of this new legal and social climate, it is important to be an advocate for yourself and for the individual with a disability. Part of this advocacy work involves lobbying your state and national legislators so that the ability of the person with a disability to participate in society will continue to expand.

Being an able advocate also means educating yourself and others about both the specifics of the law and the arrangements for obtaining help from professionals. It is this combination of understanding the individual's rights and legal standing and understanding how to contact the appropriate professionals which allows the individual with the disability to take full advantage of the legal system.

Part Two

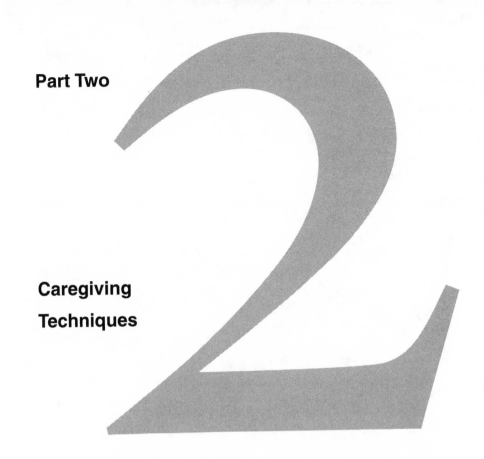

**Caregiving
Techniques**

Taking Care of Yourself When You Care for Others

Taking care of any child requires a good deal of work, time, and patience, and taking care of a child with special needs requires an abundance of all three. Oftentimes, parents feel overworked and frustrated, and they are concerned and distracted by the emotional and financial burdens that affect them as they raise a child with cerebral palsy.

STRESSORS

Beginning with the birth of the child, and sometimes even before, parents have periods of anxiety and a great deal of uncertainty. Parents and other caregivers are faced with finding answers to questions that can't always be answered. They will often need to make important decisions quickly, since conditions can change swiftly. They must find professionals who can meet their child's needs—and can communicate with the family. This process, as well as the many other things caregivers do, requires lots of time and effort.

Depression is a very common result of dealing with a child with disabilities. It can manifest itself in sleeplessness, over- or undereating, impatience, irritability, anger, or a profound sense of sadness. The physical health of caregivers is also at risk because caring for their children presents such heavy demands. Lifting children who have grown into adults can pose a tremendous physical strain, for example. Some parents find the needs of the child so overwhelming that they neglect their own health, either because it seems insignificant or because it is too costly to eat well and to get proper rest and respite from caregiving responsibilities.

Marital discord often results from the enormous stress of having a child with disabilities. Many feelings—including guilt, fear, anger, and anxiety—can cause people to lash out at each other. Sometimes a parent finds it difficult even to get in touch with personal feelings, because the day-to-day activities of caring for a child with special needs while simultaneously holding down a job and caring for the rest of the family are overwhelming.

It's not uncommon, either, for different parents to react differently to the child's problem: one may become outwardly overemotional, while the other withdraws and even appears uninterested. Partners often discover that they have less time for each other or seemingly less interest in the relationship than they used to. A single parent might not have this type of conflict, but he or she will then have to make decisions alone, which is also stressful.

Siblings are often affected by the extra needs that a child with disabilities presents to the family unit. Jealousy and attention-seeking behavior are common ways in which siblings try to make sense of the situation. Additionally, brothers and sisters may have difficulty dealing with their peers' reactions to their sister or brother who has a disability. Guilt can also be a formidable feeling in a child who is able to run, jump, and skate while his older brother is unable to walk. On the other hand, most children cope pretty well with life's surprises, as one little girl named Colleen shows in her story, called "A Special Sister":

All my life I wanted to have a sister! I imagined her to be my best friend. I always wanted to have somebody there when I needed them. I wanted somebody to hug, to laugh with, and to be myself with. I wanted a special closeness with my sister. Kind of like we always had a secret together. A sister would be with me all my life.

My dream came true!!! I did get a baby sister. Her name is Kathleen. She fooled us all by being born on April first. I was so happy my insides were jumping all around. I made a big colorful picture for her to look at in her crib.

When I held her for the first time I felt my heart melt because we loved each other so much!

In a short time we found out that Kathleen has cerebral palsy. It's only on her right side. Her arm and leg don't work too well. So we do therapy with her! I am learning a lot about how our body works so I will be able to help her! She and I work well together. She listens to me, so I listen to her. And that's the way it will be all our lives.

Kathleen is more special than I ever thought she could be. I hug her, I laugh with her, and we already have secrets together! She is very special!!

As a child with a disability grows, parents need to deal not only with the increased time commitment necessary to care for the child but also with whatever prognosis the doctor has provided. Needless to say, the other responsibilities of running a household coexist with these special responsibilities. Parents may find themselves making a multitude of visits to different physicians and therapists, and spending untold time and money.

Children frequently need surgical procedures that require a parent to spend increasing amounts of time away from family and job, and that can make life very difficult. Additionally, the financial cost of purchasing wheelchairs, braces, and various other equipment can be staggering.

HOW TO COPE

All parents have dreams for their children. Some children with mild disabilities are able to live normal lives. However, there are many children whose parents must accept that they will never walk and may never be able to feed themselves or speak. It is therefore essential that caregivers—be they mothers, fathers, grandparents, siblings, or unrelated individuals—recognize their stressors and develop and maintain coping mechanisms. They must learn, for example, to ask for advice and help, and they must come to terms with the fact that not all of their child's needs can be met. Other parents who are now or who have been in a similar situation can be of great comfort and help. Often they can provide more assistance than well-meaning friends and relatives who don't have any experience in this area.

Caregivers need to be in tune with their feelings and be on guard for signs that they might need some help maintaining their own emotional health. Parents need to communicate with each other and with health care professionals as much as possible, so that decisions are based on their true feelings. Couples need to be aware of the stress on their relationship and then avail themselves of opportunities for help. They may simply need to set aside more time for talking, or they may want to arrange for special times alone with each other. Marriage counseling can often be very helpful for couples who are having trouble coping with stress of various kinds.

Caregivers must acknowledge that they cannot be effective caregivers unless they take care of themselves. They must learn to be in touch with their needs and seek out the resources to have those needs addressed. "Resources" come in many shapes and sizes. You may develop a pool of friends who can provide respite, some time for yourself without the children. To reduce the time and strain of numerous appointments and errands, you can coordinate appointments and, if possible, obtain many services at the same facility. The various Ronald McDonald houses throughout the country are a wonderful resource for families needing to travel away from home for specialized treatment or surgery. Mini-vacations, even a day trip to the country, can provide an enormous amount of relief. You also need to cultivate individual stress-reducing techniques, such as exercise, reading, hobbies, or prayer. Religious institutions and community groups may have support groups. Finally, you may want to find a support group. There are professionals who can help guide you to an appropriate support group depending on your needs.

In some cases you may need to place your child in a group home or a similar facility, so the major responsibility for care is put in the hands of people who are able to handle the nuances of nurturing a child with a disability. This is particularly true as caregivers grow older, or if siblings are being neglected or otherwise suffering from the experience. Ultimately, the caregiver needs to care for himself or herself in order to be able to continue to care for another person.

Protecting the Caregiver's Back: Basic Body Mechanics

Many tasks in caring for a child may place the care provider's back at risk for injury. Most of these tasks involve performing the activities of daily care such as dressing, bathing, feeding, and moving the child. This section describes good body mechanics that can be used by the care provider to decrease the risk of back injury.

DRESSING

Newborn to age 3. Use a surface that is at a comfortable working level, such as a changing table. The parent should not be forced to lean over the surface in order to dress the child. At this age the crib surface should also be at a comfortable level (keeping in mind that the mattress must be lowered when it is anticipated that a child will soon be standing up), and the crib mattress may provide a good surface for dressing the child.

Ages 3 to 10. If the child is able to, he ought to be encouraged to stand up and hold on to furniture while being dressed. This is good therapy and movement toward an adult style of dressing and allows the child to be dressed with less lifting than is done when the child is dressed lying down. If the child must be dressed lying down, and the child's bed is used for dressing, then the mattress surface should be at a comfortable level for the parents to work. This can easily be achieved by placing the bed on blocks, but care must be taken to use side rails so that the child does not fall out of a high bed. If the bed is on the floor, the caregiver ought to place one or both knees on the floor rather than bend over from the back.

The older child and teenager. The same rules apply, but at this age, because of the child's larger size, it is especially important to dress her while she is standing if at all possible.

BATHING

Bathing is an activity that can involve a great deal of lifting and bending over in positions that can be very stressful to the caregiver's back. Before bathing a young child on a changing table, the caregiver should adjust the level of the table to the level of the caregiver's mid-abdomen. Children from age 2 to age 10 especially enjoy being bathed in warm water and are usually bathed in a bathtub. There are several different kinds of bathing chairs that provide trunk support for the child who has poor trunk control; an occupational therapist can help you select one that is appropriate for your child.

The main problem in tub bathing for caregivers, however, is lifting the child into the bathtub. Before he reaches about age 10 this may be difficult but can still be managed. After age 10, it becomes more difficult. Whenever possible, the child should be lifted or helped into the tub in a standing position; then he can sit down from the standing position. This is much easier for the caregiver. Also, if the caregiver sits on the edge of the bathtub with one foot in the tub before lifting the child, this reduces the stress on the caregiver's back. For the child who can stand, use a shower with a hand rail for him to hold on to. This is an excellent way to bathe an older child who can stand.

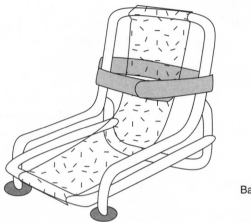

Bath chair

As the child approaches puberty and adult height, it is no longer wise to continue to lift her into a bathtub. This is hard on the caregiver's back and usually is unsafe for the child, because there is an increased risk that the caregiver will slip and drop the child when she is heavier. If she will continue to be bathed in a bathtub, a mechanical lift device that attaches to the bathtub or the ceiling should be used. Or she can be wheeled into a shower if the proper home modifications are made. There are a number of different shower chair alternatives. Ask your child's occupational therapist to evaluate her and determine the best way for her to be bathed—that is, the best way for the child, the care provider, and the housing situation.

MOVING

The small infant and child is primarily moved about his environment by being carried. As the child grows but does not begin to walk, caregivers must begin to protect their backs and not simply continue to carry the child until they are physically unable to do so. This requires planning for a home environment that is accessible to a wheelchair; planning should take place when the child is between the ages of 4 and 8. Another option is to use a rolling stool and push yourself, with the child on your lap, along the floor; alternatively, if the child can hold on securely to the stool, he may be pushed along alone. This will only work if the house is not carpeted, however.

As the child gets larger, transferring from bed to wheelchair becomes difficult. If he may be capable of bearing his own weight so that standing transfers can take place, this needs to be encouraged even at the age when the child is still small enough to be lifted. If you wait to start doing standing transfers until he absolutely cannot be lifted, then it's harder for both the child and the caregiver to learn the technique, and it's much more anxiety provoking. Both of these factors make it more likely that attempts to learn the technique will be unsuccessful. If a child cannot bear weight and is to be cared for by one adult alone, then mechanical lifts are usually needed to improve the safety of the transfers and to protect the caregiver's back.

FEEDING

Most infants are fed while being held by the caregiver. By 9 to 12 months, however, the child should be fed while sitting in a seat, with the caregiver doing the feeding sitting in front of the child. This frees both arms and allows the caregiver to position herself at a comfortable height and have an easier view of how the child is doing.

GENERAL GUIDELINES FOR PROTECTING YOUR BACK

1. Always get your body as close to the child to be lifted as possible before starting to lift.

2. Whenever possible lift by bending the knees, not by bending through the back.

3. When working standing up, adjust the work surface and the child so that he is at the level of your navel (mid-abdomen), so that you don't bend over while bathing or dressing him.

4. If you are working with a child sitting (such as feeding a child), the child's face should be almost even with yours when you sit up straight. This prevents you from slouching over and putting strain on your spine.

Making Things Easier for You and Your Child: Home Modifications

There are various ways to modify the home environment so that your child will have more independence and things will be easier on you. The cost of these modifications varies from being inexpensive to very costly. The desired modifications may involve more available space and current resources than the caregiver has, however.

Any modification must be consistent with the cognitive level of the individual for whom it is planned. In the case of individuals with significant mental retardation, the ability to be more independent in the home could remove a barrier that is a potentially useful safety net. In other words, it is undesirable to modify the home in a way that would allow the person more freedom of movement if the person might inadvertently hurt himself or herself. Therefore any suggestions must be evaluated in terms of the cognitive level of the child with the disability.

Here are several suggestions for modifications. Some involve merely placing objects differently, some involve making purchases, others involve construction. Those that involve construction range from relatively simple projects that the caregivers might do themselves to modifications that will need to be contracted out.

- Rearrange furniture in order to remove obstructions from pathways to rooms as well as to allow for a wheelchair to turn within a room. This latter requires a space at least 60 inches by 60 inches square.
- Rearrange kitchen cabinets and refrigerator to put necessary items within reach of your child. Bathroom accessories should be arranged as well. Pull-out drawers and lazy susans can increase accessibility.
- Remove plush wall-to-wall carpeting. Finish wood floors with a nonslip finish or install industrial-type carpeting.
- Widen doorways.
- Replace doorknobs with lever door handles.
- Replace entrance steps with ramps.
- Install a hinged arm support for help with toileting. A high-rise toilet is particularly helpful, as is a bidet.
- Install single mix faucets with levered handles and include an anti-scald device.
- Adjust the height of light switches and plugs to put them within reach.
- Program portable telephones to allow your child full-time access to others.
- Install an intercom system that can be used between rooms as well as at entrances.
- Replace bathtubs with wheel-in showers.
- Install an adjustable-height sink and counter with an open front in the kitchen and bathroom.
- Install an angled mirror above stove burners to allow your child a view of the contents of pots from his or her wheelchair.
- Buy a home automation system that allows your child to control the TV, intercom, and thermostat all from a central device.
- Buy a lounge chair with electrically powered positioning and lifting ability.
- Install a fire extinguisher at an accessible level.
- Make use of various adaptive devices such as bath chairs, lifts, corner

chairs (which provide support on two sides rather than only in the back), hospital beds, and eating and writing utensils.

• Increase accessibility with a properly trained service dog.

There are agencies that help plan for and carry out changes to accommodate the needs of individuals with disabilities. There are four with a national focus:

1. ABLEDATA is a database of products, devices, and equipment for people with disabilities (800-227-0216; *www.abledata.com*);

2. The National Rehabilitation Information Center (800-246-2742; *www.naric.com*);

3. The National Council of Independent Living (703-525-3406; *www.ncil.org*);

4. Americans with Disabilities Act Information Hotline (202-514-0301; *www.ada.gov*) is another excellent resource for people with disabilities

For similar local agencies, check your telephone book or call the local chapter of the United Cerebral Palsy Association.

Choosing Appropriate Seating

Strollers, feeding chairs, tumble form sets, headrests, seating supports, and corner chairs—all of these are forms of adaptive seating that may benefit children with cerebral palsy. Many companies make different types of seating in several categories.

Strollers are a universal method of seating—almost all infants and young children are wheeled about in a stroller by their parents or other caregivers. For most children with cerebral palsy who are younger than 1 or 2 years, the standard strollers that can be purchased at any department store are adequate. A 2-year-old who is having a great deal of difficulty with head control, however, and even the 1-year-old who is not able to provide any trunk support or head control, needs more support than standard strollers provide. One good temporary alternative to buying a different stroller or a wheelchair is to have an insert fabricated for the existing stroller that can provide stability, head and trunk support, and more safety.

Most of the nonmedical strollers that are available on the market are not strong enough for the slightly bigger child, between the ages of 3 and 5. At this point, a decision must be made about how much support a child needs, based on an assessment of how much head and trunk control he or she has. If the decision is made to purchase a medical stroller, the parent may be pleased to learn that there are a number of medical strollers on the market that look very much like the standard baby stroller.

Larger stroller-type chairs are useful for quick transportation such as going to the grocery store. Most of these, however, have a significant drawback

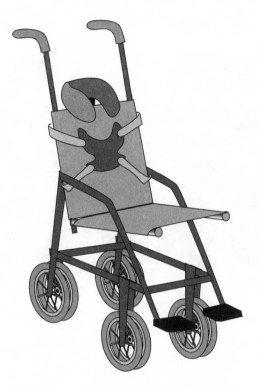

Medical stroller

for a child who is able to push a chair, since there are no wheels that the child can reach to push. Many of these larger chairs have a fairly narrow base, too, and can tip over easily if used on an uneven surface. Unlike these strollers, which usually have small wheels, there are strollers designed for outdoor use which have larger wheels. They are especially useful for parents who want to take their children on outdoor walks. These large-wheeled strollers are very stable and are easier to push on uneven terrain. There are also a few specialized wheelchairs that can be used at the beach, over sand and even by the water.

For the child who isn't walking and needs more support, generally strollers are not a good idea for long-term sitting past age 2 or 3. All of these strollers continue to have the form and shape of the infant baby stroller, a factor that appeals to parents because the public tends to pay less attention to these strollers than they do to a wheelchair. From the child's perspective, however, continuing to be pushed around in a stroller type of device is undesirable, especially when the child is bright and interested in interacting with his peers. Moving to a regular large-wheeled chair, or a more standard-appearing medical wheelchair, gives him the sense that he is now growing up and is into a "grown-up's" wheelchair. Also, as awareness catches up with technology, these wheelchairs are becoming more attractive and colorful, thus more appealing to a child and more acceptable to his or her peers. Such a chair also allows the child to push himself if his arm strength and coordination permit.

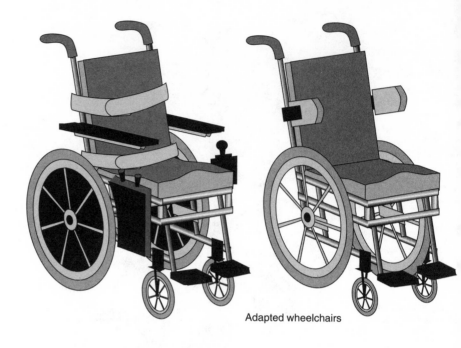

Adapted wheelchairs

There are many other advantages to having a standard type of medical wheelchair. The adaptive seating—including trunk support, solid supported seats and backs, headrests, neck supports, and chest straps—is much easier to insert. The large wheelchair is much easier to push over many kinds of terrain, and it is more stable. For this reason, certainly by the age of 5 or 6, since mobility is so important, the child should move out of the stroller into a regular type of wheelchair, perhaps a power wheelchair. If a power chair is purchased, a stroller might be an acceptable backup, if you already own one. It is certainly not necessary to order a fully adapted secondary wheelchair if a power chair has been ordered; on the other hand, it is a good idea to have a secondary type of wheelchair available, both because power chairs break down and because there are many places where power chairs can't be transported or may not be usable due to the space required for maneuvering.

There are many adaptive chairs used to improve the child's sitting posture and especially for feeding. Generally, an adequately arranged wheelchair with good trunk support, head control, and a lap tray can be the feeding chair for the child as well. Some parents or therapists prefer to have a separate feeding chair; a frequently used type is the tumble form, which is a foam-molded chair in which the child can bend forward. For the child who has a tendency to extend the head and spine, these chairs work well for feeding. However, these tumble form chairs provide very poor postural control for the child who tends to collapse forward and should not be used as wheelchair inserts or for a significant portion of the child's sitting time during the day. Corner chairs are also used, and they help the child develop sitting balance. These

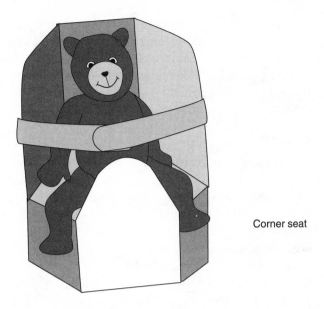

Corner seat

are very simple and excellent seating devices to allow the child to develop sitting coordination and balance on the floor.

PURCHASING A WHEELCHAIR

Parents should never walk into a medical supply store and tell a salesperson that they would like to purchase a wheelchair for their child, because even well-intentioned salespeople have received little training in assessing the child's needs. Generally the child's physical therapist, or the orthopedist or physiatrist who is seeing the child, will provide guidance about a wheelchair purchase based on the child's needs. Many pediatric hospitals have wheelchair clinics where physical therapists, rehabilitation engineers, and physicians discuss the family's and the child's situation and determine what type of chair will meet the child's, the family's, and the school's needs, and then advise the parents accordingly.

Before purchasing a wheelchair, these three factors must be examined: the child's need for postural control and support, the child's ability to push his or her own chair, and the need for any adaptive devices. In addition to these issues, which directly involve the child, it is also important to consider the child's home and school—the settings where the wheelchair will be used. This will determine how important it is to have a lightweight chair and will have a bearing on the size of the chair purchased. A chair to be used in a country environment, where there are no sidewalks or paved streets, needs to be extremely stable; in this setting, small-wheeled wheelchairs, which are difficult to push across gravel and loose dirt, are to be avoided.

The availability of service and repairs should also be considered (see

"About Wheelchair Maintenance," below). Although manual wheelchairs need repair less often than power chairs, parts of the wheelchair will eventually wear out or break and will need to be replaced. Another issue that is important for many children and for their families is the appearance of the chair: its color and structure, as well as how the child looks when seated in the chair. Certainly a child who has a colorful, well-constructed chair in good repair is more likely to receive the same kind of positive response from friends, acquaintances, and strangers as the child who is well dressed and clean. A child who is in a drab, poorly maintained, and poorly constructed wheelchair often elicits the same type of response as the child who is taken into public wearing clothes that are worn, dirty, and badly coordinated.

Insurance companies and government agencies will usually purchase one wheelchair every three years for a growing child. For this reason, growth needs to be considered when selecting a chair, and parents and the child must understand that the wheelchair will need to last for three years. If a power wheelchair is being purchased, a manual chair should be purchased as a backup using the same prescription. Social service personnel can be helpful in locating funding for purchasing chairs, but occasionally purchases will need to be organized through community groups such as the local chapter of the United Cerebral Palsy Associations or the Variety Club, or possibly by community fundraisers.

Another important aspect to consider when purchasing a wheelchair is how it will be transported. If the only transportation available is an automobile, the size of the trunk needs to be considered. All chair inserts need to be removable. If your child goes to school on a school bus and rides the bus seated in his wheelchair, you need to make sure that the wheelchair is acceptable for bus tie-down. Only a few wheelchairs have been crash-tested, and as soon as a customized seating system is added, each one becomes unique. Be sure that a headrest and an automotive-style seatbelt (not Velcro) are added to the wheelchair for safety. It is also important to understand that a wheelchair seatbelt is not certified to be a primary restraint when traveling in a vehicle. An additional seatbelt connected to the vehicle that goes around the passenger is necessary for safe transportation.

As mentioned, most wheelchairs for children can be expected to last approximately three years, though there are a number of wheelchairs that are marketed as being able to expand from age 3 to age 30; in other words, to go from infancy to adulthood. Here is the reality of this situation: it is virtually impossible to manufacture a wheelchair that fits adequately and is not overwhelmingly large and bulky for the 3-year-old which would not be inadequate by the time he is even 8 or so years old. It is extremely unusual for a wheelchair to last more than five years in childhood. Plan on making a wheelchair purchase every three to five years until your child is fully grown.

A child should be checked every six months or as needed to make sure the fit of the wheelchair meets his or her positioning needs. There are several ways growth is built into a wheelchair:

1. Most wheelchair frames are expandable in depth, and a few in width; expansion requires replacing parts and seating components if a new wheelchair frame is not recommended.

2. Inserts into a wheelchair should be measured to adjust in seat depth and back height so that only adjustments—not replacements—are needed as the child grows.

3. Wheelchair bases should be measured to be about 2 to 3 inches wider than the hip width to allow for some growth. If the base is wider than this, a child who self-propels will not have the best access to the rear wheels and will lose stability. Remember, although provision for some growth can be built into the chair, significant changes in the child's size, such as significant weight gain or a growth spurt, can't always be anticipated.

Choosing and Using Car Seats

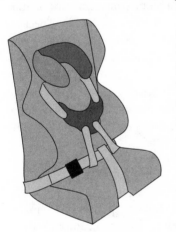

Most states have passed laws requiring that children under certain ages be transported on roads only in approved car seats. The purpose of this regulation is to provide a means of restraining children for their own safety during motor vehicle accidents. Car seats protect children with disabilities, as well; in fact, they can be vitally important for children with cerebral palsy, since many of them do not have natural protective mechanisms because of poor muscle control and coordination. For many young children with CP, the standard approved car seats provide adequate protection up to age 3 and 4. For the child with poor head control and trunk control who needs supportive seating, however, the medical and transportation department–approved car seats should be used.

Wheelchair manufacturers often state that a specific chair can be used for everything from a car seat to a bathroom seat to a feeding seat. This scenario sounds good in advertisements, but the reality is that wheelchairs are wheelchairs, and, while they may be used for feeding chairs, they do not work well as car seats, and few parents use any of the systems that are marketed as dual-purpose systems. Parents generally find these seats to be too large, too clumsy, and too complicated to remove from the wheelbase for car use. It is very difficult to lift a 50-pound child out of a wheelchair, remove and secure a 40-pound wheelchair seat as a car seat, and then lift the child back into the car seat. For the child who has significant trouble with trunk support, it is best to purchase a separate car seat that always remains in the vehicle in which the child travels.

The other alternative to using a car seat is to use the child's wheelchair by placing it in a van and tying it down. With approved wheelchair tie-downs and adequate restraints in the wheelchair, the child is extremely safe. If the child is evaluated in a wheelchair clinic, the issue of vehicle seating should be addressed with respect to the child's specific needs and the vehicles in which the child will usually be riding. Obtaining funding to purchase adequate car seats may be difficult, since very few insurance companies or government agencies will pay for an adequate car seat.

Here are several different options when considering vehicular transport:

1. Standard car seats available at department stores should be used if the child meets the size and weight criteria. Additional foam or towels may be padded inside the car seat's cover or placed along the child's body to provide extra support, especially to the head or trunk.

2. If the child exceeds the weight limit for a standard car seat, there are a number of car seats that are available through durable medical equipment dealers that may hold up to 100 pounds. Additional support can be added to these seats, too, as long as the basic structure of the car seat is unchanged.

3. If a child has good head control and fair trunk control, an option may be to supplement the standard lap/shoulder belt with a harness specially available for transport. These harnesses should not be used by the child who requires total positioning, however, since their primary function is to provide lateral and anterior trunk support.

4. The child's own wheelchair, with the proper tie-downs, may be the best alternative if a van is available. Remember, for additional safety, some type of chest harness as well as an approved seatbelt and headrest should be added.

About Wheelchair Maintenance

A wheelchair, whether it is motorized or manual, requires routine maintenance and care to keep it in the best condition, just like an automobile or a bicycle. Several parts of the wheelchair must be checked to ensure the best use. In order to maintain a wheelchair, it's important to use the recommended tools and cleaning supplies. Here are some products that you'll want to keep on hand:

- auto paste-type wax for metal frame
- mild soap
- vinyl and upholstery cleaner
- distilled water for batteries
- baking soda for battery terminals
- oil (30 weight, not designed for autos) for lubricating
- tire pump
- flat and Phillips screwdrivers
- adjustable wrench (or socket set), $\frac{7}{16}$" and $\frac{1}{2}$" common

- spoke wrench
- set of standard Allen wrenches, usually ⁵⁄₃₂″ and ³⁄₁₆″
- hammer

The guidelines presented below provide a general overview of preventive maintenance. You'll want to consult your owner's manual for specific information about how to care for your specific model.

MANUAL WHEELCHAIRS

Monthly.   Check tires for proper inflation (proper inflation specifications are usually recorded on the sidewall of the tire). Most tires require between 50 and 65 pounds per square inch; high performance tires may need as much as 120 psi. Check tires for cuts, flat spots, and wear.

After checking the tire pressure, check the wheel locks. They should engage and disengage easily. Over time, they tend to loosen and slide away from the tire (especially solid tires), and some tips that contact the wheel may also wear so the wheel locks no longer hold. *Do not use wheel locks as brakes!*

If wheels are spoked, check to see whether spokes are loose or bent. They can be tightened with a spoke wrench or replaced. Loose spokes often are the main cause of wobbly wheels.

Clean metal parts to remove dirt and to avoid rusting. Tighten nuts and bolts, especially on moving or swing-away parts.

Every six months.   If the wheelchair has a cross-brace, lubricate center bolt and tube. Wheels with quick-release axles should be popped off and lubed. Check the bearings; remove dirt, hair, and other materials from nuts and bolts (especially on removable or moving parts). Check for rust.

BATTERY-POWERED WHEELCHAIRS

Power wheelchairs should be inspected by an authorized dealer once or twice a year for a "tune-up." An authorized dealer can also check the voltage at the posts to determine whether the batteries are too old.

Wheelchair batteries should be deep cycle. They generally last for 300 to 500 charging cycles, which may be equivalent to between 10 and 18 months. When charging batteries, be sure that you are charging them at the proper setting (the setting is lower for gel batteries than for acid batteries). Most charges are automatic—they shut off when the battery is fully charged.

Unsealed acid batteries must be handled with care. Keep any unsealed battery away from flames or sparks. Don't tilt it. Wear a mask and goggles, and charge the battery in a well-ventilated area. Most power wheelchairs now come with gel batteries. These batteries are recommended because they are safer to use and require very little maintenance.

Keep the water in the battery at the correct level, adding only distilled water as needed.

Inspect case terminals and clean with baking soda, if needed, or medium-grade sandpaper or a wire brush.

Gel batteries don't require the same amount of maintenance. They charge faster and they are safer, but they usually cost more and don't last quite as long.

When replacing batteries, replace both of them at the same time.

INSERTS

If you are using a seat insert that is separate from the wheelchair, every 3 to 6 months you need to check whether all the attaching hardware is in place and is tightened, and check the insert for rips and tears. Be sure that the insert can be easily removed, that it secures to the wheelchair properly, and that the wheelchair folds smoothly when it is in place.

Pressure Management Awareness

Most of us don't think about repositioning ourselves while sitting at our computer, or getting up from our chair to simply move around, though we do it automatically. We all need to change positions to manage the pressure points throughout our bodies. For some, changing positions is not that easy. For children who use wheelchairs, the need to change positions or relieve pressure, particularly on their buttocks or ischial tuberosities, is critical. If pressure is not relieved, skin breakdown or pressure sores can occur.

A primary factor contributing to pressure sores or skin breakdown, particularly as it relates to positioning in a wheelchair, is immobility, or the lack of movement within the chair. Poor distribution of pressure across the seating surface or seat cushion can contribute to skin breakdown, as can shearing or friction forces as the child transfers in and out of the wheelchair. Denervated tissue (the loss of sensation) can also contribute to skin breakdown secondary to reduced blood flow to that area of the body, though this is not a common problem in children with CP. Far more common in children with CP is the lack of subcutaneous tissue due to poor general nutrition, meaning there is no "padding" on the child's buttocks or legs to provide some cushioning. Another contributing factor is postural changes in the body that alter the pressures distributed throughout the body. In a typical seating and mobility system, the seating components are not "dynamic." In other words, as one's posture changes, the seating components do not accommodate automatically. Consideration needs to be given to adjustment of the seating and positioning components within the mobility system to accommodate for changes in the body following orthopedic surgery.

When a child in a wheelchair has skin breakdown, seating specialists use tools to help determine the possible cause of skin breakdown when the wheelchair is considered a likely culprit. Among these tools are several pressure-mapping systems that provide pressure information relative to posture. These systems involve a mapping surface consisting of thin resistive semi-conductive polymers sandwiched between highly conductive fabric. The changes in resistance which result from the different pressures on the semi-conductor are interpreted by the Interface module and relayed to the computer, where they are displayed as an array of colors and pressure values. This provides immediate information to the clinician to help determine whether the seating surface is contributing to skin breakdown.

Pressure-mapping systems provide the clinician with the ability to compare different seating surfaces or cushions in an objective manner. In addition, they provide education to the user by graphically showing the effectiveness of weight-shifting interventions. Pressure-mapping systems provide a tool for configuration of seating systems for the child who is more prone to skin breakdown. Keep in mind that this is only an assessment tool. This is not something that is required on every evaluation or with every recommendation for a new seating system.

Ultimately, good pressure distribution and pressure relief techniques will greatly reduce your child's chances of skin breakdown. There are many variables that factor into the successful management of skin and pressure sores. Always consider the risk factors of pressure sores, including peak pressure, friction, impact injury, heat, moisture, posture, immobility, sensory loss, body type, nutrition, infection, incontinence, and disease. One or more of these factors may be the reason for skin breakdown in your child. These are better dealt with in advance of an actual breakdown, rather than trying to heal one after it has occurred.

Choosing a Stander

A stander is a device that helps a child stand. If the child is not standing between 18 and 24 months, it is necessary to start a child standing even when she does not have adequate head or upper body control to stand alone. Standing is important because it allows the child to do some weight bearing through the legs, which in turn helps make the bones stronger and stimulates the development of motor coordination and head control. It also allows the child to adopt a position different from sitting or lying, and many children interact better with their environment when they are standing up. Standing is strongly encouraged for all children, regardless of how severely involved they are. The benefits are present in many areas, from improving bone size and strength to posture, breathing, and bowel function, as well as preventing muscle tightness from sitting too long.

The length of time in the stander will vary greatly, depending on how the child responds to it. A good beginning is to start out in the stander for 10 to 15 minutes, with an attempt to gradually work the time up to an hour twice

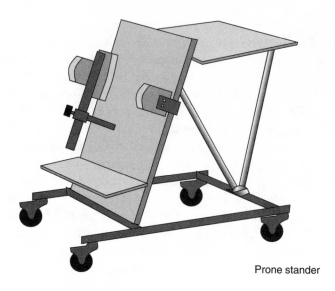

Prone stander

a day if the child tolerates it. The child should not be left in the stander if he is fatigued, crying, or uncomfortable. Music or television can often make a child's standing experience more pleasurable.

If the child has very poor control of her feet, a pair of ankle-foot orthoses (AFOs) will help support her ankles. Other bracing is not necessary, since the legs can be strapped into the stander.

Each of the different types of standers—prone, supine, sit to stand, and Parapodium standers—is used in a specific situation. Most have the ability to adjust the angle of the stander and thus add or eliminate levels of support. It is important to remember that the stander ideally should be used in the most upright position and with the least amount of support that the child can tolerate. An angle of more than 30 degrees from the vertical position allows very little weight bearing. An upright position allows the child to work with their head and trunk in the most functional position.

A prone stander has pads and support in front of the child. The amount of support can vary, coming up to the child's chest or only up to her waist. The child leans forward in the prone stander. Often a tray is attached at the front of the stander and the child can put her arms there and play with toys. Most prone standers allow the angle of standing to be adjusted from very low to nearly upright. The child who does best in the prone stander has at least partial head control. This child often has some difficulty with upper body support, but a prone stander helps her support her upper body.

In contrast to the prone stander, the supine stander has pads and support behind the child. The supine stander may be beneficial to caregivers with large or heavy children. The supine stander often allows for easy bed to stander transfers when placed in the horizontal position. Once the child is secured, the caregiver can adjust the mechanism to get the child into the

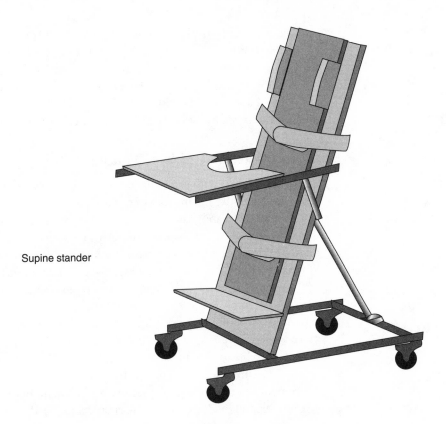

Supine stander

most tolerated vertical position. The supine stander is a good option for the child with poor head control whose head often falls forward in the prone stander. The supine stander is also a good choice for children whose knees do not straighten completely. With some padding placed behind the knees, the supine stander works well for this type of child.

A sit-to-stand stander is a new type of stander. It allows a child to be transferred into the stander from a wheelchair or bed in the sitting position. Once the child is strapped in, a mechanism is used to transform the stander from a sitting position to an upright position. Sit-to-stand standers are excellent for heavier patients. However, they tend to be very costly and do not provide the best support.

A "Parapodium" stander is a stander that has a base in which the child's legs can be strapped in up to the waist. The child stands straight upright; although the stander may provide slight support around the chest, most of these standers support only the waist or the bottom of the chest. In general, this type of stander is a poor choice for children with cerebral palsy because it provides only minimal upper trunk support. Children with CP have poor upper body control, and end up falling forward and leaning against a strap or the tray.

Standers are expensive to buy from a medical equipment dealer. However, many health insurance companies will pay for standers. Parents may wish to investigate the different designs that can easily be made out of plywood and upholstery. Physical therapists are often excellent resources for counseling parents on the best type of stander for a particular child. They also often have demonstration units. Trying out various units before deciding on which one to purchase can be extremely beneficial.

About Walkers and Gait Trainers

To help a child with cerebral palsy begin walking, a walker is often helpful. This is because the muscles of the body and extremities lack the coordination, strength, and stability needed to help keep the body upright while stepping. There are no absolute indicators for initiating the use of a walker, though there are a few motor control activities that seem to be necessary to be able to start using a walker. Being able to hold up one's head independently, sitting in a chair with minimal support, and being able to stand and accept weight through the legs are a few of the basics that are needed. The child also needs to be able to guide the direction of the walker using his hands and to see where he is going for safety reasons. It is also helpful if he demonstrates an ability to maintain some weight on one leg while stepping with the other. As with standers, the goal is to have the child walking with minimal support and, at the same time, to support some of his body weight while being properly aligned. Therefore the child's skills need to be matched to the appropriate walker. This is best done by having the child evaluated in the proposed piece of equipment. There are many styles of walker, as well as accessories for each walker, to maximize the child's ability to use it.

The most supportive type of walker is the "gait trainer." The trainer is most often used as a rear-facing walker. The design is based on the idea that the child will stand more erect if he cannot push the walker too far in front of him, and if he has to push up on the hand supports to keep his body upright. It can also be made into a forward facing walker by switching around the foot pieces. This type of walker offers a variety of levels of trunk and pelvic support. It may have a seat for a child who tends to collapse into flexion and guides to keep the legs from crossing and to control step direction and step length. Using the supports at the trunk and pelvis as well as the seat option can also help the older child who is large and difficult for the parent to control, but who has the desire to walk. These options offer trunk stability to align the pelvis over the feet. The wider base makes it less likely that the walker will tip over but it is more difficult to maneuver in the home. For the younger child these types of support may be assistive in bringing the child upright over her feet and beginning the action of stepping. To maximize the walker's usage, it is crucial that the child have the desire to walk and the ability to initiate stepping with a weight shift. The walker can also be used with just the pelvic guides and special arm supports for minimal alignment assistance. There are a few hand and forearm styles to choose from for support and guidance. There are multiple wheel features to control direction and speed. The gait trainer has many different ways for your child to use the walker, and many accessories, which can be added or deleted, as needed, to fit your child's ongoing needs.

Like the gait trainer, the more standard walker helps a child walk, but with less assistance for alignment and more help for balance and weakness of the legs. This type of walker is similar to the older person's walker that you may be familiar with. It can have from 2 to 4 wheels and may be made of metal. Many children with cerebral palsy use the walker in the rear-facing position to help keep their hips straight and their bodies upright. The gait trainer can have a pelvic guide that assists in keeping the pelvis centered over the feet. It can have a seat for a child with limited endurance, though it will not prevent her from collapsing. This seat is posterior in the walker frame and must be manually adjusted. A variety of wheel options help to control the walker's stability, speed, and direction. The wheels can have drag to decrease the walker speed for the child who relies on its stability while stepping, or it may have wheels that prevent the walker from moving backward when the child pushes on it to step forward. Increasing the number of wheels to all four posts may help the child who has the need for increased speed and efficiency. The walker can have swivel wheels to enable the user who has good balance and weight shift control to turn and adjust the walker simultaneously while walking.

Once the child is able to bear weight on her legs and demonstrates a desire to step, a walker evaluation, whether it is for a gait trainer or standard walker, is appropriate. Determining the appropriate walker for your child is crucial for her success. The correct walker is determined by knowing your child's specific needs, and matching these needs with specific equipment. Correct selection of the walker and its accessories will maximize the support, efficiency, and usage of the walker.

About Braces

When your physician prescribes a brace (also referred to as an *orthosis*) for your child, be sure to find out its intended purpose. This will help you explain to your child why he must wear the device or, if the need is not severe, will help you decide on occasion to let your child go without it. Ask the doctor how many hours each day is it to be worn, and exactly when during the day—for instance, in the daytime, at night during sleep, when standing, when sitting, or when engaged in physical activity. Ask the orthotist who made the brace to tell you how to clean it.

Other questions you may want to ask your doctor include the following: How is the orthosis to be applied? Where in relationship to the joint is the orthosis to be positioned? For instance, if my son has a knee brace, specifically where should the brace be positioned relative to his kneecap? Can the device be worn when exercising, or might that be a problem?

Skin care is very important for someone who uses an orthosis. You'll need to check your child's skin periodically for any sign of pressure, such as redness, blistering, or an opened area. Notify the doctor or the orthotist if skin problems occur. Generally if this happens the child must be examined by the doctor, who will evaluate the orthosis's fit. Because some problems that require the use of an orthosis change over time, it's possible that the child has outgrown the appliance. Sometimes, too, the materials in the orthosis break down after longtime use, which means that the orthosis is no longer capable of delivering the performance for which it was initially intended. Any sign of skin problems or problems with the brace itself need to be evaluated by the physician.

Different insurance companies have different options regarding how many orthoses they will pay for in the life of an insurance policy. To keep replacement costs to a minimum, some braces are designed to grow with the child to a limited extent. Parents can help by keeping the brace clean and in good working order.

CARE AND MAINTENANCE

Cleaning and lubrication.   A brace may be made of metal, leather, or certain plastics, or a combination of these. Braces made of these different materials require different kinds of care. Your child's orthotist and physician will give you instructions for keeping the brace in good working order, but here are some general tips to help you out.

To keep metal parts in smooth running order, keep them free of dust and dirt, and lubricate them periodically. Leather parts also require periodic cleaning. Ask your child's orthotist what cleaner he or she recommends.

Plastic braces should be washed with mild soap and cool or lukewarm water. Some plastics change shape when they are exposed to heat, so it's important to keep the brace in a cool place. Leaving it in an automobile in summer months is not recommended, because the inside temperature of a closed-up automobile in the summer may be high enough to soften the plastic brace and cause it to change shape, thereby making it useless.

Labeling.   Orthoses are very expensive, and therefore in addition to keeping your child's braces clean and in good working order, you need to make sure that they are carefully and indelibly labeled with the child's name. This is especially important if your child participates in activities with other children who have similar assistive devices, since caregivers or school personnel will find a proper label essential in returning the devices to their owners. You should also label the orthosis to indicate which part of the body it will be used on. Use labels like "inside left foot," "outside right wrist," "top of back," and so on.

Instructing others. If you know that someone else is going to apply the orthosis to your child, give that person instructions. Explain how the brace is supposed to fit and how it is to be applied. Do not assume that anyone else has been given information about your child's brace. No one knows as much about your child's particular brace as you do, so you need to share this information to be certain that your child is benefiting from wearing the brace.

Choosing the Correct Shoes

When choosing an appropriate shoe for the child with cerebral palsy, parents have many options. They will want a shoe that is as attractive as possible, of course, and one that takes the child's special needs into account, as well. Many children with CP need to wear orthopedic shoes (also called corrective shoes), but many do not. An orthopedic shoe is a special type of shoe, usually made of heavy leather extending above the ankle. It typically has a rigid sole and sturdy construction to provide support to the foot. It may have a straight last, which means that it does not have the normal inside curve. Some of these shoes are made with special arch supports.

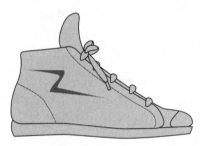

An extremely heavy and rigid and sturdily built shoe was considered essential footwear for all children just one generation ago. The theory was that these shoes would ensure that children developed well-balanced feet. It has subsequently been shown that children without disabilities have no need for special shoes or foot support. The large number of orthopedic shoe manufacturers have as a result been severely restricted in their ability to sell shoes, and to compensate they have targeted the population of people with disabilities. The well-built athletic or running shoes on the market today, however, are constructed in such a way that they provide equally good support to the foot. They are well constructed, with soft arch support and very adequate ankle support.

The main reason for a child to wear heavy orthopedic shoes is to permit him to wear a metal brace attached to the shoe. These shoes are built of very sturdy leather and can be disassembled or have lifts and other devices added very easily. If a decision is made to use metal braces instead of the more commonly used plastic, then the orthopedic shoe is usually necessary. Except for use with a brace, there are few reasons today to prescribe orthopedic shoes or any other corrective shoe for children with cerebral palsy. In fact, the shoes that are best for these children are the same shoes that are best for other children, primarily athletic shoes that have soft soles made of rubber to prevent slipping and a moderate arch support that is soft so that it won't hurt the foot.

When choosing an athletic shoe for your child, consider that the material composing the upper shoe may be soft leather, synthetic, or a nylon fabric material, all of which provide adequate support to the foot. These shoes very nicely accommodate inserts, which may be specially made in some circumstances to fit completely inside the shoe, as well as the more commonly used AFO. If you are searching to buy shoes to fit over AFOs, it is important to look for shoes with a tongue that goes as far out as possible on the toe box. Shoes can be laced out as far as possible to allow the shoe to be opened up and provide much better accommodation for the brace to fit into. This makes it much easier to take the shoes on and off with the brace. Extremely lightweight canvas shoes are ideal for this.

The main problem with standard orthopedic shoes is that they are very heavy. They also usually have leather soles that do not provide the kind of traction that rubber soles do, and they look unattractive, as well. They tend to draw attention to children with disabilities and make them stand out as being different. Regular shoes help promote an appearance of normalcy, which is especially important for children who are in regular schools, where wearing the latest style or fashion can provide a significant boost in self-esteem. Personal appearance is also important for the public impression of a child who is not walking but is in a wheelchair.

The most important concern for children's shoes is that they be large enough so that there is plenty of room at the toes. The shoes should not cause the child pain or discomfort when he walks. Whether they are orthopedic shoes, athletic shoes, or high-top hiking boots, the main goal of shoes is to keep the feet warm and provide a stable foundation for the child to walk on without hurting his feet.

Increasing Independence with Service Dogs

Well-trained service dogs provide increased independence to physically challenged individuals such as those with cerebral palsy, as well as providing an emotional outlet for the owner. These dogs are trained and supplied by a number of organizations, most of them nonprofit organizations. A person receiving a service dog is asked to make a contribution, but the cost of training the dog is far more than the contribution—the nonprofit organization makes up the difference.

Most organizations provide dogs to children as well as to adults, providing that the recipient can accept the responsibility of owning a service animal. The organizations providing dogs are very careful to select healthy dogs that are well suited for their role.

To prepare a dog for service, the organization first gives the dog lessons in obedience. Once the dog has been obedience-trained, it receives general service training, including training in retrieving dropped objects, taking items from shelves, opening doors, and paying cashiers with a specially designed wallet.

Many recipients have very special needs, such as a need for the dog to follow commands given through an electronic communicator. After an individual has been matched to a specific dog, the dog undergoes additional training to enable it to accommodate the recipient's special needs. The dog's soon-to-be owner also undergoes training in how to handle and care for the dog. The organizations that supply dogs provide counseling to help the animal's owner cope with the separation that accompanies the dog's need for retirement or the dog's death.

There are several organizations that provide and train dogs throughout the United States. Call the Delta Society at 1-425-226-7357 (Pacific time) for information about the organization nearest you. If you live in the mid-Atlantic states, you can call Canine Partners for Life, in Cochranville, Pennsylvania, at 1-610-869-4902.

Managing the System

Caregivers can be either victims of the system or survivors of the system. By "system" we mean any organization whose rules and regulations may on occasion interfere with your ability to protect your child's interests. The system might be an insurance company, your state's Medicaid policies, the school system, a community service, or even a local sports league. Individuals with disabilities have different needs for services, and their caregivers' ability to procure those services varies greatly.

Availability of services can differ amazingly, even between neighboring states. One insurance company might cover new braces for a child every six months, while another claims to allow reimbursement for one set for a lifetime! One school might inform a parent that there are no services available for a child who by federal law must have services provided; another might be providing an aide for a child with barely discernible hemiplegia. People with disabilities often have to contend with discrepancies such as these.

The first step in managing these problems is to identify the specific system that must be addressed and to represent your child wholeheartedly. If you cannot personally be an advocate for your child, find someone who can. The individual need not be a person with a special education or a prestigious position in society, but he or she does need to be willing to be persistent and patient with ongoing attempts to frustrate his or her best efforts. No matter who represents a person with a disability, the effort is made easier with good organizational skills and hands-on experience gained as the effort continues. For children who are cognitively able, this is a responsibility they may assume as they reach adulthood.

Here are some tips that will help you as you learn to manage the system.

Never make a phone call without a pencil and paper in hand. When asking questions about an issue, find out and record the name of the individual who gives you information, as well as his or her title. Record the date of every phone call made and write a brief description of the information exchanged. If the answer to your inquiry is not acceptable, persist until you are allowed to speak with the individual's supervisor. Make it clear that you are not going to give up. Try to do this calmly, because shouting only makes it appear that you are losing control. Instead, speak firmly and in a way that demonstrates that you will never get so frustrated that you'll give up and go away.

Don't stop calling. The old saying about the squeaky wheel getting the grease is extraordinarily appropriate when it comes to acquiring services. If you believe that your child's rights are being violated, do not hesitate to get legal help.

Keep an ongoing list of individuals who have been helpful and their phone numbers. Send a note to thank those who have been helpful and, when appropriate, a letter of commendation to their supervisor.

Network with other parents and other caregivers, and help each other by sharing strategies that have yielded results. It is particularly helpful to have one designated person with whom to discuss issues and strategies. This may be a therapist, a physician, a friend, or a relative.

Make use of community and church service organizations and local newspapers. Often the problem you are tackling is one that another child is facing, and the publicity you get can help others. For example, if the school system alters its treatment of your child because of your efforts, and then the local newspaper carries a story about this, other parents can learn about your efforts, the school system's response, and the rights of their own child.

More than anything, don't give up. Over and over we have experienced a situation where an "absolute no" becomes a "yes" through persistence.

Working with a Case Manager

The case manager is the person who is responsible for coordinating and facilitating the procurement of services from different provider agencies in both the public and the private sector. This person can serve as a single point of contact in helping families obtain the services and assistance that they need to care for the child or adult with cerebral palsy. The case manager may be a social worker connected to a school or agency, or perhaps may be a public health nurse or a nurse connected to an insurance company. He or she may be appointed by the state or a county agency, be a staff member of a hospital caring for a child, or be appointed by the insurance company covering the child's medical expenses. When the case manager is a government child welfare manager, it is also sometimes necessary that she or he be an advocate for the child, to make sure that the child receives appropriate medical attention.

While the case manager works to be sure that necessary care is obtained, he or she also regulates care to avoid duplication of services or provision of unnecessary services. Case managers have a good deal of control over the medical care arrangements made by many people today. For example, suppose that John Doe's company provides XYZ health insurance, and that XYZ health insurance assigns a case manager to each individual and each family enrolled in the plan. If John's spouse hurts herself when she slips on the ice, the case manager will direct her to an orthopedist whose services are approved for payment on the XYZ plan; will refer her for special studies, if necessary, at an appointed facility; and, if physical therapy is suggested by the doctor, will direct her to provider-approved therapists. The goal for this type of manager is to manage health care to ensure cost containment.

Letters of Medical Necessity

In order to reimburse you for the purchase of equipment or other durable medical goods such as braces, standers, seats, communications aids, toileting aids, and adaptive feeding devices, insurance companies or other funding agencies almost always require a letter of medical necessity from a physician or therapist. Such a letter must include the child's diagnoses and a description of why the equipment is needed, or the request will be automatically rejected.

Because the letters written by physicians who are not familiar with insurance company requirements sometimes don't include all the necessary information, we've provided a sample letter here. To help avoid delay or hassle over reimbursement, you can make sure that the physician who writes a letter of medical necessity for you includes the kind of information indicated in this sample. If the physician follows this format, you will at least get a fair hearing from the funding agency. You might want to photocopy this sample letter and give your doctor a copy. She or he will send the letter on hospital or office stationery.

Date

To Whom It May Concern (or, better, to a specific employee of the funding agency):

John Smith is a 5-year-old male with a primary diagnosis of cerebral palsy. He was seen recently at the Seating Clinic at the Alfred I. duPont Hospital for Children in Wilmington, Delaware for the prescription of a new seating system to meet his positioning needs.

John presents with the following: generally decreased tone in upper and lower extremities, and fair head and trunk control. He is dependent in transfers and mobility. He is cognitively severely delayed. He is incontinent in bowel/bladder. He has frequent respiratory complications and is subject to bronchitis and pneumonia, and he receives chest therapy. He occasionally aspirates, he has increased skin sensitivity, and he has seizures, but they're generally under control with medication. He must have a tilt-in-space wheelchair with appropriate positioning to provide safety and support, and to facilitate breathing and feeding.

His current seating system is a Zippie tilt-in-space that is 3 years old. It no longer meets his positioning needs because he has outgrown it, and the seating insert needs to be changed to meet his current positioning needs.

The goals for John for seating are to maintain posture, protect skin, provide comfort, and enhance function. Upon evaluation, the Seating Team has recommended that the following equipment be prescribed for John:

Action Tiger, desk arms, swing away detachable elevating leg rests, semi-reclining back, special seat depth, stroller handles, custom positioners and lateral hip guides, high brackets, solid seat with attaching hardware, solid back with attaching hardware, shoe holders, heavy duty straps.

The Action Tiger is prescribed because it is a manual wheelchair for total positioning, and because he is dependent in mobility. The tilt is needed because he is hypotonic in head and trunk. He also has difficulty breathing, and it will help aid in feeding. It will help with low endurance and pressure relief. The adjustable height arms are needed to support the tray at the right height, for upper body support and balance and for ease of transfers. The I-back will bring side supports in close to the trunk, and the insert will fit the full width of the wheelchair. The laterals will encourage midline trunk position, compensate for lack of trunk control, provide safety, and contour around the trunk for better control. The chest harness is needed for safety in transport by providing anterior support, preventing forward flexion, and retracting the shoulders. The headrest is needed for poor head control due to low tone, active flexion of the head, posterior lateral support, safety in transfers, and facilitation of breathing. The clear tray is needed as a functional surface for schoolwork, for stimulation, for upper arm and trunk support, and as a base for augmentative communication devices. The shoe holders are needed to control increased extension or spasms in lower extremities, excessive internal rotation, and external rotation, and to prevent aggressive behavior for safety. The anti-tippers are needed for safety.

Should you have any questions regarding these recommendations, please do not hesitate to call me at (302) 651-4000. We hope that you will be able to accommodate these needs in an expedient manner. Thank you for your cooperation and assistance in this matter.

Sincerely,

Freeman Miller, M.D.
Pediatric Orthopedic Surgeon

Make a note of the date the letter was mailed, and if after three or four weeks you haven't heard anything, it might be a good idea to telephone the insurance company or funding agency and gently inquire about the status of the claim. Make sure to find out the name of the person you speak with, and write it down. The person will probably tell you that the claim is being processed; you can ask when you might expect to receive notification of payment, and then call again if that date passes and you still haven't heard anything. It's not generally a good idea to be seen as a nuisance or, worse, as an irate client; but you will want to stay on top of the situation, and let the agency know that you are doing so. If the agency remains unresponsive, you can enlist your doctor's assistance.

Occupations for Adults with Cerebral Palsy

There are many options for teenagers and adults with cerebral palsy who wish to work. Options will vary depending on the degree and type of disability. A vocational rehabilitation evaluation may help determine the type of vocation/job for which the teenager or adult is best suited. For the high school student, vocational counseling is frequently offered through the school system. Many communities offer vocational rehabilitation programs for adults who are physically or mentally challenged. People with diplegia whose legs are affected but who are able to use both hands effectively have many options, including using a computer to place orders for a company, doing research, writing, manufacturing and repairing small engines, or teaching. For the person with hemiplegia affecting one side of the body, it's best to avoid bilateral dexterity speed tasks. Such a person would be able to perform most of the jobs listed below, as would a person with quadriplegia, especially those focusing on interpersonal verbal skills, such as receptionist, dispatcher, or shipping clerk.

The following list is by no means comprehensive and is provided only to give an idea of the variety of possibilities available. In choosing a career, any person needs to take into account personal interests and aptitudes as well as education and previous experience and other practical training.

Creative
Artist
Art therapist; director, hospital art
    studio
Freelance photographer
Caricaturist
Watercolorist

Federal government
Civil service mathematician
Social Security claims represen-
    tative

Health
Patient care coordinator
Rehabilitation coordinator
Director of volunteers, hospital
Speech pathologist; supervisor
Cytotechnologist
Clerk, hospital laboratory
Speech therapist
Radiologist
Clinical psychologist

Child psychiatrist
Community relations, hospital

Information
Communications specialist/associ-
    ate programmer
Senior computer analyst
Systems programmer
Computer programmer
Librarian, rehabilitation center
TV and radio surveyor
Systems analyst, hospital

Law and ministry
Attorney
Minister
Deputy probation officer
Private police agency, owner
Legal researcher

Merchants and manufacturing
Shop owner
Lift manufacturer

Corporate president
Film producer
Handi-Ramp, Inc., owner

Office related
Hotel personnel manager
Insurance underwriter
Office worker, auto salvage employee
Telephone salesperson
Accountant

Rehabilitation
Director, state department of rehabilitation
Rehabilitation counselor
Rehabilitation counselor, domiciliary
Psychologist
Program coordinator, adult development center
Social worker
Employment counselor
Medical social worker

Sales, home-based
Home products salesperson
Ad specialty distributor
Map dealer
Greeting card salesperson
Typist and telephone salesperson
General insurance agent
Magazine subscription telemarketer
Brokerage firm owner

Sales, office-based
Travel agency owner or agent
Radio announcer
Advertising salesperson
Account executive
Insurance agent
Cattle owner
Stockbroker

Science and engineering
Engineering supervisor, aerospace firm

Self-employed draftsperson
Meteorological technician
Technical writer, aerospace firm
Museum curator
Research engineer
Translator
Tutor
Liaison engineer, hospital

Services, home-based
Income tax preparer; bookkeeper; notary public
Police and fire dispatcher
Telephone answering service worker
Nurses' registry manager
Video documentation producer
Equipment maintenance specialist
Justice of the peace
Employment consultant
Wake-up service caller
Correspondent for small businesses

Services, office-based
Chauffeur
Private employment agency owner or agent

Teaching and education
College professor
Teaching English to deaf people
Elementary, junior high school, or high school teacher
Elementary, junior high school, or high school principal
Learning disabilities clinician
Federal aid coordinator
Hospital teacher
Junior college instructor

Writing
Technical writer and researcher
Magazine editor
Newspaper editor

About Hospitalization

A child—or anyone—may be admitted to the hospital on either an elective basis or an emergency basis. For an elective admission, you decide to admit your child to the hospital so that he can undergo tests or have a procedure or surgery done. You have some part in deciding when the admission and procedure will take place, taking into account the demands of your own life as well as the physician's busy schedule. An emergency is something over which we have little or no control—such as appendicitis or a heart attack. In an emergency, your child would be admitted immediately to the hospital for treatment.

Your child's physician will tell you why he or she wants to admit your child to the hospital. In addition to getting a detailed description from the doctor, you might also ask for any literature on the procedures to be performed, or ask for a reference list so that you can read about the procedures or tests in the library. Once you feel comfortable with the treatment plan, you should find out what's involved for your child and what your responsibilities will be after the treatment.

Ask your child's physician to sketch out very simply the test or procedure that he or she intends to perform on your child. Be sure to ask your doctor the following questions:

- Will my child be in pain during or after the treatment?
- What measures will be taken to alleviate my child's pain?
- How long will my child be in the hospital? Will she be in intensive care?
- Will medications be prescribed for use at discharge?

The purpose for obtaining an explanation of the procedure is to allow you to give informed consent—to sign hospital forms saying that you are willing for your child to undergo the procedure, and that you understand the possible risks and complications. It will also help you to care for your child at home after the test or surgical or other procedure.

THE PREADMISSION PROCESS

Most hospitals have preadmission counseling that will answer many of your questions about the admissions process, insurance issues, and accommodations. Ask specifically about the arrangements for parents visiting and staying with their child, whether you may stay at your child's bedside, and under what circumstances you may not stay at your child's bedside.

PREPARING YOUR CHILD FOR HOSPITALIZATION

Whether going to the hospital is a new experience for your child, or whether he or she has been to the hospital many times before, you must prepare the child in advance for what is going to happen. The hospitalization will be a more positive experience—will be less frightening and less traumatic—if the child has been told what to expect.

Generally speaking, the more a child knows about the reasons for hospitalization and all the details of hospitalization, the better off he will be. Also generally speaking, the more positive a parent or significant other is about the experience, the better the experience will be. With that in mind, parents should realize that their child is a unique individual and must be treated as such; in fact, professionals recommend that parents relate to their child in the way that the child can best understand and accept.

Ask if there is anyone responsible for patient education in the hospital where your child will be admitted who can advise you as to how to proceed with preparing your child for admission. Your physician may know professionals who can assist you in preparing your child. Ask the office nurse or clinic nurse for advice, since he or she may be able to help, or may direct you to others who will be able to help you.

Pediatric hospitals sometimes have a child life department, which can suggest the appropriate approach to take with your child. Nurses and social workers may be helpful in advising you in this area and may be able to give you information well in advance of the admission date to help you plan to prepare your child.

The following guidelines for different age groups are guidelines only; based on your knowledge of your own child, you can tailor them to help your child through this experience.

The young child. For a young child, preparation for hospitalization should take place as close to admission as possible, preferably only a few days before. Children between 1 and 5 years of age can handle only simple explanations of what is going to happen, no more than three days before admission. Children learn best by imitation. For young children, use dolls as models to describe the part of the body that will be affected, and play with puppets and "play" hospital equipment such as a stethoscope and a blood pressure cuff. Read books about hospitals and medical personnel, and look at pictures with your child.

Sometimes, answering your child's questions will be the best way to approach the experience. A tour of the hospital the day before admission can be beneficial for everyone. A call to the hospital's public relations department may provide specific answers to your and your child's questions about the hospital, and can disclose whether there is a program for touring the facility. You'll need to make arrangements for this tour ahead of time.

No matter how you approach communication, be honest with your child. This age group needs to know that their parents will be waiting during their surgery or hospitalization. They need to know that their parents will be present, primarily because the younger child most fears separation from family. If you must leave your child, tell your child that you will be leaving. And tell him when you plan to return. Never tell a child that you will be right back and then not return. Give your child facts. For example, tell him, "I will not be back tonight, but I will be back tomorrow to have lunch with you."

Middle childhood. Verbal explanations can be given about one week before admission for a child of 6 to 8 years. This age group also benefits from the use of puppets and playing with hospital equipment. Also, children in this age group are better able to tell you what they think will happen, and you will be in a better position to correct any misconceptions for them. This age group has a better notion of the concept of asking questions and having their questions answered honestly, and parents can provide more details for them than for younger children. Children at this age also are better able to grasp concepts such as the length of stay, separation, and postsurgery issues such as limits on activity.

Preadolescence. The child 9 to 12 years of age can handle explanations given as much as two weeks before admission. Children in this age group learn by logical thinking. They benefit from clear verbal explanations and from a variety of visual cues: films, diagrams of body outlines with minimal detail, and books and videotapes. This group enjoys handling equipment, and they can more easily formulate a question about something they do not understand. Children this age benefit from information about procedures, surgery, and specific treatments. They also comprehend information about how they can participate in their own care, and should be told about limitations in activities which will be imposed by the treatment. They often benefit from visits by family and friends.

Adolescence. Children between the ages of 13 and 18 years benefit from having all types of information shared in a variety of ways as soon as the admission is scheduled. This age group learns well in peer groups. They are able to handle many directions and rules. Use of correct medical terminology and detailed information is important for this group. Questions should be encouraged and should be dealt with in detail. The older child most fears disability and a loss of body parts. They miss their friends and are worried about death.

Try as much as possible to keep routines the same as at home, and talk with the hospital staff about this to encourage them to help. Encourage your child to bring a favorite toy or other object from home, and if possible allow him to wear his own clothing in the hospital.

ANTICIPATING DISCHARGE: WHAT YOU NEED TO KNOW TO PREPARE

The hospital may have a system in place to provide counseling regarding what the child will need after being discharged. The person providing the discharge counseling may be a social worker or a nurse, either of whom can help you with the transition from hospital to home. Ask this person or your doctor for details on the following issues as they apply to your child. You may want to write down the answers on a note pad so that you can refer to them later.

- Should I be doing anything before admission to help me prepare to manage my child at home? Should I arrange for a hospital bed, wheelchair, potty chair, or anything else before admission, or will I have enough time to prepare for special things while my child is in the hospital?
- Will there be anything different upon the discharge of my child which will cause him to be more dependent upon me than he was upon admission?
- What arrangements will be made to prepare me to manage my child at home? Will my child need specialized care upon discharge which I can provide? Will the nursing staff teach me to provide for my child's new special needs at home? If not, then who will train me? Am I permitted to invite other family members to training sessions?
- Will my child require any specialized nursing care when she returns home from the hospital? Who will help me arrange special care?
- Who should I call if my child cannot be comforted at home and I feel that I need some advice on how to help her?
- Will special therapy be required during the hospital stay? Will this therapy be required at home? For how long? How will therapy be arranged for at home, and to whom may I speak for help and advice about this?
- Will special lab tests ordered during the hospital stay be required at home too? How will I go about getting tests completed at home? Is there someone who can advise me about getting special lab tests at home? When will I see the physician for follow-up?
- Will my child be able to walk or sit as she did before? If not, how long will it be before she returns to her normal state? If not, how long will it be before we know how much difference there is?
- How long will my child's activities be limited?
- When can my child return to school? Will she be able to use the usual mode of transportation to school, or will special transportation be needed?

On the subject of schooling, we should say that it is very important that you notify your child's school when your child will be hospitalized, and that you explain the procedure that will be done. The school will probably ask you for details about the hospital stay. If surgery is going to be performed, they will want to know whether there are any limitations imposed which they should be aware of, especially any restrictions on the child's activity which would affect his activities at school.

Keeping Medical History Records

Keeping a comprehensive but concise record of your child's medical history is essential to the proper management of the child's medical care. A child with disabilities generally has a great deal of contact with health care personnel and may have undergone a series of surgeries and other procedures. The child may be on multiple medications and the medications may need periodic dose adjustments. Keeping an up-to-date description of medical care is extremely valuable in designing present and future care. A brief "parent medical record" will also provide important information to emergency room personnel in the event your child needs to be taken to the emergency room. Because of the need for accurate, readily available medical information, the American College of Emergency Physicians, in collaboration with the American Academy of Pediatrics, developed an "Emergency Information Form for Children with Special Needs." This form (reproduced on pages 332 and 333) contains essential information emergency personnel need in order to make appropriate medical decisions. If you create your own brief record, it should include the following information.

Parent's Medical Record

1. Immunizations: up to date/missing _____.
2. Allergies to medication, foods, pollens, etc.
3. Medical problems (for example, CP, seizures, cardiac, gastrointestinal, diabetes, asthma).
4. As applicable: current medications and dosages; size and type of tracheostomy; gastrostomy tube, supplier, and type and amount of feedings. This list may be lengthy but is essential.
5. Current pediatrician and other medical or surgical specialists (for example, neurologist or orthopedist) and therapists.
6. Ongoing record of height and weight/growth chart (include dates).
7. School assessments (most recent).
8. Documents to confirm legal guardianship; insurance cards.
9. Record of surgeries (most recent first):

Example:	Date	Procedure	Surgeon	Hospital	Complication
	2/2/04	spine fusion	Miller	duPont	none
	5/9/00	tonsillectomy	Stone	County	bleeding

10. Record of hospitalizations:

Example:	Date	Reason	Physician	Hospital
	2/6–2/11/03	pneumonia	Bachrach	duPont
	3/5–6/5/90	premature birth	Smith	Lourdes

11. List of names and addresses of individuals to whom you wish a copy of your child's most recent health report to be sent. For example, when your child is seen by his neurologist, the pediatrician should receive a report.

Emergency Information Form for Children With Special Needs

American College of Emergency Physicians®

American Academy of Pediatrics

Date form completed	Revised	Initials
By Whom	Revised	Initials

Name:	**Birth date:** **Nickname:**
Home Address:	**Home/Work Phone:**
Parent/Guardian:	**Emergency Contact Names & Relationship:**
Signature/Consent*:	
Primary Language:	**Phone Number(s):**

Physicians:

Primary care physician:	**Emergency Phone:**
	Fax:
Current Specialty physician:	**Emergency Phone:**
Specialty:	**Fax:**
Current Specialty physician:	**Emergency Phone:**
Specialty:	**Fax:**
Anticipated Primary ED:	**Pharmacy:**
Anticipated Tertiary Care Center:	

Diagnoses/Past Procedures/Physical Exam:

1. _____

2. _____

3. _____

4. _____

Synopsis:

Baseline physical findings:

Baseline vital signs:

Baseline neurological status:

*Consent for release of this form to health care providers

Diagnoses/Past Procedures/Physical Exam continued:

Medications: Significant baseline ancillary findings (lab, x-ray, ECG):

1.

2.

3.

4.   Prostheses/Appliances/Advanced Technology Devices:

5.

6.

Management Data:

Allergies: Medications/Foods to be avoided   and why:

1.

2.

3.

Procedures to be avoided   and why:

1.

2.

3.

Immunizations (mm/yy)

Dates						Dates					
DPT						Hep B					
OPV						Varicella					
MMR						TB status					
HIB						Other					

Antibiotic prophylaxis: Indication: Medication and dose:

Common Presenting Problems/Findings With Specific Suggested Managements

Problem	Suggested Diagnostic Studies	Treatment Considerations

Comments on child, family, or other specific medical issues:

Physician/Provider Signature: Print Name:

You should carry the parent's medical record or emergency information form at all times so it will be available during scheduled appointments as well as in an emergency.

Although it's a smart idea to carry a brief record with you, we recommend that you keep a more extensive file at home. This file should include copies of reports from medical, psychological, and developmental tests done throughout the child's life, and should be kept in chronological order.

The file should also include copies of the Individualized Education Plan (IEP) and the Individualized Family Service Plan (IFSP), as well as notes and reports from teachers and therapists, and copies of any correspondence written on the child's behalf. Without your written permission, such reports cannot be given to you or anyone else. In April 2003, privacy and confidentiality regulations of the Health Insurance Portability and Accountability Act of 1996 (HIPAA) were implemented. Health care providers and health care organizations have strict guidelines that must be followed to protect the confidentiality of "protected patient information." Protected patient information includes all identifiable information that can be used to identify a patient including paper records, electronic records, and reports (including reports from therapy, school, Individualized Education Plans, Individual Family Service Plans, and verbal communications among providers, therapists, teachers, and nurses). No information can change hands without proper authorization. Consent forms must comply with the language in the privacy and confidentiality regulations. Parents therefore need to sign appropriate HIPAA-compliant consent forms and must specifically state the name of each individual who will be allowed access to their child's health information, and specifically what information is permitted to be accessed. Note that authorization forms are now required to have an expiration date or an expiration of a specific period or event. This period can be determined by the parent. If the parent wants information released after the expiration date, a new authorization form must be signed.

In the file, include a list of contacts with their phone numbers and the nature of your interaction with them, plus the outcome of the interaction. Also keep a list of all health care and school contacts with addresses and phone numbers, as well as information about insurance carriers and vendors of equipment. Include a letter authorizing release of reports dealing with your child which you might wish to be sent elsewhere. If you leave spaces for the addressee and a description of the report and where it originates, you can photocopy this letter and fill in the blanks as needed.

There are many ways to keep all this information in order. Many parents use their computer for record keeping. You do not need sophisticated computer skills to enter this information. You can easily list medications on a simple Word document and update this list whenever changes are made. Medication allergies, feeding schedule, supplies, procedures, and appointments are easily entered into the computer and can be printed out before a doctor's visit. Personal digital assistants (PDAs), which are handheld digital computers, allow portability. The date book in your PDA can be especially helpful when making follow-up appointments. If you do not have access to a computer, you can use a file card system for telephone numbers, supplemented with a loose-leaf binder containing reports. Or you might want to keep records in a file drawer or file box. If you take the time to set up the system properly, adding new information will be easy. This kind of record keeping will help you as you advocate for your child. If you become involved in a parent support group, you might describe your system for other parents who want to get started.

IMMUNIZATION SCHEDULE

Because children are not born with a natural immunity to diseases such as polio, measles, and mumps, every child needs to be immunized against these diseases, as well as others. Your child's doctor will keep a careful record of your child's vaccinations, but you need to keep a separate record. Ask your doctor for a booklet that you can keep updated. If you move out of town or change doctors for any other reason, be sure that the doctor sends your child's vaccination record, along with other medical records, to the new doctor. The most current immunization schedule can be found on the American Academy of Pediatrics Web site under "Children's Health Topics" or by calling 1-847-434-4000.

Life Planning Process

To prepare a plan in a simple step-by-step procedure without feeling overwhelmed by the process, families should know the 10 life-planning steps. If these steps are followed with the assistance of a qualified special needs planner, the family will create a comprehensive plan that addresses the lifestyle, legal, government benefits, financial, and care needs of the person.

Regardless of the age of the child or the severity of the disability, creating a plan is critically important now.

1. **Prepare a life plan.** Decide what you want regarding residential needs, employment, education, social activities, medical and dental care, religion, and final arrangements.

2. **Write informational and instructional directives.** Put your hopes and desires in a written document. Include information regarding care providers and assistants, attending physicians, dentists, medicine, functioning abilities, types of activities enjoyed, daily living skills, and rights and values. Make a videotape during daily activities such as bathing, dressing, eating, and recreation. A commentary accompanying the video is also useful.

3. **Decide on a type of supervision.** Guardianship and conservatorship

are legal appointments requiring court-ordered mandates. Individuals or institutions manage the estate of people judged incapable (not necessarily incompetent) of caring for their own affairs. Guardians and conservators are also responsible for the care and decisions made on behalf of people who are unable to care for themselves. In some states, guardians assist people and conservators manage the estate of individuals. Many parents who have children with disabilities do not realize that when their children reach 18, parents no longer have legal authority. They must petition the courts for appointment as a legal guardian. Choose conservators/guardians for today and tomorrow. Select capable individuals in the event you become unable to make decisions in the future.

4. **Determine the cost.** Make a list of current and anticipated monthly expenses. When you have established this amount, decide on a reasonable return on your investments, and calculate how much will be needed to provide enough funds to support her lifestyle. Do not forget to include disability income, Social Security, etc.

5. **Find resources.** Possible resources to fund your plan include government benefits, family assistance, inheritances, savings, life insurance, and investments.

6. **Prepare legal documents.** Choose a qualified attorney, paralegal, or certified legal document preparer to assist in preparing wills, trusts, power of attorney, guardianship, living will, etc.

7. **Consider a "Special Needs Trust."** A Special Needs Trust holds assets for the benefit of people with disabilities and uses the income to provide for their supplemental needs. If drafted properly, assets are not considered income, so people do not jeopardize their Supplemental Security Income or Medicaid. Also, they do not have to repay Medicaid for services received. Appoint a trustee and successor trustees (individuals or corporate entities, such as banks). There are various types of Special Needs Trusts. Make sure the person preparing your documents understands the differences and provides you with the right one.

8. **Use a life-plan binder.** Place all documents in a single binder and notify caregivers/family where they can find it.

9. **Hold a meeting.** Give copies of relevant documents and instructions to family/caregivers. Review everyone's responsibilities.

10. **Review your plan.** At least once a year, review and update the plan. Modify legal documents as necessary.

Once you have decided to prepare a plan, find someone to help you or hire a professional planner. Referral sources are available through governmental agencies, organizations, or local support groups. "Who will care when you are no longer there?" is an overwhelming concern people with disabilities and their families must address. Solutions are available. The next step is up to you.

About Casts

Before taking a child in a cast home from the hospital or doctor's office, parents should receive detailed instructions in how to care for the child (and for the cast) from the child's doctor or another health care professional. For example, the parent should find out what physical limitations this cast will impose: if the child is normally ambulatory, for example, will she be permitted to walk with the cast? If she normally can sit on the toilet, will she be able to do so in the cast, or will a bedpan be needed? Other questions parents need to have answered include:

- Do I need to arrange special transportation home from the hospital, such as an ambulance?
- When can my child return to school in the cast?
- Will I need to provide special care for my child and the cast? Who will train me in how to perform this care, and when will the training begin?
- What are some problems a cast can cause that I can look for?

Once you've received instructions and training in taking care of a child in a cast, and you and your child have arrived home, the following care tips might be useful.

Bathing. The skin under the cast should not get wet. If your child can walk in the cast and get to the bathroom for a sponge bath, let him do so. If you need to bathe your child in bed, here are some tips:

1. Gather towels, a washcloth, a basin with water, soap, a soap dish, and protective towels or flannel-covered plastic bed protectors for the bed and the cast. Use a bath sheet (a large towel) to keep your child warm during the bath.

2. Wash the head, ears, and face first, then all exposed skin beginning with the chest and moving to arms, trunk, back, and legs. Wash the genitals and buttocks last. Cover exposed areas with a bath blanket or dry towels.

3. Make sure along the way that you have removed all soap residue and have dried the skin. Be careful not to get soap under the cast, since this may cause itching. Do not use lotions or creams under the cast or near the edges of the cast.

Tooth care. If your child can walk to the bathroom, allow her to brush her own teeth. If not, you will need a spit cup or emesis basin so she can spit out the contents of her mouth after she brushes her teeth in bed. If you normally brush your child's teeth, you probably have your own efficient technique and should continue with it.

Hair grooming and washing. If your child can get to the sink, help him wash his hair over the sink or tub. Protect the cast with plastic to keep it from getting wet. A plastic barber's or hairdresser's cape might serve the purpose. If the child must be confined to bed for a bath and hairwashing, you may want to invest in special equipment that is commercially available to allow water from hairwashing to drain off the bed. Check with local department stores or home care companies for a listing of the products they carry that make it easier to wash hair in bed. It may be possible to wash your child's hair in bed by funneling a plastic drape from around his neck into a plastic container (a trash can or bucket), allowing the shampoo water to run from the head, to the plastic, to the container.

Clothing.   No special clothing is needed. Do not dress a child in a cast in a way that will overheat him, however, since he may perspire and begin itching. Loose, comfortable clothing is the best choice.

Cast checks and skin care.   Casts should be checked daily. Report to the doctor any changes in the cast or the skin. To check a cast, you'll need to use a flashlight and your eyes, hands, and nose. Note the general condition of the cast, and observe for any cracks, breaks, weakness, or damp areas. Observe whether the cast is getting tighter, either because of swelling under the cast or because your child has grown since the cast was applied. A tight cast can be very dangerous and must be reported to the doctor at once.

If your child is in a large cast such as a hip spica or body cast, you can feel the skin with your hands and look with a flashlight for any signs of secretions, drainage, or skin irritation. Check for odors coming out of the cast. Pay attention if your child complains of tingling and numbness, burning or itching. Report any such complaints, as well as any sign of odor, secretions, or drainage to your child's physician.

For skin care, do not use lotions or creams under the cast, since they build up and can irritate the skin. Plain 70 percent isopropyl rubbing alcohol, with nothing extra in it, is used by many physicians to clean older children's skin. It can be used sparingly on the skin at the edges of the cast, since it will dry better than soap and water. This technique should not be used on young children, since it dries out the skin and can produce skin irritation.

Neurovascular assessment.   Probably the most important task you'll do every day in connection with your child's cast is to perform a neurovascular assessment. This involves observing all casted extremities (or, in the case of a body cast or a hip spica, all extremities) for the following: color, temperature, swelling, sensation, numbness and tingling, range of motion, and circulation. Immediately report to the doctor any of the following:
- swelling
- severe color change
- lack of capillary refill (capillary refill is indicated by the pink color returning to the fingertips after pressure is applied and then released)
- increased pain; strange feelings
- changes in skin or body temperature

Finishing the cast, or petaling the cast. This is a means of making the cast edges smooth and free from scratchy edges and of preventing pieces of the cast from falling off. If the cast is finished with stockinette pulled smoothly over the edge of the cast, nothing more needs to be done. If the cast is not finished in this way, a variety of petaling materials may be used.

Cut moleskin or waterproof tape into strips an inch or two wide by three inches long. Place these strips in an overlapping fashion with about one inch of the tape inside the cast, sticky side against the cast, and the remainder pulled tightly and placed on the outside of the cast. Carefully observe these cast edges as the days go by, because some young children have a sensitivity to the adhesive material on the petaling strips, and even though the sticky surface is against the cast, there is enough sticky material at the petal edge to cause some irritation.

Positioning. If your child is capable of changing her position on her own, encourage her to do so. In any case, make sure that your child changes position at least every two to three hours during the day and every four hours during the night, to relieve the pressure of the cast on the various skin surfaces, and to avoid bedsores. This is especially important for the child in a body or hip spica–type cast.

Bedpan use. If your child is in a body cast and must use a bedpan, follow these steps in helping your child use the bedpan successfully:

1. Elevate the head of the bed, or use pillows to elevate the child's head higher than the hips. In this way, gravity can help drain urine and feces into the bedpan.

2. Cut pieces of plastic about 8 by 12 inches which will be tucked between the skin and cast. Turn the child to one side and insert the plastic between the cast and the skin surface in the buttocks area, so that the pieces of plastic overlap each other.

3. Place the rim of the bedpan against the cast. Center the child on the bedpan. Funnel the plastic into the bedpan to prevent fecal material from soiling the cast. Urine and fecal material will be diverted into the bedpan via the plastic.

4. When your child has finished, remove the plastic from the edge of the cast as you turn your child back to the side. Clean the genital area and dry it well.

For the incontinent young child in a spica-type cast, place a sanitary napkin or folded diaper for extra absorbency over the genital area, and then place a diaper over that. For a young child, the material must be changed every two hours; for the older child, the diaper must be changed every time the child eliminates.

Using Nutritional Boosters

Because children with CP often have difficulty gaining weight and tolerating different textures, caregivers may need to find ways of supplementing their child's food intake. Concentrating the calories in the foods a child will eat is a good way to increase the calories and protein in his or her diet. As long as your child can tolerate them, you can add any of the following foods to your child's diet to increase the calorie and protein intake:

- butter, corn oil, margarine on bread, crackers, vegetables, rice, pasta, or cooked cereal
- powdered milk added to regular milk (fortified milk) or used in cooking
- wheat germ
- puddings or custards (can be made with fortified milk)
- milkshakes, ice cream, yogurts
- cream soups, cream sauces, gravies
- sour cream, cheese

A general rule of thumb is not to give your child anything plain. If your child eats blended food, add juice, gravy, or milk in place of water in the blender.

A wide selection of nutrition supplements are available on the market today. Most are milk based and lactose free. Recently, more juice-based supplements have become available. The supplements can range from 30 to 60 calories per ounce. Most can be found at your local pharmacy or grocery store. Many are flavored and can be taken orally. For many children, taste is the determining factor when it comes to deciding what formula to use. For some children who are supported nutritionally by formula feedings, the appropriate formula can be determined with the help of your pediatrician or dietitian. Some formulas are very specialized for children who have problems tolerating tube feedings. Below is a sample of some of the products available:

Milk-based formulas
- Carnation Instant Breakfast
- Boost / Boost Plus
- Ensure / Ensure Plus
- Kindercal
- Jevity
- Nutren Jr / Nutren / Nutren 1.5 / Nutren 2.0
- Pediasure / Pediasure with Fiber
- Promote / Promote with Fiber
- Resource / Resource Just for Kids
- Scandishakes
- Sustacal

Juice-based formulas

- Boost Breeze
- Enlive
- Nubasics
- Resource Juice Drink

Specialized formulas

- Neocate
- Peptamin Jr / Peptamin
- Vivonex / Vivonex TEN

Consult your insurance company to see if there is help with payment for either oral supplements or tube feedings. You may also need a prescription for the supplements and/or a Letter of Medical Necessity. If your child is eligible for The Women, Infants and Children Supplemental Food Program (WIC), this program may provide some of the formula for you. In some states Medicaid or Medicare may help with payment.

Managing Tube Feedings

If your child is unable to gain adequate weight with oral feedings, or if your child is at risk for aspiration either because of poor oral motor muscle coordination or severe gastroesophageal reflux, an alternate method of feeding may be needed. Tube feedings are given via a feeding tube surgically inserted into the stomach (gastrostomy tube or G-tube) or inserted into the beginning of the small intestine (jejunostomy tube or J-tube). Both types of tubes can come as a skin level tube ("button tube") which lies flat on the skin or as a catheter. The catheter can be secured to the undershirt by wrapping a piece of tape approximately 1 by 1 inch around a section of the tube and attaching a safety pin to the end of the tape. The safety pin can then be attached to the undershirt.

Before your child is discharged from the hospital, be sure that you understand and are comfortable with the care of your child's gastrostomy tube. There are many different types of tubes available, but you should be taught how to care for the specific kind of tube that your child is using. Health care specialists will teach you exactly how to feed your child through the gastrostomy tube, but here is an overview of gastrostomy tube feedings for you to refer to at home.

TYPES OF FEEDINGS

There are two basic types of feedings. One is the *bolus*. In this type of feeding, a specific amount of formula is given three or four times a day, much like a regular mealtime. A syringe pump or gravity system is connected to the tube, and formula flows in over a period of between 15 and 60 minutes.

The other type of feeding is *continuous*. In this setup, formula flows slowly into the stomach or small intestine over a long period. A special pump is used to measure precise amounts of feedings and to regulate the flow of food. Jejunostomy tube feedings are always given as continuous feedings.

You will need the following equipment:

- Food at room temperature. It will most likely be a commercially prepared formula. Your dietitian will determine which food is best for your child.
- tap water at room temperature (to rinse the tube)
- a syringe
- a feeding bag
- tubing
- any special adapters specific to the tube used by your child

HOW TO GIVE A TUBE FEEDING

1. Gather equipment and be sure it is in working order.
2. Wash your hands.
3. Position the child so that his head is elevated. This can be done by positioning the child on your lap. If the child is older you can elevate the child's head by raising the head of the bed with pillows, a rolled blanket, or a wedge under the child's head and shoulders. You may also position the child comfortably in his wheelchair.
4. If a feeding bag is used, run the feeding through the bag and the attached tubing.
5. Attach a syringe to the gastrostomy tube and flush with water to be sure that it is clear. (This preliminary water flush may or may not be recommended by your child's physician. Follow his or her instructions.) If the tube is occluded (blocked), consult your physician for further instructions. Do not force the flush.
6. Remove the syringe from the gastrostomy tube and attach the feeding bag and tubing to allow the bolus to go in or the continuous feeding to begin. Use the special adapter required by some button tubes for either type of

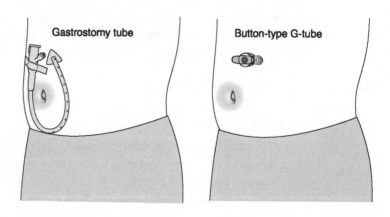

Gastrostomy tube   Button-type G-tube

feeding. You may use a 30–60 cc syringe without plunger to allow the feeding to flow by gravity. Continue adding to the syringe until finished, or you should set the rate prescribed by your physician to run automatically on a pump.

7. When the feeding is complete, flush the tube with water in the amount specified by your child's physician.

8. Pinch or clamp the tube before removing the syringe or tubing. Clamp or cap indwelling tubes. Remove the feeding adapter from the button tube and snap the plug in place.

9. Observe the child for abdominal distention and vomiting. Notify the doctor if this becomes a problem. There are certain venting procedures required for certain tubes; your child's physician will describe these to you.

10. Clean the syringe in warm soapy water. Rinse until clear.

TUBE FEEDING INFORMATION CARD

Many parents find that keeping a feeding tube information card is helpful. We suggest that you record the following information on a file card and keep it handy. This way you'll be sure to have all relevant facts ready at a glance, should you need them.

Child's name:
    Tube specifications:
        size:
        type:
        balloon volume:
        button size:
        dates tube replaced:
    Surgery date:
        surgeon: telephone number:
        specialist: telephone number:
    Feeding:
        type:
        amount:
        water:
    Feeding instructions:
        feeding times:
        amount of each feeding:
    Pump setting or rate:
    Flush with   cc water before/after every feeding

Oral Hygiene: Providing Mouth and Teeth Care

Start oral hygiene in the first year even before the child has teeth. Begin by just wiping the inside of the child's mouth with a moist cloth—this will get him used to having his mouth cleaned. Toothbrushing should start by age 18 months and can be initiated with soft brushes. Brushing should include the gums and tongue as well as the teeth.

The first visit to the dentist should be between the ages of 18 and 24 months. At this time, the dentist will review the oral hygiene program you are using and will help you resolve any frustrations you may have. Usually x-rays will not be taken until later, but the main goal of the first visit is for the dentist and the dental hygienist to understand how your child will react in the dental office and what his special needs are.

Toothbrushing is the most important daily activity in maintaining oral hygiene, and it needs to be established early. Brushing should not be a struggle for the parent or the child. Find a time of day when the child is usually in a good mood, and try to do it at the same time every day. Then you can provide some reward for the child's behaving well. Eventually, brushing becomes an accepted part of the daily routine. Although it is advisable to leave the child with a clean mouth overnight, brushing when the child tolerates it best will provide the greatest opportunity for success in the long run.

If your child has problems of head and trunk control, you need to position him so that you can control his posture. This is usually done in the best seating system the child has, such as his wheelchair. Choose a soft multi-fluted nylon brush and use both circular and up-and-down motions. If the child will not tolerate a toothbrush, use a cotton-tipped swab or a soft washcloth that has been soaked with a mildly abrasive toothpaste or with an antiseptic solution. Eliminate gagging by watching where you are brushing and avoiding areas that trigger the gagging.

As your child starts to brush his own teeth, monitor his technique and be sure that it gets done. This is exactly like other activities of daily living, such as bathing, where parents are often monitoring children between ages 5 and 10 years. Schoolteachers can also provide excellent positive reinforcement in the school setting.

Fluoride treatment is an important aspect of preventing cavities. Fluoride can be taken as a flavored liquid or chewable tablet, or as a mouth rinse. Or it can be applied directly to the teeth by a dentist. The specific need for fluoride varies, depending on the amount that is in the local water supply; however, many children with significant disabilities do not drink much tap water and will need to obtain additional fluoride. Check with your dentist or physician, since you will need a prescription for fluoride.

Cavities can also be decreased by watching the diet. For example, fresh fruits, and artificially sweetened soft drinks are preferred over cakes, candy, cookies, and sugary soft drinks for the prevention of cavities.

Toilet Training Your Child

The most important factor in successful toilet training is the cognitive or developmental level of the child, regardless of his or her chronological age. Children can be successfully toilet trained if they have the developmental and cognitive abilities of a 2 to 4 year old. Physical barriers can be overcome with adaptive seating so the child can be properly positioned on the toilet seat. The child will need the help of a parent or aide at school to assist with transferring from the wheelchair to the toilet seat.

Another important factor in successful toilet training is the attitude of the parent, who must be relaxed and positive about the process of toilet training and who must convey this attitude to the child.

Praising the child for success on the potty is crucial. But even before toilet training can begin, both the child and the parent must be ready. Your child may signal her readiness for toilet training in one of several ways. For example, while urinating or having a bowel movement (or just before), the child may become either fussy or quiet, wiggle and demonstrate the need to change position, suddenly lie or stand very still, go to the corner and squat, change facial expression, or say that she is wet. The parent needs to pay attention to these behavioral changes and be ready to interpret these gestures to mean that the child needs to eliminate. Only when all these signals and good intentions come together can toilet training begin in earnest.

ESTABLISHING A PATTERN

One thing that will help establish a pattern of elimination is keeping regular mealtimes. In this way, the stomach, bowels, and bladder will be empty and full at regular intervals. Not only that, but food tends to stimulate the bowel, and many people go to the bathroom after a meal, usually breakfast or dinner. So you may be able to predict your child's bowel habits based upon mealtimes. After you've determined the normal pattern of elimination, you'll know when to place your child on the toilet in order to achieve the best success.

GETTING STARTED

Choose a time when your child is rested and in a good mood to begin. You'll need a child's-size potty chair or potty seat.

When your child has indicated (by one of the above gestures, or something similar) that she needs to urinate or have a bowel movement, take her to the bathroom and explain in simple language what is to be done. Use very specific common words to describe the act of elimination. Place the child on the seat and stay with her until the training session is completed. After about five minutes on the toilet, the child should be wiped and rewarded with hugs and praise for the desired behaviors.

If the child was not successful in achieving the desired behavior, praise her for cooperating and sitting quietly on the toilet or potty chair. During training, the child should sit on the seat without toys or playthings, since these would divert attention from what she is supposed to be doing.

Repeat this process until the child is able to tell you in advance that she needs to go, or is able to use the bathroom or potty on her own.

BOWEL TRAINING

If your child is mentally retarded, it may be helpful to institute a bowel training program. This, too, involves establishing a regular pattern of mealtimes to help establish a regular pattern of elimination, but the difference is that routinely, about 15 to 30 minutes after one meal is finished, the child is placed on the toilet for 15 to 30 minutes. Choose either breakfast or dinner and stick with it, since the point of a bowel training program is to train the child to produce a bowel movement at the same time every day or every other day.

Make sure that the child is comfortable, with feet flat on the floor or supported by a stool. Use simple descriptive common words to describe the desired activity. Again, be positive by praising the desired results, and praise the child for sitting on the toilet as you wished, even if there is no bowel movement. Be sure there are no distractions during this time.

Many children with CP have chronic constipation, which can interfere with bowel training. If your child does not have a bowel movement at least every other day, your child is probably constipated. The treatment of constipation is described in Chapter 3.

ADAPTIVE TOILETING

Special handling techniques are used for toileting the child with cerebral palsy who is physically challenged. To protect the child (as well as themselves) from injury, care providers need to learn these techniques. Ask a physical or an occupational therapist for tips in handling your specific child.

It may be necessary for a child with CP to use adaptive seating to be properly positioned on the toilet seat. Children with CP need firm support, with handrails and feet flat on the floor or a hard surface. Proper body mechanics while lifting a child to the toilet seat are necessary to decrease stress on the caregiver's back (see page 300). Further information on adaptive seating is usually available through your child's occupational therapist.

Giving an Enema

You may have to give your child an enema, either occasionally or on a regular basis. Enemas work by distending the rectum and making the child feel the need to have a bowel movement; in addition, they clean out stool that has been held in the rectum. You can buy Fleet or Pediatric Fleet enemas at the drugstore, or you can use tap water in an enema bag. Check with your doctor about what's best for your child. Use about 1 ounce of water for every 20 pounds of the child's weight. Unless recommended by your doctor, do not use more than 4½ ounces of water. Before you give an enema to your child, be sure to explain what you will be doing, and what will happen.

HOW TO GIVE AN ENEMA TO A CHILD

1. The enema should be warm—close to body temperature, not hot or cold.
2. Position the child in one of three ways: sitting on the toilet or potty chair; lying on a rug on the bathroom floor, face down with hips and knees bent toward the chest; or positioned on the rug on the left side, with the left leg straight and the right leg bent at the hip and knee and placed on top of the left leg.
3. For a disposable enema: Remove the protective cap from the enema bottle. Gently insert the tip about one inch into the rectum. Slowly squeeze the enema container until it is nearly empty. (A small amount of the contents of the container will remain after squeezing.) Remove the tip from the rectum. For an enema bag: Put Vaseline jelly on the enema tip; gently insert the tip about one inch into the rectum and slowly squeeze the water into the rectum. Hold the bag about one foot above the child's body.
4. Hold the child's buttocks together, if necessary, to keep the water inside the rectum until the child tells you he or she needs to have a bowel movement, usually after about three to five minutes.
5. Help the child to the toilet or potty chair, or place her over a bedpan that has been placed in her bed. Or allow the enema to be expelled into a diaper, if necessary.
6. Keep a record of the results.

Giving Rectal Medications or Suppositories

For a variety of reasons, some medications may need to be given by rectum. When a child is vomiting and it's important for her to have the medication, the medication can make its way into the child's system if it is administered rectally. Medications are also given rectally to children who have difficulty swallowing, who are unable to swallow, or who are actively seizing. Finally, a child who will be having surgery within a day often must refrain from having anything by mouth. Some necessary medications can nevertheless be administered by rectum.

The medications most commonly given by rectum are antiseizure medications, sedatives, antipyretics (medications that help control temperature), antiemetics (medications that help control nausea), and bowel-stimulating suppositories, usually composed of glycerin. Rectal medications are primarily supplied in suppository form (suppositories are shaped like bullets, with one rounded end and one flat end). You can lubricate a suppository for easier insertion by dipping it in water or in a water-soluble lubricant. Do not use an oil-based lubrication, since it may interfere with medication absorption.

HOW TO GIVE MEDICATION IN SUPPOSITORY FORM TO A CHILD

1. Before getting started, ask the child to try to move his bowels, since if there is stool in the rectum, this may interfere with absorption of the medication.

2. To get started, position the child either on his left side, with hips and knees flexed, or on his abdomen with knees flexed and positioned toward the chest. Older children prefer to lie on their sides, whereas insertion is easier in infants if they are placed on their abdomen.

3. Put a non-latex glove on the hand you will be using. With a gloved finger, insert the medication beyond the sphincter. Use the pinky finger to insert the suppository in infants and toddlers. In older children, use the index finger. The usual distance for the insertion of rectal medications is as follows:
- in infants and young toddlers, about 1 to 1½ inches
- in older toddlers and preschoolers, about 2 to 3 inches
- in school age or adolescents, about 3 to 4 inches.

4. For the medication to be effective, it must be held in the rectum for 10 minutes. To prevent early expulsion of the medication—before it has been fully absorbed—it may be necessary to hold the buttocks together for 5 to 10 minutes. Older children are generally able to control their sphincter better than younger children. A suppository that has been administered to stimulate a bowel movement ought to be held for 5 minutes, or until the child states a need to move his bowels.

HOW TO GIVE LIQUID MEDICATIONS RECTALLY TO A CHILD

The goal of the procedure is to deliver by rectum an appropriate amount of medication via a catheter. We recommend using a size 15 French (Mentor) catheter for this procedure.

The following equipment may be needed:
- size 15 French (Mentor) intermittent catheter
- the prescribed medication
- a syringe to deliver the volume of medicine ordered
- tap water
- a water-soluble lubricant
- a protective pad

1. Remove the syringe from the package and attach a needle to it.

2. Draw the medication from the bottle into the syringe, taking up a little more than the prescribed amount.

3. Flick the syringe with your finger to get rid of air bubbles, and measure the amount of medication in the syringe again.

4. Remove the needle from the syringe and place the needle in a safe container for disposal. (Do not attempt to recap the needle because of the danger of sticking yourself with the needle.)

5. Draw up into the same syringe an amount of air equal to the amount of medication. The air will move to the top of the syringe when the syringe is held upright. When the medication is administered, the air will follow the medication into the rectum and will assist in clearing the syringe and delivering the ordered amount of the medication.

6. Lubricate the catheter tip in water-soluble lubricant and attach the catheter to the end of the syringe.

7. Position the child on his or her left side. Insert the catheter into the rectum. For a child weighing 22 pounds (10 kg) or less, insert it 1¼ inch; for a child between 22 pounds and 44 pounds (10–20 kg), insert it 1½ inches; for a child weighing more than 44 pounds (20 kg), insert the catheter 2¾ inches.

8. Hold the syringe upright so that the air bubbles rise inside the syringe and are delivered last. Push the medication into the tubing and follow it with the air in the same syringe.

9. Remove the catheter and hold the buttocks together for 3 to 5 minutes to allow the medication to be absorbed.

Suctioning Techniques

Note: You must be trained in suctioning techniques by your health care professional or a home health professional before you try the procedure on your own.

Some children need help in clearing their airway of mucus. Suctioning will help clear the airway, but this procedure should only be performed when the child needs it. Suction your child under the following circumstances: (1) when you hear your child make wet breathing sounds, as if air is being pushed through wet mucus; (2) when your child is having difficulty breathing and is restless; or (3) when your child's color is paler than usual and the nostrils are flaring out. The child will probably gag or cough when you use a suction catheter.

The following description of the procedure for suctioning is provided only as a memory refresher for caregivers who have already been trained to do the procedure by a doctor or another health care professional. If you do not feel comfortable performing the procedure, you should not attempt to do it alone. *Do not attempt to suction your child if you have not been trained to do so.*

You will need the following equipment for the procedure:
- suction machine and tubing
- cool salt water
- containers for rinsing the tubing

You can make up the cool salt water, or saline, solution by mixing ¼ teaspoon of table salt with 2 cups water. Boil this mixture, and then cool it. After it has cooled, place it in the refrigerator in a clean glass jar. Manufactured saline solution can also be obtained by a prescription from your doctor.

HOW TO SUCTION A CHILD

1. Gather necessary equipment and make sure the suction machine is working properly.
2. Wash hands thoroughly.
3. Connect suction tubing to suction machine tubing.
4. Measure the tube from the tip of the earlobe to the tip of the nose. Keep your fingers on this mark. This is how far the tube will need to be inserted.
5. Insert the tip of the tube into the saline to wet the tube. Place the thumb over the tube opening to check on the effectiveness of the suction.
6. Tell the child what you will be doing and what to expect, and try to enlist his help.
7. Insert the tube into the nostril to the appropriate length, with *no* suction. Keep your finger off the suction port opening in the tube.
8. With the tube in place, put your thumb over the suction port, and rotate the tube as you slowly move it out of the nostril. This should take no longer than 5 seconds.
9. Rinse the tube in saline. Let the child relax a moment.
10. Repeat steps 5–9 for the other nostril.
11. After suctioning the nostrils, you may suction the mouth. Remember to rinse the tube in saline first.
12. Insert the tube into either side of the inside of the mouth with *no* suction.
13. Once the tube is correctly placed in the mouth, place your thumb over the suction port and rotate or twist the tube out of the mouth for no more than 5 seconds.
14. Rinse the tubing by suctioning the saline through it until the tubing is clear.
15. Repeat oral suctioning if necessary.
16. Dispose of unused saline.

To clean the tubing, follow these steps:

1. Rinse very well in tap water and then place in hot soapy water.
2. Rinse inside and outside with hot water.
3. Place on paper towels to dry. When dry, place in clean plastic bag until needed for the next time.

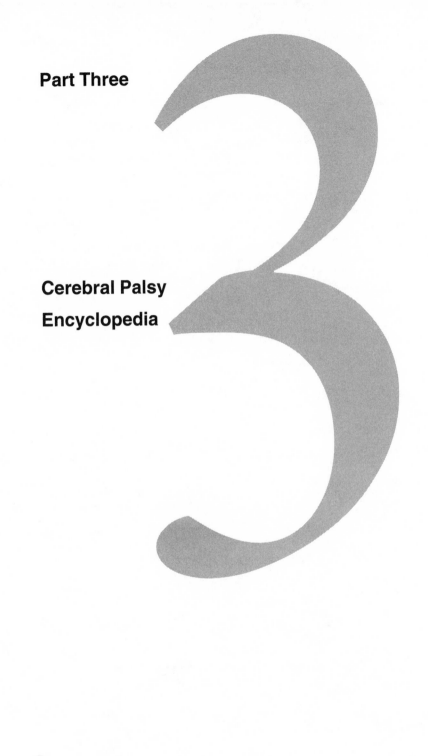

Part Three

**Cerebral Palsy
Encyclopedia**

Achilles Tendon Lengthening

(TAL, tendon Achilles lengthening, Achilles tendon contracture, equinus contracture)

The Achilles tendon is the muscle that is most commonly contracted in children with cerebral palsy. Contracture of this muscle prevents the foot from being flexed up. For the child who is able to stand, this contracture prevents him from standing with his foot flat—instead, he is on tiptoe. He may try to place his foot flat, but he will have to bend his knee back to do this. The initial treatment for an Achilles tendon contracture usually involves physical therapy combined with brace use (AFO) during the day.

Indications: Achilles tendon lengthening is indicated for children for whom the brace no longer keeps the foot flat or for teenagers trying to discontinue the use of the brace. Also, if the muscle is too tight to allow the child to use an AFO, then Achilles tendon lengthening is rec-

ommended. Occasionally, tendon lengthenings are also done for people who cannot stand or walk but who want to keep their feet flat on a wheelchair rest. In this case, the procedure is done for cosmetic reasons and to enable the person to wear shoes.

The surgery. The Achilles tendon is located behind the ankle and is attached to the gastrocnemius and soleus muscles, which are located just above and behind the knee. There are three different techniques for surgical lengthening of the Achilles tendon. *Percutaneous tendon Achilles lengthening* involves making a small stab wound through the skin in two or three different places, then stretching the tendon. The goal is to nick the tendon in several places and have the tendon tear in such a way that it stretches itself out and heals back in place. The advantage of this procedure is that it involves very small incisions; however, it provides the least control over the amount of lengthening.

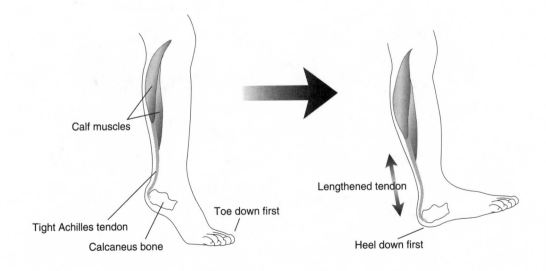

Calf muscles

Tight Achilles tendon

Calcaneus bone

Toe down first

Lengthened tendon

Heel down first

The second method, called *Z-plasty lengthening,* involves making an open incision that exposes the tendon; a Z-cut is then made in the tendon. The tendon ends slide apart and are sutured into place again. This procedure allows the most controlled lengthening of the whole tendon and muscle area.

The third method is called *Baker lengthening, gastroc recession,* or *myotendinous lengthening* and involves identifying where the gastrocnemius and soleus muscles come together in the middle of the calf to form the Achilles tendon. The gastrocnemius muscle is loosened and slid proximally over the soleus. The advantage of this procedure is that it has the lowest risk of *over*lengthening; one disadvantage is that sometimes it does not provide sufficient lengthening. This difficulty in obtaining sufficient lengthening with the Baker method explains why the Z-plasty is often the preferred procedure.

After-surgery care: After an Achilles tendon lengthening the child wears a short cast (from the toes to the knee). These casts typically have soles, which allows the child to stand and walk immediately after the Achilles tendon lengthening has been done. Following removal of the cast in 4 to 6 weeks, the child returns to a stretching program for maintenance. An AFO may also be used to maintain correction, especially for the growing child. A hinged brace may also be used, allowing the child to raise the front of the foot, but not to lower the toes to walk on tiptoe.

What to expect: The complications from Achilles tendon lengthening, especially in children who walk, may be very severe if the tendon is overlengthened. It is far preferable for the child to have a slightly tight Achilles tendon so that the child tiptoes slightly than to have the tendon completely nonfunctional. Another risk from Achilles tendon lengthening is the need to have the lengthening repeated. The child between the ages of 3 and 5 has a 25 to 30 percent chance of having the lengthening repeated between the ages of 9 and 12. Repeated lengthenings can be done three or four times, but it is seldom necessary to repeat more than once.

Agenesis of the Corpus Callosum
(Aicardi syndrome)

The corpus callosum is the structure in the brain that joins together the two cerebral hemispheres and provides a pathway from one side of the brain to the other. If a child does not have this structure, he may have seizures and mild to moderate mental retardation, as well as impaired visual and motor coordination. Sometimes children who don't have the corpus callosum are also deficient in cellular migration and proliferation, which essentially means that the brain wiring is not correct; this can be seen in a variety of chromosomal defects. Agenesis of the corpus callosum is an integral part of Aicardi syndrome, which appears to occur only in females and is characterized by severe mental retardation, generalized seizures that begin early in life, and specific abnormalities of the retina.

The absence of the corpus callosum is diagnosed with an MRI scan or a CT scan of the brain. Some individuals

Corpus callosum   Cerebral hemispheres

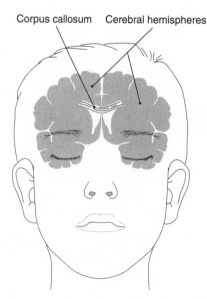

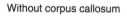
Without corpus callosum

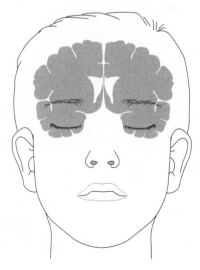

with this diagnosis are completely normal otherwise. However, children with many other congenital deformities of the brain are at higher risk for having this deformity. When it is seen by MRI or CT scan during an evaluation of a child for cerebral palsy, it suggests more underlying problems. This diagnosis by itself cannot be used to make a specific prognosis of what will happen to the child, however. Because of their brain abnormalities, these children often have cerebral palsy.

Air Swallowing

(aerophagia)

Chronic air swallowing is predominantly a problem for children with mental retardation. Its main characteristic is that it causes the abdomen to become distended. If the child has had an operation to prevent gastrointestinal reflux, so that stomach contents cannot come back up to the mouth, then she is not able to release the air pressure that develops in her stomach by burping, which may cause significant abdominal distension and pain. If she has a gastrostomy tube, the air can be vented through the tube. If she doesn't, occasionally the pain becomes severe enough that a tube is required. Usually children who have not had operative procedures to prevent vomiting or reflux are able to release the air themselves by burping. Aerophagia is usually made worse when the child is agitated or is not engaged in an activity. Treatment is predominantly directed toward keeping the child comfortable and occupied with toys or a similar activity. There are no other significant side effects from chronic air swallowing.

Airway Clearance

Respiratory complications are often a significant problem for children with CP. Respiratory infections are the most common cause for repeated admissions to the hospital for these children. One of the reasons for their susceptibility to respiratory problems is that their normal airway clearance is often compromised by their limited mobility and a weak or ineffective cough. Children who have quadriplegic CP, resulting in their inability to walk, spend most of their day in a wheelchair. Thus, they do not have the opportunity to exercise and breathe deeply, which is one of the main mechanisms for clearing one's airway. In addition, many children with CP cannot clear their airway with an effective cough. They either may be unable to take in enough air to have an effective cough, or they have poor coordination of the muscles of their throat, making their cough either ineffective or nonexistent. Without the ability to cough effectively, these children are unable to clear the secretions

that are normally produced in the lungs, and such pooled secretions can lead to recurrent pneumonia or bronchitis.

Traditionally, technique for removing mucus from the lungs of a child who cannot cough effectively has been a technique called *chest physical therapy*. Typical treatments last 20 to 30 minutes and are usually required several times a day. The caregiver or nurse administers percussion to the child's chest wall, while having her lie in a variety of different positions. Many children with CP have scoliosis and/or contractures, making the proper position difficult to achieve.

Another treatment that has been used to help mobilize secretions in the lungs is the ABI vest*. It consists of an inflatable vest connected by hoses to an air-pulse generator. The generator rapidly inflates and deflates the vest, thus compressing and releasing the chest wall. The resulting chest wall oscillation generates increased airflow through the airways, creating forces that are like a cough and mobilizing secretions. It does not require any positioning or special breathing techniques.

Amblyopia

(lazy eye)

Amblyopia is defined as subnormal vision in one or both eyes and is sometimes referred to as "lazy eye." Amblyopia is frequently associated with strabismus (crossed eyes). Because the brain sees double with strabismus, there is a tendency to suppress or tune out the image of the deviating eye so that only one image is seen. If this persists untreated in a child, such suppression can result in amblyopia and eventually lead to a significant loss of visual function in

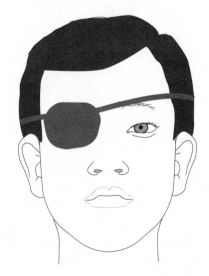

that eye. The key to successful treatment is early detection and intervention.

With an infant, amblyopia can be reversed in a matter of weeks, whereas with an older child in whom it has existed for a longer period of time, months or even years of treatment may be necessary. Treatment may include (1) providing the clearest possible image to the eye by correcting any refractive error with glasses, or removing a cataract; or (2) stimulation or forced use of the amblyopic eye by patching the better-functioning eye. Patching forces the child to use the amblyopic eye and may result in a restoration of near normal vision.

American Academy of Cerebral Palsy and Developmental Medicine
(AACPDM)

This organization was formed in 1947 by professionals from many different subspecialties of medicine with the goal of fostering the total care of children with cerebral palsy. Its membership currently includes medical specialists and therapists from all disciplines caring for children with cerebral palsy and associated conditions. There are annual meetings at which professional papers are presented. Most physicians interested and involved in the care of patients with cerebral palsy become members of the Academy, which currently has members worldwide. Membership is gained by expressing an interest in cerebral palsy and being recommended by a current member of the Academy.

Anemia

Anemia is a deficiency of red blood cells in the blood system. Red blood cells carry oxygen and are important to human physical and mental development. If anemia is severe a child may appear pale, but mild anemia can easily be missed because there are no physical symptoms. Anemia can be caused by many different conditions, the most common being insufficient iron intake. Insufficient iron is seen most often with children, who get a limited amount of iron in the foods they eat. Lack of other vitamins such as B12 and folic acid can also cause anemia, but these are less common in childhood. Children fed cow's milk during the first year of life may become anemic because of an allergic reaction to the milk, causing microscopic blood loss through the intestinal system and into the stool. It is for this reason that either breast milk or infant formula is recommended for the first year of life. Infant cereals supplemented with iron and foods like meats and spinach have a high iron content, and are excellent nutritional supplements. Anemia in children with CP is also most commonly a result of iron deficiency due to a diet lacking sufficient iron.

Anterior Midline Defects
(holoprosencephaly, septo-optic dysplasia)

There are a number of malformations that fit into this category. The most common is holoprosencephaly, which involves failure of the midline facial structure and the brain behind it to develop. In the deficit's most complete expression, the brain has a single large ventricular cavity, with the inferior frontal and temporal regions of the brain often absent and the remainder quite rudimentary. The brain stem and cerebellum are present and fully developed.

Septo-optic dysplasia is a form of holoprosencephaly that includes a lack of development of the optic nerves resulting in severe visual impairment or blindness. It also results in deficiencies of certain hormones produced by the brain. This can cause very short stature, frequent urination, and other abnormalities. Any of these brain malformations can be accompanied by cerebral palsy.

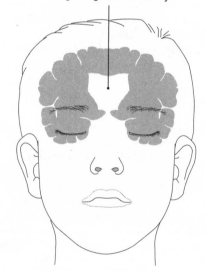

Single large midline cavity

Antiepileptic Drugs
(AEDs)

Antiepileptic drugs (AEDs) are medications used to try and control seizures. AEDs raise the seizure threshold in the brain. This process then decreases the electrical impulses in the brain to prevent a seizure or the spread of a seizure. The primary goal of therapy is to control seizures with no side effects from the AEDs. If this goal is unattainable, then the secondary goal is to decrease the number of seizures and/or the duration of seizures, prevent frequent repeated seizures, and/or decrease the side effects of the AEDs. A health care provider who is knowledgeable in seizure treatment must be involved in the management of those with epilepsy/seizures.

Arteriovenous Malformation

(AV malformation, AVM)

Arteriovenous malformation is the malformation of arteries and veins in the brain. During fetal development, the arteries and the veins, which should develop independently, may form abnormal connections. These abnormal connections most commonly form in parts of the brain, and because the abnormal vessels have very thin walls, they may rupture. Children born with AV malformation may be completely normal throughout their whole lifetime or they may develop sudden bleeding, causing a stroke, which can result in cerebral palsy. The presence of this malformation in and of itself does not usually cause any problems—it is the bleeding from ruptures of the vessels which may lead to headaches, occasionally seizures, or in the case of an acute large bleed, sudden death.

The cause of AV malformation is unknown. Depending on where the AV malformation is located, it can some-

times be surgically removed. If not, treatment is directed at the symptoms caused by bleeding into the brain, such as seizures or motor dysfunction. Often a hemiplegic type of pattern occurs because the bleeding occurs predominantly on one side of the brain, but there is significant variation depending on the location and severity of the brain damage caused by the bleeding.

Arthrogryposis

Arthrogryposis is a congenital condition in which a child's muscles and joints are stiff, often causing affected limbs to be held in extended positions. This condition may affect one, two, or all of the limbs, and varies in degree from being relatively mild to being so severe that a person is unable to walk or to use his arms for functional purposes. There are four basic causes of arthrogryposis: Muscle atrophy, lack of sufficient room in the uterus during pregnancy, malformation of the brain or spinal cord, and abnormalities of tendons, bones, or joint linings.

Children with arthrogryposis are not spastic, although their condition can be mistaken for cerebral palsy. They have normal mental development, and their surgical treatment is very different from that of children with cerebral palsy. Although the surgical treatment is different, other aspects of treatment and care are very similar. Aggressive physical therapy is the ideal treatment to maintain the joints in the best functional position and maintain the limited amount of motion that is often present.

Asthma

(reactive airway disease, wheezy bronchitis)

Asthma is defined as recurrent and reversible bronchospasm, meaning that the airways of the lungs go into spasm and narrow, obstructing air flow. This narrowing results from contraction of the muscles around these little airways, as well as from increased production of mucus and swelling because of inflammation. Both large and small airways can be involved and are responsive to a variety of stimuli, including pollens to which the patient is allergic, dander from cats or dogs, cold air, or noxious environmental agents such as tobacco smoke, aerosols, chemicals, or strong aromas. Some children develop symptoms when they exercise, or when they laugh or cry. Overall, it is estimated that between 5 and 10 percent of children have asthma at some time during their childhood.

Asthma accounts for 10 percent of emergency room visits and 10 percent of medical hospitalizations in the United States, and is the most frequent cause of school absenteeism and chronic illness in children under age 18.

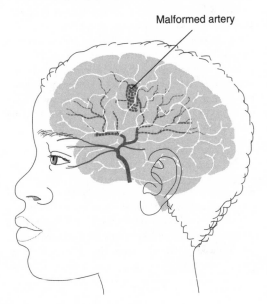

Malformed artery

Boys are affected more than girls, by a 3:1 ratio. Though many children who develop asthma early in life tend to improve during mid-childhood and adolescence, a significant proportion continue to have symptoms into adulthood. There has been an increase in hospital admissions and in deaths from asthma over the past years, for reasons that are not clear.

Asthma does run in families, but it is not strictly a genetic disease. The fundamental abnormality seems to be a hyperreactivity of the airways. A history of bronchiolitis early in life is a risk factor for the development of asthma later in childhood, as approximately one-third to one-half of the children who have asthma in adolescence had more than one episode of bronchiolitis early in life.

The hallmark of asthma is recurrent wheezing, which is reversible with the use of specific medications. Wheezing is a high-pitched sound heard when the child breathes out. Some children have only occasional episodes of such symptoms, which can vary from mild to severe, and may require medication just on those infrequent occasions. Others may have recurrent episodes every few months, yet be free of symptoms in between. Still others may have chronic or daily symptoms that interfere with their lives, school attendance, and physical activity, with frequent visits to the emergency room and hospitalizations. Many of these children require multiple medications every day.

While wheezing is a hallmark of asthma, not every child who wheezes has asthma. There are many other causes of wheezing, including tracheomalacia (a soft, floppy trachea), acute infections such as RSV bronchiolitis, cystic fibrosis, bronchopulmonary dysplasia, or aspiration of a foreign body. Children with cerebral palsy may have chronic or recurrent wheezing because they are aspirating their stomach contents, their food while eating, or even their own secretions and saliva. These items often get into their lungs rather than into their stomach and cause recurrent respiratory symptoms, such as bronchitis, pneumonia, or wheezing. Treatment of the underlying abnormality (such as preventing gastroesophageal reflux) may end the respiratory symptoms.

Asymmetric Tonic Neck Reflex

(ATNR) (see p. 438)

ATNR is an infantile automatism, or a reflex of infancy, often known as the fencer's position. The reflex is triggered by turning the head from side to side. As the head is turned to one side, the arm and leg extend on that side. On the opposite side, where the skull or the back of the head points, the arm and leg flex. This reflex is present in normal infants up to 6 months of age and should disappear after that age.

The presence of the asymmetric tonic neck reflex after age 1 is a sign of significant brain damage; if it persists past age 2, it is evidence of poor long-term prognosis with respect to walking, a significant finding in a child with cerebral palsy.

Ataxia

(balance)

Ataxia means a lack of balance. Under conditions of normal development, the body's balance mechanism evolves from three separate systems: the eyes provide input to determine the body's position in space; the semicircular canals in the inner ear work like a gyroscope to tell the brain what position the head is in or how it is changing; the position sensors in the joints, particularly those in the neck, provide important information about where the limbs are. A child with cerebral palsy has some limitation in his balance capabilities, which is often expressed as an uncoordinated gait or difficulty standing in one place without moving. Ataxia continues to improve until the child is approximately 8 to 10 years old, at which time his balance and coordination system reaches maximum improvement. Because ataxia involves the hands, it makes fine motor control activities such as writing difficult.

One of the ways a child may compensate for ataxia is to walk very rapidly, because balance tends to be better when the child goes fast, just like riding a bicycle is easier at a faster speed. The child may also adopt a very wide-based stance. Often it is easier for the child to stand with some joints immobilized by ankle braces. There are many children whose main reason for not walking independently is severe ataxia. However, there is no surgery or medication to help this problem. The best way to improve ataxia is by practicing movements similar to the methods teachers use to teach children ballet or gymnastics. A physical therapist can structure balance activities and exercises to maximize a child's abilities, and these usually involve walking on a balance beam, learning falling, and working on a therapy ball.

Athetosis

Athetosis is a movement disorder in which there are gross movements, often with fanning of the fingers. Athetosis is usually most prominent in the arms, where it causes slow, irregular, writhing involuntary movements occurring at or around the long axis of the limb, which become more intense with attempted voluntary movement. It may also make speech difficult. Athetosis does not cause contractures to develop, although athetosis and spasticity are often both present in the same person and the spasticity may cause contractures.

Care and treatment: Treatment for a child with athetosis involves finding postural positions that allow her to control the movements. Weighted vests or weighted sleeves are the ideal treatment because they may help to suppress the movements. If spasticity coexists, the spasticity forms a natural dampener on the athetosis. For this reason, suppressing spasticity in the presence of athetosis must be done very cautiously, because it may bring out athetosis, which is often worse in terms of function for the child than the combination of athetosis and spasticity initially present. Generally, surgical muscle releases are very unpredictable with athetosis, but operations that stiffen joints, such as spinal fusions, work extremely well.

Most children with athetosis are initially very floppy and often have very good cognitive function but poor upper body control. The gross movements are not present at birth, but slowly develop after the first year and increase in severity by ages 6 to 8. With the child who has normal cognitive function, communication problems, because of the impact of athetosis on speech, are the most difficult problems to overcome. Early use of augmentative communication devices should be encouraged if the child is not speaking. Power wheelchairs are also recommended for the child who is unable to walk by age 5, since the child who is unable to walk due to athetosis is seldom able to push a manual wheelchair.

Augmentative Communication

Augmentative communication is a term used to describe the technology that helps a person with a communication disability to interact with her environment. The technology used for augmentative communication is similar to a prosthesis, which is used for a person who is missing a limb; in that sense, this technology could be considered a communication prosthesis. There are many different levels of augmentative communication: the best technology is determined by the child's age, cognitive level, and level of disability, and by the environment in which she lives. Augmentative communication techniques may involve the use of sign language by one's hands; sign language by eye movement; symbol boards or picture boards; or computer-generated speech devices, which may be accessed with keyboards or scanners. Assistive writing devices such as computers with word-recognition software are also important aids in communication, especially in the school environment.

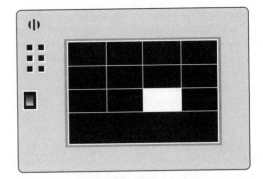

Simple communication device

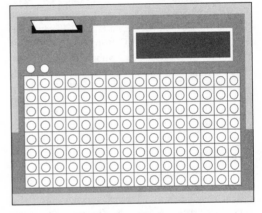

Complex communication device

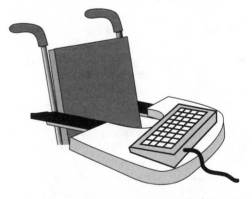

Augmentative communication device
on wheelchair tray

Indications: A child who is unable to speak or communicate by 2 to 3 years of age should be evaluated by a speech therapist or an augmentative communication specialist with the goal of trying to establish the most appropriate communication device. This initially means starting with a symbol board if the child's eyesight is good enough to allow him to point at pictures or other symbols to express his desires. Most children this age use head sign language (shaking or nodding the head, for example). Eye sign language can also often be used very effectively for a yes or no. Usually the child moves her eyes vertically to demonstrate a positive response and moves the eyes from right to left to demonstrate a no response.

As the child gets older and enters school, at 5 or 6 years of age, more sophisticated communication devices can be employed, such as computer-based speech synthesizers. Again, this is dependent on the child's cognitive ability as well as her ability to use the communication device. This may require the combined efforts of an occupational therapist, a speech therapist, an augmentative communication specialist, and a wheelchair engineer. The child who is entering third or fourth grade and is being held up because of a motor disability which makes writing slow should be assessed for augmentative writing devices. This is usually done with a laptop computer using shorthand typing in which one or two letters can be started with word recognition so that words which are typed frequently are recognized after the first two keystrokes. This significantly increases the child's typing speed and is much easier to read than handwriting, which may be difficult to read when the child is trying to write fast.

Benefits and risks: The benefits of the augmentative communication devices are in providing the child a mechanism for interacting with her environment and the development of self-confidence. The ability to be involved in a meaningful educational experience requires the ability to communicate, and often the level of communication which can be established with a child with a significant physical disability determines the level of the education which the child may achieve. This again is based on the assumption that the child has normal cognitive capabilities.

One of the risks of augmentative communication is attempting to provide and teach a child a sophisticated mechanism for communication which is above his or her cognitive capability; the difficulty here is that even determining a child's cognitive ability often requires augmentative communication devices. Sometimes the only way to determine what is appropriate is by using equipment on a trial-and-error basis. This is the only way to be certain of the child's ability or inability to use a specific piece of equipment.

Another risk with using sophisticated augmentative communication is that it requires the caregivers who are interacting with the child (usually the family) to be involved and to understand the communication device. This technology only works if both the child who is using the communication device and the person with whom she is trying to communicate understand the language. This means that parents or other caregivers are often required to be involved in the training and learning of this communication system as well.

Maintenance and care: Some of the augmentative communication technologies, such as eye or hand signing and symbol boards, require only that the people with whom the child is communicating understand the language and know how to respond. The computer-based speech synthesizers and more sophisticated access devices that involve scanning or head switches are technically sophisticated and prone to breakdown. A system for communication or a device for accessing the system should not be purchased unless there is a clear understanding of who is going to be available to provide repairs and how those repairs are going to be provided.

If an excellent communication system is purchased and the child and family invest a significant amount of energy in learning how to use it, but it is broken down and out for repair 80 percent of the time, the system is not functioning as a communication system. Most of the communication systems will only be able to be used effectively if they are used regularly for the majority of the communication.

Autism

(autism spectrum disorder)

Autism is part of the spectrum of disorders known as autism spectrum disorder. By definition, autism means that there is an impairment in the social interaction of the child with those around him, impairment in communication skills, both verbal and nonverbal, and a restricted repertoire of activities and interests. Often the child with autism performs ritualistic repetitive behaviors. Children with autism are not necessarily mentally retarded.

The cause of autism is unknown, and no medication has yet been found to be useful in treating this condition. There are children who both display autistic behavior disorders and have cerebral palsy or motor problems, but autism and cerebral palsy are separate problems even when they occur in the same child.

Back Knee Gait

(knee hyperextension)

A back knee gait, which means that the child's knee bends back when she steps on her foot, is usually due to a tight

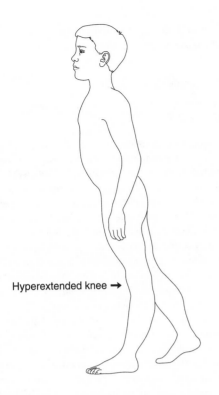

Hyperextended knee ➔

Achilles tendon and an overlengthened hamstring or weak hamstring muscles. Children with cerebral palsy and children with muscle weakness or severe hypotonia who do not have good control of their knees often have a back knee gait. The primary treatment of a back knee gait is to use an ankle-foot orthosis (AFO), which may be hinged to allow for the ankle to be lifted, but blocked so the knee cannot bend backward without lifting the toes off the ground. There is almost never a need to use a long leg brace for this condition. There is no harm in children walking short distances without their braces, if they wear their braces the majority of the time. Another treatment for a back knee gait caused by very tight Achilles tendons is surgical lengthening of the Achilles tendon followed by the use of an AFO.

Indications: The indications for surgical treatment vary; generally, however, as long as the back kneeing can be controlled with an AFO, surgery is not indicated. If the Achilles tendon is tight and does not allow the ankle to come to neutral or to be held in an AFO so that both the front and the back of the foot touch the ground, surgery should be performed to lengthen the tendon. For an adult, an attempt should be made to discontinue the AFO by lengthening the tendon. Care must be taken not to over-

lengthen because this may cause further instability in standing and more difficulty in walking.

A back-kneeing gait can result in a gradual stretching of the knee structure. In young adults, severe back kneeing often becomes uncomfortable and can significantly limit the amount of walking that can be done. In rare cases, with children with significant weakness, back kneeing is the only stable gait pattern; following surgical lengthening of the Achilles tendon, they may be unable to walk without braces.

Behavior Modification

Behavior modification may best be seen as a series of learning-based interventions aimed at developing wanted behavior or decreasing unwanted behavior. Behavior therapists typically evaluate a child's behavior within the context of where the behavior occurs. Therapists develop a "functional analysis" of the behavior to determine how the behavior "functions" in the environment. For example, a child with cerebral palsy was screaming frequently at home but not in the classroom. The therapist made observations in the home and found that the child typically screamed when mom was busy cooking dinner. Mom would stop and reprimand the child and then return to her chores. The screaming would recur and mom would reproach the child again. Here, it appeared that the absence of mom's attention during cooking chores resulted in the child's screaming, and mom may have been inadvertently "rewarding" this behavior with her attention. Recommendations for increased attention to the child when mom is cooking to "reward" positive behavior and ignoring the screaming were then made to the child's parents.

Typical strategies for increasing wanted behavior include the use of praise and attention and tangible rewards. These positives tend to increase the frequency of the desired behavior when they are delivered following the behavior. Typical strategies for decreasing unwanted behavior include the removal of positives, like "time out" (e.g., removing the child from the work table for a minute for hitting or spitting) or providing a negative consequence. Negative consequences like spanking generally should be avoided because of such unintended consequences as fear, avoidance of the punisher or modeling the very behavior that therapists would like to see decreased. Ignoring is another strategy for decreasing behavior. When behavior is not dangerous, ignoring can be a powerful way of helping behavior to decrease. Sometimes, however, with ignoring, behavior "gets worse before it gets better."

Indications: Behavior management is clearly indicated to develop particular behavior like appropriate toileting or social skills. The use of rewards to shape the development of new skills is key to all learning. As well, behavior management is indicated to increase behavior such as saying please or cleaning up after playing or to reduce unwanted behaviors such as hitting or biting. When attempting to increase or decrease the target behavior in its natural environment, the analysis of the child's behavior should find what in the environment is maintaining the behavior. When this is changed, it should help to change the behavior. Examples of common behaviors often maintained by the environment are biting, tantrums, or acting out in class.

Benefits and risks: Great benefit can be realized through the use of organized, data-driven, reward-based programs. Keeping data as to the incidence of the target behavior and how it changes with intervention allows the parent or teacher to see if the program is working and to make changes if needed. The use of punishment-based programs, even behavioral programs that emphasize the removal of positives, should be monitored closely to prevent "negative side effects." When behavior management is applied to self-harm situations such as self-injurious behavior, it is important to work with an experienced therapist who is familiar with the use of behavior modification approaches for that behavioral issue. It is always important to reward small steps, progress toward a clear goal, and be flexible about changing a program that is not effective.

Maintenance and care: When beginning a behavior change program, it is important to have consistency of approach across environments (e.g., home and school). Reward often, reward immediately directly after the behavior occurs, and specifically (not "you were good"). As the behavior changes, begin to reward intermittently to maintain the behavior change. Always adapt the behavioral program

to the child's developmental level. Find a way of rewarding parents and teachers for their good efforts as well.

Biofeedback Devices

(auditory feedback, augmented feedback, behavioral training helmet)

Biofeedback devices operate under the theory that if a child is given feedback about an unwanted position or behavior and then rewarded for changing it, the child will learn to use the more normal behavior. Biofeedback has been used in an attempt to control drooling, to encourage head control, to improve sitting posture, and to decrease foot flexion at the ankle or toe walking. Most of these behavior modification techniques use devices with electric switches. For example, a helmet is fitted with a level so when the child allows his head to drop, a switch activates and turns off his television set. When the child holds his head up straight, the television set turns on again.

Similar types of devices have been developed for many other functions. For example, another biofeedback device is the small bib or cup held under the chin. When a child drools and wets the cloth, an electric switch is tripped and the child's television set is turned off. Therefore, if he does not control his drooling, he is unable to watch TV. In still another example, a small switch may be inserted in the heel of an ankle brace and operated in such a way that if the child steps on her toe but does not step on her heel at the same time, a loud noise will be generated. In this way a child can be trained to walk with her foot flat so as not to activate the negative reinforcing noise.

Indications: At this time, there are no established clinical indications for the use of these devices, although many people continue to explore their use, especially in research environments. They have been evaluated predominantly for control of drooling, for head control, and for attempts at improving gait.

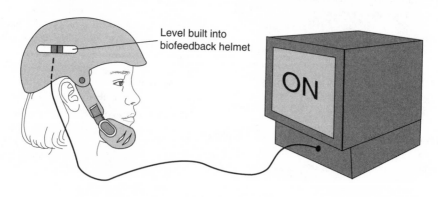

Level built into biofeedback helmet

ON

Benefits and risks: The main benefit of many of these devices such as the helmet or the drooling cup or the ankle switch is that they can change behaviors in a specific environment. The major risk is that the desired behavior may not be carried over after the device is removed. This may establish a false hope in parents and other caregivers that a certain activity can be learned, when in fact the child may never be able to make it automatic. In a sense, this situation is similar to that of the person who can sit erect with good posture but who slouches as soon as he relaxes and stops concentrating on maintaining the correct position.

Maintenance and care: Most of the devices are electrical and therefore do require ongoing maintenance. Some of this maintenance may be difficult, such as of the drooling-control devices, which require wetting a cloth to make an electrical connection. Since most of these devices are used in a research environment, the person fitting the device is usually quite familiar with their maintenance. If devices are purchased from a commercial vendor, it should be clear who will provide the service and maintenance of these devices in addition to the normal cleaning which the caregiver would provide.

Blood Transfusion

(autologous blood donation)

It is not unusual for children with cerebral palsy to require corrective orthopedic surgery. Such operations, including correction of scoliosis or hip abnormalities, may require support in the form of blood transfusions. Because these are likely to be planned or elective operations, patients have the option of donating their own blood. That is, in the weeks prior to surgery, patients can donate their own blood to be stored for use during their operation if the need arises. This type of donation is called a preoperative autologous blood donation. Blood donated for use by those other than oneself is called allogeneic blood donation.

To qualify for preoperative autologous blood donation, patients must be old enough to understand the procedure and cooperate fully. Hospitals and blood centers that collect donations typically require the patient to be of a certain weight to ensure a good quality sample. While these criteria vary, a realistic weight standard is 65 pounds or greater.

It is preferable to collect autologous blood during the weeks before surgery. Blood collected more than 6 weeks from surgery must be frozen. The last collection should occur no sooner than 72 hours before the scheduled surgery to allow the patient time to replace their own blood. The number of units donated depends on the anticipated surgical blood loss. Patients should take iron supplements during the weeks before surgery.

The main purpose for autologous donation is to prevent the transmission of blood-related infections to the patient. However, the current blood supply is very safe from the standpoint of infections caused by viruses like hepatitis and HIV. In fact, the most common causes of transfusion-associated infections are bacteria. The risk of a transfusion-associated bacterial infection is the same for both autologous and allogeneic transfusions. So, if a patient is not capable of donating his own blood for surgery, blood from an alternative donor can be safely provided.

Despite significant efforts to maintain a very safe blood supply in the United States, transfusion is not without risks. Minor complications of transfusion include fever, nausea, or hives (allergic reaction). Rare complications include: (1) transfusion of a different blood type causing blood cells to break (hemolysis), (2) patient intolerance of the fluid volume causing heart failure, (3) difficulty breathing, and (4) severe infection.

Although blood transfusions can carry risks, when children must undergo major surgery such as spinal fusion, blood transfusion can be lifesaving. Under such circumstances, the benefits of transfusion to patients far outweigh the risks.

Bone Densitometry

(DEXA, DXA)

The mineral (calcium) content of the bones can be measured by using low-level x-ray (dual energy x-ray absorptiometry or DEXA). Low bone mineral content increases the risk of the bone breaking (fracture).

Bone densitometry is performed lying on a table, while the whole body or one part of it (leg, hip, spine) is scanned with x-ray. The time needed for the study varies from one to ten minutes, depending on how much of the body is scanned. One must not move during this time. There is no pain involved, as nothing touches the patient.

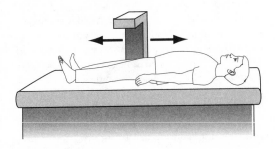

Indications: Children with CP are frequently found to have low bone density, especially when they are nonambulatory and/or have difficulty with nutrition. Many have fractures (broken bones) after minimal trauma. A bone densitometry study may be done if a child had one or more fractures, or if it is suspected that the child is at risk for low bone density based on his or her clinical condition.

Benefits and risks: The benefit from knowing about low bone density is that it can be treated with nutritional supplements and/or medication. Treatment that raises bone mineral density may reduce the number of fractures or prevent fractures. The only risk of the test is from the x-ray, which is not considered significant, because the amount of radiation from a DEXA study is less than the standard chest x-ray. If the child needs sedation to hold still for the study, then that adds the small risk associated with sedation, and the child will need monitoring while sedated.

Botulinum Toxin Injections

(Botox®, Myobloc®)

Botulinum toxin is a drug that may be injected into the muscle to weaken or temporarily partially paralyze very spastic muscles. There are two commercially available types, Botox® (botulinum toxin A) and Myobloc® (botulinum toxin B). The drug is injected through a very small needle and causes little pain. It does not cause scarring like alcohol and phenol injections, both now uncommonly used. Botulinum toxin lasts four to six months and can be given multiple times. It can be given in up to four to six involved muscles at a time with the total medication given limited by the body weight of the patient. It does not seem to prevent, but may delay the development of contractures.

Indications: The main indication for botulinum toxin is spasticity. Injections are most commonly given in the hip adductor, hamstring, and gastrocnemius muscles. In the upper extremity, the biceps, pronator, wrist and finger flexors, and thumb adductor are also commonly injected. The most common situation are circumstances in which the underlying spasticity is expected to improve significantly or there is concern about the impact of permanent weakness. In a situation where a child is improving, such as after an acute head injury or near drowning, injection of botulinum toxin provides a six-month window to see how much recovery and natural diminishing occurs in the spasticity. However, spasticity in the child with cerebral palsy does not change significantly, and it is almost certain that six months after the injection the problem will return to the same degree as before. In these children, injections are used primarily to delay surgery.

Another indication is *dystonia*, which is a movement disorder often affecting one or two muscle groups. Dystonia may cause very severe contractures of one muscle or muscle group for a short period of time and then switch and cause the opposite deformity. For this reason, surgical lengthening may be performed but is somewhat more unpredictable. Using botulinum toxin avoids a high risk of the opposite deformity occurring.

The newest use of botulinum toxin for children with CP is as a treatment for drooling. A single injection of botulinum toxin into the submandibular glands has been effective in reducing drooling, with the maximum effect from 2–8 weeks after the injection.

Benefits and risks: The main benefit of botulinum toxin injection is that it allows the physician time to observe how much natural recovery is taking place.

The risks of botulinum toxin injections are very few. The most frequent is temporary muscle weakness for up to 24–48 hours. Acetaminophen (Tylenol) can be given to relieve any discomfort. Rarely, temporary excessive localized muscle weakness and temporary generalized weakness has been reported. Allergic reaction is extremely uncommon. In addition, it is not uncommon for patients to eventually develop a tolerance to botulinum toxin requiring an increase in dosage or making the drug ineffective. This is occasionally due to true antibody formation against the drug.

Maintenance and care: After botulinum toxin injections, normal activity may be immediately resumed. If the injections are performed for contractures such as of the hip or the ankle, it is important to continue splinting and stretching to maintain the correction for as long as possible. Usually these injections will need to be repeated in four to eight months if the gain is to be maintained.

Brace, Ankle

(ankle foot orthosis, AFO, MAFO, DAFO)

These braces are the most common type of brace used in children with cerebral palsy. The brace extends from just below the knee across the ankle and includes the foot. Although some physicians may still prescribe a leather shoe attached to a metal upright, most up-to-date ankle foot orthoses (AFOs) are made of a light-weight, high-density plastic and are custom molded (MAFO) to the patient's foot and ankle. More recently, a wraparound style of ankle foot orthosis with "tone reducing" features molded into the foot plate (DAFO, Cascade, Inc.) has been very popular. Most braces fit well inside of a sneaker or shoe although a larger size is usually required to accommodate the brace.

Sneakers with a removable inlay are helpful to accommodate the AFO.

Indications: The most common indication for this type of brace is a child who toe walks or back knees due to a tight gastrocnemius muscle or Achilles tendon. The muscle or tendon can not be so tight, however, that the foot can not be positioned into the brace without causing excess pressure. This means that an AFO cannot be used in a child who has a fixed ankle deformity that is unable to be ranged into a neutral ankle position. Varus or valgus foot deformities may also require a MAFO if the foot can not be controlled with a shorter brace. Occasionally, the child with a crouched gait may require a MAFO to keep the ankle from collapsing into a dorsiflexed position.

There are many types of MAFOs, some of which are described here.

1. Solid ankle MAFO. This brace is fixed at the ankle and gives maximum ankle support. It is best for the young child who is just beginning to walk and requires ankle stability for balance, or the severely involved child (quadriplegic) with poor ankle control or severe foot and ankle deformity. There is typically a strap around the ankle and one just below the knee.

2. Articulated MAFO. This brace has an ankle hinge and typically allows dorsiflexion but stops at ninety degrees to prevent toe walking. It is best for the child who is ambulatory and is able to voluntarily dorsiflex the ankle. It should not be used in a child who crouches at the knee. Due to the extra bulkiness of the hinge, it may be more difficult to fit into a shoe.

3. Plantar flexion block MAFO. The indication is very similar to an articulated MAFO. However, movement does not occur at a hinge. Instead, it allows the ankle to dorsiflex forward out of the brace because there is no strap below the knee holding the leg in the brace. Plantar flexion is blocked at ninety degrees. It is best used in the child who can not tolerate a hinge due to rubbing or when maximum control is required to correct a severe varus or valgus foot deformity.

4. Ground reaction MAFO. The indication for this brace is the child with a severe crouch. The foot slides into the brace from behind. With each step the child takes, forces are generated up to the front of the lower leg just below the knee to help push the knee into extension.

5. Leaf spring or plantar flexion resist MAFO. This brace is best used in the child without significant contractures, who has mild toe walking due to spasticity of the gastrocnemius muscle. It resists plantar flexion but will allow for some push off at the ankle. It also helps to spring the foot back up into dorsiflexion. This is especially useful in the child with weak dorsiflexion due to tibialis anterior muscle weakness. These patients have a foot drop when their heel strikes the ground during walking.

Benefits and risks: The benefits of using a MAFO are that it gives the ambulatory child a more stable base of support to walk on by controlling the foot and ankle deformity while the brace is on. In the nonambulatory child, the brace can provide stability in a stander or gait trainer. It also helps to delay fixed muscle contractures. The risks are that with a more rigid deformity, the brace may cause pressure sores. Also the more rigid the brace is as it crosses the ankle, the less exercise the gastrocnemius muscle gets.

Maintenance and care: Most of these braces are constructed of a high-density plastic. They will occasionally break if the brace is used to correct too rigid of a de-

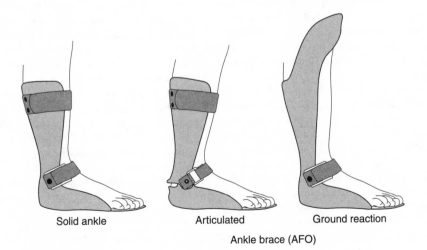

Solid ankle   Articulated   Ground reaction

Ankle brace (AFO)

formity. In general, a growing child requires a new brace approximately every twelve months. The development of pressure areas may also occur during rapid growth spurts and require adjustment of the brace. The brace should be checked every six months for the need for adjustments. The parent should check the child daily for pressure areas.

Brace, Back

(thoracolumbosacral orthosis [TLSO] spine brace, body jacket, scoliosis brace, Boston brace, Milwaukee brace, Wilmington brace)

Back braces are used to help straighten up a child who is having trouble sitting up and, in some cases, to straighten the spine, which may be developing a deformity or already have one. The correct medical designation for these braces is generally abbreviated as TLSO, which means a brace that extends from the top of the chest down across the pelvis. If there is an extension including the neck, the proper designation is CTLSO, which means that the cervical area is also covered by the brace. These are very unusual and are rarely prescribed for children with cerebral palsy. Spinal braces, body jackets, or scoliosis braces are general and older terms that are used, and there are many different designs for these braces.

The majority of current braces are made of molded plastic and open in the front or back. Some have a separate front and back that are held together with velcro straps. The specific design of these braces in different geographical areas has led to names such as the Boston, Milwaukee, or Wilmington brace. The Boston brace is a factory-made brace modified by orthotists. The standard off-the-shelf plastic brace is not particularly useful for children with cerebral palsy, since they are very difficult to fit. The Milwaukee brace is an older design that was used for bracing scoliosis. It is made with a plastic mold around the pelvis, metal uprights and pads pushing against parts of the trunk, and a circular extension around the neck. This is seldom used today and rarely has a place in the care of children with cerebral palsy.

There are many local braces such as the Wilmington brace, which are made with different minor design changes by a local orthotist. Most of these require a cast to be made of the child's body. The cast is filled to make a mold, over which the brace is then made. Most of these custom-molded braces fit much better and may be made out of very soft plastic that further prevents skin irritation, or they may be made out of a more rigid, thinner plastic that can be concealed under clothing. The process of molding and brace construction generally requires at least a 24- to 36-hour time period.

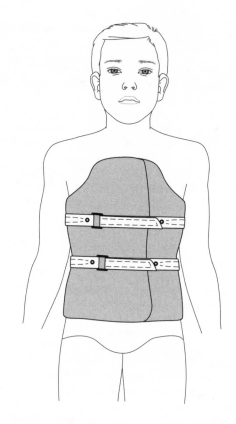

Indications: Although there is no consensus among physicians about the benefits of back brace use for children with cerebral palsy, there are two primary indications for ordering a brace. The first is for a child who has difficulty controlling his body so that when he is sitting he collapses either sideways or forward. The brace may thus be ordered for postural control. In this way it is used in place of a custom-designed and tightly fitted wheelchair insert, which provides the same function.

Using spinal braces for children with CP to maintain postural control, provide better head control, and provide better use of the arms is one option; using an adequately designed wheelchair is another. The benefits of the brace are a close fit to the body and concealment under clothing. Additionally, when the child is moved from one chair to another the brace goes along with the child. Clothes such as winter coats can be placed over the top of the brace. The advantage of wheelchair supports is easy application to the child. However, because a wheelchair is tightly fitted with regular clothes, it will not fit when heavy winter coats are worn. Also, a modified wheelchair is only useful when the child is sitting in the chair.

The second use of a back brace, and in our view a misguided use, is to treat spinal deformities, such as scoliosis.

These braces were initially designed and used most extensively for children with idiopathic adolescent scoliosis, a condition in which spinal curvatures develop in normal preadolescent or adolescent girls. This type of scoliosis is entirely different from the scoliosis that occurs in children with cerebral palsy. There continues to be controversy concerning how effective these braces are in the control of scoliosis in children with idiopathic scoliosis, but there is almost no controversy about their lack of effectiveness in children with CP. Braces have no significant effect on preventing the development or progression of scoliosis in children with cerebral palsy. There is a general, but not universal, consensus that the use of any kind of spinal brace in the treatment of scoliosis provides no impact on its eventual outcome in the child with cerebral palsy. Likewise, treating kyphosis is generally not felt to have any long-term impact.

Benefits and risks: The primary benefit of a well-fitted brace is that it provides better postural and head control, while at the same time being less cumbersome and noticeable than a wheelchair. The primary risk is that a brace that is not fitted adequately causes skin irritation with blisters and subsequent skin sores. The skin needs to be checked every day; whenever pressure areas are found, the brace should be modified.

Many of the children who need these braces for postural control either have feeding problems or have difficulty coughing. The use of these restrictive braces further restricts their lung function and may put them at higher risk for developing repeated pneumonia because they are unable to clear their lungs when they develop minor viral infections. The chest wall in a growing child is flexible, and when braces are worn tightly they can deform the chest wall, causing protruding ribs or flattening of the chest. Likewise, the application of a tight constricting abdominal brace may increase nutritional problems, such as GE reflux, poor stomach emptying, or constipation. Generally, because of these complications, which are most likely to occur in children who need the postural support, the adequately fitting wheelchair is a better option.

When a brace is needed for postural control, a brace made of a soft foamlike material is more comfortable and less likely to cause complications than the more rigid plastic material.

Maintenance and care: At the beginning, these braces should be used for short periods—at most, several hours during the day, while the child is closely monitored for skin irritation. Areas of pressure underneath the brace may be toughened by being cleaned with alcohol after the braces are removed. There is no need to use the brace at night in a child with cerebral palsy, because it will only increase pulmonary and abdominal constriction and will not benefit the child in any way, since lying in bed does not require any postural control.

If the brace is made of a low-temperature plastic, it must be carefully protected from direct sunlight and must not be left in a car in hot weather, because the brace may melt. It should not be cleaned with harsh detergents, since they may also damage the plastic. Usually a T-shirt or an undergarment needs to be worn underneath the brace so the plastic does not directly touch the child's skin.

Brace, Foot
(heel cup, UCB orthotic, arch support, SMO)

Foot braces and special shoe inserts cover part of the foot up to the ankle or slightly above the ankle. Foot braces, heel cups, and arch supports make up a group of braces that are smaller than the ankle-foot orthosis (AFO), which extends from the toes to the top of the calf just below the knee. These braces are at the highest just above the ankle-bone and are called supramalleolar orthoses (SMOs). They vary greatly, including those that are custom molded from casts, and range from the ankle-foot orthosis to the simple arch supports that may be sold over the counter (such as Dr. Scholl's arch supports).

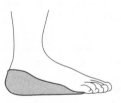

Heel cups are manufactured by a number of companies as off-the-shelf products. They are made of either hard or soft materials that cover the heel. They are meant to help control the tilt of the heel and to keep it flat inside a shoe. Generally, they are quite inexpensive and don't provide much support.

There are many different kinds of arch supports. They range from those made from casts, costing seven hundred or eight hundred dollars, to those that may be purchased off the shelf for five to ten dollars. These are constructed of leather, plastic, or metal.

A special type of orthotic that has received a lot of publicity is the UCB orthotic (the University of California at Berkeley orthotic), a foot orthosis that is made from a cast. A close mold of the heel is made, which is extended forward to the base of the toes or under the toes. In some circumstances, this brace is brought up over the anklebone to help provide further stability for the heel so it doesn't twist. Because the UCB orthotic is very tightly molded, it is supposed to correct rotation of the heel and is usually used to improve flat feet. There are a number of theories that recommend various pressure points to be molded into the braces in an attempt to decrease spasticity. Although there may be vocal local advocates of these special braces, there is very little scientific evidence that any one of these special orthotics has a significant advantage over any other.

Indications: The use of shoe inserts has no recognized standard of care or application. Frequently the specific practitioner and geographic area seem to favor a particular brace; the philosophy of a neighboring practitioner or community may be entirely different. Heel cups are usually utilized for people with painful heels in an attempt to stabilize the heel fat pad; they are often made of soft material to provide extra cushioning.

Some practitioners prescribe heel cups to improve flat feet, but in general arch supports are utilized in an attempt to correct flat feet. They are frequently prescribed to help with knee pain in runners. This is not relevant to the CP patient, and certainly no arch support will reduce knee pain in the child with cerebral palsy. The UCB type of orthotic, with its multiple variations, is the most common foot orthosis prescribed to treat flat feet in children with cerebral palsy, and is probably the second most popular brace after the full-length AFO, which provides much better support.

The specific indications for foot braces are very diverse, and none of them have well-documented scientific support. Certainly, in normal children the use of arch supports or any shoe inserts has been shown to make absolutely no difference in long-term outcome, since the foot tends to progress along whatever course the child's genetic predisposition has determined. In children with cerebral palsy, at this point it is not certain whether arch supports make any long-term difference, and there is currently no scientific evidence to suggest that they do. However, neither is there good evidence to suggest that they don't make a difference. The natural history of flat feet varies in children with cerebral palsy; for this reason, the main indication for shoe orthotics ought to be those that make the patient's feet feel more comfortable and improve the patient's ability to walk. If shoe inserts or braces detract from either of these daily necessities, then there is very little indication for continuing their use.

Benefits and risks: The immediate benefit is comfort to the wearer; similarly, the main problem is pain and discomfort—especially if the insert or brace is incorrectly fitted. This is particularly true of tightly molded braces that try to make a lot of correction in the flat foot. Frequently the foot looks nice in the brace, but the child complains that his feet hurt when he walks. Because of the uncertain benefit of these braces, any brace that causes the child pain or diminishes his ability to walk should be promptly removed or at least modified in an attempt to alleviate the discomfort.

There is never a good reason to use a brace or shoe insert that rubs the foot, causing blisters or breakdown of the skin. If these skin breakdowns are ignored, they may become infected, leading to long-term periods of "feet up" rest. Obviously the inability to walk is very detrimental to a child's continued progress in gaining mobility.

Maintenance and care: When new shoe inserts are obtained, they should be worn gradually, starting with one to two hours at a time. As they become more comfortable, as long as they are not causing any blisters, they may be worn for longer periods of time, comparable to a normal day's "shoe wear." The care of the specific brace depends on the material it is made of. Braces made of leather should be kept as dry as possible, and plastic braces, depending on the material, need to be protected from high temperatures.

Brace, Hip

(hip, knee, ankle, foot orthosis [HKAFO]; pelvic band, hip brace, hip abduction brace, A-frame brace, abduction pillow)

These braces are part of a whole family of braces that extend across the hip joint from the pelvis to the thigh, across the knee, and attach to a foot brace. The designation is hip, knee, ankle, foot orthosis (HKAFO) because it covers all of these areas. Some of the older terms include names such as long leg braces with a pelvic band or the pelvic control brace.

The typical long leg with pelvic band brace is constructed with metal uprights that are attached to shoes. There is a metal joint at the knee. The uprights extend again to the thigh cuff and then cross the hip on the outside, having a hinge at the area of the hip joint. This metal upright bar is attached to a metal, leather-covered band, which goes around the pelvis. This typical long leg brace with a pelvic band was used extensively during the polio era of the 1920s–1950s, and there are still many older people who had polio and who continue to use these braces.

Other types of hip braces sometimes used for children with cerebral palsy include twister cables, which are a type of flexible material (usually plastic or flexible metal) that is

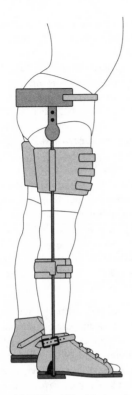

HKAFO with pelvic band

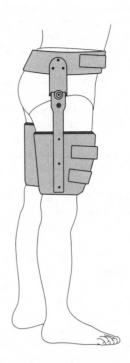

Abduction brace

attached to a brace below the knee and then extends up above the knee and hip joints to help control rotation of the leg, primarily to prevent the toes from pointing in. There are also braces that are constructed to prevent the legs from crossing. Frequently these hip abductor braces do not extend below the knee; they may have hip hinges or may be rigid, simply holding the legs apart. The standard brace has a metal band around the hip extended to metal braces along the outside and thigh cuffs just above the knee.

Some braces are constructed to fit on the inside of the legs, where they push the knees apart. Often these have the appearance of A-frames. They may extend below the knee and usually do not have hinges at the knee. This type of A-frame brace is usually constructed out of a soft material and has the appearance of a pillow with velcro straps that hold the knees against the side of the pillow.

Indications: There are a number of indications for the use of braces across the hip joints. One of the indications is to improve a child's ability to walk or to allow a child to walk. For children with cerebral palsy, the use of braces above the knee is seldom useful. Most of these long

leg braces with pelvic bands or the standard HKAFO are used today for children with spinal cord dysfunction (such as spina bifida, meningomyelocele, or spinal cord injuries). These children have normal upper body strength, motor coordination, and balance; when their lower legs are controlled, they are then able to walk by using crutches.

Children with this degree of cerebral palsy in their lower extremities almost never have enough upper extremity strength, muscle coordination, or balance to be able to profit from this much bracing. It usually only weighs the child down, making him look good while standing and taking a few steps but blocking him from functional walking. These braces may also be used to control feet that turn in, and frequently a lighter version or a twister cable as described above may be prescribed for this purpose. Likewise these twister cable braces frequently make the child look better standing but in no way improve his function. They usually greatly diminish how far and fast he can walk, and may injure the knee joints. The use of these long braces is seldom recommended for children with cerebral palsy.

Another indication for these braces is to prevent the adductor muscle from becoming tighter. These muscles are in the inside of the thigh and make the legs cross over each other. Because this process causes the hips to dislocate, there has been some sense in the past that using braces to keep the knees apart may help prevent this dislocation or keep the muscles from becoming tighter. Current guidelines, however, are not to use hip abduction bracing in any child with cerebral palsy unless muscle surgery has been done to release the tight muscle first. There is some indication that bracing against very tight muscles only injures the hip joint further, which may cause abnormal growth in the hip joint or cause it to dislocate more quickly than if no bracing were used.

There continues to be a great difference of opinion with respect to the use of braces following hip muscle surgery. There is some evidence that diligent use of night braces to keep the hips apart may help the hips develop more normally or at least avoid dislocation. If this is done, however, the opposite deformity may occur, in which the hip may become stuck in the outward direction, which is even more disabling for sitting. The consensus seems to be that there is little indication for long-term rigid bracing for hips after muscle releases. The efficacy of short-term bracing is also debatable, although maintaining the child in a good position during sleep and sitting is important and hip braces are one means of achieving this goal.

Finally, the use of hip abduction braces, A-frame braces, or abduction pillows to treat the problems of hip subluxation or tight adductor muscles after muscle surgery continues to vary greatly. It is a fairly well-established opinion among physicians treating patients with CP that bracing before muscle release surgery has no efficacy and is probably more detrimental than effective.

Benefits and risks: The benefits and risks of the use of abduction braces, pillows, and A-frames for the child with spastic hip subluxation are uncertain at this point, and there is no agreed-upon community standard of practice. Generally, the trend is that the risks and complications in bracing outweigh their benefits.

The primary complication of the use of bracing to improve gait is that it diminishes the ability of the child to walk by decreasing speed and distance at the expense of better cosmetic appearance. Any brace that is attached to a pelvic band makes sitting more difficult. It is also cumbersome to constantly apply and remove these braces, and as a consequence it is not practical for a child to wear such a brace constantly if she is sitting for long periods of time. Nor is it practical to apply the brace every time she wants to get up and walk.

The complication of using hip abduction braces to improve hip subluxation or treat tight muscles can be dislocation of the hip if braces are used before muscle release surgery. If an abduction brace is used after muscle release surgery, it may create a deformity called the *wind-blown*

deformity: one hip abducts or becomes more "stuck away from" the midline of the body while the other hip tends to drift in toward the midline. This deformity tends to make sitting and standing very difficult. Also, children who really have tight muscles or who are becoming more contracted are frequently very uncomfortable in these braces and find them almost impossible to sit in. Many of these braces also are stuck in hip flexion (legs drawn up) either because the hinge is fixed in flexion or because there is no hinge, which may contribute to the development of hip flexion contracture.

Occasionally, the very young child (less than 6 years old) with low muscle tone (hypotonia) and a hip subluxation will benefit from a hip abduction brace. The hip should be less than 50 percent subluxated and the brace worn at night time in an effort to maintain hip stability until the child's acetabulum develops and hypotonia improves. The child's hips require close observation and may require surgery at an older age.

Maintenance and care: The majority of hip braces are made out of metal and plastic. The plastic may be cleaned by a gentle detergent, but it is important to keep it out of high temperatures such as direct sunlight. Braces which are made out of leather or have leather components should have the leather kept dry and have it cleaned with a leather cleaning agent. Most of these braces have joints that should be lubricated with a small amount of lubricant such as WD-40 or the lubricant recommended by the orthotist. As children are growing, these braces need to be adjusted and should be seen by a physician or an orthotist at least every six months to check on their fit. Parents should be checking the skin daily when the brace is removed for any red areas or skin breakdown. If skin breakdown is noted, one should check for wrinkles in the stockings underlying the brace; if the same area is persistently red, the brace needs to be evaluated by the physician or orthotist.

Brace, Leg

(knee-ankle-foot orthosis [KAFO], long leg brace, twister cable, circular wrap, knee brace)

A knee-ankle-foot orthosis (KAFO) is any brace that starts just below the hip and extends to the ankle, crossing the knee joint. The braces have a number of variations. A very common older brace has a metal hinge that often has a drop lock at the knee to prevent the knee from bending. When the patient wants to sit down, she can pull the drop lock up, which allows the knee to bend. This device may be called a drop lock, double upright, or long leg brace—which is its older term. A twister cable is yet another brace: it has cables attached to a short leg brace but extends above

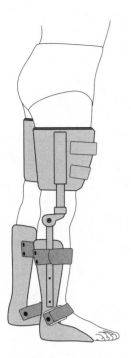

KAFO with drop-lock knee

should only be used for a period of a month to two months at the most and should *not* become permanent means of locking the knees.

Benefits and risks: Although these long leg braces have clear benefits and indications for selected patients, as mentioned above, invariably for children with CP the risks created by the braces are far greater than any benefits they bring. The primary risk in using KAFOs for children with cerebral palsy is typically a decreased functional ability to walk instead of an improved function. These braces generally create an improved cosmetic appearance while the child is standing, but at the expense of a greatly diminished functional benefit. Children who have a great deal of difficulty walking only short distances with walkers usually cannot walk any farther when they are encumbered with long leg braces. Additionally, they have difficulty sitting because these long leg braces are usually rigid under the thigh. If they are not properly fitted, they may cause skin irritation as well.

Using braces, such as twister cables or wraps, for rotational control can also lead to the possible complication of twisted stress through the knee joint, which may become painful. Certainly, the joints are much more susceptible to overstretching than the bones, and a child usually complains of pain when too much rotational stress is applied.

Maintenance and care: Some of these braces are constructed with a plastic AFO foot section, although some of them are attached to rigid orthopedic-type shoes at the foot. In newer models, the metal uprights and metal hinges at the knee have frequently been replaced with plastic uprights and hinges, which are then attached to either leather or plastic cuffs at the thigh. Care must be taken to ensure that the braces continue to fit a growing child—they should be checked every six months by the physician or therapist. After the brace is removed, the skin needs to be checked daily for pressure areas or blisters. Hinges should be kept dry.

the knee and oftentimes above the hip. A circular wrap is a soft device that is wrapped around the leg and tied above the hip to control rotation about the hip.

Indications: These braces are rarely used for children with cerebral palsy. Most children with CP who have trouble controlling their knees also have much difficulty with balance and motor coordination. The addition of long braces may make these children look better standing or walking, but in fact the braces make them walk more slowly because they have a great deal of difficulty handling the extra weight of the braces.

The use of the metal knee hinge brace is primarily for children with spinal cord dysfunction such as meningomyelocele, spina bifida, or a spinal cord injury. These children have excellent upper body strength and have no control or very little control of their legs. Using the brace to control their legs often allows them to walk because of the rigid support, but they often have a decrease in their function because of increased energy needed to handle the braces. Additionally, there is no long-term benefit.

Another indication for a long leg brace, often a knee immobilizer, is temporarily after surgery. During the period after surgery, patients often have difficulty developing control of their muscles and, as a short-term strategy to help patients learn to control their muscles, the use of these temporary braces may be beneficial. These, however,

Bronchopulmonary Dysplasia
(BPD)

BPD is a chronic lung disease that is seen primarily in premature babies who require ventilator support and oxygen therapy after they are born. (Many children who have cerebral palsy were premature.) Occasionally a baby who never required ventilation will develop chronic lung disease as well. In general, the lower the birth weight and gestational age of an infant, the higher the incidence and severity of BPD, and in these infants hyaline membrane disease (respiratory distress syndrome) is almost always present before they develop this condition. It is possible, however, for term infants to develop a BPD-like illness or chronic lung disease after neonatal pneumonia, meconium aspiration, or another severe illness in the neonatal period.

The specific criteria for the diagnosis of BPD are subject to opinion and debate. However, BPD is considered in an infant who was treated during the first two weeks of life with mechanical ventilation, continuous positive airway pressure (CPAP), or oxygen and who continues to have respiratory difficulty at the age of 28 days after birth or at 36 weeks postconceptional age. Respiratory difficulties include at least the need for supplemental oxygen therapy (some infants with severe BPD may require even more respiratory support) and symptoms such as increased work of breathing. Chest x-rays will show characteristic changes including cystic changes in the lungs, and in some cases the lungs will generally appear cloudy instead of clear.

In some children with BPD the lungs develop areas of fibrosis or scarring; atelectasis, areas of the lung that do not fill with air; and small cysts, not unlike emphysema in an older person. In other children with BPD, the lungs remain underdeveloped and lung growth is not normal, but scarring and other changes are less prominent. In severe cases of BPD, oxygenation and ventilation are more severely impaired and increased pulmonary fluid may be present. Infants with BPD may be discharged home from the nursery with oxygen, monitors, and other technological supports. In infants with BPD, growth and nutrition is extremely important to promote lung healing and the growth of new lung tissue, which occurs most dramatically during the first two years of life.

As new lung tissue grows BPD symptoms improve. However, infants and young children with BPD remain susceptible to respiratory viral infections, particularly RSV (Respiratory Syncytial Virus), and readmission to the hospital for pneumonia, respiratory distress, or other problems during the first two years of life is not uncommon. It is important that the appropriate vaccinations and other strategies to protect against infection be maintained. Other challenges that may require medical intervention include the development of asthma symptoms, including chronic coughing and wheezing, and feeding difficulties, including aspiration, oral aversion, gastroesophageal reflux, or failure to thrive.

Bronchoscopy

Bronchoscopy is a procedure in which a physician places a flexible or rigid telescope into the back of the throat and down the airway, allowing him or her to look into the airway and assess whether it is inflamed or floppy or has any other problems that are causing difficulty in breathing. The test is generally done under heavy sedation or under general anesthesia and can be performed on an outpatient basis.

Indications: Children who have difficulty breathing and possibly have some anatomical obstruction in the trachea or bronchi must have this area directly visualized with the bronchoscope. Children who may have breathed in a foreign object that cannot be dislodged must also have a bronchoscopy. Occasionally, a child may also develop fixed secretions and form a plug in one of the large airways in the lung, and the bronchoscope can be used to go into the plugged tube and remove the obstruction. Bronchoscopies are performed by physicians with special training in this technique—they are pediatricians specializing in pulmonary diseases or are ear, nose, and throat (ENT) surgeons.

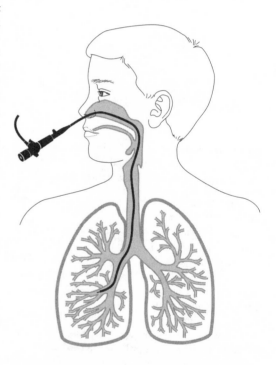

Benefits and risks: Bronchoscopy allows the direct visualization of the airway; as a consequence, anatomical problems such as obstructions or collapses of the airway can be directly seen. Sometimes scar tissue has formed from having an endotracheal tube in the trachea for long periods of time. Scar tissue can also be directly visualized through the bronchoscope. With rigid bronchoscopy, there is a small risk of dental injury. Rarely, swelling from manipulating the airway can cause a crouplike picture. The major risk of this procedure is that it does require signifi-cant sedation and is occasionally done under general anes-thesia. The airway must be carefully maintained because the child must continue to breathe during this whole pro-cedure. In general, when this procedure is performed by physicians who are trained in its use, the risks are very small.

Care after the bronchoscopy usually centers on the child's recovery from the anesthesia or sedation. If there is a risk of postoperative airway swelling, there may be the use of steroids and close monitoring to make sure that breathing continues without difficulty. The procedure may be repeated, especially if it was performed for removal of obstructions such as thick secretions.

Bruxism

(teeth grinding)

Grinding or clenching the teeth while not eating is called bruxism. This is a common problem for some children with cerebral palsy but also occurs, usually at night, in some children who are otherwise normal. Clenching and grinding can cause greater pressure on the teeth than oc-curs when the child is chewing. The increased force can cause the teeth to wear down prematurely or to become malaligned. Causes of the behavior may be ulcers in the mouth, hypersensitive gums or teeth, or it may be a learned behavior. The treatment involves identifying the cause and trying to eliminate the problem. If there is a sore or hypersensitivity, this should be treated. If the problem occurs at night, using diazepam (Valium) may help bring muscle relaxation. The most common method of treat-ment is to make a mouth insert that will stop the grinding. This treatment is usually performed by a pediatric dentist experienced in dealing with children with disabilities.

Bunions

(hallux valgus, cocked-up great toe, flexed great toe, great toe arthritis)

A bunion is a prominence that develops on the inside of the foot where the big toe joins the foot. Children with spastic cerebral palsy often develop bunions, especially if they have flat feet and tend to walk on the inside of the foot. This bunion may become sore as it rubs against the side of the child's shoe. It is usually associated with a toe that has slipped over or started bending toward the inside of the foot, often overlapping or underlapping the second toe. This deformity is called *hallux valgus*. It may also be as-sociated with a cocked-up great toe that becomes stiff and

painful. The big toe may also become flexed down and curl inside the foot.

In all of these deformities, as the toe gets stuck, arthri-tis develops in the great toe joint. Not only can the arthri-tis cause a significant amount of pain, but the deformity makes wearing shoes problematic. These deformities also occur in patients without cerebral palsy, but it is important to note that the treatment differs significantly when no spasticity is present. Treatment in patients without CP of-ten involves attempts at rebalancing muscles and correct-ing the alignment of the toe, but this approach almost al-ways fails in the patient with spasticity. The natural history of these deformities for people with spastic feet is that they gradually get worse and continue to become more problematic.

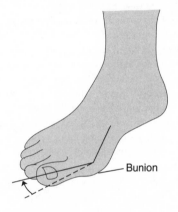

Bunion

Indications: The child should be treated if there is pain with shoe wear or with activity. Initially, some modi-fication of the shoe, if the primary problem is irritation from the shoe, may be attempted. If this is not successful, a surgical correction is indicated. The surgical correction that is performed for almost all of these types of deformi-ties is a fusion of the joint between the great toe and the metatarsal, called a great toe metatarsal phalangeal joint fusion. Often it is fixed with one or two pins or screws af-ter the joint cartilage is removed, which places the toe in a good position. The correction lasts a lifetime and elimi-nates pain.

Benefits and risks: The benefits are relief of pain and the ability to wear shoes comfortably. The main complica-tions of this surgery are the possibility that the bones will not fuse properly or difficulty with healing. Although non-fusion is rare, it requires a second procedure because pain usually persists if the bones do not heal together. Follow-ing a fusion of this nature, the child is placed in a cast that covers the lower leg from his toes to just below the knee; the cast is worn for six to eight weeks. If a pin is used and is left sticking out of the joint, it is usually removed at the time the cast is removed. No bracing or therapy is usually needed after this procedure.

CPAP; BiPAP®

(continuous positive airway pressure; bi-level positive airway pressure)

Introduction: When a person breathes in, the respiratory muscles create a negative (below atmospheric) pressure in the chest cavity causing air to flow into the lungs. Exhaling (breathing out) is normally a passive process that does not require any muscular force.

Although normal breathing depends on the development of negative pressure, occasionally it becomes necessary to apply positive pressure to the respiratory system (the airways and lungs) to assist breathing. For example, this can be needed during surgery, acute illnesses in which breathing becomes ineffective (respiratory failure), or if the airway is obstructed as occurs in obstructive sleep apnea. Positive pressure can be applied to the respiratory system via a tightly fitting face mask in what is called noninvasive ventilation, or via a breathing tube in the airway (either an endotracheal tube or tracheostomy tube) in what is called invasive ventilation.

Positive pressure support is a form of respiratory assistance used when the pressure of air entering a person's lungs needs to be higher than normal atmospheric pressure. The main reasons for using positive pressure respiratory support are unacceptably low levels of blood oxygen, unacceptably high levels of blood carbon dioxide, or unacceptably high levels of respiratory distress. With positive pressure respiratory support, air is pushed into the lungs by a machine, rather than, or in addition to being pulled in by the respiratory muscles. There are a variety of strategies to facilitate this process, but two are described here: CPAP and BiPAP®.

Definitions and indications: CPAP, continuous positive airway pressure, can be administered either invasively or noninvasively. When CPAP is applied invasively it is also called PEEP (positive end-expiratory pressure). CPAP is used to provide positive pressure at a constant level throughout the respiratory cycle, in both inspiration and exhalation. It is used acutely to support breathing for several reasons, one of which is helping to keep the alveoli (the very small air sacs in the lungs) open. The alveoli have a tendency to collapse during illnesses such as severe pneumonia and Respiratory Distress Syndrome (seen in pre-

mature infants), which often cause unacceptably reduced blood oxygen levels. CPAP can be used to support the respiratory muscles when work of breathing is increased and to keep the airway open in conditions such as tracheomalacia, where the trachea has a tendency to collapse, or in cases of upper airway obstruction. Conditions such as these can be associated with unacceptable increases in the carbon dioxide level or unacceptable levels of respiratory distress due to labored breathing. Examples of more chronic use of CPAP include obstructive sleep apnea, where positive pressure is applied to the airway during sleep to stent it open during sleep. In some very severe cases of tracheomalacia, CPAP is applied via a tracheostomy tube to keep the airway open. A final example is in cases of muscle weakness, in which extra support is needed to assist the respiratory muscles.

BiPAP®, bilevel positive airway pressure, is another form of positive pressure respiratory support, which is only approved by the Food and Drug Administration for noninvasive use. It involves the application of a constant level of airway pressure during exhalation (CPAP), but a higher pressure during inspiration. Bilevel positive airway pressure support provides a boost of pressure to either assist the respiratory muscles or to push the airway open during inspiration. During exhalation, continuous positive airway pressure at a lower level is applied to help keep the lungs or airway open. BiPAP® is applied with a mask that fits over the nose or occasionally both the nose and mouth, and is sometimes referred to as noninvasive ventilation or nasal mask ventilation.

The acute indications for BiPAP® are generally similar to those for CPAP, although since it is an increased level of support, patients who require BiPAP® may be sicker than those who need only CPAP. Bilevel positive airway pressure is not used in newborns. Patients who are recovering from surgery or other severe illnesses, and who needed invasive mechanical ventilation with a breathing tube may be placed on BiPAP® for a short time as well. The most common chronic uses of BiPAP® are obstructive sleep apnea and muscle weakness requiring more support than CPAP can provide.

Benefits and risks: Positive pressure ventilatory support, either invasive or noninvasive, is a serious therapy that is used to address significant abnormalities with airway or respiratory muscle function and gas exchange. The risks of leaving these sorts of problems untreated are almost always greater than the therapy. Positive pressure ventilation allows for greatly improved oxygen absorption and carbon dioxide elimination by the lungs and provides needed support to the airway or respiratory muscles without having to use a breathing tube and invasive ventilation. The major acute risk of all positive pressure ventilation is the development of a pneumothorax, a condition in which air escapes from the lung into the chest cavity causing the lung to collapse. This complication is extremely rare with noninvasive ventilation and even with CPAP applied via a tracheostomy tube. Pneumothorax is easily identified with a chest x-ray and a tube can be inserted into the chest cavity to drain the air if needed.

Although mask ventilation is preferable to invasive ventilation for many reasons, both CPAP and BiPAP® can be challenging therapies both in the short and long term. Tight-fitting masks are sometimes difficult to tolerate and care needs to be taken to find a mask that fits correctly and maximizes comfort and tolerance. The sensation of air being forced into the nose and/or mouth can also be difficult to adjust to and various strategies may be necessary to enhance acceptance. Nasal drying and irritation and sinusitis are possible consequences of nasal mask ventilation, and excellent skin care is needed to minimize irritation or even breakdown at the site where the mask is in contact with the skin. Each of these problems is treatable and in the vast majority of cases does not preclude the use of these useful and potentially lifesaving therapies.

Maintenance, care and discharge planning: When used acutely the maintenance, care, and administration of CPAP and BiPAP® are the primary responsibility of the medical team. It is important for the family to attend to patient comfort and tolerability of the mask and to evaluate the underlying skin in an ongoing fashion. When used chronically the maintenance, care, and administration of CPAP and BiPAP® are the primary responsibility of the family. Although this may seem overwhelming at first, with the appropriate training this can become routine and the care team should always provide supervision and medical follow-up when needed. It may also be beneficial for the patient to bring his own mask to the hospital when testing or hospitalization is required.

Carpal Tunnel Syndrome

(finger numbness, hand pain)

Carpal tunnel syndrome is a common problem that occurs most often in people who use their hands extensively in repetitive tasks, such as knitting, typing, or using hand tools. It does sometimes occur in younger individuals, especially in women during pregnancy.

The major nerve (median nerve) in the area travels to the hand through a very narrow area called the carpal tunnel, located at the wrist. The area is occupied by this nerve and eleven tendons. If the tendons are used extensively, they may become inflamed and cause tightness, thereby constricting the nerve and causing numbness, usually in the thumb, index finger, and long finger. The feeling is often worse at night when the fingers are not moving. It may be a dull ache, or a sensation of needles or pins in the fingers. Sometimes the pain also shoots up toward the elbow. With teenagers and young adults with cerebral palsy, carpal tunnel syndrome may occur from using the hands for pushing manual wheelchairs or for patients who are heavily dependent on walkers or crutches for weight bearing.

Indications: The use of anti-inflammatory medications such as aspirin, ibuprofen, or other anti-arthritic medicines is the first line of treatment. Splints should be worn at night to hold the wrist extended. If this intervention does not relieve the symptoms or if they return immediately after discontinuing splinting, the tunnel in which the nerve runs can be surgically released with a procedure called a carpal tunnel release. This is a simple outpatient procedure that can be done on adults under local anesthesia. It requires only a soft bandage for ten days. However, individuals would be restricted from weight bearing with walkers and crutches, and from wheelchair use for three weeks.

What to expect: Complications and risks of the procedure are minimal and mostly relate to possible recurrence as the tunnel heals and tightens up again. The main instructions for preventing recurrence include ensuring proper hand use with wheelchair wheels, crutches, and walkers.

Cataracts

A cataract is present when the lens, which helps focus the image on the back of the retina, is cloudy and limits the transmission of light through it. This condition has many causes, including congenital infections and congenital malformations. Cataracts are sometimes associated with other malformations that may cause cerebral palsy. The treatment involves surgery to remove the cataract and possibly to implant a new plastic lens. The earlier this procedure is done, the more likely it is that good visual function will develop.

Cerebellum

The cerebellum is the upper back part of the brain. It consists of two hemispheres and is located in the posterior cranial fossa portion of the brain. The cerebellum coordinates the action of muscle groups and times their contractions,

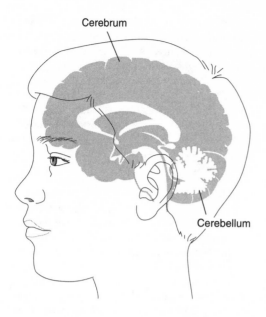

Cerebrum

Cerebellum

so that movements are performed smoothly and accurately. Clumsy and disorganized motor skills caused by damage to the cerebellum is called *cerebellar ataxia.* Sensory information may also be integrated through the cerebellum.

Cerebral Palsy

(static encephalopathy, Little disease)

Cerebral palsy is caused by malformation, scarring, or injury to the immature brain that usually occurs before age 5 and that results in difficulty with muscle movement or control. The brain damage that causes cerebral palsy does not change over a child's life; however, as the child grows and matures, the symptoms of the disability may become more apparent.

Cerebrum

The cerebrum is the major front and upper part of the brain where active coordination and voluntary muscle movement is controlled. This is also the part of the brain where consciousness, thought, and psychological functions reside and are organized (called the executive function). This part of the brain is extremely vulnerable to injury and is the area in which scars occur that lead to cerebral palsy.

The cerebrum is divided into two halves, the right and left hemispheres. The right side controls the left side of the

body, and vice versa. Injuries to one hemisphere cause dysfunction of one side of the body, called *hemiplegia* (motor involvement of one arm and one leg on the same side of the body). Injuries to both sides cause *diplegia* (motor involvement of the lower extremities with difficulty in trunk control and fine motor skills) or *quadriplegia* (motor involvement of all four limbs).

In each half, or hemisphere, there are specific areas that control specific functions. Specific areas such as the frontal lobes predominantly control emotion; speech is controlled primarily on the right side of the brain; and specific areas of the brain control the hands as compared to the feet. The different areas of function have been mapped out very well—largely by careful observation of known areas in which injury has occurred, followed by recording the deficits that patients subsequently exhibit.

Injury to specific areas of the brain explain why some children with cerebral palsy exhibit behavior difficulties or have specific problems with their motor control. Children with cerebral palsy may have full areas of the brain missing (revealed when scans are performed), but because their brain is still developing, the function ordinarily performed by that part of the brain may be taken up by a new part of the brain. This is the major reason why the outcome in cerebral palsy differs greatly from the outcome of head injuries occurring in adults.

Child Abuse

(child neglect, shaken baby syndrome)

Child abuse is defined by Public Law 93-247 as physical or mental injury, sexual abuse or exploitation, negligent care, or maltreatment of a child under the age of 18 by a person who is responsible for the child's welfare.

There is much about the abuse of children that is not understood. We do know that child abuse has a tendency to be present in certain families, especially where parents themselves were abused as children. Children with disabilities, especially severely involved children with cerebral palsy, are at higher risk for child abuse than children without disabilities. These children may be unusually irritable or difficult to comfort, which can become frustrating for parents and caregivers. Parents of children who are very difficult to care for may neglect or physically harm them as a way of dealing with their own frustration. Any stress can precipitate striking out, and parents of children with disabilities often experience a great deal of stress related to their child's care.

Parents of children with disabilities need to have someone whom they can call for help. This may be a grandparent, a friend, a neighbor, or a social worker. Parents should learn to call and admit that they are unable to handle the situation, especially when they have difficulty controlling their emotions and when their frustration level is very high.

Shaken baby syndrome occurs when a caregiver is trying to quiet a baby by shaking her back and forth. If this maneuver is done too roughly, it can cause bruises and contusions of the baby's brain, which can cause long-term brain scars and cerebral palsy. This too is a form of child abuse.

The complications from child abuse can be very severe, from bruises and broken bones to neglect, such as not being given needed medication or adequate food, and can even lead to death. Very few parents actually intentionally abuse their child, but it can become the only form of reacting to the environment that the parent is capable of at the time.

By law, suspicions of child abuse must be reported by school and medical personnel to the appropriate state agency which investigates the situation. Responses may include support for the family, or in severe situations (where the child's safety or health is felt to be threatened) removal of the child from the home on a temporary or long-term basis. The vast majority of reported suspicions of child abuse are handled by social workers who are able to provide education and supportive help to the parents so they can deal with the situation.

Chromosomal Disorders

Each human cell contains a full complement of genetic information that is encoded in 46 chromosomes, which are actually made up of 23 pairs of chromosomes, with one set of 23 donated by each parent. Chromosomes are composed of genes, which are themselves composed of DNA. Each chromosome pair contains genes coding for similar traits; we have 2 of almost every gene, one from our mother and one from our father. One chromosome pair is made up of the sex chromosomes, consisting of the XX chromosome pair in a female and the XY pair in a male.

A variety of things can go wrong so that a child has too few or too many chromosomes. In most cases the fetus does not survive, but there are specific instances where a child is born with a chromosomal disorder that is compatible with life but associated with various abnormalities, including central nervous system problems such as cerebral palsy. Over 50% of the fetuses that are miscarried before 12 weeks of gestation are found to have a chromosomal anomaly. As the fetus continues to develop and get closer to the delivery date, the chance of chromosomal anomalies and spontaneous abortion or miscarriage decreases.

When an entire chromosome is involved, there are also many genes involved. Thus, children with chromosomal disorders often have typical facial features, or birth defects such as congenital heart defects, in addition to developmental delays or cerebral palsy. Most people recognize Down syndrome in which there is an extra chromosome number 21. People with Down syndrome share certain physical features such as a flat profile, upslanted eyes, hyperextensible joints, and varying degrees of mental retardation. Heart defects and defects of the intestines are also frequent.

Another chromosome anomaly is the deletion of a small piece of a chromosome, whereby a small part of a chromosome is lost (and thus a number of genes are missing), a duplication in which a piece of a chromosome is present in 3 copies rather than in 2, or a translocation, whereby a small piece of a chromosome may be attached to another chromosome. These can be identified by preparing and examining the chromosomes under a microscope. Depending on the specific genes involved, these children may have multiple physical and cognitive problems as well. Rarely, one healthy parent of an affected child may have a rearrangement of his or her chromosomes, which predisposes to a (micro)deletion, duplication, or translocation in a child. Thus, when any chromosome deletion, duplication, or rearrangement is identified, parents are often tested.

More recently, very small submicroscopic (too small to be seen with the standard microscopic techniques) chromosome deletions have been identified. They are referred to as *microdeletion syndromes*. Once again, depending on the specific gene or genes involved, features may vary and patients are often presumed to have cerebral palsy early on until the diagnosis is made. They will not be found on standard chromosome studies, but instead require more complex DNA tests. Identifying patterns of physical and behavioral features is important for the physician deciding which syndrome, if any, should be tested for in any individual child.

Subtelomeric deletions/rearrangements involve the very ends of the chromosomes. Features of the specific chromosome abnormality vary. It is estimated that a subtelomeric rearrangement will be identified in 4–7 percent of children with a combination of developmental delay and small size. Examples of microdeletion syndromes follow.

Angelman syndrome. Angelman syndrome is associated with severely delayed or often no speech, severe sleep problems, difficult-to-control seizures, and discoordinated gait. Children have a very typical puppetlike movement of the arms and legs in walking. Most are described as very happy children who rarely cry and often laugh aloud without obvious reason.

Prader-Willi syndrome. Prader-Willi syndrome is associated with a unique unabated desire to eat; individuals with this syndrome thus become extremely obese. Children are typically very loose jointed, often with muscle weakness, and most do not have normal intelligence. Infants often appear floppy and are paradoxically poor eaters until approximately age 2, at which time they begin to eat voraciously.

Smith-Magenis syndrome. Smith-Magenis syndrome is another genetic disorder that has very typical behaviors associated with it. Children with Smith-Magenis often display an unusual self-hugging behavior. Self-injury is typical, as is poor sleep. Most do not have normal intelligence. Although often there are no typical facial features, these children can be floppy at birth and may develop a progressive neuropathy (injury to the nerves) in the legs.

Genetic syndromes. The **Fragile X syndrome** is often considered in any male with developmental delay. Females have 2 X chromosomes, while males have only one X and one Y chromosome. The genes on the X and Y chromosomes are not the same; in males, the genes on the X and Y chromosomes are the only genes for which there are not 2 copies. Thus, an abnormal gene on the X chromosome will cause symptoms in males, because there is no normal gene to take over function.

Males with Fragile X syndrome typically have mental retardation, often with autistic features and hyperactivity. There are often distinctive facial features such as a long face, large ears, a prominent jaw and after puberty, large testes. Many affected children have few features except for the mental retardation.

Because females have 2 X chromosomes, they are less likely to show symptoms of a defective gene on one of them. However, ~50% of females who carry an affected gene have learning disabilities or mild mental retardation. A blood test to measure the number of DNA repeats in the FMR1 gene can diagnose the Fragile X syndrome in both males and females.

The gene for **Rett syndrome** is also on the X chromosome. This disorder, however, typically is seen only in females, rather than males. Affected males are thought to be miscarried because of the severe effects of Rett syndrome on the developing brain. Since females have a second MECP2 gene, the presence of one normal one may help to offset the effects of the abnormal one, allowing these children to survive to birth.

Girls with classic Rett Syndrome develop normally until about the second year of life when growth, including head size, begins to decelerate. They lose speech skills and develop an autistic-like lack of interest in social interaction. Purposeful movement of the hands becomes limited and they display a characteristic hand-wringing behavior. Spasticity, seizures, progressive scoliosis, and unusual episodes of hyperventilation develop over time.

A "Preserved Speech Variant" is a milder form of the disorder in which females share features of classic Rett syndrome such as autistic qualities, but often regain some speech and hand use, and may not show growth failure.

Since the gene that causes Rett syndrome has been identified, and a test made available for the disorder, we now know of living males with the disorder. Most develop seizures, growth retardation, hypotonia, and severe growth retardation in early infancy. Some have even followed a course similar to classically affected females.

Testing for Rett syndrome involves looking for changes in the gene itself in blood or tissue samples. It is laborious and expensive, but is being offered by many commercial laboratories.

Clonus

Clonus is a symptom of spasticity. It is a special reflex from the spinal cord that is not being controlled by the normal mechanism in the brain. Rapid stretching of a muscle, such as pushing hard against the sole of the foot, causes the foot to make rhythmic movements. As the muscle is held under tension these rhythmic movements may gradually die down, but in some people they are persistent. Constant clonus is noted to be present when a certain pressure causes a constant beating of the muscle. Clonus activity that causes a beating motion at the ankle joint is very common in children with cerebral palsy. This can cause a problem for children who are sitting in wheelchairs, because their legs may jump. AFO braces used on the ankle may suppress this reflex.

Cochlear Implants

Cochlear implant is an auditory rehabilitation option for children with sensorineural (nerve) hearing loss that is not "aid-able" with conventional hearing aids. In this situation, the hearing aids are not powerful enough to bring the hearing thresholds into the normal range. Because most types of sensorineural hearing loss involve disorders of the cochlea (organ of hearing) but spare the nerve of hearing (cochlear nerve), it is possible to directly stimulate the nerve of hearing electrically and bring sound information to the brain.

The cochlear implant is a surgically placed device that takes sound information from a microphone, transforms

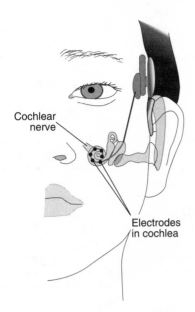

Cochlear nerve

Electrodes in cochlea

this into pulsed electrical signals that are sent along an electrode array in the cochlea to directly stimulate the nerve of hearing. Not all children with profound sensorineural hearing loss are candidates for cochlear implantation and an experienced cochlear implant team composed of audiologists, speech pathologists, deaf educators, language scientists, surgeons, and social workers evaluate each patient on an individual basis to help with this important decision.

Complementary and Alternative Medicine

(CAM)

Complementary and alternative medicine (CAM) describes a group of diverse medical practices and products that are not presently considered part of conventional medicine. While some CAM therapies have been studied scientifically, most have yet to be investigated through well-designed scientific studies, and questions remain as to whether these therapies work for the medical conditions for which they are used, and whether they are safe. Although it is often assumed that natural products such as herbs must be safe, this is not necessarily true, as many have significant medicinal properties and may have significant side effects. Because the FDA does not have any jurisdiction over these products (they are considered a food rather than a medicine), they are not tested for safety or effectiveness and may include harmful contaminants, or they may not contain the ingredients they say they have.

Complementary medicine is used together with conventional medicine, whereas alternative medicine is used in place of conventional medicine. A third category, that of integrative medicine, combines mainstream medical therapies and CAM therapies for which there is good scientific evidence of safety and effectiveness.

The federal government has established the National Center for Complementary and Alternative Medicine to explore these practices in the context of rigorous science. The center has sponsored research into many of these alternative medical treatments and disseminates authoritative information to the public and to medical professionals.

Chiropractic is an example of an alternative medical system. Chiropractors use manipulative therapy as a treatment tool. Homeopathic medicine is another alternative medical system, which uses small quantities of very diluted medicinal substances to cure symptoms, when the same substances given at higher doses would actually cause those symptoms. Dietary supplements are products taken by mouth that contain a "dietary ingredient" that is meant to supplement the diet. These may include vitamins, minerals, herbs, amino acids, and substances such as enzymes. Dietary supplements can certainly be used in a complementary fashion with conventional medicine, but have also been used as an alternative to conventional medicine.

Patients and families need to weigh the basis for the use of these products and, as with many other treatments, discuss with their medical practitioners both whether these products are effective and whether they are safe.

Computerized Axial Tomography

(CT scan, CAT scan)

The CT scan is a special type of x-ray where the computer makes pictures using information from x-rays taken around the body. A CT scan can be made of any area of the body and gives excellent definition of bone and soft tissue. Scans of the brain can define major abnormalities such as tumors, increased fluid in the brain, and major congenital deformities.

The dose of radiation is more than received from conventional x-rays, but not considered harmful. The patient lies on a table and needs to hold still. Contrast material is sometimes injected into the bloodstream to help define the blood vessels. CT scans cannot, however, detect all deformities or scars.

Indications: For children with cerebral palsy, the main reason CT scans are utilized is to define possible deformities in the brain. Often a CT scan may be used in the initial evaluation to see if there are any specific treatable deformities of the brain, such as tumors. Hydrocephalus, or increased fluid on the brain, can also be diagnosed with a CT scan. Another common indication for obtaining a CT scan is a child with a shunt for hydrocephalus. The function of the shunt is checked by obtaining a CT scan.

Benefits and risks: The benefit of the CT scan is that it provides a good view of the brain and can often be done much more quickly than an MR scan. The machine also is a smaller tube and does not give the sense of being enclosed in the way an MR scanner does. The risks of CT scan involve the fact that a low dose x-ray is used; also, because the scan still requires a child to hold still, some children may require sedation. Another problem with the CT scan is that it is limited to defining only major deformities of the brain. This means that there are subtle brain deformities that the CT scanner cannot define.

Maintenance and care: If a child is sedated, care must be taken to monitor the child until the sedation has worn off.

Congenital Infections

(cytomegalovirus [CMV], toxoplasmosis, syphilis, rubella [German measles], herpes simplex virus, varicella [chicken pox])

A number of infectious agents can infect a pregnant woman and then infect the fetus she is carrying, causing a variety of physical abnormalities and sometimes brain damage resulting in cerebral palsy. These infections may be acquired during pregnancy, during delivery, or occasionally following birth. Frequently, these infections are subclinical (meaning that they do not show any symptoms), and yet can later result in neurological damage. The infections listed here are known to cause brain damage in the fetus or young child.

Contracture, Elbow

Elbow flexion contractures are present in children with severely involved quadriplegic or hemiplegic cerebral palsy. In the severest form, the elbow is tightly flexed, and it is impossible to extend the elbow enough to clean the elbow crease. This causes a foul-smelling moist area. When the elbow cannot be extended it is also difficult to dress the child, especially to put sleeves on the arm. Elbow flexion contractures in children with hemiplegia are cosmetically unappealing, especially when the child walks, because the elbow is held flexed up.

Elbow flexion contractures occurring in young children between the ages of 3 and 6 have a tendency to get slowly worse. If good elbow motion is maintained until adolescence, generally it can be maintained throughout adult life. However, there is a tendency for muscle stiffness to increase with aging, and further contracture may develop in the late teenage years or adulthood.

Care and treatment: Children with a tendency to develop contractures may use night resting splints as well as physical therapy exercises to maintain range of motion. Since it is not certain whether contractures can be avoided in certain children, there is a wide spectrum of opinion as to exactly how aggressive the medical professional should be about splinting and stretching.

The majority of children continue to work with some combination of stretching and bracing; only in rare cases do the flexion contractures become so severe that cleaning the flexion crease or dressing the child becomes extremely difficult. In these circumstances, release of the biceps and the brachial muscles at the elbow is recommended. This is a relatively minor procedure and is frequently combined with other procedures that address specific functional care problems. For some children with severe hemiplegia, cosmetic concerns are such that release of the muscles to let the arm extend is of great benefit for the child's self-image.

Benefits and risks: The benefits of a successful procedure are greater ease in cleaning and dressing the child, and an enhanced appearance. Surgical release is a rather simple procedure with few complications. There is a risk that brace wear may cause skin breakdown, so the skin needs to be monitored daily after the brace has been removed. Also, stretching, if done too aggressively, may cause fractures of the arm. Surgical release of the elbow, if it is too aggressive, may result in the elbow's being stuck in an extended position—which is even more cosmetically objectionable and more functionally debilitating than a flexed elbow. The goal should be to have the elbow at approximately 90 to 100 degrees if the child is wheelchair bound or approximately 120 degrees if ambulatory.

Maintenance and care: The main instruction after surgery is to work with range of motion. For parents, this may involve gentle work with range of motion during bathing or at dressing time, and can often be done in the context of the normal activities of daily living rather than setting aside special exercise times. Braces used may be quite flexible and variable. If surgical release is performed, it is recommended to continue with exercise and occasionally with a bracing program for at least six months to a year.

Contracture, Finger

(flexor tendon lengthening)

Tightness of the finger flexion muscles often exists side by side with another problem: wrist drop and tightness of the muscles that pull the wrist into flexion. There are two groups of muscles that cause the fingers to flex. One is the profundus muscle, extending from the forearm all the way to the tip of each finger. This muscle does not cross the elbow and is usually the least likely to have significant shortness. The other is the flexor sublimis muscle, which starts above the elbow and goes to the first joint (PIP joint) of each finger, and is primarily involved with contractures.

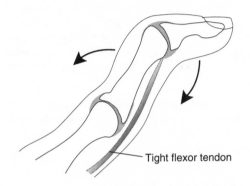

Tight flexor tendon

Often the finger flexor muscles are not tight when the wrist is in the flexed position, but if surgical procedures are done to correct the fixed flexion and put the wrist in a better position, at times the finger muscles become so tight that the fingers cannot be straightened out. The tendency over time is for these muscles gradually to get tighter, although they seldom become so tight that the fingers are clenched into the palm.

Care and treatment: The primary treatment is splinting, which is usually used in addition to the wrist drop splints that are described in the wrist contracture section. It is seldom necessary to treat the finger flexors or to brace the finger flexion contractures without also addressing the wrist flexion problem. If a decision has been made to treat the wrist flexion contractures and the finger flexors are tight, they should be treated surgically at the same time.

The surgery: There are two surgical approaches, both of which include loosening the muscles at their insertion above the elbow and allowing them to slide toward the fingers, which is generally referred to as the muscle slide procedure and involves identifying and lengthening each tendon with a Z-cut. The first procedure of lengthen-

ing the elbow involves less exact lengthening. The more commonly used procedure at the wrist is more exactly controlled, and only the sublimis tendons are lengthened. In severe deformities, the profundus tendons may need lengthening as well.

Benefits and risks: The benefits are both cosmetic and functional. Overlengthening, which removes the strength from the muscles and decreases the ability to close the fingers or to grasp objects, may be a significant complication that is best avoided by conservative, controlled lengthening. If both the sublimis and the profundus tendons are lengthened, major weakness is a higher risk. If only the sublimis tendons are lengthened, there is a risk of developing swan-neck deformities, which means that the first joint (the PIP joint) of the finger may go into extension while the joint at the end of the finger (the DIP joint) flexes. This causes the fingers to lock and makes it difficult for a person to use them for grasping.

Another complication that may occur involves scarring of the tendons, resulting in decreased motion. This can usually be treated with occupational therapy through motion exercises. Occasionally, surgery is needed. Following lengthenings, the fingers are usually immobilized, slightly flexed, in a cast, and the tendons are allowed to heal for four weeks before motion begins.

Contracture, Peroneal

(peroneus longus contracture, peroneal tendon lengthening)

The peroneal tendons and muscles are located along the outside of the leg (lateral side) and pull the foot out. When they are spastic or too tight they cause severe flat feet. These muscles are not commonly severely spastic, but some children do develop significant spasticity.

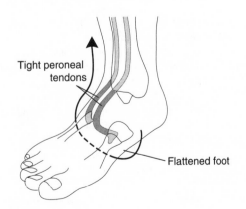

Tight peroneal tendons

Flattened foot

Care and treatment: If severe spasticity seems to be a significant cause of flatfootedness, lengthening these tendons may be necessary. The outcome of peroneal tendon lengthening, however, is very unreliable, with a high incidence of either recurrent deformity within several years or the developing of the opposite deformity if too much lengthening is done. Peroneal tendon lengthening is not a commonly performed operation because of its unreliability. Usually it is better to use a brace (AFO)—and if this is not possible, to proceed with subtalar fusion, which involves fusing the bone in the back of the foot to prevent a flat foot deformity.

Contracture, Pronator

(pronator teres transfer, pronator release)

A common contracture that develops in children with cerebral palsy is a pronation contracture, where the hand is turned palm away from the face. The primary muscle involved is called the pronator teres, which is the muscle that comes from just above the elbow to the middle of the forearm. This contracture occurs commonly in children with hemiplegia and is present in some children with moderate to severe quadriplegia. The deformity begins as the child's preferred position. With growth, the muscle frequently becomes tighter and more contracted.

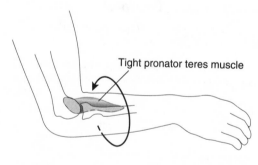

Tight pronator teres muscle

Care and treatment: Exercises to stretch this muscle should be incorporated as part of the child's elbow and hand exercises. Splinting the muscle is difficult because torsional splints require tying up the hand from above the elbow all the way down to the wrist. Splinting is generally not useful because of the difficulty of keeping the arm in a fixed position. This deformity does not cause any significant hygiene or dressing problems; however, it does cause functional problems because the palm and fingertips are turned out of sight, making it difficult to manipulate switches and joysticks because the child cannot see how his palm and fingertips are moving. It also makes picking up utensils or other objects difficult. Pronation often be-

comes a significant cosmetic deformity, especially for the child with hemiplegia who is walking and participating in normal daily activities.

The surgery: The treatment for pronation contracture involves either releasing the pronator muscle from its insertion on the forearm or transferring it to wind around the bone in the opposite direction—making the hand supine, or turned up. There are surgeons who believe that the transfer provides a better outcome. The determination of whether to release or transfer varies, and for most patients the two provide essentially the same results.

Benefits and risks: Benefits are the ability to see the palm and therefore possibly to use it better, and a more pleasing appearance. The complications from pronator release or transfer surgery include the possibility of developing the opposite deformity, but this seldom occurs. The procedure is quite minor and is usually incorporated as one of a number of procedures to deal with other deformities at the same time.

After-surgery care: Following the operation, the patient is usually in a cast above the elbow for four to six weeks. Exercises are subsequently started; bracing is not used.

Contracture, Shoulder

(pectoralis contracture, latissimus dorsi contracture)

Shoulder contractures are common in children with severe quadriplegia. However, they are seldom a problem except with the child whose shoulder is pulled down to the side with the hand across the chest—or, alternatively, with the child whose shoulder may be pulled down to the side with the arm stuck straight out. If the arm is pulled across the chest, it is called an *internal rotation contracture,* and if it is pulled out away from the body it is called an *external rotation contracture.* Internal rotation contractures are usually due to the contracture of the pectoralis major and minor muscles, and the therapy usually involves working at range of motion. External rotation contractures are often due to the contracture of the teres minor and latissimus dorsi muscles. Again, the treatment involves working on physical therapy and positioning.

The surgery: For those severe external rotation contractures that cannot be stretched out with therapy, surgery may be necessary, usually an osteotomy just below the shoulder. The arm must be turned in and held in this position while the bone heals. For severe internal rotation contractures, a pectoralis release is occasionally necessary. This is a very small procedure done at the shoulder which allows the arm to rotate externally far enough to allow for personal hygiene and dressing.

Indications: The main indication for surgical procedures for internal rotation contractures is the need to improve the caregiver's ability to dress the child, especially to place the arms in sleeves and for personal hygiene—primarily to clean the armpits. For external rotation contractures, the major problem develops in a larger child when it is difficult to get the child through doors and to sit well in a wheelchair.

Benefits and risks: The major benefit is improved range of motion, which allows the caregiver to clean and to dress the child, and increased ease of moving the child. The complications from either of these procedures may involve overcorrection. Overcorrection is a special concern with the internally rotated arm: release should not be overly aggressive, since the arm may become fixed in external rotation. Likewise, for the externally rotated arm that is surgically rotated in, too much internal rotation is possible.

After-surgery care: The postoperative treatment usually is immediate, aggressive physical therapy for the muscle releases. A period of splint immobilization of three to four weeks is necessary after the osteotomy to allow healing.

Contracture, Thumb

(adducted thumb, thumb tendon release, thumb fusion)

Thumb deformities in children with cerebral palsy are very common. The most common problem is a thumb that is drawn close to the index finger, making the web space between the index finger and the thumb very tight and narrow. This makes it difficult to get the thumb out away from the hand to grasp objects such as balls or glasses. Sometimes the thumb is flexed tightly into the palm. In some children this can make hygiene very difficult, with the palm becoming moist and foul smelling. From a functional perspective, the problem of the thumb in the hand makes grasping objects more difficult; pinching from the tip of the thumb to the index or the long fingers may also be difficult. In some children the first thumb joint (the IP joint) may also become extended, and the joint at the base of the thumb (the MCP joint) may be flexed or extended.

Care and treatment: As long as the hand can be cleaned and the palm does not become moist and smelly,

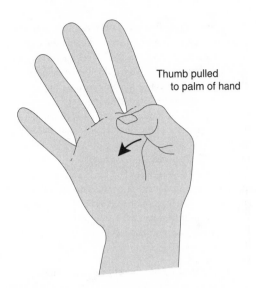

Thumb pulled to palm of hand

treatment for thumb deformities is not needed. If the thumb is tightly drawn into the hand and flexed into the palm, then hygiene is a problem, and the appropriate treatment is almost always surgical. The most common technique involves fusing the joint at the base of the thumb (the MCP joint or the IP joint), with release of the thumb flexor tendon and the adductor tendon in the palm. Sometimes a tendon transfer to help pull the thumb out of the palm is needed. These fusions are minor procedures in which the cartilage and the joint are removed, and the bone is held with a pin for four to six weeks as the bones grow together. This is a permanent correction.

Initially, hands that are functional but causing difficulties should be splinted. Either rigid plastic splints to deepen the space between the index finger and the thumb or a splint that is made as part of a hand or wrist splint is appropriate. Soft splints are available which hook over the thumb and pull it back. These are useful to pull the thumb out of the palm to improve use of the hand and prevent development of contractures. This type of splinting is especially useful during childhood from the ages of 2 to 10. Adolescents almost never accept splinting because of the attention drawn to the hand's appearance. Functionally, the splinting usually is more of an impediment to the teen than a benefit. If thumb deformities continue to be a functional problem they are generally best handled with surgical correction, which is usually done as part of multiple other procedures either on the same arm or on the legs. The timing is related in part to the timing of other procedures.

The surgery: The simplest surgical procedure is the release of the thumb adductor muscle with a small incision in the palm, which often needs to be augmented with the addition of transfers to help increase the strength or power of the thumb-extending muscles. The usual muscle that is used is the muscle in the palm called the palmaris longus. There are multiple other muscles such as finger flexor muscles or wrist flexor muscles that may be used for this purpose as well. Occasionally, with a severely involved hand, fusion of one of the thumb joints may also be indicated.

The surgical procedures used to treat thumb deformities vary among surgeons. The same surgeon may use many different combinations because thumb deformities are quite different from one hand to the next. The decision about which muscles to transfer and if fusions are indicated is determined by physical examination and the surgeon's specific experience.

Benefits and risks: Benefits include improved use of the hand and better hygiene. One risk is that bracing thumb deformities may cause skin irritation. Observation of the skin and well-fitting braces can prevent this complication. The surgical complications are related to overcorrection of deformities, the severest being the thumb stuck far out of the palm, which creates significant cosmetic problems and difficulties with dressing, such as getting a hand through a sleeve. Although complications are rare, the more common complication is the deformity that is not completely corrected. It is much better to have some residual tightness with the thumb in toward the hand than to have the opposite problem.

Maintenance and care: After surgical correction, casting is usually required for four to six weeks, sometimes followed by splinting. In a functional hand, some occupational therapy aimed at achieving the maximum benefit from the surgery is usually necessary for one to three months.

Contracture, Wrist

(wrist tendon transfer)

Wrist flexion is a common deformity in children with hemiplegia and severe quadriplegia. The wrist is dropped in position and is sometimes referred to as a *dropped wrist*. Occasionally, the child is able to bring the wrist up to a neutral position. In this flexed position it is difficult to get good finger grasp because the wrist position makes the finger flexion muscles much weaker. This flexion contracture develops in the middle childhood period between the ages of 3 and 6. Initially, it is flexible and does not cause any problems, but tightness develops as the child continues to grow into the early teens; during the adolescent growth spurt, the muscles become shorter relative to the bone.

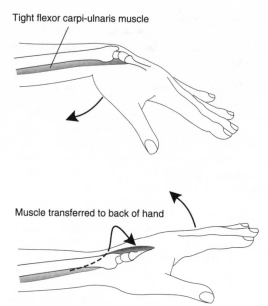

Tight flexor carpi-ulnaris muscle

Muscle transferred to back of hand

At this point, correction of the deformity becomes more difficult. In its severest form, the hand may be folded completely onto the forearm, making skin care and hygiene difficult and creating a moist area that may start to smell. For those children who have a mild case of cerebral palsy and are more functional, as the wrist flexion becomes more contracted, more difficulty with hand use—especially with finger grasps—is encountered.

Care and treatment: The primary treatment for wrist flexion contracture is an exercise program with gentle stretching and the use of resting splints. If splints are used to cover the hand, the child may lose interest in using the hand, and its ability to stay limber diminishes. For this reason, some combination of splint use and functional use is best. For wrists that are not developing significant contractures and can be brought completely into an overcorrected position, overtreatment with braces should be avoided. For the child with severe quadriplegia and no functional hand use, the goal should be to create sufficient flexibility to allow for good hygiene and ease of dressing. The development of some contracture in this situation is not detrimental.

For the child with functional use of the hand, attempts should be made to keep the wrist in a functional position. If this is not possible, as the child grows into adolescence surgical correction should be considered. Usually no earlier than age 6 and generally between the ages of 9 and 12 is the best time for surgery. Children with significant wrist flexion contractures and hemiplegia, even if they are nonfunctional, often have cosmetic appearance concerns and should be considered for surgical corrections. An awkward-looking hand draws much less attention if it is corrected, even if its function is not changed. The best age for the surgery is at or just before the adolescent growth spurt in the early teen years.

The surgery: Surgical treatment typically involves transfer of the muscle on the little finger side of the wrist called the flexor carpi-ulnaris. It is attached to the muscles that lift the wrist, usually the extensor carpi-radialis brevis. For children who have difficulty lifting their fingers, the muscle is transferred into the extensor digitorum communis muscle, which helps to extend the fingers. This transfer, along with tightening the muscles that lift the wrist, improves the straightening of both the fingers and the wrist at the same time.

The exact tendon that is transferred into each muscle varies and is determined by clinical examination. There are some laboratory tests available that use electromyographs (which involve inserting small wires into the muscle) and observation of the hand as it functions, thus determining which muscles are functioning and in what fashion. These tendon transfers are well established and are not new or experimental.

Benefits and risks: Benefits include improved cosmetic appearance and better hygiene; often function is improved as well. The main problem associated with splints is the possibility of causing skin irritation and diminished function. Overly aggressive stretching of very tightly contracted muscle may cause fractures and should be avoided. The major surgical complications are overcorrection or undercorrection. It is best to end up with less than perfect correction if one needs to consider making an error in one direction.

One severe complication is an overextension, backward, of the wrist. This could occur with too much tendon release at the palm side of the wrist or if the tendon transfer on the wrist is too tight. This is especially detrimental if the transfer is into the finger-extending tendons, which means the fingers cannot be bent. It could also make grasping difficult. These problems can be corrected by lengthening the transfer tendons, but it is best to avoid them by not placing the transfers too tightly. Occasionally the transferred tendons may tear out, leaving the person with essentially the same deformity he started with.

After-surgery care: After surgical transfers for correction of this problem the person usually has to wear a cast for four to six weeks, followed by a positional brace, usually worn at night. After one year all bracing is stopped. Intense occupational therapy aimed at improving function and mobility is recommended after the surgical healing period is over, usually beginning at four to six weeks after surgery.

Cotrel-Dubousset Instrumentation
(CD rod, TSRH instrumentation)

CD rods are metal rods and hooks that are attached to the spine to correct and maintain correction of spinal deformities until bone fusion occurs. This instrumentation system involves rigid rods with a number of hooks that attach to the vertebrae. A very popular method of fixing the rods to the spine involves the use of screws in the vertebra called pedicle screws.

Indications: This system of spinal instrumentation is currently the one most commonly used for idiopathic scoliosis, which is side curving of the spine in otherwise healthy children or adolescents. It has the advantage of giving a better correction than the Harrington rod, the old system, which has only two connections to the spine. CD rods provide a better cosmetic result and are stronger, thus having less risk of breaking. Some surgeons are experimenting with their use in children with cerebral palsy, but the indication for use in scoliosis in this population remains uncertain at best.

Benefits and risks: The benefit of these rods is that they are very strong and seldom break; therefore, braces or casts are not usually used after instrumentation. The com-

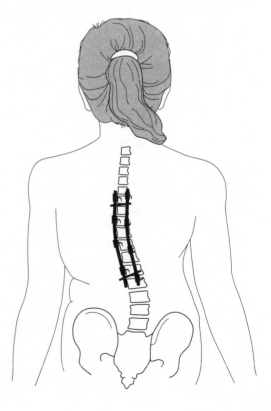

plications of CD rods are mainly those related to posterior spinal fusions. Some of the hooks may slip off the vertebrae. Pedicle screws have less risk than hooks of becoming dislodged. However, there is a risk of nerve injury when they are inserted. Because of the multiple hooks, for a few patients the bone fusion does not heal or an infection may develop around the metal.

Maintenance and care: After the posterior spinal fusion with CD rods, the patient may usually return to nearly normal activity except for contact sports, which the child should wait six months before pursuing.

Crossed Extension Reflex

The crossed extension reflex is present at birth; in normal children, it disappears between the fourth and sixth week of life. If the reflex is present much beyond this age, it indicates brain abnormalities and spastic cerebral palsy. This reflex is elicited by applying a noxious stimulus (such as a pinprick) to the sole of one foot, which is held in complete extension. The reflex consists of the other leg first flexing, then being brought forward, and finally extending, as if to push away the noxious stimulus.

Crouch

(crouched gait, tight hamstring, tight hip flexor, overlengthened Achilles tendon)

A crouched gait is commonly seen in children with diplegia: they stand with their knees and their hips flexed, and often with their ankles dorsiflexed, so that their weight is resting on the heels. Children with a crouched gait may also stand up on tiptoe. When it is mild, this natural pattern works quite well and there is no need to correct it. However, if the crouch becomes severe, for example with knee flexion of 45 degrees when standing, then it becomes a very energy-consuming gait and it is extremely difficult to walk. When a child gains weight, often the crouching becomes more severe, especially during a growth spurt.

A crouched gait is usually caused by a combination of factors, the primary cause being a tight hamstring muscle. Tight hip flexor muscles are another cause, and oftentimes an overlengthened Achilles tendon may be a contributing factor.

Care and treatment: The treatment of a crouched gait initially involves physical therapy, with therapist and child working at stretching the hip flexors and the hamstring muscles. In younger patients, botulinum toxin injections into the hamstring muscle and hip flexor muscle

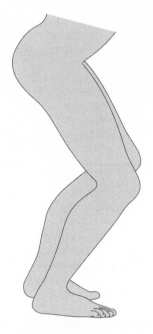

(iliopsoas) may be helpful when the tightness is due primarily to tone. If the crouched gait is getting worse in spite of therapy, a ground reaction ankle-foot orthosis which locks the ankle may be necessary. If this fails and the crouching continues to get worse or the hamstring and hip flexors are very tight, lengthening the hamstring muscles and hip flexors, especially the iliopsoas muscles, should be considered. If the Achilles tendon is tight it may need to be lengthened, but with extreme caution, since an overlengthened Achilles tendon will certainly make the crouching worse.

The complications of a long-term crouch are knee pain and the gradually reduced ability to walk. The knee pain is caused by increased pressure on the kneecap and may become severe enough to prohibit walking. If muscles are lengthened early in a child's life (before age 8), this often needs to be repeated at adolescence, since growth will again cause shortness in the muscle. If, as the child reaches full maturity, the degree of crouching is mild, it generally does not get worse. If it is severe, however, it tends to get slowly worse. Overlengthening the muscles, which may cause the knee to bend backward, may be another complication of treatment. This gait pattern is even worse than crouched gait, and it should be avoided by conservative lengthening of the muscles with the risk of needing repeat lengthening.

After surgery, some surgeons use long leg or hip spica casts for three to six weeks, followed by physical therapy exercises for stretching and teaching an improved gait pattern. Many surgeons don't use casts, but instead use removable splints that are worn part time in conjunction with physical therapy that is started immediately, usually on the first or second day after surgery. Braces, either standard nonhinged or ground reaction AFOs, are often used to help reduce the crouch for the first 6 to 12 months after surgery.

Crutches

(canes, quadcanes, Lofstrand crutches, walking sticks)

"Crutches" make up a group of devices that may be used to help a child with mild cerebral palsy walk. The standard crutches that go under the armpit, which are often used after people break their legs, are seldom used for children with cerebral palsy because there is a tendency for the child to hang on with the armpit. This incorrect use usually leads to very poor standing posture. If crutches are recommended for a child with CP, most physicians prefer the Lofstrand or forearm crutches, which have a ring through which the arm goes and a handle for the child's hand. This discourages leaning on the crutches and requires the child to hold onto the crutches, putting the weight on the hands.

Indications: Crutches are most useful for those children who are having a great deal of difficulty balancing. There is also a small group of children with severe leg involvement but excellent arm function who become excellent crutch users. There is a tendency, however, for the child to lean forward when using crutches. In this case, she might try one of the many different kinds of canes that are only held onto by the hand and do not have any other contact with the arm. The quadcane has small feet and stands on its own, but isn't much more helpful than a standard cane. A good choice is the use of a straight stick, which allows the child to hold it slightly higher, giving her extra balance. Canes are not used as much to lean against floors as they are for the additional weight they provide for the child to hold in front of herself.

The resulting bent posture should not prevent a child from trying crutches or canes. For most children with cerebral palsy, the use of crutches or canes is temporary, and most children who are able to walk eventually abandon all assistive devices. However, a few children do permanently need the extra assistance for balance, and the device that

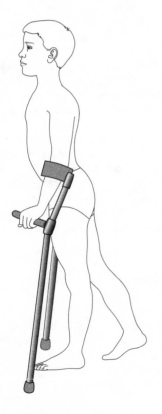

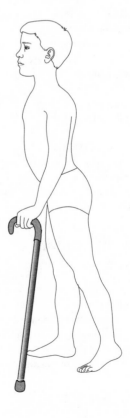

they are most comfortable with is generally the correct one. Trying out multiple devices such as Lofstrand crutches and different types of canes allows the child to find the one that he is most comfortable with. If a child refuses to use a specific crutch or cane, it usually is his way of telling you that either he doesn't need it or he is uncomfortable with it.

Benefits and risks: Greater balance is the most obvious benefit of using crutches or a cane, but often there are risks involved when a child is moved from a walker to crutches or canes. The child may initially have a cosmetically poor forward-bent posture, sometimes crouching further with his knees bent. It is best to have a therapist work with this transition at the outset and then move to using the new device around the house.

Moving from a walker to canes or crutches often makes the child more unstable, so practice use should be done in a safe environment. The child may also feel less efficient and slower with crutches compared to a walker. If there are any questions about the child's frequent falling, the use of a helmet should be encouraged to avoid head injuries. Practice falling should be strongly encouraged and rehearsed under the guidance of a physical therapist in a safe therapy environment.

Maintenance and care: All crutches and canes should have rubber tips where they contact the floor to prevent slipping. These rubber tips should be inspected frequently to make sure that they have not worn through; as soon as there is significant wear and the rubber starts slipping, the tips should be replaced. Every six months while the child is still growing, the length of canes and crutches should be evaluated by the therapist or physician who is following the child, so that adjustments appropriate to the child's growth can be made. Most crutches and canes have a fixed life expectancy of two to three years, especially if they are used heavily by an active child. As soon as connections become loose or start to slip, the device should be repaired or replaced.

Cyanotic Extremities

(blue hands, blue feet)

When skin color is a light to dark blue and the skin somewhat cool, this is called cyanosis. This blue discoloration may be due to poor oxygen saturation in the blood and may indicate heart and lung trouble. In the child with cerebral palsy, cyanosis in the hands and feet, is almost always due to poor regulation of blood flow, rather than to heart or lung problems.

Because of nervous system difficulties and poor control of circulation, the extremities are often cold to the touch and can show marked changes in color. These circulatory problems are not the same as those seen in individuals with diabetes or cardiac abnormalities, or in elderly individuals. The individual's feet should be kept as warm as possible with appropriate socks and shoes. They are not at risk for skin breakdown due to this poor circulation. In the child with cerebral palsy, these changes in color and temperature are only cosmetic and do not cause discomfort for the child. Except for making sure that the feet don't get too cold, there should be no other restrictions or concerns.

Cytomegalovirus

(CMV)

Cytomegalovirus is a relatively common viral infection among the general population. A person infected with CMV may simply have symptoms of a mild cold and not realize that she has this particular virus. Approximately 15 percent of women who are infected for the first time during pregnancy will have a baby with some physical symptoms at birth, while the rest will have no symptoms at all. Approximately 5 percent of infants with congenital CMV infection will have profound involvement, with growth retardation in utero, brain damage, jaundice, enlarged spleen or liver, microcephaly and severe hearing impairment.

Even among the 85 percent of infected infants with no symptoms at birth, some will ultimately have hearing or vision problems, mental retardation, or dysfunction in school as a result of the CMV infection. The CT scan or magnetic resonance image of the baby shows calcifications in the brain if the infection did involve the brain. A baby born with congenital CMV infection may continue to carry and shed the virus in his urine for months or even years. However, exclusion of such children from schools or institutions is not justified, since infection without symptoms is common to newborn infants (approximately 1 percent of all newborns are infected in utero and excrete CMV at birth). Instead, careful handwashing, especially after changing diapers, is recommended in caring for all children.

Decubitus ulcers

(bedsores)

Decubitus ulcers, or bedsores, are breaks in the skin which occur due to pressure or friction over areas of bony prominences. The most common sites for these ulcers are over the sacrum, or tailbone area, from lying or sitting; over the ischial tuberosities, or the prominences on the bottom of the pelvis, where one puts most of the pressure when sitting; or over the side of the hip from lying on one side too much. Other places that may develop ulcers are over prominent areas of metal rods or plates that have been used to correct alignments of bones. Also, the bony areas about the ankle or knee can occasionally develop skin breakdown. Bedsores are caused by lying in one position for too long without turning or changing positions.

The best treatment for decubitus ulcers is prevention. Prevention requires that the skin be inspected daily, and any areas that are red or appear to be developing increased pressure need to be carefully protected. This means these areas should be carefully padded to avoid pressure and that the position in which the child is lying needs to be avoided. In prevention, the most important element is the length of time involved. In other words, a child lying for five minutes on an area at risk for developing skin breakdown may be able to do so safely. However, if the child lies on this area for eight hours during sleep, skin breakdown will occur rapidly.

If the breakdown has started, then the primary treatment is keeping the area clean and dry and avoiding pressure on it. This may mean lying in a different position or avoiding sitting, if that was the cause. Oftentimes, changes in wheelchairs or mattresses are necessary. Careful attention to the seating system must be paid when this problem starts to occur. Pressure mapping may be used to assess the child while sitting in his wheelchair.

If the skin breakdown becomes very deep (which occurs only rarely), using special medicated creams and avoiding pressure on the area sometimes will still allow the wound to heal. These deep wounds often, however, need surgical treatment, which involves removing all of the dead tissue and adding new tissue with a good blood supply. This procedure is usually performed by a plastic surgeon.

Children with cerebral palsy usually have good sensation and are at low risk for developing decubitus ulcers. However, some children who have more severe involvement and are very thin may have prominent bones and are thus at high risk, especially when they are inside casts or if they are very ill and lack their normal ability to move or respond. For such children, it is essential that the caregiver inspect the skin every day during bathing and diapering to make certain that no skin breakdown is occurring.

Developmental Delay

This term is used to describe a child who has not attained normal development when compared to the standard population. There may be a delay in physical development (such as the ability to walk), or a delay in cognitive development (such as the ability to recognize shapes or stack blocks), or a delay in language (both spoken words and understanding of language).

Many children who are developmentally delayed at a young age eventually develop physically and cognitively so that by the time they enter school they are within the developmental norm. Thus, the term does not generally imply a permanent condition. When properly used, the term indicates that there is some expectation that the individual may eventually reach normal developmental milestones. When the developmental lag continues into late childhood or the teenage years, then developmental delay should not be used as a diagnosis; instead, a specific term such as *cerebral palsy* or *mental retardation* should be applied.

Developmental Disability

Any disability developed during childhood which impacts on the child's normal development is considered a developmental disability. This is a very broad category that includes such diverse diagnoses as autism, cerebral palsy, mental retardation, genetic conditions associated with delays (such as Down syndrome) and many other conditions.

Developmental Dysphasia

The development of language and speech is delayed in many children with cerebral palsy. When this delay is due to neurological problems originating in the brain, it is termed developmental dysphasia. This is a common problem in children with athetoid pattern cerebral palsy and is treated with speech therapy and augmentative communication.

Developmental Milestones

The normal development of a child includes a specific growth process that involves progress reaching specific milestones, which are often used to monitor and chart the child's normal development. These include a child's ability to crawl, to walk, to understand what is said to them, and to speak in sentences.

In a child with CP, however, the typical developmental milestones are often delayed. The specific age at which developmental milestones are reached is unique to each child with cerebral palsy. It is very difficult to make long-range predictions for an individual child about how rapidly these developmental milestones will be reached or even whether they will be.

Diplegia

(paraplegia)

Diplegia and paraplegia are terms used to describe children with cerebral palsy who have difficulty using their legs. Generally the term diplegia is applied to children with cerebral palsy who, in addition to the leg problems, have some difficulty with upper body control, including use of their arms and fine motor skills. If the motor problem is secondary to a spinal cord injury or spina bifida, the term generally applied is paraplegia, which means that the child has minimal or no limitation of the arms above the area of injury. Most children with diplegic cerebral palsy walk either independently or with assistive devices, such as crutches or canes.

Discretionary Trust

This is a legal term. It means that the trustee (the person responsible for a trust) has the authority or the ability to use the funds from the trust toward the goals outlined in the definition of the trust. Specifically, the parent who has a discretionary trust in his or her child's name may be required to use funds from that trust for the care and benefit of the child, but the parent is given the discretion to define what care and benefits mean for their child.

Dislocation, Elbow

(radial head dislocation)

Dislocation of the whole elbow is rare in children with cerebral palsy but does occasionally occur in a child who has an extremely severe spastic pattern and whose function is limited. Although the dislocation causes a cosmetic deformity, usually the arm can easily be placed into a sleeve. An isolated radial head dislocation, where the small bone just below the elbow becomes dislocated, is much more common. This deformity has the appearance of a lump on the outside of the elbow and may limit bending, but not

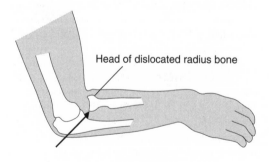

Head of dislocated radius bone

enough to prohibit driving a wheelchair or using eating utensils. There is also significant limitation in the degree to which the hand can be turned palm up. Because the deformity is subtle, often these dislocations are not noticed for many months and sometimes years, and when they are noticed they are usually functionally well compensated for by the child.

Generally, the disability caused by a dislocated elbow is so minimal that risking a surgical procedure is not warranted. In the late teenage years or early adulthood, pain develops from the dislocated radial head, which can be removed surgically, ending the pain while not limiting motion. After surgery, the elbow should be splinted for three weeks, and a gentle range of exercises should be completed. Complications from the surgery are rare, but there may be some persistent pain and a small loss of movement.

Dislocation, Hip

(spastic hip subluxation, spastic hip dislocation, acquired hip dislocation, congenital hip dislocation, migration index, Reimers Migration Index, developmental hip dislocation, CDH, DDH)

The terms congenital hip dislocation and developmental dislocation of the hip (DDH) refer to conditions in which the hip has already started to come out of the joint or is already out of the joint when the child is born. If this is treated early and aggressively with splinting, a normal hip usually develops and is functioning perfectly by 6 to 9 months of age. If the hip dislocation is discovered later in a child's life, it can be quite a difficult problem, often requiring surgery, especially if not discovered until 18 months of age or later.

Experts don't know the exact causes of congenital hip dislocation, but evidence suggests it is related to the mother's pelvic anatomy, family history, and, most of all, how the child is lying in utero. These factors are further influenced by how the child is positioned and cared for as an infant.

Congenital hip dislocation is an entirely different condition from the hip dislocation developed by children with cerebral palsy. It is possible for a child with cerebral palsy also to have congenital hip dislocation. Usually, though, hip dislocation related to cerebral palsy occurs in middle and late childhood, from age 2 to 10 years. Almost always these children have normal hips until 18 to 24 months of age, but then, under the influence of bone growth and short, spastic muscles, the ball of the hip joint is gradually pulled out of the socket. The process occurs slowly, taking from many months to years.

There are many different terms for hip dislocation in

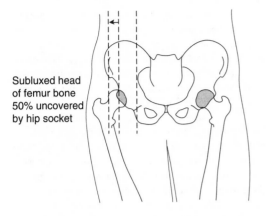

Subluxed head
of femur bone
50% uncovered
by hip socket

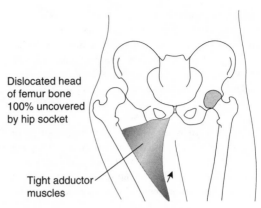

Dislocated head
of femur bone
100% uncovered
by hip socket

Tight adductor
muscles

children with cerebral palsy. The most widely used is *spastic hip dislocation* because this term conveys the idea that spasticity causes the dislocation. Another widely used term is *acquired hip dislocation*, which distinguishes it from congenital hip dislocation—"congenital" implying that the child is born with the problem.

The term *subluxation* means that the hip joint is partially out of the socket but is still in contact with it. Because this is a slow process, a child's hip goes from being a normal or reduced hip to a subluxated hip, and at the point of severe subluxation the ball moves completely away from the socket. It is then dislocated.

Indications: Spastic hip dislocation is the most common and most physically disabling muscle and bone condition that children with cerebral palsy develop. The first signs of hip subluxation are an increasing spasticity in the legs and the inability to spread the legs. Because hip subluxation cannot be detected by physical examination alone, especially in its early stages, by 2 years of age all children with cerebral palsy who have tightness in their legs should have an x-ray of their hips. As the child grows or the spasticity gets worse, the legs often become tighter; at some point, it may be difficult to diaper the child because of the degree of tightness. As the hip starts migrating out of the joint and becomes more subluxated, this tightness generally increases.

By the time the hip has become dislocated, it is extremely tight; often, the dislocated leg appears to be shortened. Because of the tight contractures, perineal care, diapering, and wheelchair seating are difficult, especially if both hips are dislocating. During the time in which the hips are becoming subluxated and dislocated there may be some mild to moderate discomfort for the child, especially during periods of attempting to diaper the child or to bathe him, which is often the first sign parents notice of any problem with the hip. Frequently the child does not

indicate discomfort until late in the subluxation phase and perhaps not until the hips are actually dislocating.

After the hips become dislocated they are no longer in a nice smooth cup, and abnormal wear on the end of the bone starts taking place. Arthritis sets in and, over a number of years, gradually becomes worse. Children with cerebral palsy who have an untreated dislocated hip can expect a 50 percent chance of developing severe pain from degenerative arthritis by their early twenties. Seating and nursing care are also more difficult. For children who are walking, the pain from arthritis often significantly limits their ability to walk.

All children with cerebral palsy are not at equal risk for developing hip subluxation. Children with hemiplegia have almost no risk of developing it, but those with moderate or severe diplegic cerebral palsy have approximately a 20 or 25 percent risk of developing hip subluxation or dislocation. Therefore, this group needs to be closely observed. Because these children are walking, hip subluxation or dislocation is especially debilitating for them. As they become young adults, it frequently limits or diminishes their ability to walk. Children with quadriplegia are at the highest risk of developing hip dislocation, with both moderately and severely involved children having a 75 or 80 percent chance of developing this condition.

Hip dislocation in children with cerebral palsy can be avoided by early close monitoring coupled with appropriate treatment for the young child, with the goal of having normal hips by the time the child becomes a teenager. Almost all hip dislocations in children with cerebral palsy are preventable.

Care and treatment: Care and treatment options for spastic hip subluxation in children with cerebral palsy are still somewhat variable but are becoming more standardized. The primary treatment is early detection, and the standard early detection method involves a physical examination and an x-ray of the hips. Every child who is unable to spread his legs to at least 45 degrees on each side when the hips and knees are extended needs to have an x-ray. Between the ages of 2 and 8, x-rays need to be taken approximately every six months to one year. All children with cerebral palsy ought to have at least one x-ray of their pelvis between the ages of 2 and 5 to make certain their hips are normal.

Most experts agree that bracing for the prevention of hip subluxation prior to surgery is not helpful. There is a subgroup of children who do not have spasticity, are extremely floppy, and develop hip subluxation or dislocation. It is possible that this small subgroup of children who

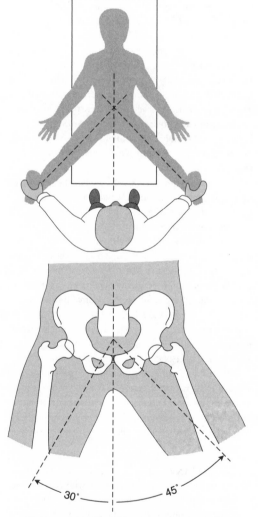

Tight muscles if <45° leg spread on each side

have what is called *hypotonic hip dislocation* may benefit from bracing to allow the development of normal hips, but even this is uncertain at this point.

The standard measurement of hip subluxation on an x-ray is the *migration index*. It defines how much of the ball of the hip joint has moved out of the socket. Generally children whose migration index is between 30 and 60 percent should be considered for adductor muscle-lengthening surgery (the adductor muscles are the muscles on the inside of the thigh). For higher migration indexes or older children, varus osteotomies, or cutting and redirecting the bone, should be considered. These surgical procedures reliably prevent hip dislocation and are far superior to anything available to treat hips that are dislocated and painful. Once the hips have become dislocated and painful, the treatment requires either resection of the hip joint, which frequently does not alleviate the pain, or implanting a total hip replacement, which is often difficult.

The complications of hip dislocation arise in three areas. Fifty percent of children who develop hip dislocations develop significant and debilitating pain at some point in young adulthood. The treatment of this disabling pain is extremely difficult and unrewarding. The dislocated hip becomes contracted, which often makes nursing care, specifically perineal care and diapering, difficult. Dislocated and contracted hips often put the body in positions that make seating difficult. Although seating difficulties may be addressed with wheelchair modifications, they often continue to present problems. Some dislocated hips cause the pelvis to tilt and thus may initiate scoliosis because of the posture required for sitting. This is a controversial issue: some professionals believe that a sitting position may cause scoliosis and others do not believe that it can cause this condition.

Dislocation, Shoulder

(shoulder subluxation, shoulder instability)

Shoulder dislocation means that the shoulder is coming out of its joint. The humerus is the bone in the upper arm that can completely come out of its socket at the shoulder joint; this is a fairly common occurrence in teenagers and is frequently associated with athletic injuries. Children with cerebral palsy who have significant spasticity and have vigorous physical therapy for mobilization of the shoulder can suffer a shoulder dislocation as a result of aggressive therapy. Picking up children who have abnormal muscle control by their arms can also cause a dislocation, and lifting should be replaced by picking up children by the chest. Another group of children with cerebral palsy who have frequent trouble with shoulder dislocations are those with significant athetosis, whose movements involve pulling the arm out and back. These movements stretch out the shoulder joint capsule, as well as the muscles that hold the bone in joint.

Children with cerebral palsy who have shoulder dislocations often have specific postures that lead to the dislocations. One common posture is while holding the arm overhead during sleep, particularly in children with significant athetosis. By removing circumstances under which the shoulder dislocates, the joint will frequently tighten back up again and resolve without further treatment. The caregiver should consider the possibility of tying pajama sleeves down to waist belts if the shoulder is dislocating during sleep. During waking hours, it may be necessary to use straps to hold the arm down by the side, especially if athetosis is part of the problem. Keeping the arm in place may also be accomplished by using lead-weighted arm sleeves to keep the arm on a wheelchair tray. If there is sufficient muscle control, working with exercises to strengthen those muscles that pull the arm down to the side of the body and to the midline are helpful.

Shoulder dislocations are seldom significant long-term problems for children with cerebral palsy. Usually the discomfort is minor and temporary, and when the activity has been eliminated for a period of time the dislocation is resolved. It is uncommon for a shoulder to become dislocated and stay dislocated, and in those circumstances where it does remain dislocated the shoulder is not usually painful. However, the shoulder should not be left in a dislocated position if it can easily be reduced. There are rare occasions during which recurrent dislocations become painful, and these require surgically tightening the muscles around the shoulder joint. Surgery to reduce a dislocated shoulder should only be considered if the shoulder is painful.

Disorders of Cellular Migration

(schizencephaly, lissencephaly [agyria], macrogyria, micropolygyria)

During the first seven months of fetal life, the brain and central nervous system undergo both growth of new cells and migration of these cells to their correct location. Failure of these cells to reach their proper location results in various abnormalities of the brain, which are categorized under the term disorders of cellular migration. They can cause cerebral palsy.

The failure of brain cells to migrate correctly can be caused by chromosomal defects, fetal alcohol syndrome, or fetal hydantoin syndrome (the exposure of the fetus to a medication used to treat epilepsy in the pregnant mother, called hydantoin or Dilantin). However, most cases have no known cause.

There are a number of types of defects in this category, which can be distinguished on CT scans or MRI of the brain. One type of migrational disorder is schizencephaly, characterized by clefts within the brain, extending from the surface of the cortex to the underlying ventricles. The region of the brain that has a cleft is usually underdeveloped. This can result in mental retardation and/or cerebral palsy, specifically hypotonia (decreased muscle tone—see

Normal, bumpy brain with gyri

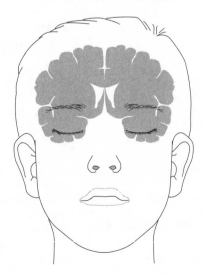

Smooth brain surface without gyri

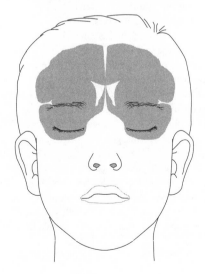

"floppy infant"), hemiparesis (weakness of one side of the body), or spastic quadriplegia (whereby all four limbs are affected), and may be accompanied by seizures and microcephaly.

Another type of migrational disorder is lissencephaly (also called agyria), which literally means smooth brain. The surface of the brain ordinarily has indentations called gyri, and their absence results from defects that keep the migrating nerve cells from reaching their proper location. In about half the patients, lissencephaly is characterized by severe mental retardation, marked hypotonia, and microcephaly. Seizures tend to be difficult to control.

Other types of migrational defect include macrogyria, where the indentations on the surface of the brain are very coarse and too few, and micropolygyria, where the brain is characterized by an excess of indentations, which are both too small and too numerous. Macrogyria gives a similar clinical picture to lissencephaly, but with cerebral palsy of the hemiplegic type. The clinical picture in micropolygyria is one of mental retardation and spastic or hypotonic cerebral palsy.

Dorsal Rhizotomy

(rhizotomy)

Spasticity is a predominant condition in children with cerebral palsy. There have been many attempts to correct spasticity with neurosurgical procedures. A successful procedure has been developed called selective dorsal rhizotomy in which nerves are cut along the spinal cord, but not in the spinal cord itself, to reduce this spasticity: "dorsal" means that the operation is done on the nerves that are most posterior, or toward the back of the spine; "selective" means that only some of the nerves are cut; and "rhizotomy" means cutting of nerves.

There are some physicians who believe that rhizotomy is a completely experimental procedure and has more complications than benefits. There are many physicians with intermediate opinions who say that rhizotomy does have promising possibilities but that it should be considered an operation about which much is not known and, as a consequence, should be applied with great caution. There is also a group of neurosurgeons whose whole practice consists of performing rhizotomies and who believe that a rhizotomy should be done on almost every child with cerebral palsy because it provides unending benefit for the child. Because of the medical community's tremendous spectrum of opinion, it may be difficult for parents to reach a decision about whether their child should have a rhizotomy or not.

As a parent, your first step should be to talk to your child's physician. You may also want to speak with other parents whose children have had rhizotomies, as well as physical therapists who have had experience with children with rhizotomies.

In fact, a major indication for a dorsal rhizotomy is the parent's own temperament—parents willing to take risks and try the newest techniques will be much more inclined to choose rhizotomy than parents whose approach to life is to choose procedures that have well-defined outcomes and risks, in both the short and the long term. There are no data on the long-term outcome of dorsal rhizotomy; the medium-term outcome data are extremely limited; and professionals aren't even certain that there is any benefit 5 to 8 years after surgery.

In general, the major indications for performing dorsal rhizotomies are on younger children between the ages of 3 and 7 years who are able to walk but are significantly limited in their walking by spasticity. The relative merits of undergoing rhizotomy surgery versus orthopedic surgery need to be considered, but in these children it is generally recommended that if the rhizotomy is done, orthopedic surgery follow in one year to fine-tune the problems that the rhizotomy did not address.

The child with severe involvement who is having difficulty sitting in a wheelchair because of spasticity or posturing is also a candidate for rhizotomy surgery. If the child is under 10 years of age, the surgery does provide a significant decrease in the spasticity. However, if the child's posturing is due to pain from a dislocated hip or severe scoliosis, the rhizotomy is absolutely *not* indicated, because it will in no way diminish the discomfort. These areas of pain and discomfort should be focused on directly by addressing the painful hip or the scoliosis.

Children with athetosis should not have a rhizotomy, because the spasticity works as a shock absorber to diminish the athetoid movements. Almost always, the athetosis will become significantly worse after the rhizotomy has been done.

The surgery: The rhizotomy is performed through an incision in the spine where the nerves are identified and a stimulator is used on the muscle to attempt to identify the most abnormal nerves. The abnormal nerves are then cut, resulting in an immediate reduction of the child's spasticity.

On approximately the third or fourth day after surgery the child can start sitting up and can begin physical therapy. Intensive exercises are usually avoided for the first two weeks. Many neurosurgeons recommend that the child visit a rehabilitation center for four to eight weeks to continue intensive therapy, which should be maintained for approximately a year.

Benefits and risks: There are many benefits from a rhizotomy, but they are not very predictable. The most predictable benefit is reducing the spasticity. In the child who has been appropriately selected, this should improve the gait pattern by loosening the muscle tone in the legs. Change in arm function is reported but not predictable.

This procedure does not often have complications, but when they occur, they may be very severe. The short-term complications can include infection, and the incision can be quite difficult to close because of the cerebrospinal fluid that continues to leak from the spine. Infections can be treated with repeated closures and antibiotics. Paralysis of the bladder and bowel incontinence can occur, but these are quite rare.

Severe weakness, which is difficult to define in children with CP, is always seen after surgery, but is due in part to the fact that the muscles are no longer spastic and their underlying weakness is brought out. For awhile, the child may be floppy throughout his whole body and may have difficulty sitting up, looking rather like a limp rag doll. The greatest long-term complications are recurrence of the spasticity and some numbness, which is often present in the feet but may be difficult to define in a child with cerebral palsy. Other side effects reported following a rhizotomy are beneficial and include decreased drooling and a decrease in the "startle" reaction.

The development of kyphosis, lordosis, or scoliosis after rhizotomy surgery has not been well defined, but it has occurred. It is still not certain whether this operation increases the incidence or whether it is the normal incidence of children with cerebral palsy. Some children have also been reported to develop rapid hip dislocation after dorsal rhizotomy.

Double Hemiplegia

The term double hemiplegia is used to describe children who have a weakness in all four limbs, with more involvement on one side of the body than the other. It is also applied to children who have more arm involvement than leg involvement. The use of this term varies; it can be confusing. In general, double hemiplegia as a term for a pattern of involvement should be avoided, and more specific terms such as quadriplegia, diplegia, or hemiplegia should be used.

Drooling
(sialorrhea)

Drooling, or sialorrhea, is a result of the lack of coordination of the oral, facial, and neck muscles. An extremely common problem in younger children with cerebral palsy, it may improve as a child grows. Drooling causes the face to be frequently wet, and often results in wet clothing as well. Many parents use colorful bandanas or bibs around the neck to keep clothing dry, and then change these throughout the day as they become wet.

Although bibs keep the child's clothes dry, they do not protect the face and chin from getting wet. Wetness can cause chapped facial skin, especially in cold weather. As the child gets older and goes to school, drooling often becomes a barrier to social interaction with other children.

Treatment: The first level of treatment is behavioral. Some children can be taught to swallow their saliva more often or to wipe their mouth with a tissue when they begin to drool.

The next level of treatment should be directed at the child's sitting posture. The child should be in a well-supported seat so that his head is not drooping forward. If his head is tilted back, he will drool less. Attention to good oral hygiene and correcting severely malaligned teeth, which may prevent the mouth from closing comfortably, is important. Elimination of very large tonsils and adenoids, which may be blocking the child from swallowing his secretions, is occasionally necessary.

Some medications that cause the child to become drowsy, especially seizure medications, may make drooling worse, and these medications should possibly be discontinued if there has been a significant increase in drooling. Biofeedback mechanisms in which the saliva triggers a switch, causing some unpleasant effect for the child, such as turning off his television, can be used to help control drooling. Studies with biofeedback, however, suggest that it only works when the biofeedback mechanism is in place and does not have any carryover effect.

Medications are often the next step. A variety of medications called anticholinergics have been used to successfully reduce drooling. These include glycopyrrolate (Robinul®), atropine (Saltropin®), benztropine (Cogentin®), hyoscyamine (Levsin®), and the scopolamine patch (TransdermScop®). They have similar potential side effects, including constipation, urinary retention, behavioral changes, and facial flushing. Glycopyrrolate appears to have the lowest frequency of behavioral effects. Recent studies of botulinum toxin (Botox) injected directly into the salivary glands have shown this to be effective as well, for up to 24 weeks after injection. Only minor side effects were seen, such as temporary complaints about swallowing, but the injection is done under general anesthesia, which has risks of its own.

Surgery may be indicated for those children who continue to have significant problems after the above attempts to control drooling have been exhausted. Most of the surgical procedures to control drooling tie off some of the salivary gland ducts or reroute the drainage ducts from the glands to the back of the throat or cut the nerve of the glands. These minor surgeries are usually done by ear, nose, and throat surgeons or by oral surgeons.

The major complication of the surgery is that in some children its benefits are only temporary, and the child will begin to drool again. In rare instances, the child's mouth becomes too dry, which is uncomfortable, and can also lead to dental caries.

Due Process Hearing

A due process hearing is a legal procedure established by Public Law 94-142 to allow the resolution of disputes arising between parents and their "special needs" children, on one side, and the educational system, on the other. The law allows for a hearing before an impartial person to review the identification, evaluation, placement, and services given the disabled child.

Dysarthria

Dysarthria is a term used for people who have difficulty with their speech, specifically pronouncing (articulating) words. This condition is especially common in children with athetosis. Sometimes spasticity also affects the vocal cords and causes dysarthria, and there is a dystonic type of dysarthria as well. Many adults who have dysarthria find this the most disabling impairment because it makes communication so difficult.

Because speaking is such an integral part of our relating to others, any speech problem often makes relating to others more difficult. People with dysarthria often find that others presume they are retarded because their speech cannot be understood. It is important to teach them a willingness to confront this assumption and to explain to others that their speech difficulty does not mean that they are retarded or that they cannot understand. All efforts should be made to teach the child to communicate as effectively as possible; for many children this may mean using an augmentative communication device, such as a speech synthesizer, or using writing, if their hand function is adequate.

Treatment involves speech therapy to assist in learning better articulation. Patients with dystonia may have the small muscles in the larynx injected with botulinum toxin.

Dyslexia

Dyslexia (a specific learning disability of reading) is a condition that interferes with a person's ability to read. It may involve the cognitive inability to recognize letters, difficulty in seeing the letters because of visual problems, or difficulty with processing visual information, such as the orientation of the letters.

Dyslexia is relatively common in children with cerebral palsy who are otherwise cognitively normal. This may involve some difficulty with information processing in the brain or may be related to motor coordination problems with their eyes. For many children there may be some combination of both. It is important that this disability be recognized by the educational system, which can usually structure an educational program to accommodate and/or remediate the difficulties in learning.

Dysmetria

Dysmetria is poor coordination of the hands. The inability to follow a line or to write smoothly is a characteristic of dysmetria; indeed, a child first notices it when he is unable to stay within the lines when he is coloring. The condition may improve into late childhood or early adolescence, especially when aided by occupational therapy for fine motor control.

Dysphagia

Dysphagia is difficulty feeding oneself. Just as a person with cerebral palsy may have abnormal posturing of the head and upper body and motor disturbances of the face, lips, and tongue, so, too, can she have abnormal mobility of the throat muscles that can impair her ability to eat. Dysphagia is more often seen in people who also have other problems with face and tongue control, including speech problems and drooling, and in those who have severe mental retardation.

People with dysphagia may have chronic respiratory infections, such as recurrent pneumonias, wheezing, or repeated bouts of upper respiratory infections (sometimes called bronchitis). Others may show signs of coughing and choking when eating, especially when drinking liquids, because liquids are more difficult to swallow than pureed foods or thickened liquids.

Addressing the problem of dysphagia for the child with cerebral palsy involves identifying the texture of food which can best be handled, the best position for feeding, and any adaptive equipment needed to promote safe feeding. This may involve thickening liquids or avoiding certain textures of food, which may be difficult to handle. Different eating strategies should be evaluated and prescribed by a speech therapist. In some children with severe dysphagia it may be necessary to stop oral feeding and introduce a gastrostomy tube.

Early Intervention

(infant stimulation)

Early intervention means providing therapy for a child who is not reaching her normal growth and developmental milestones. Children qualify for such services by demonstrating greater than a 25% delay in one or more areas of development. Early intervention programs vary in the types of services they provide and can include helping parents care for their child's specific developmental needs, such as difficulty using utensils, feeding problems, or difficulty walking. Therapists work with parents to show them how to help their child develop her speech capabilities, or how to provide extra support to a child who is struggling with a specific disability. Early intervention is usually provided by a team that includes physical, occupational, and speech therapists; nurses; and physicians experienced in dealing with children with developmental delays.

Frequently, children who have cerebral palsy have motor difficulties that preclude their developing normal movements as they start growing. A 9-month-old child with cerebral palsy who is still completely immobile continues to be very dependent upon others to stimulate him. Infant stimulation therapy is directed at providing the increasingly complex stimulation that the developing child needs. It often involves play therapy, providing the child with different sitting positions, movement, and visual stimulation. Another important component of infant stimulation therapy is working with the caregivers or parents of a child with CP and encouraging them to continue the stimulation process as part of ongoing care.

Benefits and risks: The benefit of early intervention is the improved stimulation of the child by a team that continues to evaluate the child's progress. This includes close monitoring of the child's feeding, physical, language and cognitive skills. A risk of early intervention can be seen in children who are medically fragile and are unable to tolerate the significant degree of stimulation which early intervention may provide. Early intervention needs to be provided by a team approach with case management available, so parents are not overwhelmed by many different professionals, some of whom may be giving different messages to the parents.

Early intervention usually continues until the child is 3 years of age, at which time she moves into a more formal educational setting.

Echolalia

Echolalia is a technical term describing a person who repeats exactly what he hears. He may repeat a word or phrase immediately after he hears it, or he may repeat a specific phrase days, weeks, or sometimes months after he hears it. Echolalia usually means repetition of small phrases or words.

This speech pattern is relatively common in children with mental retardation who have good speaking ability. This can lead to significant frustration in parents, family members, and other caregivers. Treatment involves a behavioral approach to extinguish the unwanted behavior.

Endoscopy

Endoscopy is the introduction of a thin, lighted tube into an area of the body in order to inspect it and sometimes to collect samples. For example, endoscopy may be performed by a gastroenterologist interested in inspecting various parts of the gastrointestinal system, either from above (called an upper endoscopy) by introducing a tube through the mouth, or from below (called a lower endoscopy) by introducing a tube through the anal sphincter. An upper endoscopy may consist of esophagoscopy (inspection of the esophagus), gastroscopy (inspection of the stomach), and duodenoscopy (inspection of the duodenum, which is the first part of the small intestine). Lower endoscopy may consist of anoscopy (inspection of the anus), sigmoidoscopy (inspection of the sigmoid colon, which is the lowest part of the colon just before it exits at the anus), or colonoscopy (inspection of the large intestine or colon).

During these procedures the physician is able to inspect the designated inside part of the body and record the findings on videotape or with photographs. Biopsies of the inspected tissue may be taken or samples for culture obtained. In addition, procedures such as the removal of a polyp or growth can be done via lower endoscopy, and placement of a percutaneous gastrostomy tube can be done via upper endoscopy, thus avoiding surgery.

Indications: The most common indications for upper GI endoscopy are concern about an ulcer or stomach acid refluxing into the esophagus. Infections may also occur, which can cause pain in the abdomen. The common indications for lower endoscopy are to evaluate blood in the stool.

Benefits and risks: The benefit of endoscopy is that it can be performed with heavy sedation for most children. If major internal procedures are to be performed, such as removal of a polyp or placement of a gastrostomy tube, general anesthesia is required. The risks, however, are much less than would be required for open surgery, and the recovery period is shorter.

Maintenance and care: After the procedure the child needs to recover from the sedation; it is often several hours before he is comfortable enough to start feeding.

Esophagitis

Esophagitis means inflammation of the esophagus, the tube that leads from the mouth to the stomach. Esophagi-

tis is often seen in the person with cerebral palsy because of gastroesophageal reflux, the process by which stomach acid comes up into the esophagus.

Since the esophagus cannot tolerate stomach acid, it is very easily damaged, and the result is heartburn, pain, and bleeding. A child with longstanding esophagitis may simply refuse to eat, even if he has previously been a good eater; he shows signs of pain and weight loss, even though the site of

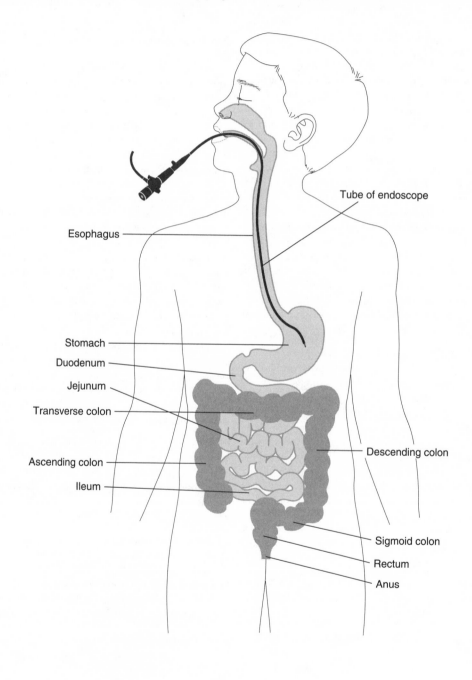

Tube of endoscope

Esophagus

Stomach

Duodenum

Jejunum

Transverse colon

Ascending colon

Ileum

Descending colon

Sigmoid colon

Rectum

Anus

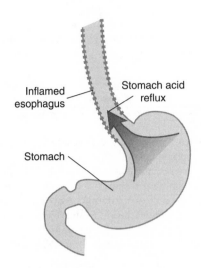

Inflamed esophagus

Stomach acid reflux

Stomach

the pain may not be clear. While acute esophagitis can be treated with medications to ease the inflammation and pain, the underlying cause such as GE reflux needs to be addressed in order to relieve the problem for the long term.

Eye–Hand Coordination

Many activities, especially fine motor activities, require being able to get a visual fix on an object and then bring one's hand to that object. This is known as eye–hand coordination. Feeding oneself, for example, requires being able to fix visually on the food and then bring the spoon to it and into one's mouth. Some children with cerebral palsy have difficulty coordinating daily tasks in that they can only perform one of the two required actions: either they can fix visually or they can attempt the motor coordination activity of bringing their hand to an object. They cannot do both. The lack of eye–hand coordination makes some activities, such as feeding oneself, brushing one's teeth or operating a computer, very difficult.

The treatment for this lack of coordination requires repeated training, especially in finding the specific movements or techniques that allow the child to reach for an object while looking at it. Optimal seating is very helpful, especially systems that provide maximum trunk and head control.

Facilitation

By definition, children with cerebral palsy have difficulty with their motor skills. Facilitation is a hands-on approach to maximizing motor skills in people with abnormal muscle control. Generally a therapist or caregiver provides hands-on guidance to promote muscle activation during a motor activity (such as sitting up from bed) in the best

alignment. Normal motor patterns are used as the ideal pattern and alignment. By repeating the technique over and over, the idea of facilitation is to create a new more "typical" motor pattern. The patient's active participation is required. The goal of facilitation is to provide the least amount of hands-on input to achieve the skill.

Failure to Thrive
(FTT)

A child who is not gaining enough weight is said to be failing to thrive. By definition, a child whose weight is below the fifth percentile for age and gender, or a child whose weight crosses more than two major percentile groups (such as from above the fiftieth to below the 25th percentile) over a relatively short period of time, is recognized by physicians as having trouble growing appropriately. A cause of failure to thrive can be almost any illness or condition of childhood, although it often reflects insufficient caloric intake. A child with cerebral palsy often does not grow adequately because he is unable to take in enough calories, mainly due to some of the swallowing problems that many children with CP have.

To treat failure to thrive, the first requirement is to identify the cause. In the child with cerebral palsy the investigator needs to compile a careful history of how much the child is eating. Often this is done with a diary in which the parents record all the foods eaten by the child over several days. A nutritionist can calculate the average number of calories per day, as well as specific minerals and vitamins that the child consumed. In addition, for many children with CP, a feeding evaluation may be helpful in identifying specific textures or liquids that the child may be having trouble swallowing. These may be causing the child to gag, or the child may actually be aspirating into his lungs, causing respiratory problems.

Treatment modalities may include the use of high-calorie foods (for example, whole milk, butter, or oil), commercial nutritional supplements; the elimination of liquids or certain textures that may be difficult for the child to swallow; or in some cases the placement of a feeding tube, either to supplement what the child can eat by mouth or to take over feeding the child who can no longer be safely fed by mouth.

Familial Spastic Paraplegia (FSP)
(hereditary spastic paraplegia [HSP])

Although this is not a type of cerebral palsy, children with familial spastic paraplegia resemble children with spastic diplegic cerebral palsy, in that they have spasticity and increased reflexes in their legs. They often are delayed in walking. The way they walk looks much like the way children with diplegia walk. The spectrum of disability is wide, from exceedingly mild to severely involved—to the point where some young adults may need a wheelchair. Genes that are responsible for several forms of FSP have been identified, and more will likely be identified in the future. FSP is a descriptive diagnosis of a genetically diverse group of disorders. While patients within this group experience similar symptoms, the genetic causes are different. Researchers have reported autosomal dominant, autosomal recessive, and X-linked recessive inheritance patterns for this disorder. Genetic counseling is strongly recommended for families with this condition.

The treatment program is the same as that for spastic diplegic cerebral palsy, although children with spastic paraplegia tend to deteriorate more quickly. For this reason, they may not make progress as well as the average child with diplegia. There are some children, however, who experience almost no deterioration over time. Spastic paraplegia is more common than many people realize; many children who are thought to have standard diplegic cerebral palsy in fact have this inherited condition, but since they are the only one in the family, familial spastic paraplegia is not suspected. It goes without saying that familial spastic paraplegia should be strongly considered as a diagnosis if two children in the same family have spastic diplegia or if a parent with spastic diplegia has a child with similar symptoms.

Femoral Anteversion

(in-toeing gait)

Femoral anteversion is a term that describes a twisted femur, or thighbone, with the knee turned in relative to the hip joint. This common twist is present at the time of birth; under the influence of normal muscle pull and walking in early years of childhood growth, it slowly corrects itself. Children with spastic muscles, however, do not develop normal muscle pull and as a consequence this rotational malalignment is *not* corrected with growth.

An early sign of this condition is the child who prefers to "W-sit"—that is, to sit with her legs in the W-position. There is no evidence that W-sitting causes femoral anteversion, nor that W-sitting causes any harm or prevents a naturally occurring correction of the anteversion. As a consequence, there is no reason to prevent the child from W-sitting if that is a comfortable sitting posture for her. In times past, W-sitting was blamed for causing in-toeing and dislocated hips. Now it is generally understood to be just another symptom of increased femoral anteversion and not its cause.

When the child starts walking, the anteversion causes her to walk with her knees and toes pointed at each other. If the condition is severe, it obviously makes walking difficult. However, there are no braces that can correct this position. Short of surgical correction, continuing with physical therapy gait training, along with the child's development of motor control, is the only method that offers a good chance of improvement.

If anteversion is a major detriment to the child's walking, is preventing her from improving her gait, or at adolescence is continuing to be a significant cosmetic or functional problem, it should be surgically corrected. At whatever age surgery is performed, the correction will be maintained. There are three methods of correcting femoral anteversion, and the operative corrections that are used vary depending primarily on the surgeon's choice.

The surgery: The procedure performed at the hip end of the femur is the most significant of the three with respect to surgical time and blood loss. The bone is cut just below the hip joint and a plate is utilized to hold the osteotomy in place. This procedure allows direct visualization of the bone and the most accurate correction with the

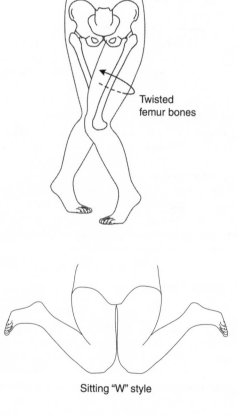

Twisted femur bones

Sitting "W" style

fewest possible complications, but it involves the placement of a plate that occasionally needs to be removed after healing. Usually casts are not necessary, and the child can immediately start walking after this correction.

The second method of correcting femoral anteversion is by operating on the middle of the femur with a surgical saw that cuts the femoral bone from the inside out. A rod is placed to hold the bone in the corrected position. With this surgical procedure, the exact amount of correction and the ability to hold the correction are more difficult, so it is primarily indicated for adults and is not widely used for children.

The third procedure is widely used for children and involves cutting the femur just above the knee through a small incision, oftentimes only the size of a small stab wound. Multiple drill holes are made and the femur is cracked and rotated into the appropriate position. Casts are applied up to or over the hip joints and are kept in place for six weeks. This is a very small operative procedure that does not take very long; however, the child is immobilized in casts and is unable to walk for at least six weeks. The correction obtained is a bit unpredictable and occasionally insufficient; at other times there is correction. Because the cut is also made in the area of the growth plate, occasionally the growth on one side of the knee or the other may stop, and an angular deformity may develop at the knee joint.

What to expect: No matter which surgical option is chosen, the postoperative care and management usually requires intensive physical therapy to try to learn a new gait pattern because, if the correction has been done properly, the knees now often point out slightly. This places the muscles in different positions. Intensive therapy can help the child learn this new gait pattern, which is especially important if casts have been used and the child has been unable to walk for several months.

Femoral Osteotomy

(varus osteotomy, varus derotational osteotomy, hip osteotomy)

Femoral osteotomy is a surgical procedure that is often performed on children with cerebral palsy. The femur (the thighbone) is cut (most commonly just below the hip joint) to make a change in the bone that will correct either of two categories of problems: hip dislocation (subluxation) and difficulties with walking.

The surgery: The osteotomies that are done for hip subluxation or dislocation involve cutting and repositioning the femur in order to place the ball of the femur more directly into the socket. Often the leg is slightly shortened, which in turn makes the hamstring muscles feel looser. The procedure is usually combined with muscle lengthenings, such as adductor and iliopsoas lengthening in the groin.

The osteotomy performed to improve walking involves turning the leg so that it points in the correct direction, which is especially helpful for children who are walking with their legs severely turned in. Some older children may have a hip flexion contracture, which causes them to walk very severely bent forward at the hips. This condition may also be straightened by a similar osteotomy and muscle lengthenings.

An osteotomy can be done in many different ways, but almost uniformly all variations involve implanting a plate to hold and fix the osteotomy. One of the most commonly used plates is called a blade plate, which is placed into the bone and fixed with screws. Another version, a screw and side plate, comes in a number of different styles: one is called a Richard's screw and another is called a Coventry plate. Each of these devices has its advocates, and the choice largely depends on the surgeon's preference. The operation is usually performed with the patient lying on his back under general anesthesia and can often be done on

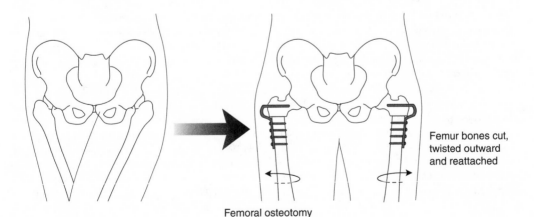

Femur bones cut, twisted outward and reattached

Femoral osteotomy

both sides without any blood transfusions. The incision is made along the outside of the hip joint.

After-surgery care: After a hip osteotomy, the child is usually placed in a hip spica cast for four to six weeks. If the cast remains in place longer than this, there is a great risk of developing soft bones and repeated fractures once the cast is removed. For children who are walking, casting for this length of time also represents a significant setback, since it is quite a while before they can get up and walk again. Generally, with modern devices such as AO blade plates, no cast is necessary, and children who were walking before the operation are able to get up after recovering from surgery. Undergoing this procedure without any casting is very helpful for families, since after-care is so much easier and rehabilitation is much quicker.

After an osteotomy, a child's hips will appear much wider, generally because he started with abnormally narrow hips. In reality, however, they are only slightly wider than normal hips. The wide hips are especially good for children who are sitters, providing them with a wider base. Also, when the child is lying down, both hips should now lie flat, and the knees and feet should point slightly out in a way that mirrors a normal child's sleeping position. Getting the rotations correct is difficult because it is important to make sure that the child can sit with his legs pointing straight down.

What to expect: Possible complications depend upon the plate that is used. When the plates are properly placed, the possibility of the realigned bones coming apart is extremely rare. However, it is possible that the child may twist his leg and break the bone just below the screws, even months or years after the osteotomy has healed. Older-style plates, such as the Coventry plate, are often quite prominent and not very strong. The plate may break, especially if there was not sufficient casting time. This plate requires a cast. The risk of nonunion or loss of fixation with older types of screws and side plates is increased. The AO blade plate and the Richard's type of screw are both significantly stronger and seldom break.

There may be other changes over the long term (meaning from one to five years). The wide hips, which the child initially has after the femoral osteotomy, gradually become less wide with growth. If the child has a significant amount of growth remaining, hip width relative to the width of the trunk decreases significantly. If the child is nearly finished growing, however, hip width does not decrease. In addition, the inward twist of the bone which may have been present will not recur in the nearly grown child. The straightening at the hip may return, however, if the child has a significant amount of growth remaining. The child

who had this surgical procedure at age 3 or 4 may have a recurrence of the hip subluxation and occasionally needs to have the femoral osteotomy repeated.

Flat Feet
(planovalgus foot deformity)

Someone with a flat (or planovalgus) foot has an ankle that rolls in. At its worst the foot turns so much that the sole is not in contact with the floor but is pointed laterally, or to the outside. When a child with flat feet walks, her weight bears down on the inside of the foot and on the great toe. This severe condition is unusual, but a mild to moderate flatfoot deformity is extremely common in children with cerebral palsy, as well as in the general population. A mild flat foot has no arch and is very wide. A moderate flat foot is clearly turned out but not to the point where the child walks on the anklebone.

The course of flat feet for a child 2 or 3 years old is difficult to predict. Normal children who have flat feet at this early age almost never have pain as they get older, and there are no braces or shoes that have any long-term impact upon this condition. For children with cerebral palsy, the natural progression of flat feet is not as clearly defined, and there is no evidence that the use of braces or shoe inserts makes any ultimate difference in the development of the feet.

Many children who have mild and moderate flat feet early in life develop better motor control as they get older, and their feet end up looking normal. In some cases the feet reverse and develop the opposite deformity, an arch that is too high. Many young children with cerebral palsy have moderate flat feet that don't ever change, function well, are pain free, and do not need any treatment, especially surgical treatment.

Indications: For other children, the flat feet get worse as they get older; as they get heavier and continue walking, the foot seems to break down more. Bracing should be tried first, using arch supports in the shoes or AFOs. If the braces cause foot pain, it is much better to discontinue them and allow the child to wear shoes that aren't painful.

If the condition is so severe that walking becomes extremely difficult, and bracing is not tolerated, then surgical correction may be necessary if the child is to continue walking. If surgery is indicated for the child under age 9 or 10 years, the subtalar (or Grice) fusion, which involves fusing the calcaneus and talus bones at the back of the foot, is classically the operation of choice. More recently, a calcaneal lengthening (lengthening the heel bone) has shown promising results in younger patients without the need to fuse joints. The older adolescent child with a more long-standing flatfoot is often treated by a triple arthrodesis, which involves fusing three joints in the back of the foot. Triple arthrodesis provides a more reliable lifelong correction of the foot. However, it does decrease the mobility of the foot below the ankle joint and may lead to long-term ankle arthritis.

Floppy Infant

(hypotonic infant)

An infant sometimes seems limp or immobile, like a rag doll. Such children are often described as floppy infants. The three main features associated with hypotonia are unusual postures, diminished resistance of the joints to passive movement, and increase in the range of movement of the joints. In the newborn period, such an infant will usually display unusual postures and little active movement. The older infant is delayed in the achievement of motor milestones.

Hypotonia may be associated with a wide variety of conditions. It may indicate a neuromuscular disorder; it may occur in children who are mentally retarded; or it may be the manifestation of a connective tissue disorder, a metabolic disorder, or the early phase of cerebral palsy. It may also occur as an isolated symptom in an otherwise normal child, with the symptom eventually disappearing.

The cause of hypotonia can be found anywhere from the brain, to the spinal cord, to the peripheral nerves, to the muscle, to the connective tissues of the extremities. Thus, the list of conditions that can cause hypotonia is a long one. In addition to conditions affecting specific parts of the nervous system, hypotonia can be seen in metabolic, nutritional, or endocrine conditions, such as rickets, hypothyroidism, or renal tubular acidosis. It can be found in genetic disorders such as Prader-Willi syndrome (where hypotonia is associated with failure to thrive early in life) or Down syndrome. As already mentioned, it can be a part of nonspecific mental retardation, of hypotonic cerebral palsy, or of metabolic disorders such as aminoaciduria or organic aciduria.

Hypotonia can also reflect a basic weakness in the muscle itself, such as is seen in various myopathies or muscular dystrophies. Lastly, it can be a normal transient condition known as benign congenital hypotonia (or essential hypotonia), which eventually disappears. These children have no underlying muscle weakness, intellectual retardation, or associated disease.

Although many children outgrow hypotonia, some children with cerebral palsy continue to be very floppy throughout their entire lives. Stimulating the child to develop and strengthen her muscles is an important means of treatment. Also, it is necessary to provide excellent supported seating postures to allow her to focus on controlling other parts of her body. For example, caregivers should provide good trunk and body support so the child with hypotonia can focus on head and hand control.

FM System

FM system is one device in a wide array of "assistive" devices to help children with hearing loss connect with their sound environment. The FM system consists of headphones, or on occasion a direct link to a hearing aid, worn by a child with hearing loss connected via a radio (FM) signal to a microphone worn by the speaker. These are typically used in the classroom and ensure that the child is receiving a consistent acoustic signal. This eliminates the vagaries of poor classroom acoustics and the problem of background noise. Because of this, FM systems have been proven to improve the school performance of all children, not just those with hearing loss, and have been used especially for children with attention deficit disorder to help them focus on what is being said by the teacher.

Fusion, Foot

(subtalar fusion, Grice fusion, triple arthrodesis, planovalgus foot deformity, severe equino varus foot deformity)

A fusion is an operation that causes two bones to grow together to form one bone. There are four bones in the back part of the foot which commonly have fusions performed on them for children with cerebral palsy, predominantly to improve position of the foot. These individual fusions can be somewhat confusing, but it is important to understand the exact reason for performing them as well as what motion will be lost after surgery.

Indications: If a child with spasticity has developed severe flat feet or the opposite deformity (a severe foot deformity with a high arch and the foot pointed down), then three joints in the foot are improperly aligned. If the child with severe flat feet is relatively young, the primary problem is between two of these joints. Initially this condition can be braced with a variety of different in-shoe braces such as arch supports or a full-length ankle-foot orthosis (AFO), especially for young children. However, if the child is unable to tolerate the brace or the deformity becomes so severe that he has a great deal of difficulty walking in spite of the brace, a foot fusion is usually necessary.

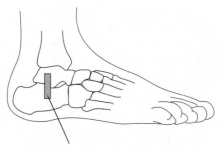

Heelbone fused with talus bone

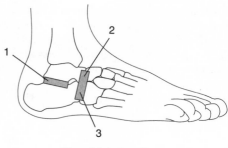

Three joints fused

The surgery: The most common surgical procedure for the 3- to 9-year-old is a subtalar or Grice fusion. This involves placing a bone block between the talus bone and the heelbone in the corrected position. Often a screw is placed across the heelbone and talus to hold the position. This procedure results in a nicely corrected foot, but in approximately 25 percent of patients, the fusion is eventually resorbed and the deformity may recur. In the adolescent with the same severely deformed foot, the triple arthrodesis allows a much better realignment of the foot and provides for permanent correction. The triple arthrodesis involves fusion of the three foot joints, so that the foot is no longer able to move in either the flatfooted or the high-arched position. However, it is not prevented from moving up and down. The triple arthrodesis is often fixed with screws and staples to hold its position until bone healing occurs. With a severely deformed flat foot it is difficult to get an excellent cosmetic correction, although a fairly normal-looking foot is usually the result for almost all teenagers or young adults.

After-surgery care: Usually short leg casting, from the toes to the knee, is applied for 6 to 12 weeks. For some or all of this time the child may not be able to step on his foot. This is determined at the time of surgery by the specific surgical procedure performed, strength of the bones, and the surgeon's experience. After the cast is removed, it usually takes approximately 4 weeks to get comfortable walking on the foot.

Benefits and risks: There is an approximately 25 percent risk of needing to have the subtalar fusion repeated as an adult because of resorption of the fusion. The primary complication from the triple arthrodesis is that there may be inadequate correction at the time of the surgery or that one of the joint fusions does not heal. Sometimes the metal is also prominent and needs to be removed. Over the long term, the fused joint may cause earlier arthritis in the ankle; however, the chance of developing arthritis is probably less than it would be from walking on the deformed foot for many years.

Although there is the risk of eventual arthritis, there are also substantial benefits in that the foot will be much more stable and be able to support the weight during standing. These fusions are performed because the feet have a tendency to collapse, and the real benefit of a fusion is that it is durable and will not give way over a person's lifetime.

Gait Analysis

(three-dimensional gait analysis, foot pressure measurements, gait videotaping, dynamic EMG analysis)

Gait has been analyzed visually by physical therapists and orthopedic doctors ever since patients with cerebral palsy have been treated. Visual gait analysis involves having the patient walk sufficiently undressed so the whole body can be carefully observed. An experienced physician identifies the major areas of concern, such as the alignment of the legs, if the knees are bending, or if the child is toe walking. There is, however, no permanent record and no numbers by which measurements can be made and recorded. For this reason, mechanical gait analysis was developed.

The simplest way to record gait analysis is by using a video camera to film what is seen so it can be viewed in slow motion, forward and backward. The videotape itself can be very helpful for assessing very subtle problems, such as the symmetry of steps, how much knee bend is present, and how the feet are used for standing. The next level of sophistication involves using markers on the body, which allows the physician to measure the angles of joint motion as the child walks. Very simple analyses are two-dimensional; only one camera is used. Markers are placed on the joints, and the angles between joints are calculated mathematically. For the child with cerebral palsy, this assessment is too simple and not very useful because of the large amount of error in the assessment.

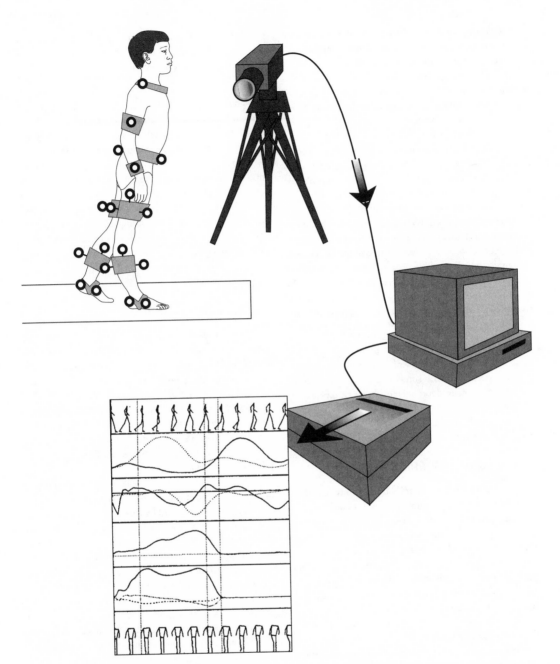

The more common and most sophisticated analysis is three-dimensional. Reflecting markers are attached at multiple points on the body, and a series of cameras are utilized to record the person's movement patterns. This analysis defines all the joints in three-dimensional space and allows assessment of all joint motions in rotation, side, and front planes. In addition, recorders with radio transmission are frequently used to record the activity of the muscle by means of small pads placed over the muscles. This concept works on the same principle as a cardiogram for the heart. A third component of the evaluation is an instrument in the floor which the child stands and walks over to give the exact amount of force placed on each leg. An additional device that helps define specifically how the foot surface is taking pressure may be inserted into the shoe, or the measurement of foot pressure is made by having the child walk barefoot on a walkway. For some children, the amount of oxygen they use for walking is also measured by having them wear a mask while they walk.

The full three-dimensional gait analysis with EMG recording, force plate recording, and foot pressure recording develops an enormous amount of information which is quantifiable and permanently recorded. The use of these data is important in determining specific orthotic prescriptions and decisions about surgical corrections. The information does not in itself, however, give immediate answers but requires the interpretation of an experienced physician. These analyses can be quite complex and are often open to differences in interpretation.

After the gait analysis is complete, there is a final interpretation, which usually includes an assessment of the predominant abnormalities and some recommendation that the physician feels would benefit the child. The presentation includes a series of stick figures that demonstrate the visual appearance of the child's walking pattern and charts and graphs that demonstrate muscle function and the range of joint motion as components of the gait pattern.

Indications: Gait analysis is indicated for a child whose physicians and caregivers are considering a major treatment decision such as surgery. Full three-dimensional gait analysis is often required before surgery, especially if the gait problem is complex. However, if the child has a relatively simple condition such as an isolated tight tendon, often gait analysis does not add any additional information, and simple videotaping with a standard format provides most of the needed information.

Benefits and risks: Besides the obvious advantage of providing a full and complete analysis of a child's gait pattern, gait analysis also allows physicians to detect unknown problems early on. However, the gait analysis should be performed in a laboratory and interpreted by a physician with experience in treating patients with cerebral palsy. Because some gait analysis laboratories are set up by people who are extremely experienced in gathering the information but do not have expertise in *interpreting* the information, proper treatment requires finding a full-service lab with qualified physicians.

Gait analysis is also expensive, with the full three-dimensional gait analysis usually costing a thousand dollars or more. The full gait analysis including joint measurements and a physical examination is also time-consuming, usually requiring two to four hours. Any gait analysis that is done in a matter of thirty minutes and only costs a fraction of the amount listed above will by definition be much simpler and less complete. The simpler analyses still do provide *some* information but are not comprehensive, and there are many variations in laboratories that provide these services, so do your homework before enlisting a particular lab's services.

What to expect: Gait analyses are often repeated following major surgical procedures, after the child's full rehabilitation has occurred. This usually means that approximately one year after the surgical procedure has been performed, the gait analysis is repeated to measure how much correction was obtained and also to set parameters for continuing to monitor the child. After the child has grown more, often four or five years later, and the deformity has recurred, a repeat gait analysis would again be performed in anticipation of a new surgical procedure or other major change.

Gastritis

(ulcers, *Helicobacter pylori*)

Gastritis is inflammation of the lining of the stomach, which can sometimes lead to an ulcer. An ulcer is an erosion of the lining of the stomach or the small intestine. Ulcers can cause abdominal pain and bleeding, which then can lead to vomiting of blood or dark "tarry" stools that contain blood that has been digested. Although many thought in the past that gastritis or ulcers were related to increased secretion of stomach acid or emotional upset, we now know that a large percentage are due to a bacteria called *Helicobacter pylori*.

H. pylori infection is best diagnosed by obtaining a biopsy during an upper endoscopy. A blood test is available but must be reviewed by a gastroenterologist, as the test can be unreliable and lead to false-positive results. This blood test can, however, help identify those children that need an upper endoscopy. In adults a special breath test for urease can be done to diagnose this infection, but this test is not currently accepted as a means of diagnosing *H. pylori* infection in children. We do not know how these bacteria get into the body, but it has been suggested that we can pass this infection to one another, as we have seen groups of children that live together in institutions become infected. Some populations have these bacteria in their stomach but do not have any symptoms.

Some other causes of gastritis and/or ulcers are surgery and medications. During the immediate postoperative period, there is a surge in secretion of acid, which can cause inflammation of the stomach. Medications such as steroids, aspirin, or ibuprofen can irritate the lining of the stomach and result in gastritis as well.

Gastroesophageal Reflux Disease

(GERD, reflux)

Gastroesophageal reflux is the process by which stomach contents come up into the esophagus, causing inflammation. These contents may include acid as well as undigested food contents. It is a common problem in young infants and is recognized when babies "spit up" following a feeding. In most infants this problem does not require any treatment. It gradually subsides as children grow and usually disappears by the time they are between 12 and 18 months of age when they are up and walking about. Many adults experience this problem as "heartburn" after a meal.

In a minority of infants, the problem causes symptoms such as failure to thrive, esophagitis, anemia, and irritability. If the reflux is more severe, the stomach contents may reach the back of the throat and may be aspirated into the lungs, causing respiratory disease. Treatment includes modification of the infant's position (keeping him upright after feeding and not lying him down for at least 30–60 minutes after a meal), modification of the diet (thickening formula with rice cereal), medications, or surgery.

In children with CP, GER is very common and usually does not go away by the time the child reaches 12–18 months of age. The treatment is the same as noted above, primarily a combination of thickening of feedings, the upright position after meals, and a variety of medications. If severe symptoms continue, especially episodes of pneumonia or chronic wheezing from aspiration, then surgery is often required to control the problem. The procedure, known as a fundoplication, can be done either endoscopically or via an open procedure (see Chapter 3 for more details).

Gestational Age

(small, appropriate, and large for gestational age [SGA, AGA, LGA])

Gestational age is the number of weeks of the pregnancy, calculated from the date of the woman's last menstrual period. Forty weeks, with a range of 38–42 weeks, is considered full-term. A child whose birthweight is within what is defined as a normal range for that length of pregnancy is considered appropriate for his or her gestational age (AGA). There are growth charts showing the normal expected weight for infants of various gestational ages ranging from very small premature babies to children born at full term. Any infant who is either below (small for gestational age, or SGA) or above (large for gestational age, or LGA) the expected weight may be showing signs of med-

ical problems. For example, a child born to a mother with diabetes may be born LGA, weighing much more than normally expected, and is at risk from a variety of problems associated with being LGA (such as hypoglycemia). A baby born SGA may also reflect specific medical problems, such as poor nutrition due to placental insufficiency or an infection suffered in utero. Babies born SGA are usually followed as at risk in early intervention programs, as they have an increased risk for developmental disabilities.

Gingivitis

(gum hypertrophy, plaque)

Enlargement and inflammation of the gums is a common occurrence in children with abnormal muscle control around the mouth. It may also be increased with the use of certain medications such as Dilantin. The main cause of this overgrowth is gingivitis, or inflammation of the gums, which is caused in part by lack of routine dental care, such as brushing and flossing. In children with spastic cerebral palsy, such dental care can be very difficult because the child may involuntarily bite down every time something is introduced into the mouth, such as a toothbrush. The main method of preventing gingivitis is good oral hygiene as well as routine dental cleaning, every three to six months.

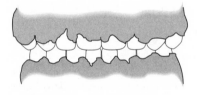

Overgrown, inflamed gums

Indications: If the overgrowth becomes large with frequent bleeding when brushing, then surgical removal of the excess gum tissue is usually indicated. This procedure must be done in the operating room under general anesthesia. Often children have to stay in the hospital overnight in case there is excessive bleeding. The main complication, however, is recurrence, if diligent cleaning is not maintained.

Another cause of gum inflammation is plaque, a hard tissue that builds up on the base of the teeth. Plaque can cause inflammation and may eventually lead to decay of the base of the tooth where it is held onto the bone. Good oral hygiene is essential, and frequent dental cleaning is needed in some individuals to control plaque.

Growth Charts

Growth charts plot the normal growth of a child from birth to age 20. Separate charts are available for boys and girls from birth to age 3 and from ages 2 to 20. These charts plot the weight, length (and later height), and head circumference of the general population, and show the distribution of values based on a percentile scale from the third percentile to the ninety-seventh percentile. Thus, a child whose weight is at the fifth percentile is smaller than 95 percent of other children his same age and gender but is still within the norm, since someone has to be in the lowest 5 percent of the population. When a child falls either below the fifth percentile or above the ninety-fifth percentile for his or her age, he or she is considered out of the normal range, and some medical investigation may be indicated.

These charts were generated using healthy children, and many children with CP do fall below the norms. It is extremely important to continue to monitor the growth of the child with CP even when he is below the third percentile, because even more important than the specific percentile is the progression and the weight gain over time. The child who grows along the third percentile over ten years is better off than one who falls from the fiftieth to the third over that same period.

Halitosis

(fetor ex ore)

Halitosis means foul or bad mouth odor. The foul odor may come from the lungs, stomach, or nose, although all of these sources are uncommon in children. Most halitosis comes from a source in the mouth—decayed teeth, ulcerated gums, or poor dental care that leaves decomposed food in the mouth. Children with cerebral palsy may be mouth breathers, which can dry out the mouth. This decreased moisture leads to less cleaning of the mouth tissues and thus to bad breath.

The treatment of halitosis starts with determining the cause. You should begin with a complete evaluation by a dentist, making sure the dentist knows that you are concerned about the child's bad breath. Filling all cavities and correcting gum problems should be the first priority. This needs to be followed by good oral hygiene. If this combination does not work, the dentist may refer you for a complete medical evaluation. Using antiseptic mouthwash may help for several hours but should not be considered the primary treatment. It can be used on a cloth to wipe the teeth and the inside of the child's mouth.

Hamstring Lengthening

(hamstring transfer, knee flexion contracture, crouched gait, tight hamstrings, hamstring contracture)

The hamstrings are a large muscle group located on the back side of the thigh. They are composed of two muscle groups, one on the inside of the thigh, which includes the semi-tendinosus, semi-membranous, and gracilis muscles, and the lateral hamstring group toward the outside of the thigh, which includes biceps muscles. These two groups have a tendency to become tight and contracted, and are especially problematic for those children who spend most or all of their waking hours sitting. The muscles become tighter as the child grows because of decreased muscle growth due to spasticity.

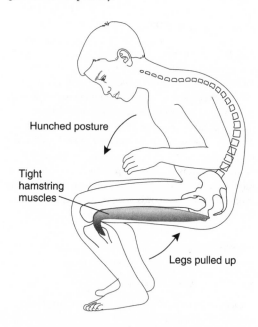

Hunched posture

Tight hamstring muscles

Legs pulled up

The major problem these muscles cause for the walking child is crouching while both standing and walking. Often the knees are bent so that the child's toes or ankle must flex upward. Children who develop severe hamstring contractures because they sit all the time eventually are unable to lie down and to straighten their knees completely. Instead, they pull their feet underneath the seat of a wheelchair.

Indications: Hamstring contractures are treated because of a child's problems with walking, sitting, general positioning, and spastic hip subluxation. Hunched posture is another possible indication of the need to lengthen hamstrings. If the muscle in the front of the knee is very tight, it pulls the knee straight; then the tight hamstring rolls the pelvis back, causing the child to sit hunched over. In certain circumstances, the tight muscles may be contributing to hip subluxation. In these situations it may be necessary, especially if the child can't stand, to loosen the muscles as much as possible. The main problem in walking for which hamstring lengthening is indicated is a crouched gait.

The surgery: To allow the child to stand up straight, the hamstrings may be lengthened. These lengthenings are usually done behind the knee; occasionally, the tendons are transferred to the femur. Currently, the transfer operation is not favored because removing tendons often causes hyperextension (the knee bending backward). It is extremely important to be conservative in lengthening the hamstring tendons because the overlengthened tendon can make walking much more difficult than does the underlengthened tendon. Occasionally the tendons may be lengthened at the buttock through an incision just below the hip. This is done less frequently because it may allow increased hip flexion. In this case, often the iliopsoas muscle needs to be lengthened on the front of the hip to balance the muscle forces about the hip.

For seating problems, the hamstring muscle may be lengthened either behind the knee or behind the hip. Again, it is important when lengthening behind the knee to not lengthen too much or the knee will be stuck straight out. For problems in lying down, muscle lengthening behind the hip involves making cuts in the muscle and allowing the muscle to slide. Lengthening behind the knee ensures that the major muscles are only lengthened an appropriate amount so they do not completely tear. This is usually done by cutting the tendinous part and allowing it to stretch, although some surgeons make Z-cuts in the tendon, allow it to slide apart, and suture it together again.

Benefits and risks: The benefits of hamstring lengthening are that the child can sit, stand, and walk more easily. There are two severe complications: The first is overlengthening the hamstrings, so the knees are stuck straight. This makes walking very difficult, and the knees eventually become painful from bending backward. It makes sitting very difficult because sitting well requires bent knees.

In correcting severe hamstring contractures, stretching of the sciatic nerve may occur, most likely during a second lengthening. Repeat lengthenings are done when a child had a hamstring lengthening four or five years earlier and now with growth has tightened up again and needs another one. Although this is the highest risk area, if the sciatic nerve does stretch it is usually only temporary. It may cause some pain and discomfort, occasionally with numbness in the foot, but it almost always resolves.

The most common but much less problematic complication after hamstring lengthening is that the hamstring continues to remain somewhat tight. However, for patients who are walking, it is much better to continue with a slightly crouched gait than to stand straight with the knee bending backward from overlengthening.

After-surgery care: The usual treatment after hamstring lengthening involves casts, splints, or just physical therapy to gain motion. Most of the time, at least some temporary splinting is used while the muscle heals in a lengthened position. If casts are used, they should not be kept on for more than six weeks as this will increase the possibility of overlengthening.

What to expect: Following the healing phase, continued stretching is important. An intensive period of physical therapy, focusing on improving the crouched gait and occasionally using AFOs, is necessary. AFOs are helpful interventions aimed at keeping the muscle stretched out while the child is relearning to walk. Additionally, night braces may be used for up to a year.

Harrington Rod
(Wisconsin wiring)

Harrington rods are the oldest spinal instrumentation still in use. The rods are attached to the spine with hooks, which can then be used to stretch out the spinal curve and hold it corrected, with the addition of bone graft, until the bones heal. This rod has a hook at each end with serrations in the rod that allow the hooks to move on the rod to stretch out the spine, similar to a simple car jack. In the past, this system was used extensively in patients with idiopathic scoliosis. It has been largely replaced with dual (two)-rod systems that are attached to the spine by screws (pedicle screws) or hooks. These dual-rod systems are much more rigid and sturdy than the Harrington rod system. These rods are sometimes used with the addition of wires through the spinal process, which is called a Wisconsin system. Sometimes the rods are used with two hooks at the top. Either system is always combined with a posterior spinal fusion (bone graft).

Indications: The use of the Harrington rod and its variations is indicated for patients with idiopathic scoliosis. This system has virtually no use for children with cerebral palsy except with the occasional child who is walking and has a very short curve.

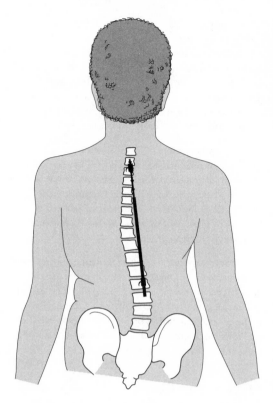

can be affected or damaged by low oxygen levels, prematurity, infections or severe jaundice. Hearing loss is more common in children born with a very low birthweight, and the child with cerebral palsy is at much higher risk than the general population for hearing problems. Detection of hearing loss is critical for all children, especially those who show signs of other problems, in particular a delay in speaking. The child with severe neurological impairment may not be responding, and testing hearing will provide important information about the child's function at an early age.

Nonresponsive, very young infants can be tested by two means: otoacoustic emissions and/or auditory evoked potentials. Otoacoustic emissions are sounds produced by the outer hair cells of the organ of hearing (cochlea) and can be measured in the ear canal indicating cochlear health. These sounds can be evoked and give a picture of cochlear function and hearing level. For the auditory evoked potential, a sound is presented to the ear, and brain waves are recorded. The auditory-evoked potential detects the lowest sound intensity capable of producing a brain wave. This test indicates whether there is an alteration in the ear's ability to perceive sound, but it does not evaluate how the child interprets this sound. Conditions such as mental retardation and attention deficit disorders may impact on the child's response to the sound. Very young children can also be tested by a well-trained pediatric audiologist, if the child can be taught responses indicating that he is hearing.

In order for a child to speak normally and learn language, he must be able to hear correctly. Often, a language delay indicates a hearing problem. All children with cerebral palsy should have their hearing screened at least once, and hearing function needs to be maximized to help the child with CP get the best possible education.

Benefits and risks: The main benefit of this system is that it is inexpensive and technically easy to use. Specific complications are that the hooks have a tendency to dislodge and that the rod may break after approximately six months if the fusion has not healed correctly. Generally additional casts, body jackets, or braces are utilized to prevent the rod from breaking, because it is not as strong as some of the other rods.

Maintenance and care: Generally children with Harrington rods need to use casts or special braces until the posterior spinal fusion has healed. Some modifications of the rods, however, are designed so that bracing is unnecessary.

Hearing Loss
(hearing impairment, auditory evoked potentials)

Several things must happen in order for a person to hear sounds. The sound must get into the ear; the inner ear mechanisms must transmit the sound impulse to the brain; and the brain must be able to interpret what the sound means. At birth, the organs and mechanisms for hearing

Hemiplegia
(monoplegia)

Hemiplegia means motor involvement of one arm and one leg on the same side of the body resulting from an injury to the brain. This term is applied to difficulties caused by any injury to one side of the brain, whether the injury is caused by cerebral palsy, a head injury, a stroke, or a tumor. The term monoplegia is used for involvement of only one leg or one arm. In reality, this is usually an extremely mild hemiplegia—occasionally a child has such a mild involvement that it affects only one limb. The term monoplegia should be reserved for those difficulties caused in one limb by a brain injury and not by nerve injuries such as a brachial plexus palsy.

Herpes Simplex Virus

Newborns infected with herpes simplex virus can have hepatitis, pneumonia, meningitis, or encephalitis, which can result in permanent brain damage and cerebral palsy. Others may have more localized infection of the skin, eyes, and mouth. Newborn infants with a herpes infection have a high risk of dying from the infection or living with severe brain damage. Antiviral drug therapy with acyclovir improves the prognosis. If a woman in labor reports signs of genital herpes infection, then delivery by cesarean section is recommended, which reduces the risk of transmitting the infection to her baby.

Hip Muscle Releases

(hip adductor lengthening, adductor lengthening, adductor transfer, iliopsoas release lengthening or transfer, obturator neurectomy, anterior branch obturator neurectomy, proximal hamstring lengthening)

Hip muscle releases include a number of similar operations on the groin to treat problems with walking or spastic hip subluxation, or both. The adductor area, which is the inside of the thigh in the area of the groin, involves a number of muscles, and these muscle groups and the nerves that drive them are the primary causes of spastic hip dislocation. They also cause scissoring problems with gait. The many different operations are directed toward balancing the effect of these muscles with the far less spastic muscles on the outside of the hip.

Indications: There are three major reasons why children with cerebral palsy may require hip muscle releases. The first is to prevent hips from dislocating. A child usually under age 8 will be examined, and when the hip muscles are noted to be tight and an x-ray demonstrates mild hip subluxation (the hip moving out of the joint), the spastic muscles should be surgically released. Children between the ages of 3 and 6 are the most likely to need this operation.

The second reason hip muscle release surgery may be necessary is to help a child who is walking but whose feet cross. Because the muscles are tight when the legs are spread apart, they work to keep the feet constantly crossed and tangled while the child is walking. This is a common problem that occurs when children with cerebral palsy are starting to walk, but often it may resolve itself without surgery. For some children, however, the problem continues and the surgery is then necessary—mostly commonly between ages 5 and 10.

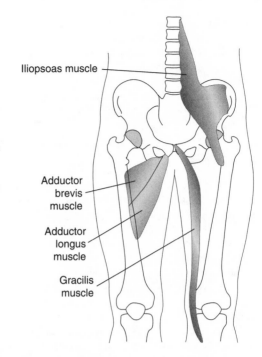

The third reason hip muscles need to be released is if the muscles become so tight and spastic that providing for toileting and perineal care becomes impossible. This is often a problem for young adult women who find it difficult to take care of the menstrual period. The most common age at which hip muscle surgery is performed to improve the ability to provide for perineal care is between 12 and 20 years of age.

The surgery: The most widely used procedure involves lengthening selected groups of the groin muscle; the muscles most commonly selected for lengthening are the adductor longus and the gracilis. Generally these two muscles are completely cut and allowed to retract. They will scar back down again to their underlying muscles. For more severe contractures, partial lengthening of the adductor brevis is indicated. Additionally, cutting the anterior branch of the obturator nerve further weakens the muscles.

It used to be common procedure to cut the entire obturator nerve, but this weakens the muscles so much that frequently the legs become stuck in a spread-open position. Almost all surgeons believe that the posterior branch of the obturator nerve should be preserved. Some surgeons advocate transferring the heads of the adductor longus, gracilis, and brevis muscles more toward the rear to help extend the hip, but this is a larger and more difficult operation, and current reports suggest that it is no more effective than a simple release.

The iliopsoas is a large muscle that contributes significantly to problems with gait and spastic hip disease. The most common procedure involves cutting the tendon and allowing it to retract. In children with severe involvement who are not going to walk, the goal should be to try to completely prevent the severed tendon from growing together again by allowing the whole tendon to retract. If the operation is done on children who are walking, only the tendon of the psoas muscle is cut, allowing the iliacus muscle to stay intact. The psoas reattaches again but is lengthened. The importance of this is not fully understood or completely agreed upon.

Through the same incision on the inside thigh the proximal hamstring muscles may be lengthened or completely released. This procedure works well in relieving hip subluxation in severely involved children who cannot walk. However, many surgeons feel that it should not be done on those who walk. Iliopsoas lengthening is by far the most widely used procedure to work with this muscle, although there are some physicians who advocate transferring the tendon and suturing it to the pelvis or the hip joint capsule. Some surgeons advocate swinging the tendon around and inserting it on the outside of the femur bone, which has been done for patients with spina bifida but is not generally felt to be a good procedure for patients with spastic cerebral palsy.

Benefits and risks: The benefits of these operations involve relieving hip dislocation, improving walking, and making it easier to care for the perineal area. The risks and complications of these procedures fall into the categories of either overcorrection or undercorrection. Determining how much lengthening is necessary may be difficult, and certainly the child may outgrow it with time. Whether there was insufficient release at the time of the first procedure or there was a sufficient release that the child outgrew so that the muscles tightened again, insufficient release eventually causes the contractures to recur.

The more serious complication is overrelease of these muscles, which causes the legs to become contracted in a spread-open position. This is very detrimental for children who are walking because it makes them walk with a wide-based gait and a large waddle. For those children who are only sitters, this abduction contracture is less detrimental, but is extremely cosmetically unappealing. It also makes side lying difficult.

A more common complication of the surgery is the combination of overcorrection on one side and undercorrection on the other, termed *windswept hip deformity,* in which one hip becomes contracted out to the side and the other hip becomes contracted across the midline. This misalignment is usually due to the asymmetry of the involvement, but the use of bracing may also contribute to the condition. Some patients will develop this deformity without any medical intervention.

After-surgery care: There are several postoperative care techniques that can be used following muscle releases. One form of management is to forgo casting or immobilization and start immediately with physical therapy. This approach generally makes it slightly harder to handle the child in the immediate couple of hours or couple of days after the surgery, but she will be largely recovered and completely back to her daily routine by three or four weeks after surgery. This method of treating spastic hip disease may have a slightly higher incidence of repeat surgery later on, although this is not well documented. There is clearly a lower incidence of developing abduction and windswept deformities. Adductor lengthening done for walking children should be immediately followed by physical therapy so that they can regain their walking ability.

Another common postoperative management technique involves placing casts on both legs with a stabilizer between to keep the legs apart. Alternatively, the casts may be extended above the hip, with the child in a full-body cast from chest to toes. Some combination of casting may be used for periods ranging from two to six or eight weeks. The advantage of casting is that the child is easier to handle in the immediate postoperative period, although she still may have many muscle spasms and need pain medicine and antispasmodic medication (usually Valium). When the casts are removed, the child is very stiff and has a good bit of discomfort when trying to move the hip and knee joints. The inability to move about easily is especially difficult for children who are walkers because they often have a more difficult time regaining their walking ability. The development of the opposite deformity (a spread-open position) is increased by this casting.

Following the casting, some surgeons prescribe long-term abduction braces that hold the legs apart, either at night when the child is sleeping, or, occasionally, full-time. The use of bracing after muscle releases, especially muscle releases done for the treatment of spastic hip subluxation, continues to remain controversial.

What to expect: After hip muscle releases, some physicians use splinting or bracing as noted above. The pain will be quite severe for the first 24 to 48 hours, but by four weeks after the surgery it is very minimal, occurring only with extreme stretching. The muscles should be substantially looser after the surgery; however, it is very important to start an exercise program to maintain flexibility because the natural tendency is for these muscles to re-tighten over time. This is especially true for a child with significant growth remaining, who may develop a repeat contracture over two or three years to the point where it is similar to what it was before the surgery was performed. Children who have had this procedure performed to improve their walking will need extensive therapy to gain the maximum benefit from the release.

Young adults who have the surgery performed to improve toileting and perineal care will find it easier almost immediately. In general, however, they will find that their hips do not open extremely widely, but that their legs will spread much more easily and will stay moderately spread.

Hyaline Membrane Disease

(HMD, RDS, respiratory distress syndrome)

Hyaline membrane disease, previously called respiratory distress syndrome, is a respiratory disease of the newborn infant. HMD is the leading cause of death in prematurely born infants in the United States, primarily affecting those born before 36 weeks' gestation. Treatment of hyaline membrane disease may include the use of a ventilator and concentrations of oxygen, either in an oxygen hood or through a ventilator.

The use of artificial surfactant, which is placed into the trachea of a newborn premature infant at risk for HMD shortly after birth has helped reduce the severity of the disease. The child born prematurely is at increased risk for cerebral palsy. This risk increases when there are additional medical problems, such as HMD. The premature baby with HMD is much more likely to suffer periodic episodes of hypoxia (low oxygen in the blood), thus increasing the chances that brain damage will occur. This could lead to CP, mental retardation, seizures, or other neurological complications.

Hydrocele

(hernia, inguinal hernia, hernia repair, herniorrhaphy)

A hydrocele is a collection of fluid that comes out of the abdomen from an open area in the abdominal lining which continues to loop down around the testicles in the male. This normally closes at the time of birth but frequently does not; a boy who develops an enlarged scrotum or appears to have swollen testicles often has a hydrocele. The fluid flows back and forth from the area around the testicle into the abdomen so that often the swelling seen in the scrotum gets larger or smaller, depending on the time of

the day and how much the child is crying or eating. If the swelling is not too large and the fluid does flow back and forth, there are usually no major problems with the scrotum or abdomen, and certainly for the first six months of life an operation is seldom necessary.

If the same abdominal lining opening and sac, which continues to be present around the testicle, is large enough so that part of the intestine falls down into the scrotum, it is called an inguinal hernia. Like the fluid, the intestine may come down into the scrotum and then disappear again. If this area develops redness, becomes swollen, and becomes very painful, it is an *immediate* emergency, and a doctor needs to see the child immediately—he may have developed a twist in his intestine, which can quickly become life threatening. If the inguinal hernia is present where the intestine descends into the scrotum it almost never disappears on its own, and a surgical procedure called a herniorrhaphy is necessary. Hernias and hydroceles are very common in children in general, but are more frequent in children with cerebral palsy.

The surgery: The hydrocele that is present after 6 months of age and continues to be quite large often should be repaired surgically. A hernia in which the bowel descends into the scrotal sac should be removed to prevent entrapment of the intestines in the scrotum, which is a surgical emergency. The surgery for the hydrocele and the hernia are similar in that a small incision is made in the lower abdomen, the sac that comes out of the abdomen is removed, and the area it comes from in the abdomen is closed.

Benefits and risks: There are few complications from this surgery, but occasionally an infection may develop. Symptoms include a temperature, loss of appetite, and a very red and inflamed incision. Occasionally the hernia or hydrocele may recur; often all that is needed for it to close up is to draw the fluid out of the sac.

After-surgery care: Hernia repairs are often done as outpatient surgeries, during which the child has a general anesthesia and then is taken home shortly after he awakens. The pain is usually minimal and easily controlled with Tylenol. The child may be somewhat uncomfortable in certain positions for a week or two but then usually recovers very rapidly. Children who undergo this procedure can be bathed after three or four days, depending upon the specific recommendations of the surgeon.

Hydrocephalus

Hydrocephalus is the enlargement of fluid-filled spaces in the brain known as ventricles combined with signs and

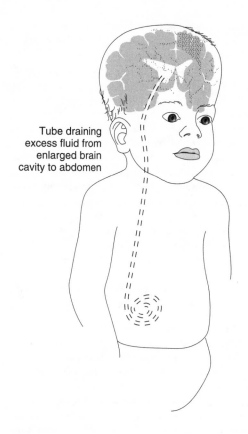

Tube draining
excess fluid from
enlarged brain
cavity to abdomen

symptoms of increased intracranial pressure. This enlargement derives from an imbalance in the production and absorption of cerebrospinal fluid, and is usually caused by blockage in the normal circulation of this fluid.

Hydrocephalus can be seen in children who have cerebral palsy. Because CP is the result of some scar in the brain, the scar may occur in an area affecting the natural flow of the fluid in the brain. When this occurs, then a blockage may develop, and the fluid builds up. Extra fluid may also be present because the brain damage is so large that there is a decreased amount of brain tissue; if it is able to drain naturally, it does not need intervention. Most of the time, however, when increased fluid is present, a shunt, or drainage tube, must be inserted.

Hyperbaric Oxygen Therapy
(HBOT)

Hyperbaric oxygen therapy (HBOT) is the inhalation of 100% oxygen inside a chamber that is pressurized to greater than 1 atmosphere (therefore described as hyperbaric because the pressure is above atmospheric pressure). HBOT is typically administered at 1–3 atmospheres of pressure.

For many years, HBOT has been successfully used to treat certain types of infections, carbon monoxide poisoning, and decompression sickness in deep-sea divers. A medical specialty known as Undersea and Hyperbaric Medicine was developed, and indications for the treatment were outlined.

More recently, HBOT has been advertised as a treatment for traumatic brain injury and stroke, as well as for more chronic brain injuries such as those associated with CP. This treatment has received a great deal of publicity despite very little scientific evidence that it works. It is not clear from a scientific standpoint how HBOT could help overcome damage to brain tissue that occurred years before in a child with CP. When HBOT was studied in a scientific manner in two groups of children with CP, with a control group placed in pressurized room air and a treatment group in pressurized oxygen, both groups improved, without any difference between the two groups. Similar results were found in a second such controlled study of children with CP.

Ear pain/discomfort and bleeding from the ear are by far the most commonly reported adverse events during HBOT. In addition, there may be an increased risk of seizures in those treated with HBOT.

In summary, HBOT is a treatment that has long been known to work for specific medical problems, but has recently been touted as a cure for CP. The limited amount of controlled scientific studies do not support these claims, and one should proceed cautiously before embarking on this treatment, which is expensive in terms both of time and money.

Hypersensitivity
(tactile defensiveness)

The brain must receive or register stimuli in order for a response to occur. For this reason, individuals with cerebral palsy can experience a number of difficulties with the sensory system as a result of their brain abnormality. The problems frequently involve the senses of touch and equilibrium as well as awareness of the body's movement and position in space.

Hypersensitivity to touch is called tactile defensiveness. Normally, infants react to touch in a self-protective manner but become more comfortable as they learn to discriminate among degrees and varieties of touch. The individual who is unable to mature in this fashion remains highly reflexive and self-protective. The goal of therapy is to enable the child to develop an adaptive response to touch. The answer is not to avoid touching, but rather to have the child be gradually able to handle the sensation of being touched. Therapists use a number of techniques, including varied textures, to stimulate the desired responses.

Hypersensitivity to external heat or cold can present difficulty for the individual with cerebral palsy because of the diminished ability to self-regulate body temperature in response to air temperature. What this means is that a child sitting in an excessively warm room will not automatically be able to discharge heat and can become seriously overheated. Similarly, the self-regulating mechanism that conserves body heat in cold weather is impaired. Caregivers must be aware of external temperatures in order to monitor the individual's comfort and safety.

Difficulties with equilibrium and position in space result from malfunction of the vestibular and proprioceptive systems. Individuals most commonly display two problems: gravitational insecurity and an intolerance of spinning or circular movement. Because of gravitational insecurity, the child may react with intense anxiety to a simple change in head position. For example, he may become very frightened when placed on an examining table, not because he fears a needle, but because he has the sensation of falling. Spinning or turning may cause excessive nausea and discomfort. Reassurance, combined with therapeutic intervention aimed at bringing about an appropriate response to these sensations, can help a great deal. Sensory integration therapy, in particular, is designed to overcome these hypersensitive reactions.

Impairment

(disability)

An impairment is a biological condition or disease, whereas a disability is the immediate manifestation of this condition as it affects behavior. Thus, cerebral palsy is an impairment that can cause the disability of limited limb movement.

A disability restricts or causes difficulty with specific functional activities. For example, a child who has an amputated foot may be disabled because he has difficulty walking. If the amputated foot, which is the impairment, is replaced by a prosthetic foot that allows the child to walk normally, the child no longer has a disability because his prosthesis is in place.

Inclusion

(mainstreaming)

Within the educational system, the practice of moving children with disabilities into regular classrooms or a regular school environment is called inclusion or mainstreaming.

Indications: A child whose cognitive abilities are age appropriate, who is able to communicate, and whose medical problems do not necessitate specialized medical care can be mainstreamed. Specifically, if a child entering first grade requires a wheelchair for mobility but can speak and is at approximately the age-appropriate cognitive level, she should be mainstreamed in almost all environments.

Benefits and risks: The primary benefit of inclusion is that it exposes a child with a disability to other children who do not have disabilities and vice versa. This can improve her circle of friends and give her an expanded, more normalized school experience. Through inclusion children without disabilities are allowed the opportunity to develop a better understanding of what it is like to have a disability.

The major disadvantage of inclusion is that frequently the staff is not as specialized, so that teachers without special experience or training will be providing education to the child with a disability. This is not a major issue if the disability does not greatly interfere with the child's regular functioning, but the child with severe motor or cognitive limitations may not be handled well by an educational staff with no specific training in educating children with disabilities.

Another disadvantage is that many public schools do not have specialized equipment that can benefit a child with a significant disability. Also, inclusion is supported by educational administrators because it is cheaper than sending a child to a specialized facility with more equipment and specialty trained staff.

Maintenance and care: The decision to mainstream a child is not made just once during a child's lifetime to apply forever. Rather, it must continually be reevaluated as the child grows and develops. For example, a child may enter kindergarten, first grade, or second grade in a specialized educational environment where additional expertise in early childhood education and additional medical services and equipment are available. As this child continues to develop, a decision may be made in middle school that he can be moved to a regular environment for part of the day, and then as the child enters junior high, he may be ready for complete inclusion. For many children it is not entirely clear whether inclusion will be a positive or a negative experience. In these cases this type of graduated, ongoing evaluation is especially appropriate.

Incontinence

(urinary incontinence, bowel incontinence)

Incontinence is defined as the inability to prevent the accidental loss of urine or feces. Incontinence is normal for the newborn baby, but most children are toilet trained by age 3. However, urinary incontinence (enuresis), especially at night while sleeping (nocturnal enuresis), is a common condition and usually does not need a medical evaluation until the child is close to age 6.

Generally, achieving normal bladder control requires the following steps: (1) an awareness of the bladder as it contracts; (2) the ability to realize the state of a full bladder and to plan ahead to go to the bathroom; (3) the ability to inhibit early contractions and postpone urination, and to facilitate the emptying reflex when circumstances are right; (4) an awareness that the bladder has emptied completely; (5) the ability to hold urine when the bladder is overfilled or during momentary stress by voluntarily contracting the muscles of the pelvic floor; and (6) the ability to inhibit emptying during sleep. Thus, a child needs to be developmentally ready before he can be toilet trained, and the child with mental retardation or a developmental delay may be toilet trained at a later age than other children.

Incontinence may also be caused by physical problems, including a urinary tract infection or an abnormality of the urinary system. In the child with cerebral palsy, the nerves going to the bladder may not be functioning normally, and may cause either involuntary emptying of the bladder or abnormal retention of urine to the point that the bladder "overflows" and urine dribbles out. These two conditions aren't common, but may occur in the child with cerebral palsy, although they occur far more frequently in children with other neurological disorders such as spina bifida.

A child who is incontinent during the day beyond the expected age of 3 or 4, and who otherwise is developmentally normal, should have a good physical examination, a urinalysis, and a urine culture. With the child with cerebral palsy with normal cognitive function, the problem may lie in his physical ability to get to the toilet or his inability to sit up on the toilet. This latter problem is not just physical but also psychological: the toilet seat may evoke fear in the child who feels as if he is going to fall, and thus he may not be able to relax enough to cooperate in toilet training. There is equipment available to help support a child sitting on a toilet.

If tests show that the bladder and kidneys are normal, then behavior modification techniques may be used to teach the child bladder control. These should include a conditioning technique such as a reward system or an alarm system. In the older child, medication is sometimes used to control enuresis.

Incontinence of stool is not an uncommon problem. Constipation is very often the cause with a child who has previously been toilet trained and then begins to have fecal soiling. What happens is that the child builds up a large mass of dry stool which is difficult to pass, and then liquid feces flow around this mass past the sphincters. Fecal incontinence caused by such an impaction is often mistaken for diarrhea, because the stool that is escaping is liquid.

Fecal incontinence may also occur when the toddler-aged child is stressed, such as following the birth of a sibling or a death in the family. If soiling begins at the time of toilet training, it is best to back off and stop the training for awhile, as this is a sign that the child simply is not emotionally prepared to be trained. Incontinence of stool is commonly seen if the child is mentally retarded or has severe constipation. Cerebral palsy by itself is almost never the cause of failure to become continent. If the child is developmentally age appropriate but is still soiling, an evaluation is in order, looking for constipation or neurological problems as the cause.

Individualized Education Plan

(IEP)

An individualized education plan is a written plan that outlines the educational program for a child in special education. It is to be reviewed annually and agreed to by the parents of the child after they meet with members of the school staff who are trained to develop the plan and explain it to parents.

The IEP for a school-aged child with CP (over the age of 3) will be based on therapists' and teachers' evaluations, as well as on a psychological evaluation. The process usually includes a physical therapist's assessment of the issues around gross motor problems, and often also includes occupational and speech therapists if the child with CP has fine motor or speech problems too. The IEP should describe the child's level of development and should specify goals for the child with CP in each of the following areas: gross motor, fine motor, speech and language, social, and cognitive skills. It also should specify who will work on each of the goals (i.e., teacher, O.T., P.T., etc.) and how often each week the child will receive each therapy. It should also specify the extent to which the child will be able to participate in regular educational programs. This should result in an educational program based on the individualized needs of the child. A suitable IEP needs direct parent involvement.

Individualized Family Service Plan
(IFSP)

An individualized family service plan is a written plan that outlines early intervention services for a child under age 3 with disabilities and his or her family. It is similar to an IEP, but the focus is on the family as a whole, rather than just the child. It describes the services necessary to enhance the development of the child with disabilities and the ability of the child's family to meet the child's needs.

The IFSP for the child with CP who is younger than 3 years of age is based on evaluations by therapists and doctors. Like the IEP, it should specify an educational program and a therapeutic program aimed to meet specific goals for that individual child. It will be based on evaluations of the child's cognitive, gross and fine motor, speech and language, and social skills, and should aim to meet goals in each of the defined areas. In addition, based on an evaluation by a social worker, it should also address family needs that are related to the child's disability, such as respite care or homemaker services for a parent who is working with the child.

Ingrown Toenail
(infected toenail, paronychia)

An ingrown toenail is a nail that has inflamed skin overlaying it. It is caused by either trimming the nail too close to the skin or having too much pressure against the side or corner of the nail. Once the tissue has become infected, it is difficult for the infection to heal. Once tenderness is felt, the primary treatment should be to prevent pressure and discontinue wearing shoes that put pressure on this area of the nail. It might be helpful to take an old pair of athletic shoes and completely cut out the top front of the shoe so the toe with the inflamed nail does not get any pressure.

A common cause of ingrown toenails in children with cerebral palsy is wearing braces that irritate the toenail or cause the shoes to be too tight for the toenail. A common cause in teenagers with cerebral palsy is the development of flat feet, so that the pressure when walking is on the side of the toe, causing the toenail to be irritated.

To prevent ingrown toenails, the toenails should be carefully trimmed straight across, and the corners and cuticles should not be touched. To treat an ingrown nail, the inflamed toenail should be soaked twice a day in warm water and dried well. Packing under the corner of the toenail

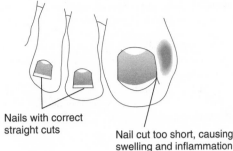

Nails with correct straight cuts

Nail cut too short, causing swelling and inflammation

with a small piece of lamb's wool helps avoid further irritating the inflamed tissue. If the skin is very red and extremely warm, antibiotics may be necessary.

If soreness does not improve within a week, occasionally surgical drainage or excision of the edge of the nail is needed to allow the toe to heal. This is often not necessary for a first- or second-time inflammation; however, after a nail has become repeatedly infected, it often develops a significant amount of scar tissue, and the only way to eliminate the problem completely is to do a surgical excision of the edge of the toenail.

Inhibition Therapy

Some disciplines of physical therapy work to prevent movements or activities that are considered damaging to a certain child; activities that avoid these pathological postures make up inhibition therapy. Examples of inhibition are placing a cast on the foot to prevent extensor posturing of the upper body, or positional changes, such as placing the child in a sitting position to prevent her hyperextending her spine and head.

Indications: Inhibition therapy is useful for children with significant primitive posturing. This is especially true for the child who is doing a lot of extensor posturing, such as trying to straighten up and pull out of a wheelchair involuntarily. It is also useful for some children with athetoid movements in which some of the unwanted movements may be suppressed by restricting distant parts of the body.

Benefits and risks: The major benefit of this therapy is that it allows the child more conscious control of the upper extremities and the head. To be able to use augmentative communication devices with hand control or head control, certain movements or postures may need to be inhibited. The major risks of inhibitive treatment involve the possibility of pain from placing too much pressure, especially with foot braces or wheelchairs that have not been fitted properly. Some children use so much force in trying to extend their hips that it can be very difficult to find the right straps or bars to hold them in the proper position.

Maintenance and care: It is important when using inhibition therapy to continue to make sure that braces and wheelchairs fit well and do not cause skin irritation. This is especially important during the child's growth, but attention to good fit may need to continue even into adulthood.

Inhibitive Casting
(tone-reducing cast, tone-reducing brace, serial casts)

Inhibitive casts are usually applied to the legs and sometimes the arms to inhibit a specific movement. Initially the cast may be used to stretch out a contracture, such as a tight Achilles tendon. The cast is used to keep the foot in a position where the sole and heel touch the ground. By keeping the ankle from flexing, other movements are improved, and the elbows flex better, fingers move more easily, and spasticity decreases in the hips or knees. The inhibitive ankle-foot orthosis (AFO) is useful in stabilizing the ankle for standing.

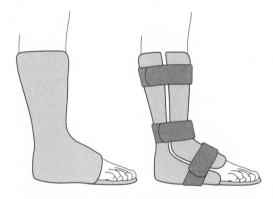

Indications: Indications for the use of inhibitive casts are not well defined. There is variable success when they are used for severe spasticity or in the attempt to stretch out tight muscles. Initially, the muscles may be able to be stretched out, but as soon as the casting is discontinued the contracture recurs. Whether inhibitive casts can decrease unwanted movements or improve function also remains uncertain. There clearly are some patients in whom immobilization of the ankle does decrease the amount of abnormal posturing. However, as soon as the immobilization is removed, the posturing returns.

In general, the use of inhibitive casts for children with cerebral palsy is rapidly decreasing, but AFOs are widely used for inhibiting movement. The AFO may be worn to immobilize the ankle, and normal shoes can be worn over the orthotic, providing a much more cosmetically acceptable approach to casting.

Benefits and risks: Using inhibitive casts, or alternatively an AFO, with the goal of inhibiting movement does improve positioning and function in some children, although as soon as the immobilization is removed the benefit is lost. Elaborate tone-reducing splints and casts with special pressure points have been developed but have not demonstrated any benefit over comfortably fitting AFOs. Inhibitive casts are most beneficial after acute head injuries because the casts prevent short-term contractures, and with time the brain heals and the tendency to contract decreases. In some clinics, serial casts are frequently used after botulinum toxin injection.

The purpose of both casting and the use of an AFO is to stretch tight muscles and provide positioning. The serial cast involves placing a cast that is removed after several weeks and replaced with another. However, the position of the body part being casted is now closer to normal from the effect of the first cast. Theoretically, one can continue with this process until the desired position is achieved. The inhibitive cast is similar but is removable by the caregivers for bathing and any other functions that the physician may recommend.

Maintenance and care: Serial casts often require changing every two to three weeks. If they are applied too tightly, they must be removed on an emergency basis. If the child has had a cast applied, and it becomes very painful, then an emergency may occur because the muscle may be in such spasm that it will not get enough blood flow.

One of the main reasons serial casts are used much less commonly now is because of the difficulty of maintaining a cast on a child, which means the child cannot be bathed, and the discomfort of ongoing cast wear. As soon as the cast is removed, within several weeks to a month all its benefits have been lost, if ongoing casting or splinting is not performed. Some physicians feel that using botulinum toxin with casts allows the gains achieved in stretching to be maintained for a longer time frame. In the long term, maintenance and care in terms of this problem is much more easily done with well-fitting AFOs.

Intrathecal Baclofen
(baclofen pump, ITB)

Spasticity is the most common motor disorder in cerebral palsy and is seen in approximately two-thirds of those with

CP. While some spasticity may be necessary for function in children with CP, it is often a problem that can be difficult to treat. Multiple approaches are available for treatment of spasticity. These include physical and occupational therapy, oral medications, Botox injections, orthopedic surgery, and neurosurgical procedures such as selective dorsal rhizotomy.

Baclofen is a muscle relaxant that when taken by mouth is not always helpful in treating spasticity in children with CP. However, when given to patients intrathecally, i.e., into the spinal fluid, it works much more consistently and efficiently to reduce spasticity with fewer side effects. The goals for treatment with intrathecal baclofen should be realistic and individualized, and they need to be agreed on by patient, family/caregiver, and medical team. Ideally a multidisciplinary team should be involved in the decision making.

Patients with dystonia have also responded to this treatment, often at higher doses. Patients with athetosis, ataxia, and myoclonus have not noted improvement. ITB can help with spasticity-related pain during the day and at night.

A trial of baclofen by mouth is not a prerequisite for patients with spasticity and CP to receive the pump. When a patient is felt to be a potential candidate for ITB therapy, a screening trial is scheduled. This involves a lumbar puncture and injection of an intrathecal baclofen test dose. Spasticity scores are recorded preinjection and at 2-hour intervals postinjection, for up to 6–8 hours. If the trial dose is felt to have benefited the child, and if the parents agree, then placement of the pump is the next step. Patients who have had a spinal fusion cannot undergo a trial, but they can have the pump implanted.

The ITB delivery system consists of a programmable subcutaneously implanted pump with a reservoir attached to an intraspinal catheter. The pump is inserted under general anesthesia. Postoperatively, the patient remains flat in bed for 48 hours.

The pump reservoir is refilled through a port in the pump that is directly under the skin, at intervals of approximately 2–6 months. Dosage adjustments are made via an external computer/programmer and transmitted to the pump by a handheld computer mouse. Doses can be programmed to deliver the baclofen in several ways. Examples include: the same dose all day long ("continuous"); the same dose all day long, with occasional extra boluses given when spasticity is highest ("intermittent bolus"); or continuous doses that vary throughout the day based on when spasticity is highest ("complex continuous").

Important issues to consider include:

- A history of seizures is not a contraindication to intrathecal baclofen therapy.
- The presence of a ventriculoperitoneal shunt is not a contraindication either. Patients with VP shunts may require a smaller dose of baclofen.
- The patient must be big enough and have enough room in his abdomen to accommodate the pump.
- The patient and family need to understand and accept the look of the pump. You typically can see and feel the pump under the skin. It is about the size and shape of a hockey puck.
- The entire team must agree on appropriate goals.
- The patient and family must be motivated to achieve these goals and be committed to the follow-up required to maintain the pump treatment.

Success of the intrathecal baclofen therapy seems to be related to appropriate patient selection, setting of achievable goals, patient and family motivation and compliance, and the help of a dedicated multidisciplinary team.

Intrauterine Growth Retardation (IUGR)

Intrauterine growth retardation is a term used to describe a fetus that is not growing appropriately in the uterus. Infants born with IUGR are small for their gestational age, with a low weight, short length, and small head circumference, and they almost always have had some significant insult that explains their growth retardation. Causes for IUGR might include congenital infections, such as cytomegalovirus (CMV) or toxoplasmosis, or malnutrition, placental insufficiency, or a variety of other conditions. Infants with IUGR are at increased risk for developing cerebral palsy because the brain is also very dependent for its full-term development on normal intrauterine growth.

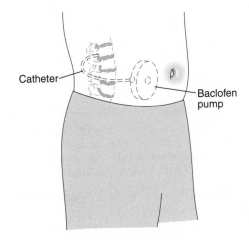

Catheter

Baclofen pump

Jaundice

(hyperbilirubinemia, icterus, "yellow skin")

Yellow discoloration of the skin and eyes is called jaundice. While jaundice can be an early sign of liver disease, in newborn infants it is a common problem and is not usually associated with any disease. This type of jaundice, called "physiological jaundice," rarely leads to problems.

When babies are born, they have a high red blood cell count. As these red blood cells are broken down in the first few days of life, a breakdown product called bilirubin is generated. If the bilirubin is not excreted through the liver and gastrointestinal system, the child will become jaundiced and appear yellow. This is common in the first few days after birth because the liver is not yet mature enough to break down all the bilirubin. If the level becomes too high, the baby is put under special lights called "bili-lights," which help break down the bilirubin as it goes through the blood vessels in the skin. If the bilirubin level continues to rise even after treatment with bili-lights, then exchange transfusions can also be done. Such a transfusion is not often done in a full-term healthy baby, but is still done in small premature babies in whom complications can develop from a lower level of bilirubin than in a full-term baby with a higher birthweight.

Sometimes jaundice in newborns is not benign. For instance, a severe infection in the blood system can cause jaundice, as can defects of the liver and incompatibility of the blood type of the mother and the infant. This last, hemolytic disease of the newborn, was a common cause of severe hyperbilirubinemia in the years before phototherapy and exchange transfusions began to be used to prevent the complications of severe jaundice. The high levels of bilirubin caused kernicterus, a staining of part of the brain with bilirubin, causing brain damage. This resulted in lethargy, poor feeding, and a shrill cry.

While many babies with severe kernicterus died, many of those who survived eventually showed signs of the athetoid type of cerebral palsy.

Ketogenic Diet

The Ketogenic Diet is a treatment for seizures. The Ketogenic Diet is a rigid, mathematically calculated, physician-supervised diet that is very high in fat and very low in carbohydrate and protein. It usually has three to four times as much fat as carbohydrate and protein combined. Fluids and calories are strictly limited. This diet allows the body to primarily burn fat for energy rather than glucose. The Ketogenic Diet can be considered in patients with any seizure type, but is most effective in absence, atonic, and myoclonic seizures. The diet should not be tried without the supervision of a health care provider and dietitian, both of whom must be knowledgeable in the diet.

Knee Immobilizers

A common problem for children with spasticity is the development of tightness in the hamstring muscles (back of the thigh). This can make it hard to stand upright and can even make sitting hard. A splint that is often used is called a knee immobilizer. The goal of this splint is to hold the knee completely straight. The splint is usually made of canvass or plastic and is wrapped around the leg and fixed with Velcro straps. This splint does not need to be custom fitted. Rather, it comes in a number of different standard lengths, one of which should be right for a particular child.

The knee immobilizers can be used to prevent or improve contractures. For this purpose they probably need to be worn approximately 8 hours a day. This means wearing them during sleep time for most children, so the splint does not prevent sitting and moving during wake times. A major side effect of the splints is that many children cannot tolerate them during sleep, and they severely restrict the child if they are worn during the day. Knee immobilizers are also frequently used after surgery, especially after hamstring lengthening.

Kyphosis

(round back)

Kyphosis is the term for a rounded spine or a severely slouched body frame. Also referred to as forward bending of the spine, kyphosis is very common in young children with cerebral palsy who do not have good upper body control. Their kyphosis completely corrects itself when they lie down. For children with cerebral palsy the deformity is due to poor muscle control, but kyphosis may also occur in adolescents in the front of the spine as a result of abnormal growth. In this case, it is called adolescent round back or Scheuermann's kyphosis.

Sometimes the bones in the front of the spine form abnormally during the child's development, in which case the child is said to have congenital kyphosis. The most common kyphosis occurs in older people, especially older women—their bones soften and the spine collapses down, and they become severely round-backed. This condition is termed senile kyphosis and is due to osteoporosis.

Care and treatment: Kyphosis in children with cerebral palsy is not well defined. It typically occurs between the ages of 3 and 8 when children with severe involvement

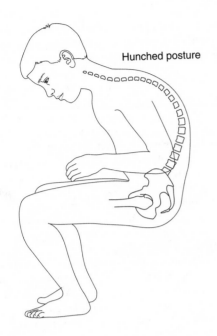

Hunched posture

ties. For this reason a body jacket or a body brace may be used for positioning comfort, and for better head control and arm use. As the large curve becomes stiff, however, children have difficulty lying on their backs. Often they end up lying on their sides. When they are sitting, the head cannot be held back, and they end up with the head dropped forward. At this point it is uncertain whether this posture has any effect on respiration or gastric function. For some children, breathing and eating habits improve when they can sit or stand in a straight position.

Laryngeal Stridor

(laryngomalacia, tracheomalacia, inspiratory stridor)

Laryngeal stridor during the first few months of life is a harsh sound heard during respiration. It can be high-pitched when the child breathes in. If stridor appears, it usually results from a disturbance in the formation of the larynx or the trachea. There are many causes of stridor. The most common of these, laryngomalacia, is caused by weak cartilage in the airway and results in partial airway obstruction.

Care and treatment: Usually no therapy is needed, since the condition improves on its own by 18 months of age. There may be difficulty feeding a child with stridor. Rarely, a child will need a tracheostomy or other procedure because of the airway obstruction. Most children with this condition seem more comfortable and less noisy lying on their stomachs.

If the child with cerebral palsy develops laryngomalacia or tracheomalacia in early or later childhood, it may be associated with severe gastroesophageal reflux. The underlying reflux is treated with either medication or surgery.

Other children with cerebral palsy can develop upper airway obstruction and stridor because of low tone of the muscles about the throat and face. The low muscle tone causes the tongue to fall to the back of the throat, which intermittently obstructs the airway. This problem does not tend to disappear with time, although positioning the child on the stomach sometimes resolves the problem. If not, some children need a tracheostomy to relieve the airway obstruction.

have difficulty with trunk control. When treating a young child with kyphosis, it is necessary to modify the wheelchair so that the child sits up straight. At this age, often the best treatment is the use of an adequately contoured wheelchair with shoulder straps and a reclining seat. A prone stander that stimulates the child to pull her spine up straighter and lift her head is another useful device; a stander that does not support the child's upper body and allows her to slouch forward without any support for the chest should not be used. Seats that are contoured with a round back, such as the plastic molded tumble frames, should also be avoided, as they can make kyphosis worse. Special exercises are not very helpful, since the child mainly needs to mature.

As children increase their trunk control, this type of kyphosis is generally corrected, although a few children enter adolescence with the head drooped forward and shoulders rolled severely forward. Sometimes this posture becomes stiff, which makes sitting up and looking forward difficult. It is also very difficult for children to sit in a chair, especially if the kyphosis starts stiffening, and they are unable to lie down except in a ball shape. For the rare child whose deformity stiffens, a posterior spinal fusion and instrumentation to straighten the spine is recommended in order to allow the child to sit up straight, look forward, and interact with the environment.

Complications due to the kyphosis are not well defined. Children between ages 3 and 8 with flexible kyphosis have no known complications, except that they roll forward and have difficulty holding the head up to participate in activi-

Laryngoscopy

(bronchoscopy)

Laryngoscopy is a simple procedure that involves inspection of the larynx and upper airway. An indirect laryngoscopy is done with the aid of a mirror; a direct laryngoscopy, in the office, involves a small, flexible bronchoscope that is passed through the nose. Rigid bronchoscopy with a metal telescope requires general anesthesia. Bronchoscopy is an examination of the lower airway, including the trachea and mainstem bronchi.

Benefits and risks: Bronchoscopy and laryngoscopy are useful procedures for inspecting the airway and obtaining a culture or biopsy. Also, a foreign body can be removed via bronchoscopy. Complications of bronchoscopy can include transient hypoxia (a decrease in oxygen in the blood) and spasm of the larynx or bronchus. Less commonly oral or dental injury can occur. A child can also contract a post-bronchoscopy croup, which is usually short-lived and can be treated with medications and mist.

Latex Allergy

Latex is a natural rubber produced by the rubber tree. Some people develop allergic reactions after repeated contact with latex. Allergic reactions can be localized, such as rash and itching after wearing latex gloves, or generalized, such as sneezing, runny nose, or wheezing. Rarely, life-threatening reactions (anaphylaxis) can occur.

Latex allergy usually affects people who are routinely exposed to latex products such as health care workers and people who have had multiple surgeries or medical procedures. This includes children with medical conditions, such as myelomeningocele or occasionally cerebral palsy, that result in multiple surgical operations or repeated bladder catheterizations.

Latex can be encountered in medical equipment such as latex gloves, blood pressure cuffs, drains, tourniquets, urine catheters, and adhesives used for dressings. Latex can also be found in common household items such as rubber bands, computer mouse pads, and balloons. Several allergenic proteins have been identified, some of which are similar to and "cross-react" with proteins in certain foods, such as bananas, kiwi fruit, and avocados.

If a latex allergy is suspected, a blood test can be done that tests for latex-specific antibodies. Once the diagnosis is confirmed, avoidance is the best way of treating a latex allergy. Most health care products are now made with latex-free alternative materials, and most hospitals and many physician offices now have a latex-free environment, thus reducing the likelihood of developing a latex allergy.

Least Restrictive Environment

If a child with cerebral palsy or other disability is found to need early intervention services or special education ser-vices, these should be provided in the least restrictive environment. This means that the child receives services in settings and facilities in which children without disabilities would participate, unless the Individualized Family Service Plan (IFSP) or the Individualized Education Plan (IEP) indicates a need for a special setting.

An example of a least restrictive environment is the regular classroom, in which a child who can speak and has an age-appropriate cognitive level, but requires the use of a wheelchair, should be included with age-matched peers in almost all environments. On the other hand, a child who has severe mental retardation with severe motor disability would not be expected to be in a regular classroom with age-appropriate children, because the least restrictive environment for this child would not be able to meet the child's needs as identified by the IEP.

For a significant group of children with cerebral palsy, determining the least restrictive environment that best meets a child's needs may be very difficult. In fact, there may be a combination of environments that would meet the child's needs, which has to be clarified by the IEP.

Lordosis

(swayback)

Lordosis refers to the spinal curvature that is normally present in the small of the back. In the person with sway-back, the spine arches to such an extent that it causes the abdomen to protrude. If a person spends a large amount of time sitting, lordosis can be beneficial because it projects the weight of sitting forward onto the thighs where the likelihood of developing pressure sores is decreased.

An abnormal amount of lordosis as an isolated problem is the most rare spinal deformity in children with cerebral palsy. Severe lordosis may be a long-term complication after a dorsal rhizotomy procedure. It is frequently associated with scoliosis, but usually scoliosis is the most predominant deformity; the lordosis is an additional difficulty. Some children with lordosis roll so far forward that their abdomens rest on their thighs; this makes seating almost impossible. It is extremely difficult to modify wheelchairs to correct for increased lordosis, although the main method is to recline the wheelchair to about 45 degrees.

Indications: Once increased lordosis becomes a significant condition, it tends to get slowly worse until a spinal fusion is performed. The indications for spinal fusion are rare in this deformity. Fusion should be considered when lordosis makes sitting difficult or impossible or if it causes intractable back pain. Unfortunately, bracing or wheelchair modifications do not benefit or change severe lordosis.

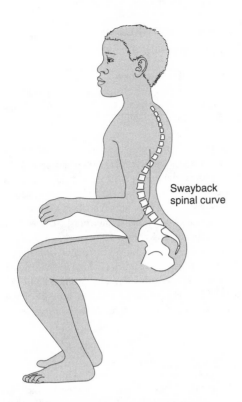

Swayback spinal curve

Magnetic Resonance Imaging

(MR, MRI)

Magnetic resonance imaging is an imaging method used extensively for examining brain tissue, though it may also be used to image the spine or other areas of the body. It involves being placed in a very large magnet that temporarily magnetizes body water. Radiofrequency pulses are used to measure the properties of the water in body tissue. The computer uses this information to create a series of pictures. There is no radiation involved in the MRI scanner, but the child is required to lie very still, which often means sedation will be needed. Sometimes intravenous contrast material is injected to learn more details about the body tissue.

This machine is the most sophisticated imaging method available. It can detect most major brain problems such as tumors, large congenital deformities, increased fluid, and many degenerative conditions. However, many children with cerebral palsy can have normal MRI scans. The reason is that MRI picks up anatomic defects. Very tiny abnormalities or functional problems present in the brain cannot be seen on MRI.

Indications: Many children with cerebral palsy will have one MRI scan, unless there is clear evidence as to the cause of the cerebral palsy. This is mainly to rule out such problems as brain tumors, major vascular abnormalities, or other treatable conditions.

Benefits and risks: MRIs currently have the highest ability to pick up disorders of the brain of any imaging test available. The major risk is in requiring the child to hold very still for a prolonged period of time, from 15 to 30 minutes. This requires heavy sedation for many children, and because there is some risk of breathing problems, the child needs to be closely monitored. There is no pain involved with the study, though patients who are uncomfortable in small spaces may feel very anxious inside the machine, which looks like a large tube.

Malformation of the Central Nervous System

Three percent of newborn infants have major malformations of the central nervous system. Some are caused by genetic conditions and others by environmental factors, including maternal infections or drugs. However, the majority do not have a known cause.

Such malformations can fall into a number of broad categories, including neural tube defects, anterior midline defects, spinal cord dysraphic states, disorders of cellular migration, and agenesis of the corpus callosum. The last two are often found in association with cerebral palsy. Disorders of cellular migration are often a direct cause of CP, whereas agenesis of the corpus callosum frequently causes seizures.

Medical Home

A medical home is an approach to providing comprehensive primary care to children with special needs. Ideally, such a medical home is defined as primary care that is accessible, continuous, comprehensive, family centered, coordinated, compassionate, and culturally effective. This concept has been developed by the American Academy of Pediatrics with the hope that many pediatricians and family physicians will serve as medical homes for chronically ill and physically disabled children.

In a medical home, the clinician works in partnership with the family and patient to assure that all of the medical and nonmedical needs of the patient are being met. Such services might include specialty care, educational services, family support, and other community services that are important to the health of the child.

Though the American Academy of Pediatrics proposed this definition of a medical home in 1992, efforts to establish such medical homes for all children have encountered many challenges. One of the major ones is a lack of adequate reimbursement for the kinds of services that physicians provide to children with complex medical problems. In contrast to care provided in a medical home, care provided through emergency departments, walk-in clinics, and other urgent care facilities, though sometimes necessary, is more costly and often less effective.

Meningitis and Encephalitis

Meningitis is an infection of the covering over the brain (called the meninges); encephalitis is an infection of the brain substance. Although there is a difference between these two conditions, the net result can be very similar. The most common cause of viral encephalitis is the herpes simplex virus. Meningitis may also be caused by a virus (in this case, it is called aseptic meningitis), but it is more commonly caused by bacteria, such as meningococcus, hemophilus influenza, and pneumococcus.

Generally children with meningitis develop a fever and stiff neck; they may also have difficulty eating, and they may vomit. Older children often complain of sensitivity to light and a headache. Infants stop feeding. A child with meningitis may fall into a coma.

Care and treatment: Although the incidence of meningitis has fallen dramatically since the introduction of the Hemophilus influenza (Hib) vaccine, and more recently the pneumococcal vaccine, many children in the United States still contract bacterial meningitis each year. When a physician suspects meningitis, a lumbar puncture (called a spinal tap) is done, and samples of spinal fluid are sent for laboratory examination. If the infection is diagnosed and found to be bacterial, antibiotics are used to treat the infection. There is no medicine that treats most kinds of viral meningitis, and most patients with viral meningitis recover without treatment. Infection of young infants with herpes virus can be treated with a medication called acyclovir. Infections with polio, rubella (German measles) and mumps, all of which can cause encephalitis or meningitis, are preventable with immunizations.

The aftereffects of meningitis or encephalitis include brain damage or death, though most children recover without severe complications. Those with brain damage may have cerebral palsy and/or mental retardation. Up to 40 percent of children with bacterial meningitis (especially meningitis caused by pneumococcus) suffer hearing impairment in one or both ears.

Mental Retardation

(cognitive impairment)

Mental retardation is a term used for intellectual functioning which is at least two standard deviations below the norm; it is usually categorized as mild, moderate, or severe. It may exist concurrently with cerebral palsy or by itself without a motor disability. It is generally diagnosed during the developmental period from 2 to 8 years of age. It is nearly impossible to make a firm diagnosis or determination of mental retardation in the very young child, because tests of intellect are not valid until age 3. Treatment involves recognizing the child's functional level and placing him in an educational environment where he is able to maximize his natural learning abilities.

Approximately two-thirds of children with cerebral palsy also have mental retardation. One-third have mild to moderate MR, one-third severe to profound MR, and one-third have normal intelligence. The presence of mental retardation is often the most disabling factor for the child with CP.

Metabolic Disorders

There are many types of metabolic disorders, which vary considerably in their clinical and pathological aspects. However, all are due to single gene defects that result in abnormal or deficient enzymes or proteins. Thus, their pathology is typically the result of an inability to properly make or break down compounds necessary for normal body functions.

When an enzyme is not working properly, the substance it is to metabolize builds up in excess, as do other associated compounds. Disease can result from these excess metabolites, which can in many cases be toxic to the brain and other organs. In other cases, it is the absence of the compound that would have been produced by the deficient enzyme that causes disease. Many children with metabolic disease thus appear normal at birth and may not be identified with cerebral palsy until the pattern of metabolic disease becomes apparent.

Treatment for a very few metabolic disorders involves replacing the necessary enzyme. For most, however, treatment is limited and consists of dietary manipulation and the use of dietary supplements to decrease the buildup of injurious compounds and maximize the function of any enzyme available. The success of these interventions varies widely.

The number of disorders identified as metabolic has dramatically increased over the past years. Despite this, they are still relatively rare. In many, but not all states in the United States and in several other countries, newborns are screened for a number of metabolic disorders for which early identification and treatment is often successful in preventing irreversible injury.

Aminoacidopathies: Amino acids are components of protein. Disorders of the breakdown of many different amino acids have been identified. The features vary, once again depending on the type and specific toxicity of the compounds involved.

One of the best known of the aminoacidopathies is phenylketonuria (PKU), which results from the inability to break down the amino acid phenylalanine. It causes seizures, mental retardation (often with autistic features), and spastic cerebral palsy. Features worsen with age. However, treatment in the newborn period with a diet low in phenylalanine is effective in preventing these features from developing in most patients. Diet is generally suggested for life, though the risk for development of severe features decreases after childhood when brain development is occurring. However, decreases in IQ have been reported even in adults with PKU who go off of diet. Women with PKU who become pregnant put their children at risk for birth defects and mental retardation if they do not follow the diet strictly during pregnancy.

Urea cycle defects: Organic acidemias involve the metabolism of certain amino acids and fats, which become acids in their breakdown processes. In these disorders, children typically have episodic symptoms, often with catastrophic outcome due to the buildup of large amounts of acid, and often ammonia, in the blood. In the disorders involving fat metabolism hypoglycemia is typical. Symptoms often occur in the early newborn period, with an illness, or with a fast when our bodies are actively trying to break down these substances for energy. Many die during this first episode.

Most of these children have very little enzyme and symptoms occur very early and are not likely to be misdiagnosed as cerebral palsy. However, there are children with some functional enzyme who have milder symptoms. These children may have unexplained vomiting, poor growth, and developmental delays. Presumably, they are experiencing high acid levels, ammonia levels and/or hypoglycemia episodically, but to a lesser degree than those with very little enzyme. Often, the abnormalities go unrecognized, and developmental delays and even cerebral palsy worsen over time, as these children may lose developmental skills with illnesses. These children may eventually be diagnosed when a more severe illness or a prolonged fast causes what little enzyme they have to be overwhelmed and the classic severe symptoms develop.

Diets limited in certain amino acids, the provision of vitamins or cofactors to aid in the function of any available enzyme, and the avoidance of fasting in the fatty acid disorders, can help to prevent or limit the injury in these disorders. For several of the fat metabolism disorders, children may be healthy and developmentally normal if these measures are taken early.

Energy production disorders: Energy production disorders involve enzymes that convert the foods we eat into a useable form of energy for our bodies. Protein, fat, and carbohydrates all require breakdown by specific enzyme pathways such as those mentioned above. However, all utilize a final shared pathway of enzymes to finally generate energy.

These disorders may be similar to the organic acidemias in that the most severely affected children often become ill at or shortly after birth. Others, typically those with more enzyme, may have episodic symptoms, usually, but not always associated with high levels of the acids lactate and often pyruvate. In some of these disorders, children have specific symptoms during episodes, such as ataxia (discoordinated walking), confusion, and liver abnormalities. Like in the organic acidemias, they often display slow regression in skills over time with a picture of cerebral palsy and mental retardation.

Lysosomal storage diseases: Lysosomal storage diseases comprise a number of hereditary diseases marked by deficiencies of enzymes involved in the metabolism of complex lipids involved in the formation of the membranes that surround cells. These enzymes are housed in organelles within the cells called lysosomes. They result in accumulation of the unmetabolized or poorly metabolized compounds trapped inside the lysosomes. Unlike the organic and amino acid disorders, these accumulated materials cannot easily get out of cells. As they build up in higher and higher quantities, they cause the cells to swell and impair their function.

Some of these disorders primarily involve cells in the central nervous system such as Tay-Sachs disease. Others can involve other organs such as the bone marrow, heart valves, liver, spleen, and the soft tissues such as skin, tendons, and airways. Hurler syndrome and Hunter syndrome are the best known of this type. Children may be mistaken early on as having cerebral palsy because joints become tight and fixed due to storage in the tissues around them, and mental retardation is common. An enlarged liver and or spleen, and a "coarsening" of the facial features due to thickening of the skin, as well as a course of regression in development are clues to the diagnosis. Over time, these disorders worsen; death usually occurs in childhood. No treatment has been available until recently. Currently, intravenous infusion of the missing enzyme is available for some, but not all of these disorders.

Peroxisomal disorders: Peroxisomes are similar to lysosomes in that they house certain enzymes in our cells. Most peroxisomal enzymes are involved in fat metabolism or in making components of cell membranes. When one or more enzymes are deficient, neurological problems are typical such as low muscle tone, hearing loss, seizures, and mental retardation. Some children have unusual facial features, short limbs, and unusual findings in their bones on x-ray. Depending on the enzyme affected, the liver may become enlarged and function poorly. Cataracts and other eye abnormalities can be seen. Because low muscle tone is usually present at birth, these children may be presumed to have CP until other features develop. Unlike the energy production or organic acid disorders, these children typically do not have episodic symptoms, but their course is progressive and usually leads to early death.

X-linked adrenoleukodystrophy (XALD) is one such disease. It involves a peroxisomal enzyme necessary to break down a particular form of fat. Onset of symptoms in most cases is between 5 and 10 years of age, with behavioral changes (often tantrums, irritability) and then regression in motor skills, which is severe and involves the white matter of the brain.

Disorders of glycoprotein metabolism: Disorders of glycoprotein metabolism (also known as carbohydrate-deficient glycoprotein syndrome or CDG) are a relatively newly identified group of disorders with a very broad range of symptoms. Glycoproteins are chemicals that activate or depress the brain and nervous system, the clotting components of the blood, and hormones to name a few of their functions. Many enzymes involved in making the glycol or carbohydrate portion of glycoproteins have been found to be deficient. For this reason, there have been varying symptoms in this disorder. Liver disease, seizures, bleeding and clotting problems, poor control of blood sugar with hypoglycemia or hyperglycemia have been seen, along with spasticity and all ranges of developmental delay. Some patients have one or more symptoms. Those children with spasticity may be mistaken for having cerebral palsy. The presence of more than one unexplained feature of this disorder, such as a clotting problem, with CP would make consultation with a metabolic specialist worthwhile to consider CDG.

Cholesterol metabolism disorders: The best known syndrome in this group is the Smith-Lemli-Opitz syndrome (SLOS). Typical children have an unusual pattern of facial features, limb abnormalities, cataracts, malformations of the genitals, kidneys, and brain, growth retardation from very early on, mental retardation, and spasticity. Within the past few years, SLOS has been found to be caused by an enzyme defect causing impaired cholesterol formation, which affects the child's development in the womb. Indeed, these children often have very low cholesterol levels in their blood.

A blood test has been developed to detect SLOS, and as is often the case, once we have a test for a disorder, we come to know the full range of features. Children have been found to have the disorder who have only mild developmental delays. Cerebral palsy could be an accompanying feature in a mildly affected child with presumably more functional enzyme than the classically affected children. Very high doses of cholesterol in the diet have been associated with some measurable improvements in some studies.

Purine and pyrimidine disorders: Purines and pyrimidines are components of DNA. Purines are important in energy transfer. Deficiency of several of the enzymes involved in purine metabolism can cause hypotonia and other neurologic problems. Seizures, growth problems, muscle weakness, and unusual problems such as recurrent infections, kidney stones, and symptoms of gout may be seen in some of these disorders. Of this group of disorders, the best known is Lesch-Nyhan disease. Children tend to be normal at birth. Often within the first year, spasticity and severe choreoathetosis (involuntary movements of the face, tongue, and limbs) develop. Seizures are quite common and a very distinct involuntary self-destructive biting of the fingers, arms, and lips is seen. Many children have mental retardation, but normal intelligence can be seen. High uric acid levels can lead to kidney stones and kidney disease, though not typically to gout. Drugs such as valium may help with the self-mutilation but are not a cure.

Pyrimidine disorders typically have more nonspecific features such as spasticity, growth retardation, and seizures. Some types have an unusual anemia and autistic features have been seen.

Microcephaly

Microcephaly is the term used when a child's head circumference is more than two standard deviations below the mean measurement for children of the same age and gender. Normally the circumference of the head is measured on a regular basis, during the first few years of life during a pediatrician's routine exam and beyond that age if there is a problem. While there are genetic conditions leading to microcephaly without any brain damage, usually microcephaly reflects poor brain growth from some damage to the brain, such as an intrauterine infection, severe hypoxia at birth, or meningitis during infancy. Those with the severest forms of microcephaly are usually severely retarded, and many others may have spastic cerebral palsy.

Motor Synergy

(co-contraction of muscles)

Motor synergy, or co-contraction of the muscles, means that muscles that have opposite functions contract at the same time. For example, the quadriceps muscles on the front of the thigh may contract at the same time as the hamstring muscles behind the thigh. Therefore, neither muscle is able to function upon the knee to cause it to bend, and the net result is a stiff knee. Although this may feel similar to spasticity, motor synergy usually occurs with specific activities, such as walking. During walking, the muscle contracts at inappropriate times, so the muscle, which normally would not be contracting, is actively blocking the normal joint movement.

Exaggerated muscle synergy is a significant problem for many children with cerebral palsy. Treating the underlying spasticity will not stop muscle synergy, although physical therapy to improve muscle coordination and to develop the ability to control these co-contractions is often beneficial. With appropriate treatment, a child's muscles will continue to improve until the age of 8 or 10. With gait analysis, the specific contraction patterns can be identified, and occasionally a muscle can be moved into an area where it functions appropriately, such as with the rectus and hamstring muscles.

Movement Disorders

This term is used to describe various abnormalities of movement. They are divided into different types, based on the kind of movement that is seen.

Ballismus: Ballismus involves extremely large recurrent, rapid, flapping, involuntary violent movements of the arms, often in a circular pattern, but may occasionally involve the legs as well. These appear to be large flailing movements which may be so eruptive and strong that they throw the person off balance and cause him to fall. This movement disorder is extremely rare and can be very difficult to control when it is present. The prime treatment is a neurosurgical procedure on the brain to remove the part of the brain that controls this type of movement. In the early stages this movement disorder may look like athetoid cerebral palsy; however, unlike CP, ballismus gets progressively worse.

Chorea: Chorea is a movement disorder that primarily involves the distal joints, mostly toes and fingers. It is characterized by small, irregular, nonstereotyped jerky types of movements. These small, uncontrolled dancing movements cannot be controlled very well and usually cause significant problems with fine motor control. Unlike tics, they cannot be voluntarily suppressed. Although similar movements occur in children with cerebral palsy, CP is rarely the main component of the movement disorder.

Dystonia: Dystonia is a movement disorder involving prolonged muscle contractions that may cause twisting and repetitive movements or abnormal posture. Usually, the arm is drawn up and may be held in the air in a flexed position, and sometimes the face or neck is affected, too. Dystonia may also involve the legs. When a child first shows signs of having dystonia, contractures do not develop; over long periods of time, however, the muscle becomes contracted from remaining in the same position. Generally, the body relaxes when the person sleeps or is at rest. Dystonic movements may then occur when movement is initiated, producing "motor overflow."

The treatments for dystonia include medications and nerve injections. The drug Artane is usually used but does not often effectively reduce the abnormal movement. Botulinum toxin injections work well for small muscles around the neck, face, and eyelids. Surgical releases of dystonic muscles can be very unpredictable, and, even without treatment, one dystonia pattern can suddenly change into another one.

This pattern change may mean that suddenly the problem that had predominantly affected one arm may start affecting a foot. More commonly, however, it means that the arm or foot was twisted in a way that pulled it into flexion, and then suddenly it switches so that the arm is held in extension. When a child with dystonia is seen briefly by a physician, the posture may look like typical hemiplegic pattern cerebral palsy. Based on one short examination, a mistake can be made that could lead to very bad outcomes following surgical procedures.

There are certain components of this pattern, however, which should not be missed, such as the relatively little amount of muscle contracture which is usually present and the postural changes that the family may complaint about. Dystonia may be present without significant changes over many years; however, some children get progressively worse over a matter of four or five years.

Tics: Motor tics are abnormal movements that tend to be frequently repeated and usually follow the same pattern. Examples of motor tics include sniffling, swallowing, throat clearing, coughing, eye blinking, facial grimacing, or neck stretching. In fact, any part of the body may become involved. However, most individuals who experience such tics do so only for a short time, and only 10 percent of the population may experience a tic lasting one month or more. Usually the onset is during childhood or early adolescence, with the transient tic disorder lasting anywhere from one month to one year, beyond which time it is considered to be a chronic tic disorder.

In addition to motor tics the child may have vocal tics as well, such as grunts, barks, or clearly articulated words and phrases. When words or phrases are used as part of a tic, this often leads to the diagnosis of Gilles de la Tourette syndrome. Although tics are not a sign of cerebral palsy, tics occur more frequently in children with CP.

Muscular Dystrophy

Muscular dystrophy: The muscular dystrophies are a group of disorders that cause progressive weakness of muscle. They are divided into various types based on the physical features an individual presents with, the severity of weakness, the characteristics of the muscle when looked at under a microscope, and how they are inherited. There are a number of genes which are now known to cause different forms of muscular dystrophy. One of the most common forms is Duchenne muscular dystrophy. This form is characterized by progressive weakness of muscles throughout the body due to a deficiency of a protein called dystrophin in the muscle itself. Boys are mainly affected because the gene for this disorder is located on the X chromosome which they receive from their mother. Genetic counseling is indicated in families with a member identified as having muscular dystrophy. Boys are usually diagnosed between the ages of 3 and 5 because of problems with walking, running, and frequent falls. These symptoms can also be seen in cerebral palsy. However, these children have a very typical pattern of walking and rising from a seated position. When these signs and symptoms are seen, a blood test for a muscle enzyme called creatine kinase (CK) may be done. CK is significantly elevated in Duchenne muscular dystrophy and usually elevated in the other forms of muscular dystrophy as well. If CK is elevated, genetic testing or muscle biopsy may be recommended to confirm the diagnosis. The weakness in Duchenne is progressive and most children are wheelchair bound between the ages of 8 and 12. The respiratory muscles and the heart are affected as well and the cause of death is usually from complications with their breathing or heart function in the late teens or twenties. Progress in managing these problems has improved the quality of life for individuals with this disease.

The various forms of muscular dystrophy can have a wide range of variability in terms of the severity of the disease. Issues such as muscle contractures and scoliosis need to be addressed as they are in cerebral palsy.

Myopathy

Myopathy is a family of diseases described by muscle weakness based on underlying muscle (not nerve) problems, most of which are quite rare. However, a child with a myopathy can appear very similar to one with hypotonia, which can be an early symptom of cerebral palsy. Thus, a child with a myopathy may initially be thought to have CP. There are often specific congenital errors of metabolism or metabolic problems that cause the myopathy. The term is used in association with many different diseases whose symptoms vary from only mild weakness to severe weakness at birth and a short life expectancy. The causes of myopathies vary; specific causes should be investigated, because some forms can be treated with medications and significantly improved. The treatment is dependent on making a specific diagnosis; once a specific diagnosis is made, genetic counseling is usually indicated.

Myositis Ossificans

Myositis ossificans is inflammation of muscle tissues, especially voluntary muscles, in which bone forms in muscles or soft tissue where it is not supposed to. Rarely, the cause of this abnormal bone formation is genetic, but by far the most common cause of myositis ossificans is a head injury. Typically, extra bone forms in the first 2 to 6 months after the injury, then gradually subsides as the child becomes more functional. In rare situations, bone may form in the muscles of children with cerebral palsy who have had their muscles lengthened, and there have been reports of children developing bone formation around the hip after spinal fusions or other large surgeries. Usually, however, the bone slowly resorbs after its initial development. With a small group of children, the bone formation is so excessive that it completely fuses the hip joint or the elbow joint. It is rare around the knee and rare around the shoulder but may occur at these joints, as well.

Care and treatment: The typical treatment is gentle physical therapy focusing on range of motion, coupled with anti-inflammatory medications. In rare situations, after physical therapy has been completed and a year or so has passed, surgical excision of this bone may be attempted. If a surgical procedure is done, the child needs radiation treatment to prevent the bone from reforming.

Neural Tube Defects

(anencephaly, encephalocele, spina bifida, meningocele, myelomeningocele)

The term "neural tube defects" (NTDs) refers to a group of malformations of the spinal cord, brain, and vertebrae that occur during early pregnancy.

The three major forms of neural tube defects are spina bifida, encephalocele, and anencephaly. The most common form is spina bifida, which is the second most common disability in childhood after cerebral palsy. Spina bifida occulta is the most common and also the most benign form. This form involves a defect in the vertebrae only, with no protrusion of spinal cord tissue or of the meninges (the membrane tissue covering the cord). Meningocele involves a defect in the vertebrae with protrusion of meninges, while protrusion of both meninges and malformed spinal cord tissue through the bony defect is called mylomeningocele. The defect is most common in the lumbar or lumbosacral area, though it can be anywhere along the spinal cord.

Ninety percent or more of those with lumbosacral myelomeningocele also have hydrocephalus (increased fluid on the brain) and Arnold-Chiari malformations (improper folding of the base of the brain). An infant with a meningocele has little to no central nervous system malformation, rarely develops hydrocephalus, and usually has a normal neurological examination. Those with myelomeningocele, depending on the level of the lesion, are often paraplegic, incontinent for urine and stool, and have various abnormalities of the genitourinary tract, which can lead to infections and kidney damage.

The other two forms of neural tube defect are both more severe but less common. Encephalocele refers to malformation of the skull through which a portion of the brain protrudes. Affected children have mental retardation, hydrocephalus, spastic weakness in their legs more than their arms, and seizures. Anencephaly refers to an even more severe malformation of the skull and brain with no brain tissue developing above the brainstem. About half of these fetuses are spontaneously aborted. Infants born with anencephaly do not survive beyond the first few days to weeks of life.

While the cause of neural tube defects is not fully understood, a high percentage seem to be caused by a deficiency of folic acid. Doctors recommend that women who are contemplating becoming pregnant should begin prenatal vitamins, including 400 micrograms of folic acid, before they conceive, or as early in pregnancy as possible.

Although children with spinal cord deformities are similar to children with cerebral palsy in that both must cope with a major disability, children with paralysis from spinal cord deformities have problems unique to their condition. On the surface, their problems appear similar to those seen in children with cerebral palsy; however, in general the medical and long-term care is different and should not be confused.

Children with paralysis have no sensation in the paralyzed area, which puts them at great risk for developing skin ulcers from high pressure on the skin. A second major difference is that the bowel and bladder are paralyzed, which means that they must follow a very specific bowel program and the bladder must be managed with a catheter. Repeated bladder and kidney infections can lead to kidney failure. Increasing spasticity may also be caused by the spinal cord being caught as a result of the child's growth or being scarred down in the congenital deformity. Often these children combine severe leg weakness with good arm strength. This allows them to walk with special long leg braces, but the type of braces used for children with spinal paralysis often differs from those used with children with cerebral palsy. Children with CP also seldom have a paralyzed bowel and bladder or insensate skin.

Neurofibromatosis

In this genetically inherited disease, the nerves develop large, tumorlike lesions. There are brown spots on the skin called cafe au lait spots and some underlying nerves are enlarged. Neurofibromatosis may be severe, involving significant distortion of the face and head, and some people develop severe tumors causing blindness and retardation. If a child shows retardation or a gait disturbance, he or she may initially be thought to have cerebral palsy instead of neurofibromatosis. If a parent has neurofibromatosis, there is a 50 percent chance that any child of that parent will also have it. The treatment involves removing very large neurofibroma lesions that cause difficulty with leg movement or that are painful. Sometimes radiation or chemotherapy are used to decrease the size of the growths. Genetic counseling is indicated for parents and for anyone with the disease who is contemplating having a child.

Neurogenic Bladder

Neurogenic bladder means a bladder that is functioning abnormally because of damage to the nerves that control bladder function. Since cerebral palsy affects the brain above the spinal cord, if there is bladder dysfunction, it is of the upper motor neuron type. This means that the bladder will most likely be spastic and the sphincter tone abnormally increased, with uninhibited contractions. The sphincters may contract tightly but are not under normal voluntary control. This means that the bladder may frequently empty, even when not full, and at times not convenient for the child.

Care and treatment: Treatment, under the care of a urologist, is based on urodynamic findings. Anticholinergic medications are often used to minimize uninhibited contractions, the most common of which is oxybutynin (or Ditropan).

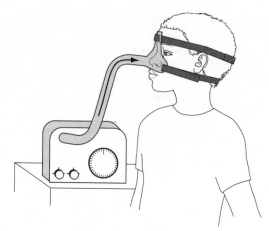

Nystagmus

Spasticity may cause the eyes to have a rhythmic jerking or jumping movement, called nystagmus. Nystagmus appears in several forms: in vertical nystagmus, the eye moves up and down; in horizontal nystagmus, it moves sideways; in rotary nystagmus, it tends to move around in a circle. Nystagmus is frequently triggered by a certain gaze, such as gazing up or to one side. Because position orientation often initiates nystagmus, many children learn to control it by avoiding looking in those directions.

Care and treatment: It is difficult to treat nystagmus when it is consistent and significant, and it may cause difficulty with eyesight. Children with cerebral palsy may have nystagmus, which causes significant problems for fine eye movement skills such as eye tracking, which is required for reading. Sometimes the nystagmus can be suppressed by immobilizing the head or preventing some head movement. Trial-and-error investigation with the individual child is required to determine what works best.

Obstructive Sleep Apnea

Obstructive apnea occurs when, despite breathing movements, no air flows in or out of the lungs. Obstructive apnea is different from central apnea in that during a central apnea event, no breathing efforts or airflow is apparent. Obstructive sleep apnea occurs when there are episodes of obstructive apnea during sleep.

Despite the impression that snoring, restless sleep, and sleep apnea are adult problems, obstructive sleep apnea is actually common in children. Snoring, the most common symptom of obstructive sleep apnea, occurs frequently in children as well. It is estimated that up to 10–12 percent of children snore and that up to 1–3 percent of healthy pre-

school children have obstructive sleep apnea. Obstructive sleep apnea is much more common in children with abnormal muscle tone (such as those with cerebral palsy), as well as those with muscle diseases or abnormalities of the upper airway or the skull bones (craniofacial abnormalities).

Symptoms of obstructive sleep apnea include snoring and labored breathing during sleep. Family members might notice the child's chest caving in or abdomen (belly) moving vigorously during sleep. Sometimes the child may actually gasp for air and arouse or seem to wake up during these episodes of labored breathing. Color changes may occur as well. Some children sleep in unusual positions, with the neck extended or may even sleep sitting up.

It is important to remember that even in children with severe symptoms at night, breathing is usually normal during the day. Some children will be congested or be chronic mouth breathers, while others (most) will have no symptoms at all.

When breathing is labored at night and sleep is disrupted, behavioral symptoms or excessive daytime sleepiness can result. Some children with obstructive sleep apnea and severely disrupted sleep may be hyperactive and there is growing evidence that school performance or learning can be affected by poor sleep quality. Sleep disruption can occur in obstructive sleep apnea for several reasons including the natural "arousal" response to airway obstruction and to abnormalities of the blood oxygen or carbon dioxide level. A pattern of disrupted sleep may occur many times during the night, resulting in inefficient, poor-quality sleep. Other night time symptoms can include bedwetting, sweating and of course, snoring and labored breathing.

Other than behavioral and learning difficulties, obstructive sleep apnea can have other effects as well. In severe cases it can lead to growth failure (failure to thrive), hypertension, and, even less commonly, heart failure.

Taking a careful sleep history and doing a sleep study to detect the presence of obstructive apnea help diagnose obstructive sleep apnea. A sleep study is a test that is safe, painless, and highly accurate in making the diagnosis. In all cases a careful airway evaluation is indicated, since in otherwise healthy children, the most common cause of obstructive sleep apnea is enlargement of the tonsils and adenoids, and removal of the tonsils and adenoids almost always cures the sleep apnea. In children with cerebral palsy however, abnormal muscle tone may be the major problem and this is more difficult to overcome. Treatment may be tried with continuous or bilevel positive airway pressure (CPAP or BiPAP®), supplemental oxygen or rarely a tracheostomy.

Orthodontics

(malalignment of teeth)

Sometimes when a child's teeth come in, they don't meet each other in a way that best facilitates chewing and speech. Malaligned teeth can also spoil a person's appearance (this is more important to some people than to others).

Indications: Children with significant spasticity around the mouth are at risk of developing malaligned teeth from this abnormal pull. Treatment involves, first, deciding whether the malalignment presents a problem serious enough to require treatment. This determination involves considering the severity of the child's neurological defect as well as the potential effect on the child who must wear braces for several years.

For any brace to work, the child must be able to cooperate which may be very difficult for the child with spasticity, who may bite down every time something is put in his mouth. Other considerations are the family and child's concern about cosmetic appearance, the availability of an experienced orthodontist, and the willingness and ability of someone to pay for the treatment. While orthodontic treatment may be desirable, it should have relatively low priority on the list of health-care priorities established for an individual child. Certainly, other dental needs such as maintaining healthy gums and preventing and treating cavities are more important. Nevertheless, each child must be evaluated as a separate individual and his case considered with regard to other medical needs, family desires—and, most important, the child's desires.

Osteogenesis Imperfecta

Osteogenesis imperfecta is a genetic condition. A child with this condition has very fragile bones and suffers frequent fractures. There are a number of variations of this condition, the most severe of which occurs in children whose bones fracture even when the child is simply picked up. Many of these children live no more than several weeks because of their severe bone fragility. There are other children with osteogenesis imperfecta who essentially live normal lives except that they may have two or three fractures throughout their growing years. Many children must significantly limit their activity because of their bone fragility; nevertheless, they continue to walk—or they use wheelchairs part of the time.

Treatment with a class of medications called bisphosphonates has helped improve the bone density in these children, to the point that many of them are able to function far better and have far fewer fractures. The most commonly used medication has been Pamidronate, an intravenous form of bisphosphonate, which is given every 3–4 months for a number of years. As they go through adolescence and develop adult hormonal levels, the bone fragility diminishes significantly to the point that, as adults, they seldom have fractures. On the surface, many children with OI may seem similar to children with cerebral palsy. They may need to use braces, may have angular deformities, and may have difficulties with ambulation. However, children with OI always have normal balance, coordination, and muscle control, which are almost never present in children with CP.

Osteopenia

(low bone mineral density, osteoporosis)

Low bone mineral density, or osteopenia, in children is defined as a bone mineral density that is two standard deviations or more below the mean for age and gender. In adults, bone mineral density is compared with that of a 25-year-old woman as the standard, because that is the age at which bone mineral density peaks. The number of standard deviations above or below the mean is written in shorthand as a T-score. In children, the bone mineral density is compared with children of the same age and gender, and the number of standard deviations above or below the mean is referred to as a Z-score. Thus, a Z-score of −2.0 or lower is considered osteopenic, as the bone density is two or more standard deviations below the mean. The Z-score below which a child would be at risk for fractures, however, has not been defined.

A number of conditions in childhood can lead to osteopenia, such as osteogenesis imperfecta (OI), various medications (such as prednisone), and various conditions that lead to lack of weight bearing (such as astronauts in space). Those children with quadriplegic CP who are not able to walk and are primarily in wheelchairs for most of the day are at a very high risk to develop osteopenia. If, in addition, they are taking certain anticonvulsant medications that interfere with Vitamin D metabolism, such as phenobarbital or phenytoin, if they get little sun exposure, or if they are unable to eat adequate amounts of Vitamin D and calcium containing foods, then their risk is even greater. These children are then at risk for osteoporosis, at risk to develop nontraumatic or pathological fractures, meaning that their bones break from a degree of trauma that would not ordinarily cause a fracture. Such activities as dressing a child, or picking them up, can result in a fracture in children with severe osteoporosis.

As children with CP become young adults, the risk of osteopenia increases. Peak bone density occurs by age 25 for everyone and then begins to decrease over time. If these children have not built up their bone density sufficiently by that age, it will fall into the low range very quickly, thus exposing them to the risk of pathological fractures. We also know that once a child with CP has had a pathological fracture, her risk for having more such fractures increases significantly. Just as described for children with OI, children with quadriplegic CP who have developed severe osteoporosis and recurrent fractures, are being treated with a class of medications called bisphosphonates, which has been shown to improve their bone density, and hopefully will also decrease their risk of fractures.

Otoacoustic Emission Testing

Otoacoustic emission testing (OAE) is an objective method of ascertaining ear-specific hearing thresholds. The outer hair cells of a healthy cochlea actually both receive and *produce* sounds. A probe placed in the outer ear canal can measure these sounds. These sounds are produced spontaneously and can be elicited by a delivered sound. This enables an audiologist to place a small probe in a child's ear canal, deliver a sound, and measure the OAEs. If they are present, it typically signifies that the cochlea is healthy and hearing normally. Because the OAEs are very quiet, the child must be quiet or asleep during the test. OAEs are being used to screen hearing in young infants and children who cannot cooperate either because of age or disability, as it does not require any behavioral response on the part of the child.

If the audiologist cannot measure the OAEs this can mean that there is a hearing loss in the involved ear, but it could also mean that there is something blocking the sounds (like ear wax, fluid in the middle ear, etc.). Because of this, a child who "fails" his OAE test will often be examined by a pediatrician or an ear, nose and throat special-

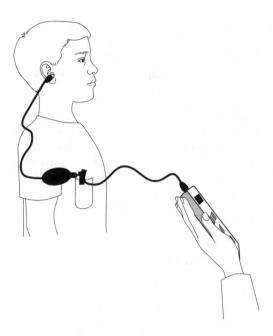

ist to be sure nothing is wrong with the outer or middle ear to prevent the sounds from being measured.

Pancreatitis

Pancreatitis is an inflammation of the pancreas that is characterized by abdominal pain, nausea, and vomiting and by an increase of the pancreatic enzymes, amylase and lipase. It is usually self-limiting. Some medications that can cause pancreatitis include valproic acid and certain diuretics. Pancreatitis can also be seen after a posterior spinal fusion, a surgical procedure used for the treatment of scoliosis, which results from the pancreas being trapped in front of the spine. Treatment includes: pain management and bowel rest for 1 to 2 weeks, while intravenous feedings are given. This is followed by a low-fat diet or placement of a special feeding tube beyond the stomach so that feedings are delivered into the small intestine, thus bypassing the pancreatic opening in the duodenum. The pancreatitis usually resolves between 4 and 6 weeks after the onset of the elevated enzymes.

Passive Motions

Passive motions are exercises performed upon a child without the child's assistance. Passive stretching involves someone else stretching a child's muscles. These are common exercises that physical therapists use for children with cerebral palsy.

Patellar Pain

(chondromalacia, stress fracture of the patella, Osgood-Schlatter disease, osteochondritis of the patella)

The patella is the kneecap. Patellar pain, or pain in the front of the knee, occurs in children with cerebral palsy, almost exclusively in those who walk with a severe crouched gait, due to hamstring tightness. Spasticity in the quadriceps muscle may also be present. Pain may be due to chondromalacia (excessive pressure behind the kneecap), stress fracture of the patellae, osteochondritis of the patella, and uncommonly, from instability (dislocation) of the patella. A child with a crouched gait stands with knees bent; the muscle in the front of the knee and kneecap is extremely tight, allowing him to stand. However, the large amount of pressure against the kneecap causes pain; if the pressure is great enough, it may cause a stress fracture through the bone and actually pull the patella apart. This pain can become quite severe, and if not treated properly may prevent the child from walking. This is especially true for children who develop stress fractures of the patella or significant stretching of the tendon.

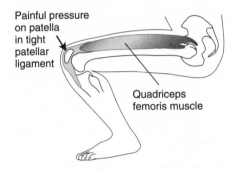

Painful pressure on patella in tight patellar ligament

Quadriceps femoris muscle

Osteochondrosis of the patella occurs if the tendon at the insertion in the patella pulls off. A similar situation, an inflammatory response called Osgood-Schlatter disease, occurs where the patellar tendon hooks onto the tibia. These are common problems in active, growing adolescents, and especially as well in children with cerebral palsy and spasticity. As the child continues to grow, both of these conditions eventually resolve if the stress is not too high.

Care and treatment: The treatment of a crouched gait, osteochondritis of the patella, and Osgood-Schlatter disease involves stretching the hamstrings in an attempt to get the child to stand up straighter and place less strain on the knees. If the knees cannot be adequately stretched out with physical therapy, surgical hamstring lengthening should be considered to get the child to stand up straighter. Stress fractures through the bone, causing the patella to pull apart, are treated with casting until healing occurs.

Instability of the patella may be caused by a combination of hamstring and quadriceps tightness, a high-riding patella (too highly placed on the knee), and torsional problems (external tibial torsion and femoral anteversion). Therapy to stretch and strengthen muscles should be attempted first but is often unsuccessful in the child with cerebral palsy. Chronic instability causing pain should be treated surgically by correcting the causes above if they are present.

Pelvic Osteotomy

(Chiari osteotomy, Salter osteotomy, Pemberton osteotomy, Dega osteotomy, acetabular shelf procedure)

The pelvic bone may be cut in a number of places, usually with the goal of redirecting or reshaping the acetabulum, which is the cup or socket part of the hip joint.

Indications: This procedure is performed on children with spastic hip disease because the socket is deformed from abnormal pressure and has not developed normally. The socket needs to be reshaped in order to provide better coverage if the hip is to stay in the socket.

The surgery: A variety of procedures have been developed (each named after the person who developed it), but each surgery involves making a cut in the pelvis above the hip joint socket, or the acetabulum. Briefly, the Chiari osteotomy involves cutting just above the socket straight across the pelvis and then sliding the pelvis in and allowing it to heal with a ledge over the socket. The Salter osteotomy involves a cut at approximately the same location, but instead a wedge of bone is placed into the cut in the pelvis and the pelvis is rotated forward. This operation is done for congenital hip dislocation but is not indicated for patients with cerebral palsy.

A Pemberton osteotomy involves a cut made in the front of the socket, which is then bent down and held in place with a block of bone. This procedure may be used for children with cerebral palsy, but is more commonly used for children with congenital hip dislocation. The Dega osteotomy is similar to the Pemberton, except that a cut is made halfway through the pelvis around the whole socket and the whole upper half of the socket is folded down and held with a wedge of bone. This procedure results in a useful reduction in the size of the acetabulum,

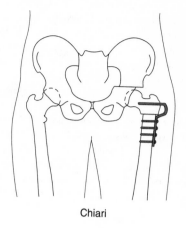

Chiari

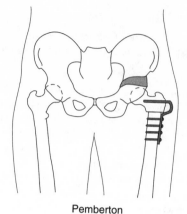

Pemberton

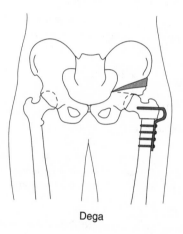

Dega

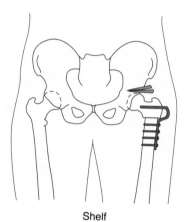

Shelf

and the acetabulum continues to grow well. The acetabular shelf procedure involves placing bone chips at the edge of the socket in an attempt to build a bigger socket. This may work well in children who are older, but if it is done on very young children it will completely stop the growth at the edge of the socket, causing the child to outgrow the socket.

After-surgery care: For those pelvic procedures that cut completely across the pelvis, such as the Chiari or Salter osteotomies, postsurgical treatment usually requires a hip spica cast. The acetabular shelf procedure requires healing to develop strength because the bone is not strong initially; therefore, it usually requires a cast as well. The Pemberton and Dega osteotomies can easily be done without using a cast. If no cast is used, the child may return to full weightbearing for walking or to full physical therapy. Casts, when used, are needed for 6 to 12 weeks, followed by extensive physical therapy because stiffness has devel-

oped. If no cast is used, full activity is usually resumed by 4 to 6 weeks after surgery.

What to expect: There may be difficulty in healing after the Chiari and Salter osteotomies, and the shelf procedure may be absorbed by the child's body or may destroy growth so that there is no further improvement after the operation. The Pemberton and Dega procedures may cause the joint to fracture or the bone wedge to be displaced. Generally, however, one can expect that the socket will successfully hold the ball of the hip joint.

Perseveration

When an activity is repeated over and over, it is called perseveration. Perseveration is a common symptom in children with mild to moderate mental retardation, who may become fixated on one concern and continue to pursue and talk about only that. This can be an annoying problem for caregivers. Behavior modification techniques that fail to reward the child for continued perseveration should be attempted as a form of treatment. This involves verbally disciplining the child to stop that focus, and then redirecting his or her thoughts to a different activity.

Pneumonia

Pneumonia, or pneumonitis, means inflammation of the lung, primarily caused by infection. The diagnosis of pneumonia is usually a clinical one, with fever, increased respiratory rate, retractions of the chest wall muscles, and, if measured, a drop in the oxygen saturation in the blood. Often a chest x-ray is done to confirm this clinical impression. The infection is most commonly either viral or bacterial, though some cases of infectious pneumonia can be caused by fungi. In children with CP, many cases of pneumonia are caused by aspiration of material from the throat, causing either infectious or chemical pneumonitis.

Most of the pneumonias in infancy are of viral origin. Bacterial infections are treated with antibiotics, whereas viral infections usually are not. Aspiration pneumonia is usually treated with antibiotics to prevent either a primary infection caused by whatever was aspirated, or by a super-infection, which is a bacterial infection that follows injury to the lung caused by the aspiration.

Children with CP, who also have problems with their swallowing, are much more likely to aspirate their own saliva, food that they are eating, or stomach acid and food that may be refluxing from their stomach. The resulting pneumonia can be quite severe, but sometimes children have mild subclinical symptoms on a chronic basis, such as chronic wheezing or congestion without typical symptoms of fever and respiratory distress.

If the child is not having severe respiratory distress, he or she can often be treated as an outpatient with oral antibiotics if there is a suspicion of bacterial infection. If the pneumonia is felt to be viral, such as that caused by influenza or RSV, then antibiotics are of no help and treatment is of the symptoms alone, such as Tylenol for fever and nebulized medications for wheezing. For children with more significant respiratory symptoms, admission to the hospital and treatment with intravenous antibiotics is often necessary, and for severe respiratory distress some children may end up in the intensive care unit on a ventilator. While an acute episode of pneumonia can happen to any child, a history of two or three such episodes in a child with CP would make one very suspicious that the child is aspirating and needs some investigation to see if there is either severe reflux or aspiration of food or secretions from the mouth.

Porencephalic Cyst

A porencephalic cyst within the brain results from the breakdown of dead brain tissue. These cysts usually result from an acute trauma to the brain, such as a stroke or an infection, during late fetal or early infant life. Sometimes they cause no problems at all, and the child develops normally. Other times they can cause neurological deficits localized to one limb or side. Porencephalic cysts are quite common in children with cerebral palsy. These cysts sometimes progressively enlarge and eventually impinge on the ventricles (the fluid cavities) of the brain, causing hydrocephalus, which is the increased accumulation of cerebrospinal fluid within the ventricles. Shunt surgery may be indicated in the unusual circumstance that porencephaly is causing abnormal enlargement of the head and progressive loss of motor skills.

Prematurity

The normal gestational period is considered 40 weeks from the first day of the mother's last menstrual period. By definition, normal gestation can vary by two weeks, that is, anywhere from 38 to 42 weeks. Prematurity is defined as birth before 38 weeks. Many children with cerebral palsy were born prematurely. Being born prematurely puts the child at risk for a variety of medical and neurological problems. However, with the improved care for premature infants that is delivered in intensive care nurseries, many of these problems are now rare except in the smallest of premature babies. Those born between 24 and 32 weeks of gestation are at the highest risk for CP, attention deficit disorder, and various learning disorders, with the most immature infants at the greatest risk.

Pressure Mapping

Children who do not have normal movement ability often develop pressure sores, also called bedsores or decubitus ulcers. This skin breakdown occurs because of too much pressure over too long a period. A tool that is used to determine where this high pressure is coming from is the pressure-mapping mat. This is a soft mat or blanket with sensors embedded in it to measure the pressure when the child sits or lies on it. The mat is attached to a computer, which shows an image of the contact area and measures the amount of pressure in any small area.

The pressure mat can be used in a wheelchair to see whether there is a problem with the seat back or the seat that is causing the skin ulcer. It can also be placed under the child while the child is lying to see if the pressure is caused

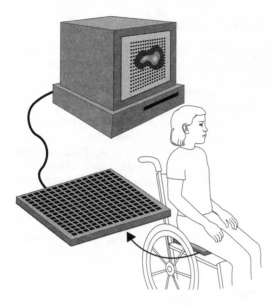

by a specific position. Pressure mapping is an important part of the treatment of pressure sores, since the goal of treatment should be not only to heal the sore, but also to determine what caused it, and hopefully prevent it from happening again.

Psychological Evaluation

Psychological evaluations typically include various testing activities, an interview with parents or guardians regarding a child's history, and direct observations. Teacher interviews, behavioral/social-emotional rating scales, developmental questionnaires, and a review of relevant medical and/or educational records are also often completed. Testing activities can involve a variety of problem-solving tasks including answering questions, hands-on activities, using a computer, and paper and pencil tasks. A comprehensive psychological evaluation could provide information regarding a child's intellectual abilities, learning and memory, attention and executive functioning (organization, planning, self-monitoring, cognitive flexibility), language, academic achievement, motor coordination, behavioral and emotional functioning, and/or general adaptive behavior.

Children with cerebral palsy, however, often present with unique testing requirements. Sensory, motor, or language limitations may make it difficult to utilize common standardized measures. For example, a child with manual motor difficulties may find it difficult to efficiently complete a timed activity requiring motor skills. Children with limited language may find it challenging to produce verbal

responses reflective of their knowledge or problem-solving capabilities. This makes it difficult to ascertain whether a weakness is due to a cognitive or an output deficit. Further complicating testing with children with cerebral palsy is the way that tests are normed. Standardized norm-referenced assessment measures require a "standard" administration to allow comparison with appropriate age norms. While many children with cerebral palsy have adequate expressive language capabilities and motor skills, others do not and require modified testing activities. This makes some psychological findings difficult to interpret. Yet, with a skilled evaluator, many assessment measures can be "adapted" to provide a reasonably reliable and valid indication of a child's capabilities. For example, nonverbal measures of reasoning and problem solving can be utilized when there is limited speech output. Many of these measures also allow for creative administration methods and response modes, so that the clinician has a better understanding of a child's capabilities. In addition to nonverbal assessment techniques, evaluators can choose test measures that allow pointing, multiple choice formats, voice output devices, or other forms of technology. Sometimes having a child's teacher, aide, or parent participate in the evaluation makes for the most comfortable environment in which the child's skills can be demonstrated.

Quadriplegia

(pentaplegia, total body involvement)

The term quadriplegia is used for children with cerebral palsy when all four limbs are involved, with difficulty in motor control and tone imbalance. Occasionally, the term pentaplegia is used for those people who also have significant difficulty with motor control of the face or head. Another commonly used term is total body involvement, which also implies difficulty with motor control of the face, head, and neck, in addition to the four limbs. All of these terms may be used interchangeably and do not have strict independent meaning.

Rectus Femoris Transfer

(rectus femoris release, stiff leg walk, knee extension contracture, quadriceps contracture)

When spasticity in a child involves the quadriceps muscle (the large muscle in the front of the thigh), the rectus femoris muscle, which lies across the front of the knee, is usually responsible. Spasticity of the rectus muscle causes stiff knee. The knee can be stiff when the child walks, specifically as he picks up his foot and attempts to bend his

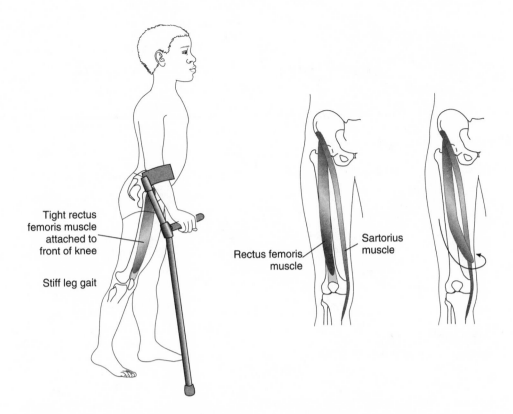

Tight rectus femoris muscle attached to front of knee

Stiff leg gait

Rectus femoris muscle

Sartorius muscle

knee to swing the foot forward, which causes a stiff-legged gait; or the knee may be completely incapable of bending, causing difficulty sitting. If someone is unable to bend the knee in order to sit in a wheelchair, then the leg sticks out in front.

Care and treatment: Initially, treatment for spasticity of the rectus muscle should involve stretching exercises, which frequently aid problems with seating. However, walking typically does not help in stretching this muscle when it is tight. Surgical lengthening or transfer of this muscle is the most common treatment of this problem, but it is usually not an isolated procedure. Instead, it is part of a number of other surgical procedures that improve the gait or the ability to sit.

The surgery: The procedure is done at the knee; it involves defining the rectus muscle and separating it from the three other muscles. It may simply be lengthened and allowed to slide; however, the muscle usually reattaches and becomes a problem again. Instead, the operation should involve transferring the muscle to the inside of the thigh and attaching the tendon to the sartorius or semitendinous muscles. This transfer helps the hamstrings to bend the knee. Some surgeons transfer the rectus muscle

to the outside of the knee to control rotational problems of the legs; the outcome of this procedure is unpredictable—though it is generally unsuccessful. This same procedure is done for those patients who have difficulty bending the knee enough to sit. Some severely involved patients require lengthening the three muscles underlying the rectus muscle; this should be done if the knees do not bend.

Benefits and risks: The major benefit lies in reducing spasticity in the rectus muscle. The complications from this surgery are minor, and the risk of overlengthening to the point of developing the opposite deformity is minimal. Treatment after this surgery may involve the use of a cast for two to four weeks; alternatively, no casting may be used.

Reflexes

(normal postural reflexes, primitive reflexes, deep tendon reflexes)

The function of the central nervous system with respect to motor behavior is coordinating the ability to move while maintaining posture and equilibrium. Every movement and change in posture produces a shift in the relationship

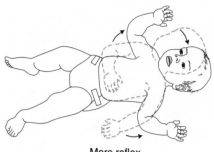

Moro reflex

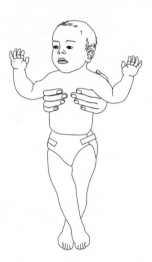

Palmar grasp reflex

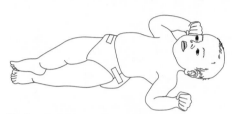

Tonic labyrinthine reflex (supine)

Crossed extension reflex

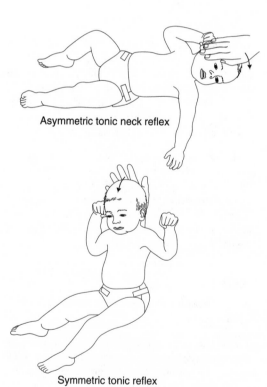

Asymmetric tonic neck reflex

Symmetric tonic reflex

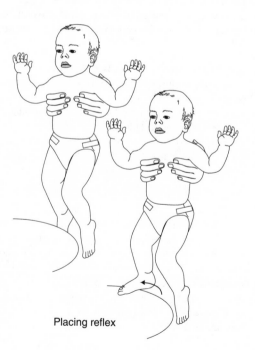

Placing reflex

of the body to the ground. Therefore, if we are not to fall, there must be a fluctuation of tone throughout the musculature to maintain our balance while moving. These changes and patterns, known as normal postural reflexes, are brought about automatically. These reactions can be grouped as *righting reactions* and *equilibrium reactions*. Righting reactions are automatic but active responses — they maintain the normal position of the head in space and the normal alignment of the head and neck with the trunk and of the trunk with the limbs. Equilibrium reactions restore balance through complex responses to changes of posture and movement. They show themselves in slight changes of tone throughout the muscles and by visible counter movements to restore the disturbed balance. These reactions are needed to maintain balance and thus to achieve, first, sitting balance, and later the ability to stand and to walk.

In the child with cerebral palsy, the delay or interference with the development of these reactions causes delay in achievement of these motor abilities. The three main reasons for the delay in the appearance of the righting and equilibrium responses are the persistence of primitive reflexes past the age at which they are normally present, the presence of a primitive reflex to an abnormal degree, and the presence of hypotonia (low tone). All three factors are present to some degree in cerebral palsy. The postural reflexes do not usually appear until the latter half of the first year, that is between 6 and 12 months of age. They include the neck-righting reaction and the labyrinthine-righting reaction, among others. The parachute reaction is an equilibrium reaction that is often looked at clinically, because it is delayed or asymmetrical in cerebral palsy. (The parachute reaction is what should happen when the child is thrust head first toward the examining table: she should extend both arms in front as if to break the fall.)

Primitive reflexes (see pages 438, 440–1) are essentially brainstem-mediated responses that develop during fetal life and are present at birth. The majority of them disappear between 3 and 6 months of age. At any age, if a primitive reflex is obligatory, it is always considered pathological because it signifies the presence of a motor disability, most likely cerebral palsy. A primitive reflex is described as obligatory if the reflex is sustained for more than 30 seconds and head movements control both upper and lower extremity positioning, with the child unable to break out of the pattern, even with crying. *Absence* of reflex activity at a time when it is normally present is also an important indicator: it may reflect generalized hypotonia that could be secondary to severe central nervous system dysfunction. Asymmetry of these reflexes (that is, an abnormal reflex on one side of the body and a normal one on the other) is ab-

normal and may indicate developing hemiplegia. Discrepancy between upper and lower extremity activity may aid in the subclassification of cerebral palsy.

Deep tendon reflexes are stretching reflexes in which the muscles are suddenly stretched by a sudden tap with a finger or rubber hammer. In a medical examination, these reflexes are tested at the knees, ankles, elbows, and wrists. In people with cerebral palsy, the reaction is typically stronger than normal.

Rehabilitation
(continuum of care)

Rehabilitation means teaching a child to regain a function that he formerly had, such as the ability to walk or to perform activities of daily living. Teaching a new activity is technically called *habilitation,* although when speaking of the care of children, habilitation and rehabilitation are not usually separated. Rehabilitation may take place inside or outside the hospital. Hospital stays for rehabilitation purposes generally last between two and six weeks. In the hospital, the child is handled by an integrated team involving a physician trained in rehabilitation (usually a physiatrist), physical, occupational, and speech therapists, and specially trained nurses. Rehabilitation is offered in a continuum from hospital, to outpatient, to school, and finally and most importantly, to the home. Therapies are given as close to home as is medically possible.

Indications for inpatient rehabilitation include a recent illness or injury which acutely alters a child's capabilities for function, or when there are new medical issues that need to be sorted out. Goals might include feeding techniques, teaching parents the new care needs of their child, attention to safety in the environment, and mobility.

There are benefits from inpatient rehabilitation immediately after some surgical procedures, such as dorsal rhizotomies and some orthopedic procedures, because the child needs intense physical therapy to regain and maximize function. This may be done with the younger child, even as young as 2 or 3 years of age, though it may be very difficult emotionally for such a young child to be left by a parent for several weeks.

There are also specific special needs that may be best addressed on the inpatient unit, such as the need for high-technology communication aids and mobility aids. The focus is not only on the child performing the activities themselves, but also on teaching the parents to direct their care.

In recent years, more and more programs have developed outpatient or day programs that provide comprehensive physician-directed rehabilitation. Length of stay

Table 10   Primitive Reflexes (see page 438)

Name	Brief Description		Age at Which Normally Appears and Disappears
	How to Elicit	Response	
Moro	Place the infant in the supine position (on the back); lift by the arm, raising the head a bit off the table, and then let go.	Extension followed by abduction of the arms with partial flexing of the elbows, wrists, and fingers.	Birth–5 months
Tonic labyrinthine	Extend the infant's head and neck 45 degrees in the midline by placing a hand between the shoulder blades.	The shoulders retract, resulting in flexion of the arms. The legs also assume a slight extensor posture. Two types of obligatory responses are always abnormal: the "decorticate" posture, in which there is primarily shoulder retraction with flexion of the arms at the elbows, and the "decerebrate" posture, where the arms assume full extension and pronation.	Birth–9 months
Asymmetric tonic neck (ATNR)	Turn the head 45 degrees to the right or left side while the infant is in the supine position.	The arm on the chin side will go out into extension, while the arm on the other side (facing the back of the head) becomes more flexed. This is known as the fencing reaction. The legs may assume a similar posture to a lesser extent.	Birth–6 months
Symmetric tonic neck (STNR)	(a) With infant held in sitting position, extend the neck backward. (b) With infant held in sitting position, flex the head.	(a) Upper extremities extend outward and legs flex. (b) The arms flex and the legs extend.	Rarely present in normal children; may be seen intermittently until 4–6 months in some normal children
Crossed extension	Apply a noxious stimulus such as a pinch or a pinprick to the sole of one foot while holding that leg in complete extension.	The other leg first flexes, followed by adduction (crosses over toward the other leg), and finally extension as if to push away the noxious stimulus.	Birth–2 months
Stepping reflex	Hold the infant in vertical position and touch the sole of one foot to the ground or tabletop. The other foot flexes, adducts, and extends.	While the second foot is flexing and adducting, the examiner immediately turns the infant so that when extension occurs that foot receives the weight, thus producing a walking or stepping response.	Birth–6 weeks
Palmar and plantar grasp	Put pressure on palm of hand or sole of foot.	Hand grasps and holds; foot flexes and grasps.	Hand: Birth–3 months (blends into voluntary activity) Foot: Birth–9 months
Upper placing	Press the back of the hand against the edge of a table.	The hand is initially lifted above the extension of the arm, thus placing the hand on the tabletop.	3 months–no stated age. These reflexes gradually merge into volitional behavior, and disappearance can't be easily assessed.

Continued on next page

Table 10 — Continued

Lower placing	Press the top of the foot against the edge of a table while holding the infant upright.	The leg initially flexes and then extends, "placing" the foot on the tabletop.	Birth–no stated age. These reflexes gradually merge into volitional behavior, and disappearance can't be easily assessed.
Positive support	Hold the infant in a vertical position under the arms with head in the neutral position. Bounce the child 3–5 times on the balls of the feet.	Three findings are possible: (a) absence of any response; (b) momentary extension of the legs, thus supporting the weight momentarily, followed by flexion; or (c) full extension, thus supporting the body weight.	Birth–no stated age. These reflexes gradually merge into volitional behavior, and disappearance can't be easily assessed.

for inpatient programs has decreased, and children often finish their acute rehabilitation as outpatients. Some children return for a few weeks of outpatient care each year, rather than being hospitalized away from their family. Children do better sleeping in their own beds and coming in to a center for their therapies. Such centers need to have a strong multidisciplinary program, which addresses the unique needs of the child living at home. The program remains in close contact with the school, and at the appropriate time, the child resumes their program in their own school.

Rehabilitation involves partnership between the child, the family, and rehabilitation specialists, with the goal of maximizing the child's function in their own community.

Retinopathy of Prematurity

(Retrolental Fibroplasia, ROP, RLF)

Retinopathy of prematurity (ROP) was previously known as retrolental fibroplasia (RLF). It is a condition seen primarily in premature infants exposed to high concentrations of oxygen and is one of the leading causes of blindness in the United States in young infants, especially infants who have cerebral palsy because of prematurity. It leads to varying degrees of abnormality of the retina, the severest form of which can lead to total retinal detachment and blindness.

When ROP was first discovered, medical professionals believed that limiting oxygen exposure would prevent this condition, but as more premature and smaller infants are surviving, it is becoming clear that ROP can develop even in infants in whom oxygen concentration in the blood is well controlled. Various modes of treatment have been attempted to prevent the severest form (that is, retinal detachment), including cryotherapy and laser treatments. These have improved the visual prognosis.

Rigidity

The term rigidity is generally synonymous with stiffness. Some children with cerebral palsy become very stiff, especially in the joints. This stiffness can be due to spasticity, in which the muscles pull extremely tightly but then suddenly relax. If the stiffness does not suddenly relax but slowly stretches out, with the feeling of bending a lead pipe, then the correct term is rigidity. There are other conditions in which rigidity occurs, more specifically arthrogryposis, which is the fixation of a joint in a flexed or contracted position. Some children with cerebral palsy have rigidity as a main component of their motor problem; however, it more commonly becomes a mild but common feature in early adulthood of individuals with severe spasticity.

Rubella

(German measles)

Rubella, or German measles, is a viral illness that causes mild symptoms in adults or children. When pregnant women are infected, however, the virus causes very severe deformities in the fetus. Congenital rubella in the past had been a common cause of severe quadriplegic pattern cerebral palsy. Common symptoms of congenital rubella may include microcephaly, cataracts, small eyes, deafness, heart defects, and mild to severe retardation.

The congenital rubella syndrome has nearly disappeared over the past years with the use of rubella vaccine to immunize pregnant women against German measles. Unfortunately, some women are now reaching childbearing age without having been immunized. If they are infected during their pregnancy, their infants may have the deformities listed above. All children should be immunized against rubella, both to prevent their spreading it to pregnant women who might be exposed to them and, for girls, to prevent their becoming infected when they are old enough to become pregnant.

Scoliosis

(posterior spinal fusion, anterior spinal fusion, Harrington rod, Cotrel-Dubousset [CD] rod, Luque rod, unit rod, Zielke rod, Dwyer instrumentation, TSRH instrumentation)

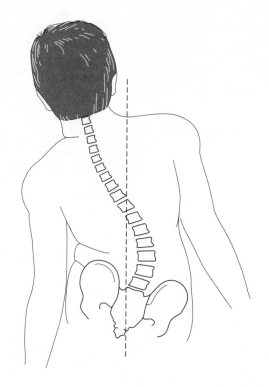

Scoliosis is a side bending of the spine that occurs in many diseases. The type of scoliosis a person has is dependent on the cause. It is important to recognize that scoliosis resulting from one cause has very little relationship to scoliosis resulting from another cause. Scoliosis is a symptom or the effect of some underlying disease process, just as abdominal pain, nausea, or vomiting are symptoms of underlying problems in the abdomen that may range from stomach ulcer or gallbladder problems to appendicitis. For the condition to be resolved, the treatment must be directed to the cause.

The incidence of scoliosis in children with cerebral palsy varies. It is uncommon in children with hemiplegia but slightly more common in patients with diplegia. The incidence for these two groups varies from 1 in 100 to 1 in 1,000. There may be some overlap because having cerebral palsy does not preclude also having idiopathic scoliosis, and it may be difficult to separate the two in some patients. The predominant group of children who develop scoliosis are the children with total involvement quadriplegia, and specifically those children who are unable to walk. The severely involved children have a 75 to 85 percent chance of developing severe scoliosis, which requires treatment.

Scoliosis in children with cerebral palsy is caused by poor muscle control, poor coordination, or asymmetrical muscle pull. The muscles in the spine function to keep the spine straight, similar to the guide wires around a radio tower which keep the tall, slender tower standing straight. Initially, the scoliosis in young children with cerebral palsy (between the ages of 2 and 8) is postural. At this age, when children sit up and do not have postural control they bend one way one time and in the opposite direction the next time. This scoliosis should be of very little concern, since it is flexible, and as soon as the children lie down their spines straighten out.

During the adolescent growth spurt, which occurs between the ages of 8 and 14, the spine becomes much longer, and it is then that the side bending develops a more permanent structured curve, so that the child starts to bend only on one side. The spinal vertebrae at this time not only bend sideways but also rotate and start to stiffen into place. During this period of adolescent growth, an increasing

curve combines with stiffness or resistance of the curve, and the spine no longer straightens out when the child lies down. This is now termed *structural scoliosis,* and is the type that continues to get progressively worse.

There was a time when doctors believed that applying body braces would help to prevent the progression or development of scoliosis in children with cerebral palsy. The general consensus now is that braces have no impact in either delaying the time at which the scoliosis develops or affecting the curve's severity. For this reason, there is no reason to prescribe spinal braces with the goal of treating the scoliosis. A brace made of a soft foamlike material can be used to help with sitting posture only in smaller more flexible scoliosis curves. However, it should not be expected to actually keep the curve from worsening.

As the scoliosis gets worse, sitting often becomes much more difficult. Wheelchair modifications need to be made, and soon a large degree of pelvic obliquity develops, so that the child sits only on one side of the pelvis or hip. If the scoliosis becomes worse, the pelvis slips inside the chest cage and the ribs start causing irritation as they rub against the pelvis. This is usually the condition that causes pain. As the scoliosis gets worse, it becomes more difficult for the abdominal muscles and diaphragm to work, which makes breathing more difficult. Scoliosis that becomes very severe can affect the blood flow through the lungs and cause heart problems. There may be difficulty with the swallowing mechanism and with stomach function. As the scoliosis continues to progress and becomes very severe, sitting for any period of time becomes difficult. Frequently there are only one or two positions in which lying down is comfortable.

Other types of scoliosis include idiopathic scoliosis, congenital scoliosis, and the scoliosis associated with muscular dystrophy. The most common of these is idiopathic scoliosis, which occurs predominantly in preadolescent or adolescent girls. Scoliosis in children who do not have cerebral palsy is treated very differently from scoliosis in children with CP. Scoliosis screening is used to attempt to identify the idiopathic form early in the normal child. The exact causes of idiopathic scoliosis are unknown. Idiopathic scoliosis is the type for which body braces and jackets are prescribed to prevent the further progression of the curve. This type of scoliosis is also treated with a spinal fusion when it becomes sufficiently severe that the risk of the curve's progression into adulthood is anticipated. Currently, the spinal fusion instruments used for this type of scoliosis are the Cotrel-Dubousset (CD) rod or the TSRH instrumentation, involving placing rods in the back of the spine with multiple hooks and fusing the spine over the area of the scoliosis. A similar design utilizing only two hooks is called a Harrington rod and has been used for many years, but is less sturdy and requires more postoperative support.

Care and treatment: For treating scoliosis in children with cerebral palsy, the choice is between a posterior spinal fusion and no treatment at all. The latter means accepting the consequences of the scoliosis. Other treatments such as exercises, therapy, braces, and manipulations have no impact on the outcome.

If the scoliosis is permitted to develop naturally, there is no certainty that it will become severe enough to prevent sitting, although this does occur in the majority of cases. If the patient is in an institutional care facility, then keeping him on his back, but with frequent changes of position so that bedsores don't develop, may be a reasonable alternative. One also needs to consider that some loss of respiratory and gastric function may occur.

For those children who can see well enough to watch television or to interact with their peers or family members, a full-time reclining position makes such activities difficult, if not impossible. It also makes feeding, as well as respiratory care and function, more difficult. In addition, transporting the child as well as having him take part in functions outside the home becomes difficult, if not impossible.

Indications: The indications for a posterior spinal fusion involve consideration of the child's remaining growth as well as the severity and stiffness of the curve. For a child who still has a lot of growth remaining, the curve may be allowed to progress further up to 90 degrees if it is not too stiff, because after the posterior spinal fusion is performed spinal growth will stop. This is usually not of major concern, since at most the procedure will remove an inch or two from the child's ultimate adult height. The posterior spinal fusion is usually performed when the child is between the ages of 10 and 15. It is best to avoid having the curve become very large, and especially very stiff, because this will necessitate two operations.

If the decision is made to proceed with a spinal fusion, the goal should be to correct malalignment so the child will sit straight with a normal appearance. There is very little place today for the type of spinal fusion whose only goal is to prevent the scoliosis from progressing, since the child who sits all the time needs to be placed straight upright with the pelvis and shoulders in a parallel position. Current technology allows this to be performed without a great deal of difficulty; generally, spinal curves between 60 and 90 degrees are considered candidates for fusion in children with cerebral palsy.

The surgery: The operation usually takes approximately four hours to complete, and the patient often needs to spend time on a ventilator and in the intensive care unit. This is a major operation that often requires a significant amount of blood to be transfused, frequently one to two times the child's blood volume. The second or third day after surgery, the child sits up in a wheelchair. Braces or casts are not necessary with modern instrumentation systems such as Luque rods or unit rods. Luque rods are two single rods wired together on each side of the spine. The unit rod is very similar, except it is one continuous rod or two rods solidly connected; it is a better means of correcting the scoliosis and controlling rotation of the spine.

Benefits and risks: After the fusion, the child may be handled in the same way as before surgery. Frequently parents find handling their child much easier after surgery because he is straight, can sit much better, and is stiff in the midsection. Significant complications and risks associated with the spinal fusion include a very large blood transfusion, which brings with it the small risk of contracting an infection. The large amount of blood needed in debilitated patients usually means they are not able to donate their own blood. Infection of the back is also a possible complication, but is fairly easy to treat and does not generally affect the outcome. Injury to the spinal cord is a possibility, especially when the curve is severe. For the experienced spinal surgeon, this risk should be quite small. A complication that is seen fairly commonly after a posterior spinal fusion is pancreatitis. This inflammation of the pancreas can cause abdominal pain, abdominal distension, and vomiting. It can result in significant delays in being able to resume feeding through the stomach, making intravenous nutrition the only route for calories for days to weeks after the surgery.

Many children with CP who undergo a spinal fusion are slender with very little body fat, and marginal nutrition can make healing large surgical wounds difficult. It is beneficial to increase feeding prior to surgery in order to have the child gain weight. Immediately after surgery, the child needs nutritional support. Either the use of intravenous total nutrition through specially placed IV lines or placing feeding tubes into the intestines is a way of starting extra feeding almost immediately after surgery. This is especially important for those severe curves that require surgery in the front of the spine. After this operation, which is a much smaller procedure, it may be a week before the posterior spinal surgery is done. If great care is not taken with nutrition, the child may go 10 to 14 days without adequate intake, a length of time that a slender child is not able to tolerate. Frequently, this type of child develops complications such as poor wound healing, infection, or pneumonia.

What to expect: After surgery, parents usually need to plan for approximately four weeks out of school, as two weeks is the average stay in the hospital for a child undergoing a posterior spinal fusion. For those who need both front and back surgery for severe scoliosis, three weeks in the hospital, and another week or two at home, will be necessary. Following the surgery no special care is needed, and the child may start standing or even walking if he is able.

Seizures

(epilepsy)

The brain normally has electrical activity going on within it in a controlled manner. A seizure is a sudden "out of control" event that can cause involuntary movements and/or behavior changes, and changes in awareness. It occurs when there are bursts of abnormal electrical activity in the brain, which interfere with normal brain functioning. Epilepsy is a group of disorders, characterized by recurrent seizures. Epilepsy is not a disease.

Sensorimotor Experience

(sensorimotor perception)

The ability to perceive and feel the movement of a limb as certain muscles are activated is a sensorimotor perception

or experience. For example, as a child moves her arms or legs she is able to perceive this movement by the positional senses that are present in the limbs. Also, as a child grasps an object she can perceive its shape and the weight of the object in her hand.

The sensory feedback that is necessary for sensorimotor perception is often diminished in children with cerebral palsy. In addition, their inability to move in space in the way a nondisabled child of the same age moves further diminishes this experience. A caregiver often discovers just how much difficulty a child with CP has when trying to teach the child to operate a motorized wheelchair. The deficit will often be more noticeable in wide-open areas outside, such as moving along a sidewalk, than it will be within the narrow confines of a hallway or a small room. In narrow areas the child has learned to perceive movement based on her eyes alone, but this is more difficult in wide-open areas, where additional feedback is required. This deficiency can be overcome with practice and training in the use of the power chair—gradually the child incorporates the available sensorimotor experience into a functional mechanism for perceiving the body's movement in space.

Spasticity

(spasm)

When muscles contract involuntarily or because of an activity such as a stretch, this action is said to be a spasm. When these involuntary contractions are persistent and cannot be voluntarily stopped, the child is said to have spasticity. When a caregiver attempts to move the child's joints, they appear to be stiff; however, with gentle stretching, the muscles suddenly relax. This form of stiffness caused by spasticity is substantially different from that caused by rigidity, which is a related term. With rigidity, the muscles do not suddenly relax and free the extremity but remain stiff, regardless of any attempts to move the joints.

Spasticity is present in children with spinal cord injuries, occasionally in those with spina bifida; it may also develop with some other nerve conditions such as multiple sclerosis. In the infant with cerebral palsy, spasticity is seldom significant in the first 6 months, but sometime between 6 months and 24 months, it starts becoming apparent. Initially, the child may be very floppy, but spasticity may develop with maturity. Proper positioning and postural control can decrease spasticity to some extent.

Care and treatment: Treatment of spasticity involves many different options, from nerve injections and medications to several surgical procedures. Medications used are of the diazepam family, Lioresal, Tizanidine or Dantrium. The side effects of each of these medications when given by mouth, especially drowsiness, make them unsuitable for continuous use in children with cerebral palsy. An exception is the use of an intrathecal Baclofen pump.

Treatments that are directed at the nerves involve injections with botulinum toxin. The efficacy of these treatments is limited because their effects don't last. Nerves may be surgically sectioned or crushed, but spasticity may recur in spite of this deliberate damage unless very large nerves are destroyed.

A *dorsal rhizotomy* is another surgical treatment, in which the nerves as they exit from the spinal cord are identified and the ones found to be most involved with the spasticity are cut. The result is a great decrease in spasticity, at least for a short period of time. However, the long-term implications of this procedure are still uncertain. Another option is that specific muscles whose spasticity is causing problems may be lengthened, released, or occasionally transferred; however, care must be taken that the antagonistic muscles are not also spastic, because the opposite deformity could then develop.

Speech Therapy
(feeding therapist)

Speech therapy is the professional discipline whose practitioners diagnose and treat problems of the oral motor system including feeding and speech issues. In the child with CP, they often evaluate the mechanical process of eating, which involves understanding how the mouth handles food, in what positions a child is best able to control the mouth muscles, how the food is moved in the mouth to the back of the throat, and how well the swallowing mechanism works.

The speech therapist often conducts a detailed examination using different food textures, often taking special x-rays in order to observe the swallowing mechanism on the x-ray screen. Based on this detailed examination, the speech therapist can decide whether oral feeding is safe for the child and can make specific recommendations concerning how to place the food in the mouth, what textures of food to use, and what position the child should be in to eat best. Speech therapists specialize in different areas, so it is important to be certain that the therapist who is evaluating the child for feeding problems has experience specifically in that area.

The second major effort of speech therapy is directed at teaching phonation (how to breathe and to use the vocal cords to make sounds) and speech. The communication component may also involve evaluating the child to see if she or he is capable of using means of communication other than oral speech, such as electronic computerized devices, symbol boards, hand speech, or eye communication.

Indications: Speech therapy is recommended for a child who is having difficulty with feeding, especially difficulty with swallowing, or for a child who is having difficulty speaking clearly or speaking at all.

Benefits and risks: There are several benefits of speech therapy: the valuable assessment that may determine the specific cause of the child's feeding and communication problems; the instruction and education provided to the caregiver; and the techniques that may help the child to eat more easily and safely and to communicate with those around her. There are no expected risks with therapy.

Maintenance: Speech therapy usually requires repeated evaluation, because feeding, swallowing, and speaking have a tendency to change as children mature. Often their abilities improve as they get older, but for some children swallowing difficulties may get worse during their adolescent growth spurt, and monitoring by a speech therapist is important during this period.

Spinal Fusion
(posterior spinal fusion, anterior spinal fusion)

A spinal fusion involves roughening the bone surfaces and removing the joints to allow the individual vertebrae to heal together; a fused spine becomes in essence one long bone. The area that is fused can no longer move, and once this has healed, it lasts an entire lifetime. The most commonly performed surgery is done from the back and is called a posterior spinal fusion, but the surgery may be performed from the front of the spine, in which case it is called an anterior spinal fusion.

Indications: A posterior spinal fusion is indicated if a spinal curvature is worsening and becoming functionally unmanageable or if a curvature is certain to progress at some point and to become severe. A posterior spinal fusion may be performed for scoliosis, kyphosis, or lordosis. For children with cerebral palsy, posterior spinal fusion almost always involves inserting spinal rod instrumentation. Any procedure that does not involve the use of instrumentation is very unlikely to provide a good result, primarily because it is extremely difficult to hold the spine straight during the healing time. If the fusion is successful, the child will be fused in a very deformed position, which is obviously not beneficial at all.

The surgery: The posterior spinal fusion involves an incision made in the middle of the back. The bone surfaces are roughened and extra bone is applied, which may be obtained from the patient's pelvic bone—or, with the patient with cerebral palsy, from bone graft from the bone bank. The procedure is usually combined with the implantation of rods to hold the spine straight and in the correct position while it is healing. This surgical procedure may include the use of Harrington rods, Luque rods, unit rods, or CD rods.

The anterior spinal fusion is performed for very severe scoliosis and involves removing the intervertebral discs in the front of the vertebrae. This both allows much better correction and improves the ability of the spine to fuse together. Usually, an anterior spinal fusion is a smaller operation than the posterior spinal fusion, takes less time, and involves less blood loss.

Benefits and risks: The benefits of fusion surgery are that it halts the progression of the curvature and straightens the spine as much as possible. Complications from a posterior spinal fusion include the possibility of infection and the need for blood transfusions. Blood loss is usually significant in spinal fusions; transfusions are almost always required. Permanent paralysis can occur but is very rare; minor nerve irritations do occasionally occur but usually resolve over several months.

Adequate nutritional intake is a problem, especially when an anterior spinal fusion is followed by a posterior spinal fusion. The nutritional requirements of the child should be very carefully watched, and often demand the insertion of a tube into the intestine for immediate feeding after the surgery or the insertion of an IV line in which protein, carbohydrates, and fats may be given immediately after surgery. Problems with seizure control are seldom encountered, although frequently parents are concerned because sometimes their child is taking a seizure medication.

After-surgery care: With most instrumentation systems, the child is usually up in a chair, in a shower, and back to school within four weeks. For a specific routine, consult the section on the specific instrumentation that was utilized.

What to expect: Children with cerebral palsy who have a spinal fusion are usually in the intensive care unit for several days and in the hospital for approximately two weeks. They should expect to be out of school for a total of four weeks, after which they should be able to return at their normal level of function. There is seldom a need for a cast or brace after this surgery, and they should be back to their normal activities of daily living within four weeks.

Splint, Elbow

(resting arm splint, extension elbow splint, spring-loaded extension splint)

Elbow splints are usually made by occupational therapists with the goal of straightening the elbow. Many children with cerebral palsy have a tendency to flex the elbow and to remain in this position. The two patterns of cerebral palsy in which this is most likely to occur are severe quadriplegia and moderate to severe hemiplegia. These splints are usually made of plastic and are directly applied to the arm. Sometimes these splints may be made from casts that are split in half and held together with velcro straps. There is a commercially available elbow splint that has a spring, its goal being to stretch the tight elbow by constant pressure from the loaded spring.

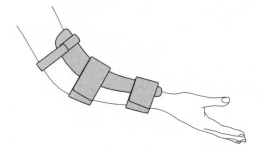

Indications: The purpose of using elbow extension splints is to try to stretch out tight elbows. They should keep the elbows sufficiently loose to allow for cleaning and easy dressing of a child. For a child with cerebral palsy with hemiplegia, the goal may be to improve function, if some function already exists. Although experts disagree on which splints to use and for what length of time, children with spasticity and cerebral palsy should use splints that are rigid and not spring-loaded. Spring-loaded splints are specifically contraindicated in children with spasticity because they further magnify the spasticity and cause the muscle to pull even harder.

Benefits and risks: The splint may improve the ability of the hand to function, but its main benefit is to prevent progressive contracture. Complications from the use of splints are primarily skin breakdown from poorly fitting splints or pain that is caused by having the elbow or wrist stretched too tightly. Generally the splints should be comfortable and should fit well. Any difficulty with pain or skin breakdown needs to be addressed by the therapist who made the brace.

Maintenance and care: Most of these braces are made out of low-temperature plastics and as a consequence

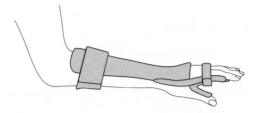

need to be kept out of direct sunlight or areas that become very warm. They should not be washed in hot water and should only be cleaned with gentle soap. They are usually applied directly to the skin or over a sleeve, and are used for several hours at a time. If the child is very comfortable, they may occasionally be worn all night.

Splint, Finger
(swan-neck splint)

A finger splint prevents hyperextension or the bending backward of the middle joint of the finger (PIP joint). The splint is made of metal and is applied very like the way one puts on a finger ring. Some plastic models of this splint are also available.

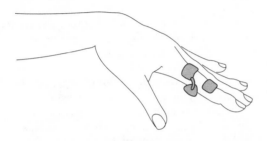

Indications: This splint is used primarily for patients with athetosis who have developed some laxity (looseness), in which the fingers bend back over the center and then become stuck. This causes difficulty because the fingers cannot bend to grasp or pick up objects. The splints may be used for specific activities such as typing, using a joystick, or picking up eating utensils, and are usually not worn full time.

Benefits and risks: The major benefit is to keep the finger from locking in the extended position. If there is too much pressure, the major risk is skin breakdown. If the splint causes a significant problem and cannot be modified, it may need to be discontinued.

Maintenance and care: The splints should be kept clean and fitting well.

Splint, Hand
(wrist splint, cock-up splint, resting hand splint, functional hand splint)

Hand splints extend below the elbow across the wrist, and are used to position the hand to prevent muscle contractures from developing. Made by an occupational therapist,

they are often custom-made out of low-temperature plastics or a nylon material. Alternatively, there are a number of off-the-shelf, ready-made models that may be used.

Indications: The indications for hand splints vary, from attempts to improve function to attempts to position the hand to prevent further contractures. The use of splints to improve function is often not very fruitful. Generally, when the splint is applied it covers the skin, which means that the hand has less sensation. This lack of sensation usually leads to less use of the hand. There are certain circumstances in which a correctly positioned splint does place the hand in a better position and *improves* function, and the functional improvement may specifically allow the fingers to hit trip switches or to use joysticks, enabling a child to drive a chair or manipulate a computer. These uses are very child-specific and frequently require a great deal of trial and error by an experienced occupational therapist to find the right splinting position with the right material to benefit the child. If a significant attempt to try different splints does not improve the child's function, then splinting ought to be abandoned.

A second reason for the use of hand splints is to keep the hand supple as the child grows and to prevent further contractures, which make dressing and hygiene difficult. Resting hand splints or cock-up splints are often used. Covering the hand with these splints is not detrimental if the hand is nonfunctional. The length of time these are used varies greatly—from short periods of 30 minutes or an hour to all night long. The child should, however, spend some time out of the splint each day, which is necessary to keep the skin healthy and to prevent hypersensitivity. There are no recognized or generally accepted protocols for the use of this type of splinting; instead, a parent needs to be guided by the philosophy and functional approach of the physician and therapists treating the child.

Benefits and risks: If a splint is used properly, it can help prevent contractures and can potentially increase function by improving hand position. The complications with hand splints occur with those used for functional purposes. The main problem is that they decrease instead of improve function because they decrease sensation. There may also be discomfort or skin breakdown; the skin under the brace should be checked daily to make certain that there is no irritation.

Maintenance and care: Most of these splints are made out of low-temperature plastics and as a consequence need to be protected from direct sunlight and high temperatures, specifically hot water. They should be cleaned with gentle soap.

Splint, Thumb

(thumb-abduction splint)

Thumb splints are used to pull the thumb out of the palm, a very common deformity in children with cerebral palsy. These braces may either be custom-made by an occupational therapist or purchased commercially.

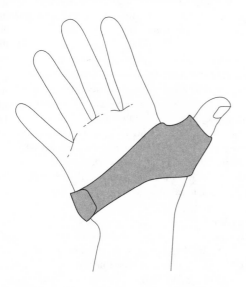

Indications: These splints have two purposes: to improve the function of the hand and to prevent a further deformity. The functional splint pulls the thumb out of the palm so that the fingers can be used for grasping large objects or manipulating joysticks or switches. The test of whether there is functional improvement is improved hand use. The second indication is to stretch the thumb muscle to prevent it from contracting, so that proper cleaning is possible.

Benefits and risks: The main benefit is preventing further contraction: children can use their fingers better when the thumb is kept out of the palm. The complications associated with these splints are related to skin breakdown from poorly fitting splints. Some of the splints can

cause pain and discomfort from too much stress, if a physician or therapist attempts too much correction. In these cases, the splint needs to be modified.

Maintenance and care: These splints are usually made of low-temperature plastics and need to be kept away from hot water, direct sunlight, or other heat that may melt them. Nylon splints should not be washed, in order to avoid damaging the material.

Split Tibialis Posterior Tendon

(STPT, tibialis posterior transfer, varus foot deformity, posterior tibialis lengthening, Frost lengthening)

Below the knee, the second largest and most commonly involved muscle with significant spasticity is the tibialis posterior muscle. When this muscle is spastic or short, it pulls the foot in and down. This spasticity is frequently associated with spasticity of the Achilles tendon. For children who walk, the most common problem caused by this spastic muscle and its contracted tendon is that the toes drag and most of the pressure is placed on the outside edge of the sole. Also, in some children with severe involvement, it may cause the foot to turn almost completely sideways, so that every attempt to stand has the child standing on the outside of the foot.

Care and treatment: In the young child, the main treatment for a spastic tibialis posterior muscle involves using a molded ankle-foot orthosis (AFO) to hold the foot flat and to prevent it from rolling in. As the child gets older, however, the condition usually does not resolve, and can get so severe that the child is not able to tolerate the AFO. At this time, surgical correction is indicated.

The surgery: The most common surgical correction utilized today is the split tibialis posterior tendon transfer, which involves taking one-half of the tendon, splitting it longitudinally, and swinging it across the back of the ankle over to the peroneal tendons on the outside of the ankle, which pull the foot out in the opposite direction. This procedure works like a bridle, so that the spastic muscle pulls on both sides of the ankle and generally keeps the foot flat. This correction works well, remains stable, and is usually not outgrown by the child.

Lengthening of the tibialis posterior tendon, also called the Frost procedure, is a slightly less involved surgery; however, it has a much higher risk of over- or undercorrection and is frequently outgrown. Although it is still used by some surgeons, the split transfer is more common.

Transfer of the entire tibialis posterior tendon is com-

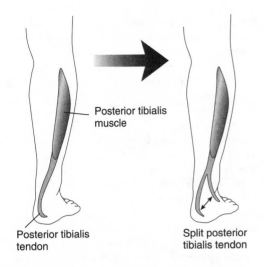

Posterior tibialis
muscle

Posterior tibialis
tendon

Split posterior
tibialis tendon

mon in peroneal nerve palsy, Charcot-Marie-Tooth disease, and muscular dystrophy (all conditions that affect the nerves or muscles) but should not be utilized for children with spasticity because it frequently causes severe deformity in the opposite direction.

Benefits and risks: The major benefit of the split tibialis posterior tendon transfer is that the foot is now kept flat so that the child can stand and walk much more adequately than before. The complications are usually minor. The most common one occurs when the transferred half of the tendon tears out where it is inserted, causing the deformity to recur. If this happens, the surgeon can attempt to resuture the end that tore loose. This procedure is usually successful. Overcorrection by developing a deformity in the opposite direction is extremely unusual with this procedure. The major complications of the Frost procedure are that children often outgrow it, and that if too much lengthening is performed the opposite type of deformity, known as severe flat foot, develops.

After-surgery care: The usual care after the split tibialis posterior transfer procedure is to place the child in a short leg walking cast for four weeks, although some surgeons prefer using a long leg cast. Most surgeons allow the child to walk. An AFO may be used temporarily after the cast is removed, but frequently this is not necessary. Special physical therapy exercises are not needed after this procedure.

Stereognosis

Stereognosis is the specific sensory capability to define the shape of an object by touch. Children with cerebral palsy

often lose this ability in the affected hand; the loss is often most dramatic in the hemiplegic affected hand. As a result, the child usually ignores that hand, and uses the functioning hand exclusively.

Swan-Neck Fingers

(locking fingers)

In swan-neck (locking) fingers, the end joint (DIP joint) becomes flexed and the middle joint (the PIP joint) extends. The fingers lock into this position and cannot be moved unless another finger is used to unlock them. This problem occurs in patients with athetosis, as well as in a hand in which the finger flexor sublimis tendons have been overlengthened.

Care and treatment: The primary means of treating swan-neck fingers is to identify the movements that cause the fingers to lock and to try to teach the child to avoid moving in this fashion. If the child cannot refrain from these movements, there are small figure-eight splints that may be worn. They are usually made of metal or plastic and surround the middle joint (PIP joint), preventing it from becoming extended. If the problem is related to certain activities, the use of splints is an excellent alternative. However, if the splints are needed all the time but cause skin irritation and discomfort, surgery should be considered.

The surgery: Surgical repair involves taking the sublimis tendons and either suturing them into part of the tendon sleeve to prevent the joints from extending or transferring the muscles so the sublimis muscles are strengthened and do not allow the middle joint to extend. Sometimes the deformity recurs because the repair stretches out, or muscle power imbalance is so great that it causes the deformity to recur.

Frequently, splints are used after surgery following the initial cast immobilization. Finger splints may be used for three to six months to protect the repair while it matures.

Syndrome

A syndrome is a constellation of physical findings that tend to occur together. Sometimes these are due to a chromosomal defect, such as with Down syndrome, which is caused by having three copies of chromosome number 21 instead of two copies. Other syndromes are associated with specific agents that can cause a birth defect. Probably the most common of these is fetal alcohol syndrome, associated with the ingestion of alcohol by a pregnant woman. Numerous other syndromes have been described and are grouped together by having similar physical findings. Many of these are known to be genetic, but many others are simply a description of a constellation of abnormalities that seem to occur together in more than a random fashion—and may or may not be genetic. Many of these are associated with mental retardation and seizures; others may have physical problems not unlike the child with cerebral palsy.

Syphilis

Congenital syphilis is contracted from an infected mother at any time during pregnancy or at birth. Among women with untreated early syphilis, 40% of pregnancies result in death of the fetus or newborn. Other infants can be born prematurely. At birth, infants may or may not have signs of disease. Such signs may include enlargement of the liver and spleen, enlargement of lymph nodes, lesions of the skin and/or mucous membranes, deformity of the bones, hemolytic anemia and/or a low platelet count. Untreated infants, whether or not they have such early signs, may develop late signs of disease, including brain damage, cranial nerve deafness, and a variety of other abnormalities. All pregnant women should be screened for syphilis early in pregnancy with a blood test and preferably again at delivery. If a pregnant woman is known to have syphilis, she can be treated with antibiotics, specifically penicillin, which should eradicate the infection. A newborn who is diagnosed with active syphilis can also be treated with antibiotics, though the brain injury may have already occurred. Although currently rare, congenital syphilis infection is a cause of cerebral palsy.

Syringomyelia

(diastematomyelia, tethering of the spinal cord)

Syringomyelia means that a cyst is present in the spinal cord. These cysts may be isolated, but are frequently associated with other conditions. They may cause scoliosis, and are often detected at adolescence when a girl is thought to have idiopathic scoliosis. The cyst may get larger and cause decreased joint sensation, weakness, or poor sensation in either the arms or the legs.

Diastematomyelia means that there is fibrous tissue, cartilage, or bone within the spinal cord. This can lead to problems as the child grows, with the spinal cord getting caught on the fibrous substance (tethering), resulting in loss of function of the legs or the bowel and bladder.

The cause of either one of these spinal cord abnormalities is usually a congenital malformation. However, occasionally the cyst is actually a spinal cord tumor that is deteriorating into a cyst, or manifesting itself as a result of a spinal cord injury. There is no known genetic cause of either condition, and both may be associated with other anomalies (including myelomeningocele), although not cerebral palsy. The presenting symptoms of syringomyelia easily mimic CP.

The advent of the MRI scan has made it possible to diagnose many syringomyelias and diastematomyelias, even when not causing any symptoms. A common recommendation is to continue to observe the child with these cysts; if the cysts do not enlarge or cause other problems, no active treatment is given. If treatment is necessary, it might include a shunt, to drain the cyst into a vein or the abdomen. Unless exceedingly severe, these cysts do not cause significant difficulty with movement or use of the legs. Surgical excision is suggested for a diastematomyelia when it is causing symptoms due to tethering, to prevent further loss of spinal cord function.

Therapy

(physical therapy, occupational therapy, sensory integrative therapy, neurodevelopmental therapy, NDT, conductive education, M.O.V.E. curriculum, myofascial manipulation, hippotherapy, aquatherapy, Adeli suit)

The goal of any therapy is to maximize each child's functioning to all that it can be. Therapy may be performed by many people, including parents, grandparents, schoolteachers, and even the child himself or herself. The professional therapists most often encountered are physical, occupational and speech therapists, who are trained and licensed practitioners under whose expertise the therapy is directed or personally given. (Speech therapy is described on page 445).

Physical and occupational therapists' approach overlap because their focus is to help the child develop motor skills. Areas in common include seating assessments, early intervention therapy, and developmental testing. Physical therapists, however, focus mainly on gross motor or large muscle activities involving the legs, such as walking, bracing, using crutches, and rehabilitation after surgery. Occupational therapists focus primarily on fine motor activities involving the upper extremities, and functions such as feeding, writing, and using scissors; they also splint the arm as necessary. As the child grows older, occupational therapists stress activities of daily living such as self-dressing, bathing, and preparing food.

In choosing a specific physical or occupational therapist, it is usually best to find one who is trained and experienced in dealing with children with developmental problems.

The following is a discussion of several of the therapeutic approaches available for a child with a physical disability. Many have not been scientifically tested in groups of children with CP. However, as any given child may respond to a specific type of intervention, parents can investigate these therapies. Parents, however, need to check with their traditional medical providers to make sure that the approach has the potential to help, and will do no harm.

Sensory integration therapy was developed by Jean Ayres to help children who do not understand how to execute normal movements because of decreased sensory input. The theory behind sensory integration suggests that movement disorders are caused by poor input from the sensory system, thus allowing primitive reflexes to persist and preventing children from developing normal motor movements. The treatment protocol involves a large amount of active and passive touching and muscle movement stimulation to encourage the brain to initiate better movement patterns. This technique employs swinging movements in swivel chairs as well as direct, hands-on exercises.

Neurodevelopmental therapy (NDT) was developed by Drs. Karl and Bertha Bobath. It has become one of the most commonly used intervention strategies for infants and children with developmental disabilities, including CP. As our understanding of how the brain controls movement has evolved, so has the theory of NDT. NDT-trained therapists use a variety of specialized techniques that encourage active use of appropriate muscles and diminish involvement of muscles not needed for the completion of a particular task. Therapists set individual functional goals that build on each other to facilitate new motor skills, or improve the efficiency of previously learned skills. In NDT the child takes an active role in treatment design. The therapist must constantly reevaluate their input into the child's movement, as they reassess and redesign the goals for the child. NDT can be used by occupational, speech, and physical therapists, as well as educators.

Conductive education was developed at the Peto Institute in Hungary and is now being provided in many countries throughout Europe as well as the United States, Canada, Australia, and others. It is a system of teaching and learning for children with motor disorders. It is a method of exercises and education that are broken down into basic functional movements. The exercises are performed intensively for five hours per day, five days per week, in small groups.

The *M.O.V.E.* *program,* which stands for Mobility Opportunities Via Education, is an activity-based curriculum designed to teach basic functional motor skills. It combines special education instruction with therapeutic methods. The M.O.V.E.* curriculum provides a framework for teaching the skills necessary for individuals with disabilities to gain greater physical independence. It combines functional body movements with an instructional process designed to help people acquire increasing amounts of independence in sitting, standing, and walking. The goal is to teach especially those functional motor skills needed for adult life. The program is for any child or adult who is not independently sitting, standing, or walking, and includes those with mental retardation. The M.O.V.E.* curriculum can be applied in a special school or a regular classroom setting and provides students with increased opportunities to participate in life activities with their peers without disabilities.

Myofascial release therapy is a gentle blend of stretching and massage. It is often used to treat musculoskeletal pain such as long-standing back pain, fibromyalgia, recurring headaches, or sports injuries. However, it has also been offered to children with birth trauma, head injuries, and CP, with little evidence that it changes the course of these conditions. It is an outgrowth of chiropractic techniques. The basic therapy consists of stretching and manipulation, with the goal of stretching out the connective tissues involved in joint capsules and in the fascia overlying the muscles.

Equine therapy, also known as horseback riding therapy, or hippo-therapy has become quite popular. The underlying theory is that the positioning and large movements provided by horseback riding are very helpful in establishing balance and relaxation of spastic muscles. The vertical motions of horseback riding are thought to provide sensory stimulus, which decreases muscle tone. Sitting on the horse helps with stretching hip adductors and improves pelvic tilt and trunk positioning. This allows better muscle movement and range of motion for the therapist to work with after the child finishes the session. Another benefit is that many children enjoy horseback riding therapy because they have friends or siblings who ride horses too.

Aquatherapy or hydrotherapy is therapy performed in water. The effects of the water give children a feeling of weightlessness, which helps to reduce tone and allow these children better motor control. Aquatherapy is used for postoperative rehabilitation to allow children to start walking with reduced weightbearing. It is also a good modality for gait training, especially in an overweight child who may be able to walk in water with relative weightlessness. In addition, swimming as a recreational activity is excellent for children with CP. For many children for whom walking consumes a great deal of energy, learning to swim, and using this as physical conditioning is an excellent option.

Spacesuit therapy was first investigated in Russia and later became very popular in Poland, using the ADELI* suit. The suit was originally designed to help cosmonauts maintain their muscle tone in a weightless environment. It was then modified to help children with CP. It is a form-fitting suit with adjustable elastic bands designed to put the body into proper alignment. An intensive physical therapy program focuses on improving sensory stimulation and allows children to learn movement, standing posture, and balance strategies. A similar approach has been started in the United States, though it is not affiliated with the European program. It utilizes multiple therapeutic tools meant to promote the performance of independent and controlled movements while strengthening an isolated muscle group. The therapy program may involve up to 20 hours per week of intensive therapy.

Indications: With such a large number of different and often conflicting types of therapy available, parents frequently have trouble deciding what is best for their child. There are many therapists, parents, and other advocates for each therapeutic modality who embrace that method with an almost religious fervor. It is generally best to take these overenthusiastic perspectives with a grain of salt, because each therapeutic method has some bit of truth to it, and no one approach can miraculously "cure" a child, especially one who is not physically predisposed to change.

Parents should choose a therapist in whom they have confidence and who seems to relate well to their child. It is better to focus on the child's progress than on the specific theory or modality.

Benefits and risks: Most pediatric physical and occupational therapy specialists who work with children with cerebral palsy use a general approach in which they choose individual techniques from many therapies for the greatest benefit to the child. Most experienced therapists try working with different methods until they find the one to which the child seems to respond best. Generally speaking, if a child is responding both physically and psychologically, then the therapeutic modality is working for her.

Tibial Torsion

(internal tibial torsion, external tibial torsion, in-toeing gait, out-toeing gait)

When a child walks, his or her foot may point slightly in (called in-toeing) or slightly out (called out-toeing). There are several causes of this, one of which is tibial torsion. Tibial torsion means that there is a twist in the tibia (the bone between the knee and the ankle) causing the knee and the ankle joint not to line up in a parallel manner. This torsion is generally due to the way a child was born or the way a child was lying in utero during the last trimester. In normal children under the influence of normal muscle pull and walking

in early childhood, torsional problems almost always completely resolve themselves. In children with cerebral palsy, however, under the influence of spastic muscles that do not develop normal rotational pull, these torsional problems have a great tendency to persist and cause problems.

Internal tibial torsion refers to the internal rotation of the ankle with respect to the knee joint, causing the foot to point in when the child walks. This can be present with femoral anteversion (a similar twist in the femur, or thighbone, and another common cause of in-toeing) which causes the knee to turn in. The in-toeing may be exceedingly severe—in some cases, the heel may be in front of the toes as the child walks, causing the feet to turn backward. However, a child may have femoral anteversion, where the knee is pointing in, and have compensatory external tibial torsion, so that the foot is pointing out. In this situation, the foot looks like it is pointing in the right direction, but the knee appears to bend in the wrong direction when the child walks, causing the knees to knock together. There are some children who have normal alignment above the knee joint but have foot problems such that they are almost rolling over the inside of the foot instead of walking with the normal heel-to-toe movement.

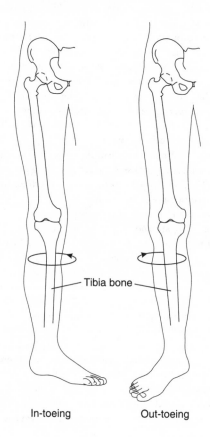

Tibia bone

In-toeing   Out-toeing

Indications: These torsional problems tend not to improve in children who have spasticity, although as they mature they may get better motor control and growth may improve their appearance. A child who is learning to walk and having severe difficulty because of rotational problems of the legs ought to have surgery. There are no braces, exercises, or other devices that have a permanent impact upon these rotational problems. However, surgical correction of these rotational malalignments at any age is usually permanent, with recurrence very rare.

The surgery: Tibial torsion is usually corrected just above the ankle joint: a small stab wound is made, and a drill bit is utilized to drill a number of holes across the tibia and the small bone (the fibula) on the lateral side. The bone is then cracked and rotated into the proper alignment. Another technique for making this correction is to make a small incision just below the knee joint and cut the bone at this level. Holding the bone in proper alignment is slightly harder in this area, and the osteotomy above the ankle joint is generally favored.

Benefits and risks: The primary benefit of this surgery lies in improving the child's ability to walk, by improving his alignment. The complications of tibial torsional osteotomies are few; however, either insufficient correction or overcorrection is possible. Further, there needs to be some way to make sure the correction is maintained during healing: if insufficient casting is applied, the proper alignment may be lost. Generally a pin is placed through the tibia just below the knee, and the foot and knee are placed in the cast to maintain the correction. This method also allows the child to start walking as soon as the pain subsides. Casting above the knee with the knee bent at 90 degrees is a method used by some physicians. However, the child is not able to walk immediately, and may develop hamstring contractures from being in a cast.

Another complication of torsional osteotomies done to correct severe torsional problems may be the stretching of nerves. Any correction of over 40 degrees requires great caution because the procedure is like wringing a dishcloth: this "wringing-out effect" can cause both nerves and arteries to be stretched, causing difficulty with nerve function or blood flow to the foot.

After-surgery care: Postoperative management depends on the type of cast used, but if a short leg cast and pin are used, the child may start walking immediately. If a long leg cast is used with the knee bent, at four weeks it is frequently converted to a short leg cast, at which time the child may start walking. Casts must be kept dry. Physical therapy is usually prescribed to work on teaching the child a new gait pattern after the cast is removed. After the cast

comes off, it usually takes three to four weeks for the foot to have normal sensation and for the child to really feel comfortable walking.

Toe Walking

(toe dragging, idiopathic toe walking, Achilles tendon contracture)

Toe walking is a very common condition in young children as they start to walk, and it is normal for children up to 2 years of age. However, by the time a child is 2½ years old, he should be walking with his heel down and the remainder of his foot flat. Persistent toe walking can be an early sign of cerebral palsy, but there is a condition called idiopathic toe walking in which children do not have any other signs of cerebral palsy but are persistently far up on their toes.

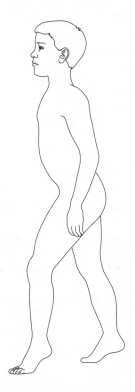

Indications: By 2½ to 3 years of age, this pattern should be treated with a brace, such as an ankle-foot orthosis (AFO). If it is ignored, some children who do not have CP gradually develop a flatfooted walking pattern; others develop such tight Achilles tendons that they need surgical lengthening by age 7 or 8. The child with cerebral palsy should be treated with an ankle-foot orthosis also, especially if the toe walking is causing difficulty with balance and muscle coordination. Initially, an AFO that does not have a hinge is best; as the child gains more muscle control, coordination, and balance, he can use an AFO with a hinged joint, which lifts up the foot so that the toe does not drag. For children with spasticity, the Achilles tendon becomes tight because the muscle does not grow adequately, and manual stretching often improves this. For some children, using the AFO may help the muscle grow.

Once the Achilles tendon contracture becomes too tight to wear an AFO, surgical lengthening of the Achilles tendon should be considered. The use of the ankle-foot orthosis is also necessary for toe dragging; however, even for adolescents with cerebral palsy, if the Achilles tendon is not too tight, they should be able to pick up the foot sufficiently so the toes do not drag. Occasionally, there are children and young adults who continue to wear AFOs because they cannot pick up their feet due to weak muscles in the front of the calf. Toe dragging is also often caused by knee stiffness and is significantly improved with rectus transfer surgery at the knee.

Toe walking fosters further contractures of the Achilles tendon and also limits balance and motor coordination, since the child does not have a rigid foundation on which to stand. With the older child, toe dragging mainly causes rapid wear of shoes, can make the child look very clumsy, and causes the child to trip.

Toes

(claw toes, hammer toes)

Small toes can develop deformities from spasticity, and usually a claw or hammer toe deformity develops when toes flex severely. Inside the shoe, the end of the toe may become very sore from digging down into the sole, or alternatively one of the toe knuckles may become sore from pushing against the top of the shoe. Padding or modifying shoes may be helpful, but these toes may cause lifelong pain that can only be improved with very simple surgical procedures.

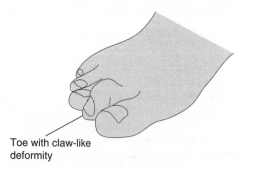

Toe with claw-like deformity

The surgery: If the patient is relatively young and the toes are not too stiff, releasing the tendons on the underside of the toes is sufficient. If the toes, however, have become very stiff, the middle toe joint often needs to be removed to fuse the joint, and a small pin is placed across the joint for approximately four weeks. In cooperative teenagers or adults, this procedure is done under local anesthesia, often in the doctor's office. General anesthesia is needed for children.

Benefits and risks: In most cases, the procedure gives a nice correction that is maintained for a lifetime. The complications from these procedures are relatively minimal, with the worst being recurrence of the deformity in the rare situation where not enough correction was initially obtained. Operations on the small toes usually do not require casts, only soft dressing, and the wearing of open-toe shoes for approximately four weeks.

Total Parenteral Nutrition

(TPN, hyperalimentation)

TPN is an intravenous infusion of nutrients that we normally would get from the foods we eat. It contains protein as amino acids, carbohydrates as dextrose, and fat as lipids, as well as vitamins and minerals. This intravenous (IV) solution is usually given centrally, meaning through a catheter that is placed into a large vein in the chest and ends in the heart. It can be given peripherally, meaning through a regular IV in the arm or leg, but only for a few days, and with much lower concentrations of nutrients. Some children will require TPN if their gastrointestinal (GI) tract is not working properly, or if they are not able to eat by mouth. While there are many different reasons that a child might need TPN, it would typically be used in a child with CP following surgery for scoliosis, after abdominal surgery, or if the child develops pancreatitis, which would result in vomiting and intolerance to feedings. Rarely, children (including those with CP) develop severe dysmotility of their gastrointestinal system, meaning that their system no longer works well, and they cannot tolerate feedings through their stomach or even small bowel. Such children might need TPN for a long time or even chronically if their system does not resume normal function.

Tracheostomy

(laryngotracheal separation)

A tracheostomy is an operation which creates an opening from the neck into the trachea (windpipe). One of the reasons it is done is to bypass a tracheal obstruction and provide an airway. It is occasionally performed on children with cerebral palsy, since they frequently aspirate (inhale) food or liquids into the windpipe. This condition leads to frequent bouts of pneumonia, a chronic cough or bronchitis, and sometimes asthma. Over time, it may cause permanent damage to the lungs and be life-threatening.

Indications: If the condition is persistent and not improving, the growing child may require that the trachea be opened in the front of the neck. A tube is then placed in

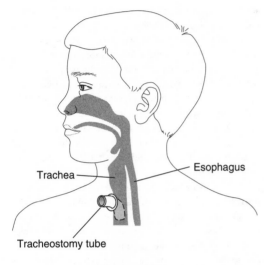

Tracheostomy

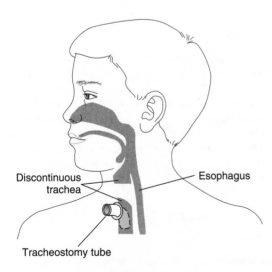

Laryngotracheal separation

the neck through this opening so that air can directly enter into the lungs. If the aspiration is severe, then a laryngotracheal separation or diversion may be needed. This is a procedure where the trachea is divided, permanently separating the lower windpipe from the mouth. This prevents saliva from entering the lower airway. A laryngotracheal separation or diversion is generally considered for children that cannot speak.

The surgery: The procedure involved is a very short operation usually requiring less than 30 minutes. It involves opening the trachea and inserting a plastic tube.

After-surgery care: A tracheostomy may seem like an intimidating procedure to a parent. Caring for a child with a tracheostomy, however, need not be complicated. It is generally easy for parents and school personnel to learn to manage a tracheal tube, including cleaning and changing it when necessary. Usually, however, the first change of the tracheostomy tube should be done by the surgeon. The tracheostomy makes suctioning easy to help the child deal with the large amount of secretions. A laryngotracheal separation prevents aspiration of secretions. A tracheostomy, however, makes finding respite care and care in some facilities more difficult because the person needs to stay with someone trained in caring for the tracheostomy. Although it is not difficult, training is mandatory.

What to expect: Increased care is usually necessary for the child who has a tracheostomy or laryngotracheal separation. The air now bypasses the mouth and is not moisturized, so some type of additional moisturizing is often necessary. A parent or other caregiver must also be trained to clean and change the tube after a tracheostomy.

Transition of Medical Services

There are two major transitional milestones that must be achieved by the adolescent or young adult, whether or not they have a disability. These are the transition from the pediatric health care system to the adult health care system and the transition from school to whatever lies after school, whether it be further education, a job, or a change in living situation.

As adolescents become adults, they need to assume responsibility for their own health care. For the adolescent with special health care needs, such as cerebral palsy, this may be difficult. It is often hard to find an adult care provider who is trained in caring for a pediatric condition such as CP or willing to assume primary responsibility for that care. Many pediatricians and pediatric hospitals will transition patients from their care either at age 18 or 21, or sometimes even 25. However, at some age this transition needs to happen, and it can be emotionally difficult for the physician, the family, and the child.

A summary of the child's health history is often a good place to begin. It is a summary form of a child's health and medical history, and if possible should be filled out by the teen herself, or with help from parents if necessary. It should include a description of the child's special needs, the medications she is currently taking and why, any allergies or adverse reactions to medications or foods, past hospitalizations or surgeries, and any serious illnesses she may have had. This is a tool for the teen to learn more about her general health and specific health care needs and how to articulate knowledge of her own condition when meeting with new doctors. It is also a chance for the parents to understand what gaps in knowledge and experience must be learned before the teen is ready to transition to adult health care and more independence. For the child with CP who may not be able to assume this kind of responsibility, for instance, because of cognitive limitations, the parents themselves may want to complete such a form.

One of the first priorities of the child transitioning her care will be to find a primary care provider who hopefully can provide a "medical home" for the young adult. This may be a family doctor who has monitored the child since infancy, or it may be the parents' own doctor who has cared for them but not for the child, and who may now be willing to assume that responsibility as well. Or it may be someone entirely new to the child and family. This primary care doctor would then help in identifying which specialists will be needed and who they might be. Alternatively, the pediatric subspecialists who have cared for the child until now may be able to identify colleagues of theirs who treat adults.

Healthy People 2010, a plan generated by the United States Department of Health and Human Services in 2000, established a goal that all young people with special health care needs will receive the services needed to make necessary transitions to all aspects of adult life, including health care, work, and independent living. There continue to be significant barriers to this goal, which can be divided into three major components that promote or impede the movement from child-centered to adult systems: service needs, structural issues, and personal preferences. Service needs refers to the availability or absence of treatment services and the degree to which these services will satisfy the young adult and his family. Such services must be developmentally appropriate and address the changing and maturing needs of young adults, including services that address his reproductive issues and concerns. Structural issues refer to insurance coverage, institutional policies, and

medical practice that either promote or impede the transition. Many youths and young adults lack the health insurance they need because family health insurance coverage typically ends for dependent children between 18 and 23 years of age, and the young adult may not have a job that provides health insurance. Many health insurance safety-net programs that are available to children are not available to young adults. The third is personal preferences and interpersonal dynamics. On the one hand, young adults often want to make the transition because they no longer want to be treated as a child. Barriers include the fact that the adult health providers may not recognize the family and young adult herself as being knowledgeable members of the treatment team in the way that the pediatric team did. In addition, many families and pediatricians have built up a very close personal relationship through the years and will have a hard time separating as this phase approaches.

Although not all these problems can be addressed, the following are suggestions to help make the transition a bit easier: The family, young adult, and provider must have an awareness that the child will likely live into adulthood (which is certainly true for most children with CP) and the transition process should be started early, meaning before adolescence. This includes planning for insurance coverage, providers, and equipment. Family members and health care providers need to foster as much personal and medical independence as the child is capable of. The pediatric health care workers and families need to learn to "say goodbye" and to celebrate transitions as they occur. As part of this process, develop a written transition plan that anticipates future needs and use the plan as a means to document what has been completed and what still needs to be done.

Triplegia

Triplegia is a term that may be confusing. There is not a typical pattern of involvement, although it is best used to describe children who have significant involvement in three limbs and have one limb that is much more functional. Usually it describes involvement of both legs and one arm. There is tremendous variation in this pattern—it is usually a combination of hemiplegia overlaying diplegia. However, some children have quadriplegia, with much less involvement in one arm.

Ultrasonography

(ultrasound)

Ultrasonography is an imaging technique employing high-frequency sound waves (above the level that we can hear) that bounce off body tissues. When sound waves are sent through body tissue, some bounce back and can be used to make a picture, which can then be viewed on a video screen. The echo pictures that show solid and fluid structures in the body are interpreted by a radiologist who has been specially trained to recognize them. The ultrasound apparatus consists of a console about the size of a desk and is equipped with one or more video monitors. Only the transducer actually comes in contact with the patient. This device emits and receives the sound waves and is connected by a cable to the console. The technologist doing the scan puts a clear gel over the area to be scanned, which helps form a better connection between the transducer and the patient. The technician then slides the transducer around until the appropriate images have been seen and recorded on the video monitor. There is no pain or discomfort when having an ultrasound exam.

Indications: Ultrasound is used extensively for imaging the fetus during pregnancy and is used to evaluate the brain in newborn infants when the skull is not completely closed. It is also used to evaluate hip dislocation in infants and to view the liver, spleen, and kidneys.

Benefits and risks: The major benefit of ultrasound examination is that it involves no radiation and is performed quickly without requiring sedation. The major risk is that the images obtained are often difficult to interpret; the outcome may depend on the skill of the technician or physician doing the examination. For this reason, ultrasound is most helpful when it is used by technicians and physicians with special training.

Umbilical Hernia

An umbilical hernia occurs when the muscle in the abdomen around the umbilicus (or belly button) has a weakness that allows the intestines to come through the opening. This type of hernia is very common and rarely causes problems in children. It is often present in very young children; as they grow, the area becomes tighter and the hernia does not bulge as much.

Unless the hernia becomes very sore, surgery is seldom recommended before age 5. If the hernia is present after age 5, it is not likely to improve on its own and a surgical repair is indicated, to tighten the muscles around the umbilicus. Complications from the surgery are rare, since it is a small procedure (usually performed on an outpatient basis) which involves suturing some of the muscle and skin. If an infection occurs, it can easily be identified and treated.

Tylenol is usually sufficient for after-surgery care. The child may be as active as he wants and is usually allowed to take a bath after three or four days.

Undescended Testicles

(testicles, testicular torsion, orchidopexy)

When a male fetus is growing in his mother's womb, his testicles form high up in his abdomen. Gradually, in the last trimester of pregnancy, they move down from the abdomen into the scrotum, where they normally are at the time of birth. If the testicles do not come down in the scrotum, they are considered undescended. Premature infants are more likely to have undescended testicles than fullterm infants because this migration process has not fully occurred. Both testicles should be descended into the scrotum by the first birthday.

Some boys have testicles that are called "retractile," because they are not in the scrotum most of the time but can be felt high at the top of the scrotum at the edge of the groin. But when they are pulled, they come down into the scrotum without any discomfort or much tension. Generally, retractile testicles do not become undescended but with growth relax and come down into the scrotum. These should be monitored by the pediatrician, however, because occasionally they can become stuck in the high position, which is technically a form of undescended testicles.

Boys with spasticity due to cerebral palsy have a high incidence of undescended testicles, which may be due in part to the frequency of prematurity at birth, but is probably also due to the spasticity, which is present in the muscles and pulls the testicles back into the abdomen.

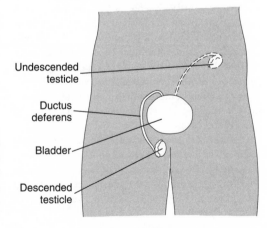

Undescended testicle

Ductus deferens

Bladder

Descended testicle

The surgery: The operation to bring the testicles down into the scrotum is called an orchidopexy; it is usually recommended for boys whose testicles have not descended into the scrotum by age 1. The surgical descending of the testicles is performed to keep the testicle from becoming entrapped or twisted, thereby cutting off its blood supply and causing it to die, which requires an emergency operation. There is also an increased risk of developing testicular cancer later in life if testicles are not descended into the scrotum. Bringing the testicle down into the scrotum, however, does not necessarily reduce the risk of cancer, but it does make the testicles much easier to examine for the presence of any lumps or masses. Also, boys who are active are much more likely to injure the testicle if it is partially descended, as it often sits right in front of the pubic bone, so any pressure in that area can damage the testicle. Another reason for surgically bringing the testicle down into the scrotum is to enhance the boy's self-esteem, especially when he grows older.

The surgery is usually performed on an outpatient basis: the child comes to the hospital, has general anesthesia, and then leaves the same day. An incision is made in the groin, the testicle is identified and brought down into the groin, and a suture is placed, holding it down to the bottom of the scrotum. Afterwards, boys are often limited in their activities, partially because of the discomfort and partially because the procedure needs time to heal.

Benefits and risks: The procedure has a very high success rate, and complications are rare. The boys usually recover very quickly and by two weeks are back to full activity without any problems. Parents should follow up with a physical examination every year until puberty to make certain that the testicles continue to grow normally. When complications occur, infection is the most common, and can easily be treated with antibiotics. Infection is identified by the child's having a fever, not wanting to eat, and having an inflamed incision. Occasionally, the blood supply to the testicle is insufficient, and the testicle has to be removed. If this occurs, a simple procedure, called *frame plantation of a testicular prosthesis,* is recommended at puberty. Occasionally, the testicle may remain undescended even after the surgical procedure, and a repeat operation is sometimes necessary.

Children with one undescended testicle have a slightly lower fertility rate than the general population. Infertility, however, is very common when both testicles are undescended. It's debatable whether the operation to descend the testicles improves fertility, but a significant number of doctors believe that it does not do so.

Unit Rod
(Luque rod, segmental sublaminar instrumentation [SSI])

A Luque rod is a smooth, stainless steel rod that is attached to the spine with wires that are passed between the spinal lamina in the back and the spinal cord beneath it. It provides very strong fixation because wires are passed at each vertebra. Usually two rods are used, one on each side of the spine in the back.

This system was originally designed to be used with patients who have neuromuscular problems; it is still utilized by a number of surgeons. However, the Luque rod has been superseded by the unit rod, an improved version that has only one single rod bent in a configuration that is ideal for enabling a child to sit. This rod may be a single unit, al-

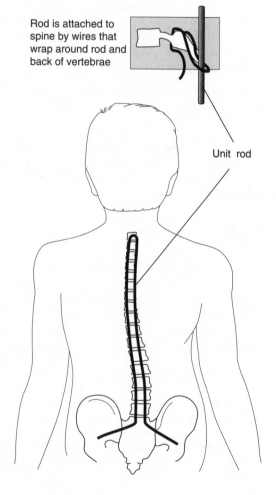

Rod is attached to spine by wires that wrap around rod and back of vertebrae

Unit rod

though some surgeons use two rods and connect them with rigid plates to make a unit rod. The unit rod is more stable than the two individual Luque rods and is far better at maintaining correction and correcting pelvic obliquity. This is the current preferred instrumentation for children with cerebral palsy.

Indications: This instrumentation is indicated for patients who have progressive scoliosis, kyphosis, or lordosis because of neuromuscular problems. One of the main indications is for children with spinal deformities due to cerebral palsy.

Benefits and risks: The benefit of the unit rod is excellent correction of the spinal deformity, which is held strongly enough so that no cast or brace is needed after surgery. Complications and risks are those of a posterior spinal fusion. The major problem with the individual Luque rods is their instability, which can prevent adequate correction of the curve at the time of surgery. In addition, the rods can shift, causing a loss of the original correction. The rods may need to be revised, since the curve can become large enough so that the child has a great deal of difficulty sitting. Also, if the spine does not heal, the rods may break and need to be revised.

Maintenance and care: Generally, after instrumentation with these systems the child is able to sit in a chair, take a shower after two weeks, and return to school after four weeks with no special restrictions or instructions. No special maintenance is necessary.

Urinary Tract Infections

Urinary tract infections include a range of infections by microorganisms in the urinary tract. Fever may be the only symptom of a urinary tract infection, especially in young children. Boys are affected far more often than girls during the newborn period, and it has been found that uncircumcised boys are affected far more frequently than those who have been circumcised. This has led to a change in thinking regarding circumcision—which until recently was felt to be an unnecessary procedure that was done for cultural but not medical reasons.

After the newborn period, urinary tract infections are far more common in girls, but, for both boys and girls, there needs to be further evaluation of the urinary tract system if an infection occurs. A major contributor to infections may be vesicoureteral reflux, which means that when the bladder attempts to empty, some urine goes back up into the ureters toward the kidney, rather than out of the body. Other predisposing factors are incomplete drainage

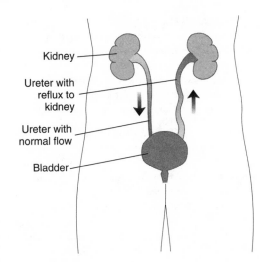

Kidney
Ureter with reflux to kidney
Ureter with normal flow
Bladder

and/or stasis in the urinary system, which means that the bladder does not empty completely and some urine remains in the bladder, allowing bacteria to multiply. In addition, if infected urine comes back up from the bladder into the kidney, because of vesicoureteral reflux, it can cause kidney damage. This is the situation in some patients with cerebral palsy, whose neurological condition has caused poor bladder functioning.

Patients with urinary tract infections should undergo radiological studies to evaluate the anatomy of the kidney and bladder and to determine whether there is vesicoureteral reflux present. Ultrasound examination of the kidney, ureters, and bladder shows the anatomy of this system. The evaluation for reflux is done by a procedure called a voiding cystourethrogram (VCUG), which consists of placing dye into the bladder and watching to see if it is all emptied out or whether some is pushed up toward the kidney.

The degree of reflux is graded on a scale from 1 to 5, with 1 being the mildest and 5 the most severe. Mild forms of reflux are usually managed with the use of prophylactic antibiotics (perhaps one dose a day of an antibiotic to prevent a urinary tract infection), whereas more severe reflux may need to be treated with surgery, by a urologist. If both the ultrasonogram and the VCUG are normal, then no further evaluation is necessary. If the VCUG shows reflux or if the ultrasonogram of the kidney is abnormal, then a renal scan is performed. This is the most sensitive means of detecting scarring of the kidney.

Urodynamic Testing

For patients with cerebral palsy who are not able to be toilet trained, the incontinence may be due to the dynamic function of the bladder, which can be evaluated by urodynamic testing. This test consists of measuring the pressure and volume of the bladder as well as the sphincter muscles, which should relax and contract at various times during urination. If these various processes are not working normally, testing will aid in assessing the problem and may indicate the right medication to help relieve these symptoms.

Indications: Children who are 5 years of age or older and have the mental capacity to understand the concept of going to the bathroom, but who are unable to control their bladder, should have urologic evaluation including uroflometry and urodynamic testing. Children who have periodic incontinence, which they do not seem to be able to control, should also undergo urologic evaluation. The child who has to urinate very frequently may have a very small bladder volume, and this too can be measured and detected with urodynamic testing. A comprehensive urodynamic evaluation includes noninvasive assessment of urination (uroflometry and post–void residual measurements) and invasive testing (a catheter in the bladder measures bladder pressure).

Benefits and risks: The benefit of this test is that it can measure the bladder's capacity and the functioning of the sphincter muscles, so that the cause of incontinence can be determined. The major risk is that it requires inserting a catheter, which has a very small chance of causing an infection in the bladder.

Maintenance and care: If the child develops burning upon urination or a fever after urodynamic testing, it may indicate an infection. In this case, the child may need antibiotics for several days. There is no other aftercare required.

Vagus Nerve Stimulator

The FDA approved the vagus nerve stimulator (VNS) in July 1997 for use in the treatment of uncontrolled seizures. The precise mechanism of action is unknown. However, it has been shown to effectively control seizures in some patients and significantly reduce seizure frequency and/or duration in many others. The device also gives the patient/family/caregiver an active part in the reduction of seizures.

The child/adolescent has an evaluation with a neurologist and health care team that is trained in the use of the VNS. Tests may be conducted, such as video electroencephalograms (EEGs) and medical imaging studies. Once it is determined that the child is a candidate for surgery, a surgical evaluation is done by either a neurosurgeon or cardiovascular surgeon, who usually do this procedure. Once these evaluations are complete, the child/adolescent is scheduled for surgery. The device is placed under the skin,

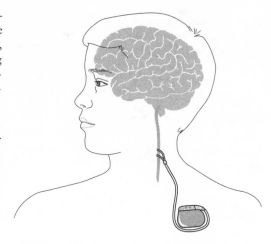

usually in the left chest area. It has wires that are threaded up under the skin and wrapped around the left vagus nerve in the neck. The vagus nerve has a link to the brain. The device is programmed by a special computer to stimulate the left vagus nerve throughout the day, which ultimately stimulates the base of the brain. This stimulus helps to control seizures in some individuals. The VNS also comes with a special, very strong magnet. This magnet can be moved over the device in the chest by the patient/family/caregiver to cause an additional stimulus to try to prevent or stop a seizure.

The VNS can be effective for all seizure types. It is available to all patients who have failed or are unable to tolerate other modalities (i.e., antiepileptic drugs, the ketogenic diet) and are not candidates for epilepsy surgery. Side effects are few. In regard to the surgical procedure, there are the risks that accompany any procedure, such as infections and bleeding, as well as anesthesia risks. There is also the rare possibility of the body's rejection of the device. In addition, some individuals experience hoarseness, coughing, gagging, and/or tingling when the device is activated.

Once the individual has the device implanted, they must keep routine appointments with a health care provider who is knowledgeable about the VNS device. The health care provider will continue to manage the individual's response to the device and its effectiveness. In some situations, antiepileptic medications may either be reduced or discontinued completely.

Valgus

(valgus foot, valgus hip, valgus knee)

Valgus is an anatomical term used to mean that a part of the body is bending away from the midline. The term valgus is generally applied to the legs. At the hip it means an increased angle of the femoral head and neck with the shaft of the femur (thighbone). At the knee it means that the leg below is bending away from the midline; or, in other words, the child is knock-kneed. At the foot and ankle, the term is used to define the foot's turning away from the midline and is approximately synonymous with the term *eversion,* which means that the sole points away from the midline of the body.

Varicella

(chickenpox)

Congenital infection of infants with varicella, due to the mother's infection early during pregnancy (up to 20 weeks gestation), is quite rare. Affected infants may have a low birth weight due to intrauterine growth retardation. In addition, they may have distinctive skin abnormalities, incomplete development of certain fingers or toes, abnormalities of the brain such as cortical atrophy or dilated ventricles, macrocephaly, small eyes, seizures, mental retardation, and neuromotor abnormalities that are treated similarly to cerebral palsy.

Varus

(varus hip, varus knee, varus foot)

Varus is an anatomical term meaning that a part of the body is bending toward the midline. When varus affects the hip, it means that the angle between the femoral head, neck, and femoral shaft is decreasing. When varus affects the knee, it means that the leg below the knee is bending toward the midline (also known as bowlegs). At the foot the sole is pointing toward the midline of the body; varus foot is synonymous with inversion of the foot.

Visual Impairment

(low vision, legal blindness)

Low vision technically means that a person may need optical aids or other modifications, i.e., TV monitor, Braille, or special lighting to be able to recognize objects that the normal person can see just with room light or normal glasses. Children with low vision qualify for state assistance, but a patient who is defined as legally blind will get additional benefits. Even if the child has CP and/or other impairments, having the ophthalmologist designate legal blindness may provide more services and benefits than just having the child diagnosed with low vision.

A person who cannot recognize the large E at a distance of 20 feet is considered legally blind. Also, if the visual field is markedly decreased even with fairly good central vision, one can be considered legally blind. For the child with CP who cannot see or speak and who may also be mentally retarded, the designation of legal blindness may seem insignificant. However, being designated legally blind does provide a number of benefits such as disability payments and additional educational services. The legal definition of blindness may be difficult to apply to a noncommunicative child, but a clinical diagnosis can usually be made by an ophthalmologist.

Vocational Rehabilitation

(job training)

Vocational rehabilitation is a program of evaluating teenagers or young adults to define their strengths and to determine vocational possibilities that will use these strengths. It generally starts in high school; most states have vocational rehabilitation training programs for young adults as well. In order to succeed with a given individual, rehabilitation must take into account the whole person, including her or his specific interests; visual, cognitive, and physical abilities; and psychological and behavioral stability. The goal is to develop a realistic plan that will match the individual with a job that is appropriate for his abilities.

Resources: Support Groups, Foundations, and Government Agencies

Advocacy Groups

American Association of People with Disabilities (AAPD)
1819 H Street NW
Suite 330
Washington, DC 20006
Works to further the productivity, independence, and integration of people with disabilities into all aspects of society. The AAPD offers financial benefits to its members in the form of services to help people with disabilities move toward achieving consumer and economic power.
1-800-840-8844
1-202-457-0046 (Fax)
www.aapd-dc.org/
aapd@aol.com

The ARC of the United States
1010 Wayne Ave
Silver Spring, MD 20910
1-301-565-3842
1-301-565-3843 (Fax)
www.thearc.org

Center on Disabilities at the California State University, Northridge (CSUN)
18111 Nordhoff Street
Northridge, CA 91330-8340
Conducts research and demonstration projects into new technologies and service models, develops and publishes materials of interest to the field of disability, assesses and trains persons with disabilities and those who serve them, and conducts conferences, seminars, and workshops in the United States and around the world.
1-818-677-2578
1-818-677-4929 (Fax)
www.csun.edu/cod
ltm@csun.edu

Citizens United for Research in Epilepsy (CURE)
505 North Lake Shore Drive
Suite 4605
Chicago, IL 60611
1-312-923-9117
www.cureepilepsy.org

Epilepsy Foundation
4351 Garden City Drive
Landover, MD 20785
1-800-332-1000
www.epilepsyfoundation.org

Family Village
Has a list of chat sites for children with CP or their parents, links to information in a variety of languages, and other organizations that deal with CP.
www.familyvillage.wisc.edu/lib_cerp.htm

Family Voices, Inc.
2340 Alamo SE
Suite 102
Albuquerque, NM 87107
1-505-872-4774
1-505-872-4780 (Fax)
www.familyvoices.org

March of Dimes Birth Defects Foundation
1275 Mamaroneck Avenue
White Plains, NJ 10605
1-914-428-7100
www.modimes.org

Movement Disorder Society
611 Wells Street
Milwaukee, WI 53202

Provides international forums to disseminate information on recent advances in both clinical and basic science pertinent to movement disorders, to encourage research related to movement disorders; and to enhance the education of physicians and the quality of care of patients with movement disorders.
1-414-276-2145
1-414-276-2146 (Fax)
www.movementdisorders.org/
jreichertz@movementdisorders.org

National Dissemination Center for Children with Disabilities (NICHCY)
P.O. Box 1492
Washington, DC 20013-1492
1-800-695-0285 (V/TTY)
1-202-884-8441 (Fax)
www.nichcy.org

National Organization on Disability (NOD)
910 Sixteenth Street, NW
Suite 600
Washington, DC 20006
A national disability network organization concerned with all disabilities, age groups, and disability issues. NOD works to promote the full and equal participation for people with disabilities in all aspects of life.
1-202-293-5960
1-202-293-7999 (Fax)
www.nod.org/
ability@nod.org

National Rehabilitation Association (NRA)
633 S Washington Street
Alexandria, VA 22314
NRA was founded in 1925 to promote the rehabilitation of persons with disabilities through legislative activity, professional development, and public education.
1-703-836-0850
1-703-836-0848 (Fax)
www.nationalrehab.org/
info@nationalrehab.org

SCOPE
Scope is a disability organization whose focus is people with cerebral palsy in England and Wales, providing information and education.
www.scope.org.uk/

TASH—Disability Advocacy Worldwide
29 W. Susquehanna Ave.
Suite 210
Baltimore, MD 21204

TASH is an international association of people with disabilities, their family members, other advocates, and professionals fighting for a society in which inclusion of all people in all aspects of society is the norm. It actively promotes the full inclusion and participation of persons with disabilities in all aspects of life.
1-410-828-8274, ext. 101
1-410-828-6706 (Fax)
www.tash.org/
nweiss@tash.org

United Cerebral Palsy Association (UCPA)
1660 L Street, NW
Washington, DC 20036-5602
The mission of UCPA is to advance the independence, productivity, and full participation in society of people with cerebral palsy and other disabilities.
1-800-USA-5UCP
1-202-776-0414 (Fax)
www.ucpa.org/
ucpnatl@ucpa.org

Americans with Disabilities Act (ADA)

Disability Rights Education and Defense Fund
ADA Technical Assistance Information Line
1-800-466-4232 (V/TT)

Equal Employment Opportunity Commission
1-800-669-3362 (V)
1-800-800-3302 (TT)

Job Accommodation Network
1-800-526-7234 (V/TT)
1-800-232-9675 (V/TT; ADA Information)

U.S. Architectural and Transportation Barriers Compliance Board—Access Board
1-800-872-2253 (V)
1-202-728-5483 (TT; in DC metro area)

U.S. Department of Housing and Urban Development—HUD User
1-800-245-2691 (V)

U.S. Department of Justice
ADA information line
1-202-514-0301
www.ada.gov

Assistive Technology/Devices

Able Net
1-800-322-0956 (V)

ABLEDATA
1-800-227-0216
www.abledata.com

Adaptive Mall
1-800-371-2778
www.adaptivemall.com

Apple Office for Special Education Material
1-800-732-3131, ext. 950 (V)

AT&T Accessible Communications Product Center
1-800-233-1222 (V)
1-800-833-3232 (TT)

Family Center on Technology and Disability (FCTD)
www.fctd.info

IBM Special Needs Information Referral Center
1-800-426-4832 (V)
1-800-284-4833 (TT)

TECHKNOWLEDGE
1-800-726-9119 (V)
1-404-894-4960 (V; in Atlanta metro area)

Blindness/Visual Impairment

American Council of the Blind
1-800-424-8666 (V/TT)
www.acb.org

American Foundation for the Blind
1-800-232-5463 (V)
www.afb.org

Blind Children's Center
1-800-222-3566 (V)
1-800-222-3567 (V; in CA)

Job Opportunities for the Blind
1-800-638-7518 (V)
1-410-659-9314 (V; in MD)

Lighthouse National Center for Vision and Child Development
1-800-334-5497 (V)
1-212-808-5544 (TT; in New York City)

National Association for Visually Handicapped
www.navh.org

National Association of Parents of the Visually Impaired
1-800-562-6265 (V)

National Federation of the Blind
www.nfb.org

National Library Service for the Blind and Physically Handicapped
www.loc.gov/nls

National Society to Prevent Blindness
1-800-331-2020 (V)

Recording for the Blind
1-800-221-4792 (V)

Communication Disorders

National Institute on Deafness and Other Communication Disorders Clearinghouse
1-800-241-1044 (V)
1-800-241-1055 (TT)

Deafness/Hearing Impairments

American Society for Deaf Children
1-800-942-2732 (V/TT)
www.deafchildren.org/home/home.html

Beginnings
1-800-541-HEAR (V/TTY)

Better Hearing Institute
1-800-327-9355 (V/TT)
www.betterhearing.org

Deafness Research Foundation
1-800-535-3323 (V/TT)
1-212-684-6559 (V/TT; in New York City)

Hear Now
1-800-648-4327 (V/TT)

John Tracy Clinic
1-800-522-4582 (V/TT)
1-213-748-5481 (V; in Los Angeles)
1-213-747-2924 (TT)
www.johntracyclinic.org

National Association of the Deaf
www.nad.org

National Hearing Aid Society
1-800-521-5247 (V)

National Institute on Deafness and Other Communication Disorders Clearinghouse
1-800-241-1044 (V)
1-800-241-1055 (TT)

Where Do We Go from Hear?
www.gohear.org/index.html

Dental Care

Video titled, "Your Smile"
Write or call:
HMS School for Children with Cerebral Palsy
4400 Baltimore Avenue
Philadelphia, PA 19004
1-215-222-2566

Developmental Disability (DD) Councils

National Association of Councils on Developmental Disabilities
Each state has a "DD" council that serves as an advocate for persons with developmental disabilities. The National Association of Councils on Developmental Disabilities Web site has a link to councils in all 50 states.
www.nacdd.org

Disability Awareness

Kids on the Block
1-800-368-5437 (V)
www.kotb.com

Education

American Association for Vocational Instructional Materials
1-800-228-4689 (V)

Association for Childhood Education International
1-800-423-3563 (V)

Center for the Study and Advancement of Disability Policy (CSADP), Special Education, 2003.
www.disabilitypolicycenter.org

Council for Exceptional Children (CEC)
An international organization that is dedicated to improving educational outcomes for individuals with exceptionalities, students with disabilities, and/or the gifted. Excellent site for up-to-date information on Individuals with Disabilities Education Act (IDEA).
www.cec.sped.org

Disability Rights, Education and Defense Fund (DREDF)
A national law and policy center dedicated to protecting and advancing the civil rights of people with disabilities. Excellent site for recent legislative activities relating to Individuals with Disabilities Education Act (IDEA).
www.dredf.org

HEATH Resource Center of the American Council on Education
A national clearing house on postsecondary education for individuals with disabilities. Excellent site for information and referral services for parents with children with disabilities.
1 DuPont Circle, Suite 800
Washington, DC 20036-1193
1-800-544-3284 (V/TT)
1-202-939-9320 (V/TT; in DC metro area)
www.acenet.edu/programs/HEATH/home.html

National Center for Research in Vocational Education
1-800-762-4093 (V)

National Center for School Leadership
1-800-643-3205 (V)

National Challenged Homeschoolers Associated Network (NATHHAN)
Christian Families homeschooling special needs children
P.O. Box 39
Porthill, ID 83853
1-208-267-6246
1-208-267-6246 (Fax)
www.nathhan.com
nathanews@aol.com

National Committee for Citizens in Education Clearinghouse
1-800-638-9675 (V)
1-800-532-9832 (V; Spanish)

National Dissemination Center for Children with Disabilities
The dissemination center is funded by the Office of Special Education Programs (OSEP) at the U.S. Department of Education to connect individuals with the resources they need in their efforts on behalf of children with disabilities.
www.nichcy.org

National Home Education Network
Provides information, fosters networking, and promotes

public relations for local and state homeschooling organizations. Has a special needs section on its Web site.
www.nhen.org

Office of Special Education and Rehabilitative Services
(OSERS)
Administering programs and projects relating to free, appropriate public education of all children, youth, and
adults with disabilities, from birth through age 21.
www.ed.gov/about/offices/list/osers/index.html

PACER Center
A nonprofit organization that provides workshops and
individual assistance and disseminates materials to
help parents become informed and effective representatives for their children with disabilities in early-
childhood, school-age, and vocational settings. Excellent site for publications on support services.
www.pacer.org

The Special Ed Advocate
This organization provides parents, educators, attorneys,
and other helping professionals with the information
they need to be effective advocates for special needs
children. This site contains current articles, cases, and
links related to special education. Excellent site for
current cases on special education issues.
www.wrightslaw.com

U.S. Office of Educational Research and Improvement
1-800-424-1616 (V)

Employment

Equal Employment Opportunity Commission
1-800-669-3362 (V)
1-800-800-3302 (TT)

Job Accommodation Network (JAN)
West Virginia University
918 Chestnut Ridge Road, Suite 1
Morgantown, WV 26505
1-800-526-7234 (V/TDD)
1-304-293-7186 (V)

Job Opportunities for the Blind
1-800-638-7518 (V)
1-410-659-9314 (V; in MD)

Mainstream, Inc.
3 Bethesda Metro Center, Suite 830
Bethesda, MD 20814
1-301-654-2400 (V/TDD)

National Industries for the Severely Handicapped
(NISH)
2235 Cedar Lane
Vienna, VA 22182
1-703-560-6800 (V/TDD)

Financial Counseling

ABC's of Special Needs Planning Made Easy, by Bart
Stevens, ChLAP
Barton Stevens Special Needs Planning, LLC, Phoenix,
AZ, 2002

Estate Planning for Special Needs
www.metlife.com/desk
1-877-638-3375

GO GET BENEFITS: An excellent reference guide that
teaches you your health care and disability rights. Ms.
Guren, who is disabled herself, writes a resource book
that can only help the user.
Nancy Guren
10714 Kings Riding Way
T-3
Rockville, MD 20852
RQX@AOL.com

National Foundation for Consumer Credit
1-800-388-2227 (V)

Health Care

Children's Hospice International
P.O. Box 20050
Alexandria, VA 22320-1050
1-800-242-4453 (V)
1-703-684-0330 (V)

Independent Living

Accent on Living Magazine
P.O. Box 700
Bloomington, IL 61702
1-309-378-2961

Independent Living Research Utilization Program
(ILRU)
2323 S. Shepherd Street, Suite 1000
Houston, TX 77019
1-713-520-0232 (V)
1-713-520-5136 (TDD)

National Council on Independent Living (NCIL)
2111 Wilson Boulevard, Suite 405
Arlington, VA 22201
1-703-525-3406 (TT)
www.ncil.org

Society for the Advancement of Travel for the Handicapped and Elderly
347 5th Avenue, Suite 610
New York, NY 10016
1-212-447-7284 (V)

Information Services

ACCESS ERIC
1-800-538-3742 (V)

BRS Information Technologies
1-800-289-4277 (V)

Date Able
1-301-657-DATE (in Chevy Chase, MD)

Easter Seal Society
1-800-221-6827 (V)
1-312-726-4258 (TT; in Chicago metro area)

National Center for Youth with Disabilities
1-800-333-6293 (V)
1-612-624-3939 (TT; in Minneapolis metro area)

National Information Clearinghouse for Infants with
Disabilities and Life-Threatening Conditions
1-800-922-9234, ext. 201 (V/TT)
1-800-922-1107, ext. 201 (V/TT; in SC)

National Rehabilitation Information Center
1-800-346-2742 (V/TT)
www.naric.com

ODPHP National Health Information Center
1-800-336-4797 (V)

Office of Minority Health Resource Center
1-800-444-6472 (V)

Legal Assistance

American Bar Association Center on Children and
the Law
1800 M Street NW, Suite 2005
Washington, DC 20036
1-202-331-2250 (V)

Disability Rights Education and Defense Fund (DREDF)
2212 Sixth Street
Berkeley, CA 94710
1-800-466-4232 (V)
1-510-644-2555 (V)
1-510-644-2556 (V/TDD)

Legal Rights of the Catastrophically Ill and Injured:
A Family Guide
Joseph Romano
www.josephromanolaw.com
info@josephromanolaw.com

National Association of Protection and Advocacy Systems (NAPAS)
Has background information and links to all state Protection and Advocacy (P&A) systems on its Web site.
Every state has a P&A agency which provides advocacy and legal services to persons with disabilities,
usually for free.
www.napas.org

National Center for Law and Deafness
Gallaudet University
800 Florida Avenue, NE
Washington, DC 20002
1-202-651-5373 (V/TDD)

Partners in Policymaking Program
This is an innovative leadership training program for
adults with disabilities and for parents of young children with developmental disabilities.
www.partnersinpolicymaking.com

Medical Home

National Center of Medical Home Initiatives for Children with Special Needs
The state resource pages provide information on state
medical home initiatives, key partners, related grant activities, and local resources for families and providers.
www.medicalhomeinfo.org/resources/state.html

Mental Retardation

American Association on Mental Retardation
1-800-424-3688 (V)
www.aamr.org

The Arc: National Organization on Mental Retardation
500 East Border Street, Suite 300
Arlington, TX 79010

1-817-261-6003 (V)
1-817-277-0553 (V/TDD)
www.thearc.org

Nutrition

Axcan Scandipharm Inc.
1-800-4-SCANDI
(1-800-472-2634)

Beech Nut Nutrition Hotline
1-800-523-6633 (V)

Gerber Consumer Information
1-800-443-7237 (V)

Mead-Johnson
1-800-BABY 123
(1-800-222-9123)

Nestle
1-800-422-ASK2
(1-800-422-2752)

North American Growth and Cerebral Palsy Program
www.med.virginia.edu/~mon-grow/

Ross Laboratories
1-800-FORMULA
(1-800-367-6852)

Parents and Family Care

Families of Children under Stress (FOCUS)
P.O. Box 941445
Atlanta, GA 31141
1-404-270-5072 (V)

National Parent Network on Disabilities
1600 Prince Street, Suite 115
Alexandria, VA 22314
1-703-684-6763 (V/TT)

Parent Care, Inc.
9041 Colgate Street
Indianapolis, IN 46268-1210
1-317-872-9913 (V)

Parent to Parent
1-404-451-5482 (V; in Atlanta metro area)

Siblings for Significant Change
United Charities Building
105 East 22nd Street, Room 710
New York, New York 10010

1-800-841-8251 (V)
1-212-420-0776 (V)

Siblings Information Network
A. J. Pappanikou Center on Special Education and
    Rehabilitation
62 Washington Street
Middletown, CT 06457-2844
1-203-244-7500 (V)
1-203-344-7590 (V/TDD)

Professional Organizations

American Academy of Cerebral Palsy and Developmental
    Medicine (AACPDM)
6300 North River Road
Suite 727
Rosemont, IL 60018-4226
This organization is a multidisciplinary scientific society
    devoted to studying cerebral palsy and other child-
    hood onset disabilities, to promoting professional ed-
    ucation for the treatment and management of these
    conditions, and to improving the quality of life for
    people with these disabilities.
1-847-698-1635
1-847-823-0536 (Fax)
woppenhe@ucla.edu
http://aacpdm.org/

American Academy of Physical Medicine & Rehabilita-
    tion (AAPMR)
One IBM Plaza
Suite 2500
Chicago, IL 60611-3604
The American Academy of Physical Medicine & Rehabili-
    tation is a national medical society, representing more
    than 6,000 physicians who are specialists in the field
    of physical medicine and rehabilitation. The associa-
    tion provides continuing education opportunities,
    increases awareness of the specialty, and advocates
    public policies.
1-312-464-9700
1-312-464-0227 (Fax)
www.aapmr.org/
info@aapmr.org

American Congress of Rehabilitation Medicine (ACRM)
5987 East 71st Street
Suite 111
Indianapolis, IN 46220-4049
The mission of the American Congress of Rehabilitation
    Medicine (ACRM) is to promote the art, science, and
    practice of rehabilitation care for people with disabilities.

1-317-915-2250
1-317-915-2245 (Fax)
www.acrm.org/
acrm@acrm.org

American Health Care Association (AHCA)
1201 L Street NW
Washington, DC 20005
The American Health Care Association (AHCA) is a federation of 50 state health organizations, together representing nearly 12,000 nonprofit and for-profit assisted living, nursing facility, long-term care, and subacute care providers that care for more than one million elderly and disabled individuals nationally.
1-202-842-4444
1-202-842-3860 (Fax)
www.ahca.org/

American Occupational Therapy Association (AOTA)
4720 Montgomery Lane
Bethesda, MD 20814-3425
1-301-652-2682, ext. 2012
1-301-652-7711 (Fax)
www.aota.org/
lesliej@aota.org

American Physical Therapy Association (APTA)
1111 North Fairfax Street
Alexandria, VA 22314
1-703-684-2782
1-703-684-7343 (Fax)
www.apta.org/
svcctr@apta.org

Association of Rehabilitation Nurses (ARN)
700 W. Lake Avenue
Glenview, IL 60025-1485
ARN's mission is to promote and advance professional rehabilitation nursing practice through education, advocacy, collaboration, and research to enhance the quality of life for those affected by disability and chronic illness.
1-800-229-7530
1-847-375-4777 (Fax)
www.rehabnurse.org/
info@rehabnurse.org

National Academy for Child Development (NACD)
PO Box 380
Huntsville, UT 84317
1-801-621-8606
nacdinfo@nacd.org

National Association for Home Care (NAHC)
228 Seventh Street, SE
Washington, DC 20003
NAHC is a trade association that represents the interests of more than 6,000 home care agencies, hospices, and home care aide organizations. Its members are primarily corporations or other organizational entities in addition to state home care associations, medical equipment suppliers, and schools.
1-202-547-7424
1-202-547-3540 (Fax)
www.nahc.org/
clc@nahc.org

National Institute of Neurological Disorders and Stroke (NINDS)
NIH Neurological Institute
P.O. Box 5801
Bethesda, MD 20824
1-800-352-9494
www.ninds.nih.gov/

National Organization for Rare Disorders (NORD)
100 Route 37
P.O. Box 8923
New Fairfield, CT 06812-8923
An organization with a database on over 1,000 rare diseases, with educational materials for parents and health professionals. It also has links to parent support groups and hundreds of organizations that can help families deal with these rare conditions.
1-203-746-6518
1-203-746-6481 (Fax)
www.rarediseases.org
orphan@rarediseases.org

Rehabilitation Engineering and Assistive Technology Society of North America (RESNA)
1700 North Moore Street
Suite 1540
Arlington, VA 22209-1903
RESNA is as an interdisciplinary society that promotes the transfer of science, engineering, and technology to meet the needs of individuals with disabilities.
1-703-524-6686
1-703-524-6630 (Fax)
www.resna.org/
info@resna.org

Rehabilitation

Canadian Rehabilitation Council for the Disabled (CRCD)
45 Sheppard Avenue East, Suite 801
Willowdale, Ontario
CANADA M2N 5W9
1-416-250-7490 (V/TDD)

Clearinghouse for Rehabilitation and Technology
    Information
1-800-638-8864 (V)
1-800-852-2892 (TT)

National Clearinghouse of Rehabilitation Training Materials
1-800-223-5219 (V/TT)

Religious Organizations

Christian Council on Persons with Disabilities
36272 County Road 79
Warsaw, OH 43844
1-614-327-2311 (V)

Keshet
Jewish Parents of Children with Special Needs
3210 Dundee Road
Northbrook, IL 60062
1-708-205-0274 (V)
1-800-526-0857 (TDD relay voice)
1-800-526-0844 (TDD)

Respite Care

ARCH National Resource Center for Respite Crisis Care
    Services
800 Eastowne Drive, Suite 105
Chapel Hill, NC 27514
1-800-473-1727 (V)
1-919-490-5577 (V/TDD)

Service Dogs

Canine Partners for Life
1-610-869-4902

Delta Society
580 Naches Avenue SW
Suite 101
Renton, WA 98055
1-425-226-7357

Fidos for Freedom
1-410-880-4178 (in MD)

Independence Dogs
1-610-358-2723 (in Philadelphia metro area)

Special Needs Adoption

Adoption Exchange Association
8015 Corporate Drive
Suite C
Baltimore, MD 21236
This private, nonprofit association operates an on-line
    national photolisting of children called AdoptUSKids.
    The photolisting can be viewed on-line at
    www.adoptuskids.org
1-888-200-4005

Children Awaiting Parents, Inc.
700 Exchange Street
Rochester, NY 14608
This organization helps with special needs adoptions and
    publishes the CAP Book, which has photolistings of
    children in the US who need adoptive families.
1-716-232-5110

National Adoption Information Clearinghouse (NAIC)
This provides a comprehensive resource on all aspects of
    adoption.
http://naic.acf.hhs.gov/

Sports, Travel, and Recreation

In addition to the national organizations listed below,
you can call the Department of Tourism and Travel or the
Department of Commerce in your state, and ask for information about accessible services, accommodations,
attractions, and tourist destinations.

Adventures in Movement for the Handicapped, Inc.
1-800-332-8210 (V)
1-425-226-7357

American Camping Association
www.acacamps.org (click on Find a Camp, then on Spe-
    cial Needs)

Boy Scouts of America/Scouts with Special Needs
1325 West Walnut Hill Lane, P.O. Box 152079
Irving, TX 75015-2079
1-214-580-2000 (V)

Echoing Hills Village, Inc.
36272 County Road 79
Warsaw, OH 43844
1-614-327-2311 (V)

Girl Scouts of the USA/"Serving Girls with Disabilities"
  Program
420 5th Avenue
New York, NY 10018
1-800-223-0624 (V)
1-212-852-8000 (V)

Magic Foundation
1-800-362-4423 (V)

Mobility International, USA
P.O. Box 10767
Eugene, OR 97440
1-503-343-1284 (V/TDD)

North American Riding for the Handicapped, Inc.
1-800-369-7433 (V)

Special Olympics
1133 19th Street NW
Washington, DC 20036
1-800-700-8585 (V)
1-202-628-3630 (V/TDD)
www.specialolympics.org

Sunshine Foundation
1-800-767-1976 (V)

Travel Information Service
Moss Rehabilitation Hospital
1200 West Tabor Road
Philadelphia, PA 19141
1-215-456-9600 (V)
1-215-456-9602 (V/TDD)

United States Cerebral Palsy Athletic Association
  (USCPAA)
25 W. Independence Way
Kingston, RI 02881
1-401-792-7130
uscpaa@mail.bbsnet.com

Very Special Arts
1331 F Street NW, Suite 800
Washington, DC 20004
1-800-933-8721 (V)
1-202-628-2800 (V)
1-202-737-0645 (V/TDD)

Supplemental Security Income (SSI)

National Organization of Social Security Claimants Representatives (NOSSCR)

560 Sylvan Avenue
Englewood Cliffs, NJ 07632
This is an organization of attorneys who specialize in social security.
1-800-431-2804
1-201-567-1542 (Fax)
www.nosscr.org

Social Security Administration
1-800-772-1213 (V)
1-800-325-0778 (TT)
1-800-392-0812 (TT; in MD)

Zebley Implementation Project
1-800-523-0000 (V)
1-215-893-5356 (V; in Philadelphia metro area)

Transition to Adulthood

Center for Children with Special Needs
Children's Hospital and Regional Medical Center
Seattle, WA 98101
www.cshcn.org

Disabled and Alone
Life Services for the Handicapped, Inc.
352 Park Avenue South, Suite 703
New York, NY 10010-1709
1-212-532-6740/1-800-995-0066
1-212-532-3588 (Fax)
http://disabledandalone.org/
info@disabledandalone.org

National Collaborative on Workforce and Disability
This is a source of information about employment for
  youth with disabilities.
www.ncwd-youth.info

The Consortium for Children and Youth with Disabilities and Special Health Care Needs
Health care transitions
http://hctransitions.ichp.edu

The Healthy and Ready to Work (HRTW) National
  Center
To stay healthy, young people need an understanding of
  their health and to participate in their health care decisions. The center provides information and connections to health and transition expertise nationwide.
www.hrtw.org/

Recommended Reading and Toys, and Where to Go to Chat with Others

There are many excellent available books for children with disabilities and their parents. The following lists cite reading materials that we think are good, along with some toy manufacturers that make toys that appeal to children with disabilities.

One resource that we want to recommend strongly for parents of children with disabilities is the monthly magazine *Exceptional Parent*. This magazine provides up-to-date information on resources for parents and children, and has annual issues dedicated to educational concerns, the most recent legal changes pertaining to children with special needs, and other subjects of interest. A subscription to the magazine entitles you to receive the Annual Resource Guide. Request a complimentary copy and subscription information from:

Exceptional Parent
EP Global Communications
551 Main Street
Johnstown, PA 15901
1-877-372-7368
www.eparent.com
epar@kable.com

Books for Parents

Winifred Anderson, Stephen Chitwood, and Diedre Hayden, *Negotiating the Special Education Maze: A Guide for Parents and Teachers,* second edition

Mark L. Batshaw, M.D., *Children with Disabilities,* fifth edition.

Eugene E. Bleck, M.D., and Donald A. Nagel, M.D., eds., *Physically Handicapped Children: A Medical Atlas for Children*

Charles R. Callanan, *Since Owen: A Parent-to-Parent Guide for Care of the Disabled Child*

Lynn Clark, Ph.D., *SOS! Help for Parents*

V. Mark Durand, Ph.D., *Sleep Better! A Guide to Improving Sleep for Children with Special Needs*

Richard M. Eckstein, *Handicapped Funding Directory: A Guide to Sources of Funding in the United States for Programs and Services for the Disabled,* seventh edition

Lydia Fegan, Anne Rauch, and Wendy McCarthy, *Sexuality and People with Intellectual Disability*

Dr. Richard Ferber, *Solve Your Child's Sleep Problems*

Nancie Finnie, *Handling the Young Cerebral Palsied Child at Home*

Jacqueline Freedman and Susan Gersten, *Traveling Like Everyone Else: A Practical Guide for Disabled Travelers*

John M. Freeman, M.D., Eileen P. G. Vining, M.D., and Diana J. Pillas, *Seizures and Epilepsy in Childhood: A Guide for Parents,* third edition

James J. Gallagher and Peter W. Vietze, *Families of Handicapped Persons*

Robert Gaylord-Ross, ed., *Integration Strategies for Students with Handicaps*

Elaine Geralis, ed., *Children with Cerebral Palsy: A Parent's Guide*

Helen Harrison and Ann Kositsky, R.N., *The Premature Baby Book: A Parent's Guide to Coping and Caring in the First Years*

Neil J. Hochstadt and Diane M. Yost, eds., *The Medically Complex Child: The Transition to Home Care*

Stanley D. Klein, Ph.D., and John D. Kemp, eds., *Reflections from a Different Journey. What Adults with Disabilities Want All Parents to Know*

Harold S. Kushner, *When Bad Things Happen to Good People*

Ginny LaVine, *Computer Access/Computer Learning: A Resource Manual in Adaptive Technology*

Jane Leonard, Margaret Myers, and Sherri Cadenhead, *Keys to Parenting a Child with Cerebral Palsy*

Barbra Lindberg, *Understanding Rett Syndrome*

Debra J. Lobato, *Brothers, Sisters, Special Needs*

Mary Male, *Special Magic: Computers, Classroom Strategies, and Exceptional Students*

Charles T. Mangrum II and Stephen S. Strichart, eds., *Peterson's Guide to Colleges with Programs for Learning Disabled Students*

William C. Mann and Joseph P. Lane, *Assistive Technology for Persons with Disabilities: The Role of Occupational Therapy*

Carolyn Martin, *I Can't Walk, so I'll Learn to Dance*

Steven Mendelsohn, *Reducing the Cost of Disability: A Guide to Financial and Tax Planning for Disabled People and Their Families*

Robert Moss, M.D., *Why Johnny Can't Concentrate: Coping with Attention Deficit Problems*

Christopher Nolan, *Under the Eye of the Clock*

Arthur Prensky and Helen Palkes, *Care of the Neurologically Handicapped Child*

Wendy Roth and Michael Tompane, *Easy Access to National Parks*

Karen Schwier and Dave Hinsburger, *Sexuality—Your Sons and Daughters with Intellectual Disabilities*

Victoria Shea and Betty Gordon, *Growing UP: A Social and Sexual Education Picture Book for Young People with Mental Retardation*

Larry Silver, M.D., *The Misunderstood Child: A Guide for Parents of Learning Disabled Children*

Charles T. Straughn II and Marvelle S. Colby, *Lovejoy's College Guide for Learning Disabled Students*

Andrew P. Thomas, Martin C. O. Bax, and Diane P. L. Smyth, *The Health and Social Needs of Young Adults with Physical Disability*

Charlotte E. Thompson, M.D., *Raising a Handicapped Child: A Helpful Guide for Parents of the Physically Disabled*

Christine Wright, O.T.R., and Mari Nomura, O.T.R., *From Toys to Computers*

Brookes Publishing Company publishes many books on a variety of disabilities, including cerebral palsy, Down syndrome, mental retardation, autism, etc. PO Box 10624, Baltimore, MD 21285-0624. www.brookespublishing.com

DisABILITIESBOOKS.com "sells top quality books, and videotapes, and provides information about products, services and resources." It also features a used equipment exchange bulletin.

Books for Children

Michelle Emmert, *I'm the Big Sister Now*

Joan Fassler, *Howie Helps Himself*

Mel Levine, *Keeping Ahead in School*

Ages 4–8

Mary Elizabeth Anderson, *Taking Cerebral Palsy to School*

Jamee Heelan, *Rolling Along: The Story of Taylor and His Wheelchair*

Paul Pimm, *Living with Cerebral Palsy*

Ron Taylor, *All by Myself*

Ages 9–12

Thomas Berman, *Going Places: Children Living with Cerebral Palsy*

Marilyn Gould, *Golden Daffodils*

Shelley Nixon, *From Where I Sit: Making My Way with Cerebral Palsy*

Doris Sanford, *Yes, I Can! Challenging Cerebral Palsy*

I'm Joshua and Yes I Can can no longer be ordered from Vantage Print. It's out of print, but copies are available by contacting the author directly.

Joan L. Whinston
406 Viking Lane
Cherry Hill, NJ 08003
1-856-428-8311
Jonay01@AOL.com

Toys

There are companies that specialize in toys for disabled children. The individual interests of the reader will vary, but a few of the larger sites are listed here. You can surf the net for days and probably not see all the sites available.

By far, the most informative list of toys and products that is available for the child with disabilities is this toy catalogue for children with special needs from Wisconsin First Step: www.nas.com/downsyn/toy.html

Other useful sites include: www.Disabilityworld.com; www.enablingdevices.com; www.independentliving.com; www.kidability.com; www.Gbkids.com; www.iphope.com/; www.nraf-rehabnet.org/

Adaptive Clothing
Special Clothes, Inc.
www.special-clothes.com

Adaptive Toys for Special Needs Disabled Children: www.scienceshareware.com/toys.htm

Family Village
www.familyvillage.wisc.edu/at/adaptive-clothing.html

Where to Go to Chat with Others

- Brain-injured child
http://health.groups.yahoo.com/group/BrainInjuredChild/
  KidPower
http://groups.yahoo.com/group/KidPower/

- Cerebral Palsy Club
http://groups.yahoo.com/group/cerebralpalsyclub/
Parents of any children are welcome to chat here

- Cerebral Palsy Network Chat Pad
www.geocities.com/Heartland/Plains/8950/enter.html

- Cerebral Palsy Webring Chat
www.geocities.com/HotSprings/Spa/1778/cpringchat.html

- CPPARENT—For parents who have a child with
  Cerebral Palsy.
http://maelstrom.stjohns.edu/archives/cpparent.html

- Massachusetts General Hospital Department of Neurology Cerebral Palsy Web Board
http://neuro-www.mgh.harvard.edu/forum/
  CerebralPalsyMenu.html

Index

Page numbers in *italic* type indicate illustrations; those in **boldface** type indicate Encyclopedia entries; those followed by t indicate tables.

Head control, poor, 5, 168, 172; oral hygiene for child with, 344; standers for child with, 174, 315

Head rolling, 60

Head trauma, 4, 11; seizures due to, 47; time to initiate therapy after, 171–72

Health care costs, 247. *See also* Financing of health care

Health care system, 229–45; case manager in, 231; financing of care in, 232, 247–55, 286–88; medical care providers in, 237–45; newborn care in, 234; primary care providers in, 232–36; transition of services in, **455–56**; who to see for specific medical needs, 234–37

Health insurance, 247–50; for adaptive equipment, 175; Americans with Disabilities Act and, 285; for augmentative communication devices, 186; for braces, 318; case manager employed by, 231, 272, 323; conditions not covered by, 249–50; difficulties in obtaining, 210, 213; letters of medical necessity provided for, 175, 323–24; limitations of, 248–49; medical care for child without, 232; policies for, 249; State Children's Health Insurance Program, 252–53; for wheelchair, 308

Health Insurance Portability and Accountability Act (HIPPA), 230, 260–61, 334

Health maintenance organization (HMO), 250

Healthy and Ready to Work National Center, The, 472

Healthy People 2010, 279, **456**

Hearing, of newborn, 23, 66

Hearing aids, 68, 179

Hearing assessment/screening, 21, 45t, 66, 234–35, **410**; in child with quadriplegia, 178–79, 189; otoacoustic emission testing, **432**

Hearing impairment, 5, 7, 11, 18, 41, 65–69, **410**; causes of, 65–66, 68–69; cochlear implants for, 68, **378–79**, *379;* conductive, 67, 68; determining type and degree of, 67; FM system for, **403;** incidence of, 65; language delay and, 68; otitis media and, 68, 70; ranges of, 67, 67t; resources for information about, 465–66; risk factors for, 66; sensorineural, 67, 68, 69, **378–79;** treatments for, 68

Hear Now, 465

HEATH Resource Center of the American Council on Education, 466

Heel cord, 129, 184

Heel cups, 135, 184, *367,* **367–68**

Height, 71–74. *See also* Growth

Helicobacter pylori infection, **406**

Helmets: behavioral training, *362,* **362–63;** protective, 50, 61, 159, 172

Hemiatrophy, 37

Hemiplegia, 5, 6, 37, 123–43, **410**; in adulthood, 209; at ages four to six, 133–36; at ages one to three, 126–33; at ages seven to twelve, 136–41; at ages thirteen to eighteen, 141–43; appearance of, 123; arm and hand surgery in, 132–33, 137–38, 142; at birth to one year, 124–26; diagnosis of, 124, 126; double, 5, 123, **395;** early signs of, 124–25; foot and leg involvement in, 123, 129–33, 135–36, 139–41; hand and arm involvement in, 125, 126, 128, 134, 137–39; lower extremity surgery in, 132–33, 135–36, 140–43; physical activity for child with, 137; spasticity in, 134–35

Hemispheres, cerebral, **376**

Hemorrhage, intraventricular, 9, 47, 58

Hepatitis B vaccine, 43

Herbal remedies, for seizures, 52–53

Hereditary spastic paraplegia (HSP), 8, **399–400**

Hernia, 41, 88–89, 234; inguinal, 88–89, **413;** umbilical, **457**

Herniorrhaphy, **413**

Herpes simplex virus, **380, 411**

Hip, knee, ankle, foot orthosis (HKAFO), **368–70**, *369*

Hip abduction brace, **368–70**, *369*

Hip adductors, 156, *411;* lengthening of, **411–13**

Hip flexors, tight, **386**

Hip muscle releases, *411,* **411–13**

Hippo-therapy, **451**. *See also* Horseback riding

Hip problems: in adolescents, 165, 196–97; antiinflammatory medications for, 191–92, 196; arthritis and, 225; braces for, **368–70**, *369;* in child with diplegia, 150, 156, 161, 165; in child with hemiplegia, 123; in child with quadriplegia, 176, 183, 191–92, 196–97; dislocation, 7, 150, 156, 161, 176, 183, 191–92, 196–97, **390–92**, *391, 392 (see also* Dislocated hip); hip fusion for, 197; prevention of, 176, 183, 197, 225; scoliosis and, 197; subluxation, 150, 156, 161, 165, 176, 183, 196, **391;** surgery for, 156, 176, 183, 192, 196–97; valgus hip, **460–61;** varus hip, **461;** windswept hips, 197

Holoprosencephaly, **356**

Home: medical, 230, **423–24, 456;** modifications of, 214, 301, 302–4

Homeopathic medicine, **379**

Hormonal contraception, 91, 92

Horseback riding, adaptive, 34, 157, 188, **451**

Hospitalization, 327–30; preparing child for, 327–29; for rehabilitation, **439**

Hunter syndrome, **425**

Hurler syndrome, **425**

Hyaline membrane disease (HMD), **413**

Hydrocele, **413**

Hydrocephalus, 4, 12, 41, 58–59, 169, **413–14**, *414*

Hydrotherapy, **451**

Hyoscyamine (Levsin), 83, **395**

Hyperalimentation, **454**

Hyperbaric oxygen therapy (HBOT), **414**

Hyperbilirubinemia, 4, **420**

Hyperextension of knees, **360–61**, *361*

Hypersensitivity, **414–15**